Current Progress in Nephrology

Current Progress in Nephrology

Edited by **Tanya Walker**

hayle medical

New York

Published by Hayle Medical,
30 West, 37th Street, Suite 612,
New York, NY 10018, USA
www.haylemedical.com

Current Progress in Nephrology
Edited by Tanya Walker

International Standard Book Number: 978-1-63241-426-7 (Hardback)

Printed in China.

Contents

Preface

Nephrology is the branch of medicine that is concerned with the diagnosis and treatment of diseases related to kidney. It also encompasses different health conditions that directly or indirectly affect the kidney. The end stage of a kidney disease results in kidney failure and the only alternative left is kidney replacement. This book includes studies on topics of utmost importance such as dialysis, chronic kidney disease, renal transplant, vasculitis, etc. It unravels the recent studies in the field of nephrology. It also includes researches and studies performed by experts across the globe. The objective of this text is to provide a comprehensive overview of nephrology and glance at the various advancements in this discipline. Researchers, nephrologists and students in this field will be assisted by this book.

This book has been the outcome of endless efforts put in by authors and researchers on various issues and topics within the field. The book is a comprehensive collection of significant researches that are addressed in a variety of chapters. It will surely enhance the knowledge of the field among readers across the globe.

It gives us an immense pleasure to thank our researchers and authors for their efforts to submit their piece of writing before the deadlines. Finally in the end, I would like to thank my family and colleagues who have been a great source of inspiration and support.

Editor

1

Mycophenolic Acid Absorption Profiles in Patients with Kidney or Combined Pancreas-Kidney Transplantation

Jan M. Fertmann[1], Helmut P. Arbogast[1], Wolf-D. Illner[1], Walter Land[1], Karl-W. Jauch[1], Johannes N. Hoffmann[1,2*]

[1]Department of Surgery, Klinikum Grosshadern, Ludwig-Maximilians University of Munich, Munich, Germany
[2]Department of Surgery, University of Duisburg-Essen, Duisburg and Essen, Germany
Email: *johannes.hoffmann@uk-essen.de

ABSTRACT

Background: Mycophenolate Mofetil (MMF) is widely used in organ transplant patients to avoid calcineurine inhibitor-associated side effects. Therapeutic monitoring of MMF is up to now perform by using trough level measurements (measurements before drug administration). The present study was designed to characterize potential differences in MMF absorption kinetics between patients with allogenic kidney transplantation [kidney Tx] and simultaneous pancreas kidney transplantation [PK Tx], which might for example occur due to diabetic gastrointestinal atony. **Methods:** A total of 64 pharmacokinetic profiles were prospectively studied in 44 adult kidney Tx and 20 PK Tx patients. To calculate AUC by the trapezoidal rule, mycophenolic acid (MPA) levels were measured in EDTA-plasma by an EMIT assay at 0, 0.5, 1, 2, 3, 4, 6, and 12 h after oral MMF administration between postoperative day 14 to 28 in stable patients. **Results:** Substantial differences between kidney Tx and PK Tx patients were evident concerning: donor age, recipient age, number of mismatches, and kidney function (serum creatinine). Despite these dissimilarities pharmacokinetic absorption profiles did not significantly differ between patient groups as measured by AUC, C2, maximum MPA concentration (C_{max}), and time until maximum absorption (T_{max}). Astonishingly, concomitant cyclosporine and tacrolimus medication did not influence adsorption profiles. Only MPA concentrations 6h post administration correlated closely with AUC in both patient groups, whereas trough levels failed to be predictive for AUC. **Conclusions:** In our study population, MMF absorption kinetics did not differ between kidney and PK Tx patients and did not seem influenced by concomitant immunosuppressive medication. Therefore, MPA measurements during the absorption phase could be useful to better estimate AUC in patients with kidney Tx and PK Tx.

Keywords: Mycophenolate Mofetil; Mycophenolic Acid; Pharmacokinetics; Kidney Transplantation; Pancreas-Kidney Transplantation

1. Introduction

During recent years mycophenolate mofetil (MMF), the prodrug of the immunosuppressant mycophenolic acid (MPA), has replaced azathioprine in cyclosporine A (CsA) or tacrolimus (Tac)-based immunosuppression for renal transplant patients, but also after liver, heart, and simultaneous pancreas-kidney transplantation [1,2]. The combination of cyclosporine and MMF for initial immunosuppression in renal transplant patients significantly reduced the incidence of acute rejection episodes when compared to standard therapy with cyclosporine in combination with azathioprine and methylprednisolone [3]. MMF is commonly administered in fixed doses of 3 g (two-times 1.5 g)/day or 2 g (two-times 1 g)/day without taking pharmacokinetic measurements into consideration.

Recent clinical studies in renal transplant patients, however, provide some evidence that steady-state complete MMF area under curve (AUC) measurements are well-correlated with the likelihood of acute rejection independent from the applied MMF dosage [1]. Besides, it has been argued that transplant patients show a substantial variability in MMF absorption [4,5] partly caused by concomitant disease (e.g. renal dysfunction or liver disease) [6]. Also monitoring of inosine monophosphatase dehydrogenase (IMPDH) activity in lymphocytes as an indirect parameter of pharmacodynamic activity has been recommended [7].

Especially when changes in the immunosuppressive regimen (e.g. steroid withdrawal) are planned during the later course in stable patients, a careful evaluation of immunosuppressive MMF efforts is obligatory [7]. Besides, there is some evidence for a relationship of area

*Corresponding author.

under curve MMF concentrations and specific early absorption parameters with gastrointestinal side effects, especially during the initial absorption phase.

The present study investigates MMF absorption in non-diabetic kidney recipients and patients with simultaneous pancreas/kidney transplantation. The effect of concomitant immunosuppressive medication as well as the correlation between MMF AUC measurements and MMF absorption values was compared to investigate potential differences in MMF pharmacokinetics in these two groups which might for example be due to the gastrointestinal atony of the late diabetic syndrome.

2. Materials and Methods

2.1. Patients and MPA Measurements

A total of 64 pharmacokinetic profiles were studied in 44 adult non-diabetic kidney recipients [kidney Tx] and in 20 previously diabetic patients after simultaneous pancreas-kidney transplantation [PK Tx] from 1/2000 until 7/2002. Pharmacokinetic profiles were obtained between postoperative day 14 to 28 after reaching a clinically stable situation. A standardized daily dose of 2 g MMF (CellCept®, Hoffmann-La Roche, Grenzach-Wyhlen, Germany) (2 × 1.0 g) was given on the day of investigation as well as the day before. Pharmacokinetic profiles were evaluated while patients were still hospitalized during routine drug monitoring for standard care. Blood samples were taken immediately before oral MMF application (trough level) and 30 min, 1 h, 90 min, 2 h, 3 h, 4 h, 6 h, 8 h, and 12 h after the morning dose of MMF. EDTA-anticoagulated samples were analyzed on-line using a commercially available test system (EMIT 2000 mycophenolic acid assay, Dade Behring, Liederbach, Germany) for measurement of MPA, the active metabolite of MMF. Calibration and quality controls were performed according to the manufacturer's recommendations. Thereafter, MPA-AUC_{0-12} was calculated using the linear trapezoidal method. C_{max} was taken as the largest observed MPA plasma concentration, whereas trough levels were defined as the morning predose. T_{max} was defined as the time to attain C_{max}.

2.2 Concomitant Immunosuppressive Medication

In addition to MMF, 24 patients received oral cyclosporin A (Neoral®, Novartis, Nuernberg, Germany), and 26 patients received oral tacrolimus (Prograf®, Fujisawa, Munich, Germany). CsA-dosing was performed to achieve approximate trough levels of 150 ng/ml, whereas FK 506 was applied to achieve a trough level around 10 ng/ml. In the remaining 14 patients, only MMF in combination with steroids was administered. Concomitant immunosuppressive drugs were chosen according to local standard protocols, e.g., addition of FK 506 for kidney recipients considered to be transplanted with an elevated immunological risk (previous transplantations with rejecttion episodes, high panel reactivity) or MMF in combination with steroids for renal transplantations in the Eurotransplant senior program. All patients received methylprednisolone in a dosage of 20 mg/day at the time of sampling.

2.3. Side Medication

Among the drugs given to the patients in addition to their immunosuppressive regimen, no substances known to interfere with MPA blood levels were identified [8,9].

2.4. Statistical Analysis

Baseline and demographic characteristics were compared between groups by the unpaired Student t-test, or the unpaired Wilcoxon test where appropriate. Correlation coefficients were calculated by using SPSS software (SPSS version 11.0, Chicago, USA).

3. Results

PK Tx and kidney Tx patients did not differ with respect to gender, body weight, hematocrit, total fluid intake, total urine volume, serum albumine, and parameters of liver function (**Table 1**). However, patients in the PK-Tx group were significantly younger and received significantly younger transplant organs. Serum creatinine was

Table 1. Demographic parameters and organ function in patients with kidney Tx and pancreas-kidney Tx.

	Kidney Tx (n = 44)	Pancreas-kidney Tx (n = 20)	p
Sex (male/female)	31/13	13/7	NS
Donor age (ys.)	48 ± 3	32 ± 3	*
Recipient age (ys.)	50 ± 2	43 ± 2	*
Incidence of insulin-dependent Diabetes	2/44	20/20	*
No of mismatches (n)	2.6 ± 0.2	3.8 ± 0.2	*
Serum Creatinine (mg/dl)	2.7 ± 0.3	1.3 ± 0.2	*
Body weight (kg)	70 ± 2	68 ± 3	NS
Hematocrit (%)	28 ± 1	30 ± 2	NS
Total fluid intake (ml)	3218 ± 225	3791 ± 413	NS
Total urine volume (ml)	3230 ± 277	3495 ± 388	NS
Body temperature (°C)	36.7 ± 0.1	36.8 ± 0.1	NS
Serum albumine (g/dl)	3.8 ± 0.1	3.5 ± 0.2	NS
AST (U/L)	10.5 ± 1.4	7.5 ± 0.9	NS
Plasma cholinesterase (U/L)	3425 ± 207	3122 ± 240	NS

All values are mean ± standard error. *indicates $p < 0.05$ for patients after Kidney Tx vs. combined pancreas-kidney Tx.

significantly lower in PK Tx patients who showed primary kidney function in 18/20 patients. Despite the MMF dosage applied being identical (2 g/day), pharmacokinetic profiling showed a large interindividual variability within patients with kidney Tx and PK Tx: Using this fixed dose application regimen, MPA area under the curve ($AUC_{0-12\,h}$) ranged from 22 - 144 µg × hour/ml and resulted in trough levels from 0.25 - 13.16 µg/ml in kidney Tx patients. Patients with PK-Tx also showed a high variability in MPA area under the curve ($AUC_{0-12\,h}$) that ranged from 13 - 100 µg × hour / ml and in trough levels (C_0 range 0.49 - 4.95 µg/ml).

When comparing pharmacokinetic parameters obtained in kidney Tx and PK Tx patients, we could not detect any statistically significant differences (**Table 2**). Thus, C_{max}, C2 (2-h levels), C6 (6-h levels) and interestingly also T_{max} (time until maximum MPA concentration is reached) did not differ between groups, subsequently resulting in comparable AUCs.

When now comparing patient groups receiving different concomitant immunosuppressive medications (cyclosporine and tacrolimus) with MMF monotherapy (**Table 3**), we found that kidney function was significantly improved in patients receiving a combination of MMF

Table 2. Pharmacokinetics in patients with kidney Tx and pancreas-kidney Tx.

	Kidney Tx	Pancreas-kidney Tx	P
	(n = 44)	(n = 20)	
C max (µg/ml)	12.4 ± 0.8	11.3 ± 1.2	NS
C2 (µg/ml)	7.3 ± 0.7	6.5 ± 0.9	NS
T max (min)	77.2 ± 7.6	86.9 ± 14.7	NS
AUC (µg × hour/ml)	54.2 ± 3.8	52.7 ± 5.9	NS

All values are mean ± standard error.

Table 3. Pharmacokinetics in patients with MMF monotherapy and concomitant Cyclosporine/Tacrolimus (FK 506) medication.

	MMF monotherapy	MMF plus cyclosporine	MMF plus tacrolimus	p
	(n = 14)	(n = 24)	(n = 26)	
Body weight (kg)	70.1 ± 4.2	71.9 ± 3.1	68.2 ± 2.4	NS
Creatinine (mg/dl)	2.9 ± 1.0	2.7 ± 0.4	1.8 ± 0.2	*
Recipient Age (ys.)	56.3 ± 3.6	46.4 ± 3.0	44.1 ± 2.1	*
AUC (µg × hour/ml)	53.8 ± 4.1	49.1 ± 5.2	56.3 ± 5.3	NS
C max (µg/ml)	12.1 ± 1.8	12.0 ± 0.8	11.9 ± 1.2	NS
C2 (µg/ml)	9.3 ± 1.7	7.1 ± 0.6	7.0 ± 0.8	NS
T_{max} (min)	80.0 ± 12.0	72.9 ± 9.8	91.1 ± 13.1	**

All values are mean ± standard error. * indicates $p < 0.05$ for MMF + Tac vs. MMF monotherapy. ** indicates $p < 0.05$ for MMF + Tac and MMF + CsA vs. MMF monotherapy.

plus FK 506. This observation is likely to be caused by the fact that 20/26 patients receiving this combination had undergone PK-Tx that is in general associated with shorter duration of cold ischemia, and, therefore, results in a nearly 100% primary kidney function. Combined transplantation was performed in significantly younger recipients, therefore patients receiving the combination of MMF plus FK 506 were significantly younger. Despite these intriguing differences between patient groups, we could not detect statistically significant changes in the pharmacokinetic parameters AUC, C_{max} and 2 h-post dose levels (C2). Immunosuppressive comedication did only influence the time until maximum absorption (T_{max}). Whereas CsA comedication reduced T_{max} from 80 min. during monotherapy to about 73 min, combination with FK 506 even prolonged T_{max} that amounted 91 min.

Interestingly, trough levels were not found to correlate significantly with AUCs representing total drug exposure, neither in kidney transplant patients nor in PK Tx patients (**Figure 1**). A more close relationship was found when C2 levels were correlated with AUC (**Figure 2**). However, only C6 levels (6h after MMF application) showed a very close correlation with AUC, which resulted in r^2-values above 0.8 (**Figure 3**). Interestingly, there was again no difference found between kidney Tx and PK Tx patients in absorption profiles.

4. Discussion

The present study was designed to compare pharma okinetics of mycophenolate mofetil (MMF) in patients after solitary kidney transplantation (Kidney Tx) withprofiles obtained in patients with simultaneous pancreas-kidney transplantation (PK Tx). Despite significant differences in donor and recipient age, occurrence of diabetes mellitus, and plasma creatinine levels, MMF was absorbed comparably in both treatment groups. Thus, there was no significant difference in maximum MMF concentrations, time until maximum absorbance, and area under curve concentration (AUC) between patients with Kidney Tx and PK Tx. This finding is in line with a recent prospective study in kidney recipients showing no existing correlation between MPA exposure and donor/recipient age as well as renal allograft function expressed as serum creatinine [10]. MMF pharmacokinetics did also not differ between patients receiving concomitant Cyclosporin A (CsA) or Tacrolimus (Tac) therapy when compared to MMF monotherapy. Interestingly, trough levels were not correlated with AUC concentrations or respective oral MMF dosage, whereas 6 h absorption levels after oral application showed a markedly better correlation with AUC in patients with Kidney Tx and PK Tx.

In contrast to earlier studies that report low variabilities of MMF absorption in healthy volunteers [11,12], our postoperative kidney Tx and PK Tx patients showed

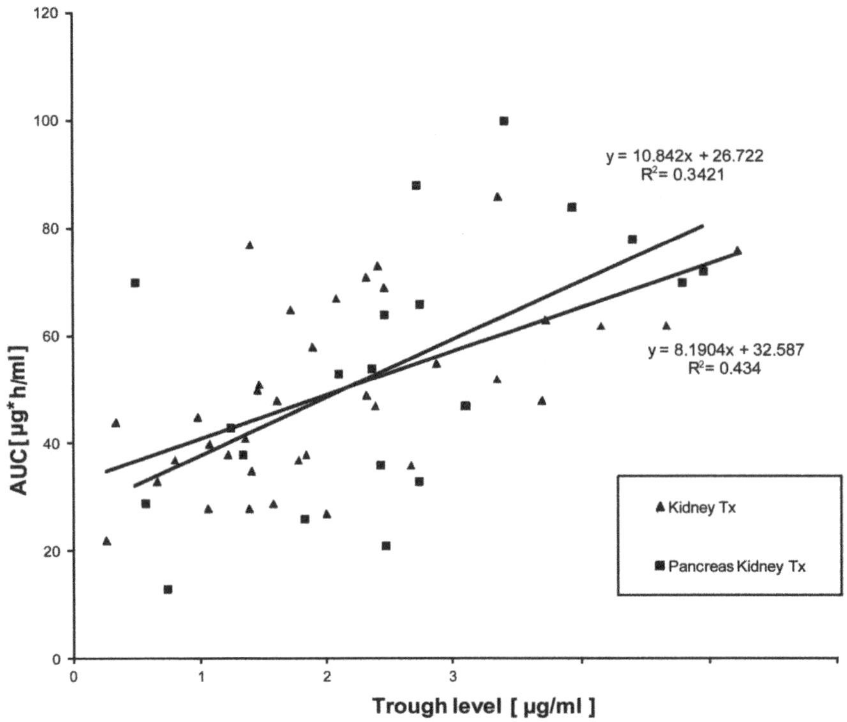

Figure 1. Correlation between trough level MPA measurements and AUC in patients with kidney Tx and pancreas-kidney Tx who were treated by a fixed dose regimen of 1 g MMF twice daily. Only a weak correlation was found between trough level measurements and AUC.

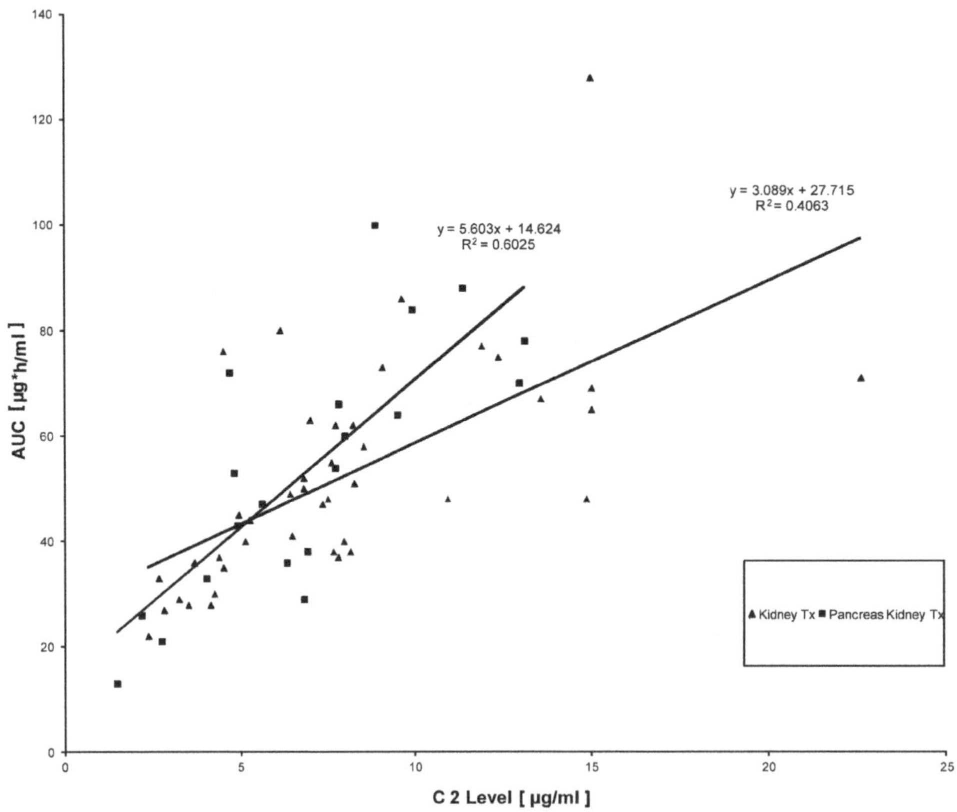

Figure 2. Correlation between 2 h post dose MPA measurements and AUC in patients with kidney Tx and pancreas-kidney Tx who were treated by a fixed dose regimen of 1 g MMF twice daily.

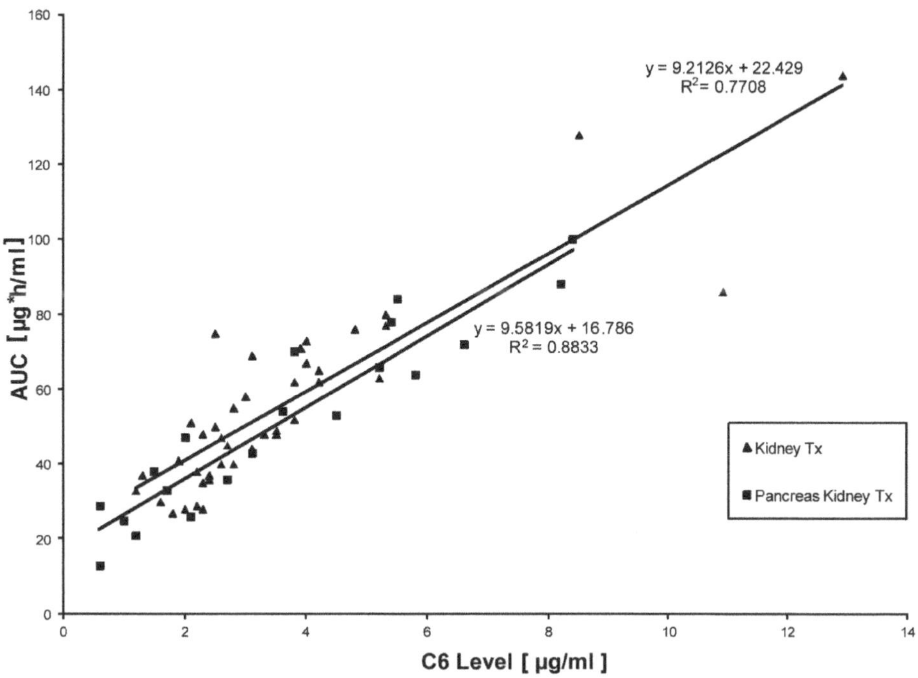

Figure 3. Correlation between 6 h post dose MPA measurements and AUC in patients with kidney Tx and pancreas-kidney Tx who were treated by a fixed dose regimen of 1 g MMF twice daily. An excellent correlation of 6 h post dose MPA measurements with complete AUC was found independent from the respective absolute 6 h-post dose MPA concentration.

high interindividual variabilities in MMF absorption resulting in a broad range of AUC despite the fact that all pharmacokinetic profiles were withdrawn under stable clinical conditions (no ongoing infection or rejection episode, no detectable gastrointestinal side effects) and with a sufficient time span between transplantation and the pharmacokinetic profiling (after postoperative day 14). This finding is in line with several recent reports in patients with kidney Tx who provided high interindividual variability in MMF absorption despite receiving comparable MMF dosages [1,13-15]. A similar wide range of MMF dose-adjusted MPA values has been reported for other transplant populations like heart and liver transplant patients [16]. The mechanisms of these initial differences in MMF absorption and metabolism are not yet completely understood. Furthermore, changes of MPA pharmacokinetics over time after transplantation [6,17] have been demonstrated, which might be dose-dependent [10].

MMF pharmacokinetics in kidney Tx and PK Tx patients have not been directly compared, thus far, as evident from the available literature. However, it is well known that MMF absorption is highly dependent from the transplantation procedure itself, at least in some patient groups. Thus, a recent study found impressive differences in MMF pharmacokinetics when comparing renal and heart transplant recipients with a comparable daily dose of MMF [18]. Differences in MMF absorption could also be clinically significant when comparing kidney Tx and PK Tx patients, since the latter group could be expected to show delayed absorption when compared to kidney Tx patients. We particularly assumed differences in absorption in patients with late diabetic syndrome who are simultaneously transplanted due to postoperative gastrointestinal atony and diabetic malfunction of the gastrointestinal system, but also due to differences in the concomitant medication. Additionally, at least during the initial postoperative phase, differences in the severity of the surgical trauma that is more pronounced during PK Tx could have been related to major changes in kidney and liver function with subsequent changes in drug metabolism. Possible changes in the enterohepatic circulation that are known to be responsible for the secondary 4 - 8 hrs MMF peak, could vary significantly between groups [19]. Therefore, we decided to compare both patient groups with respect to MMF levels after oral treatment.

Interestingly, we could not detect a significant difference in MMF profiles between kidney Tx and PK Tx patients. MMF was absorbed comparably independent from age, sex and combination treatment. Concomitant FK 506 medication did not significantly change the pharmacokinetic profile when compared to Cyclosporine medication. This result was unexpected, since it is in contradiction to several reports that indicate a higher MPA exposure in renal transplant patients when given in combination with FK 506 as compared to a combination treatment with cyclosporine [20]. Also MPA trough levels were shown to be lower in combination with CsA than in kidney recipients treated with MMF and steroids alone [21,22]. In a study performed in rats, it was suspected that this finding was due to an inhibitory effect of CsA on bile excretion of MPA glucuronide (MPAG), to which MPA is metabolized in hepatocytes [23]. In a recent report on MMF absorption in patients after orthotopic liver transplantation, higher MPA levels were found under Tacrolimus comedication [24]. However, in the latter patients postoperatively reduced liver elimination of MMF might have been responsible for the higher trough MPA levels and even increased toxicity under the combination of MMF with FK 506. In addition to MMF, CsA or FK 506, all patients received methylprednisolone, which is also thought to influence MPA bioavailability [25]. However, the dose administered at the day of AUC sampling was identical in all groups (20 mg/day).

Measurements of trough MPA levels have been propagated to reflect at least in part drug absorption and metabolism in various transplant patients, and are currently used in transplant centers to estimate MMF drug exposure [5,26]. Therefore, it seemed to be interesting to investigate, whether these measurements at 12 hrs after drug exposure could in fact help to assess MMF exposure. Whereas MPA trough measurements may be applicable in the non-transplant setting [27], our results clearly show that they cannot uncritically be recommended to estimate MPA drug exposure in Kidney and Kidney-Pancreas transplant patients. This finding is in line with reports showing high intra- and interindividual variabilities by using this method [28]. Using other immunosuppressants, plasma concentration measurements during the absorption phase have been introduced with increasing success [29,30]. Thus, Cyclosporine absorption profiling and therapeutic drug monitoring using absorption measurements 2 h after oral Cyclosporine application has been shown to be clearly superior to trough level monitoring in kidney Tx patients [29]. It seemed, therefore, attractive to investigate whether these 2 h-absorption measurements could also be helpful monitoring oral MMF application. We found a significantly improved correlation of 2 hrs. post dose (C2) MPA levels when compared with trough level measurements. However, only 6 h post dose (C6) MPA levels showed an excellent correlation with AUC that could be likely to be used instead of complete AUC during pharmacokinetic MMF monitoring. Especially in patients with pancreas-kidney-transplantation, a very close relationship between AUC and C6-levels was found. Since AUC is considered to be important as a predictive factor for the incidence of rejection episodes [5], this observation could indeed contribute to a simplification in MMF monitoring. Absorption levels of MPA 6h after oral application could serve as easily available surrogate parameters. Especially when compared to a limited sampling-AUC strategy ($AUC_{0\text{-}6\,h}$) we found a comparable good prediction of AUC [19].

5. Conclusion

In conclusion, we could show comparable MMF absorption in diabetic and non-diabetic patients receiving pancreas-kidney or kidney transplantation. Combination with Tacrolimus or Cyclosporine did not change MMF pharmacokinetics. Since plasma MPA concentration 6 hrs, after application (C6) correlates better than trough level with AUC, measurement of this parameter seems useful in patients who do not allow performance of complete AUC sampling. Based on our findings, we would recommend further studies on this subject.

REFERENCES

[1] L. M. Shaw, B. Kaplan, D. DeNofrio, *et al.*, "Pharmacokinetics and Concentration-Control Investigations of Mycophenolic Acid in Adults after Transplantation," *Therapeutic Drug Monitoring*, Vol. 22, No. 1, 2000, pp. 14-19. doi:10.1097/00007691-200002000-00003

[2] T. van Gelder, L. B. Hilbrands, Y. Vanrenterghem, *et al.*, "A Randomized Double-Blind, Multicenter Plasma Concentration-Controlled Study of the Safety and Efficacy of Oral Mycophenolate Mofetil for the Prevention of Acute Rejection after Kidney Transplantation," *Transplantation*, Vol. 68, No. 2, 1999, pp. 261-266. doi:10.1097/00007890-199907270-00018

[3] H. W. Sollinger, S. Cho, G. Danowitch, *et al.*, "Mycophenolate Mofetil for the Prevention of Acute Rejection in Primary Cadaveric Renal Allograft Recipients," *Transplantation*, Vol. 60, No. 3, 1995, pp. 225-232. doi:10.1097/00007890-199508000-00003

[4] G. Filler, M. Zimmering and I. Mai, "Pharmacokinetics of Mycophenolate Mofetil Are Influenced by Concomittant Immunosuppression," *Pediatric Nephrology*, Vol. 14, No. 2, 2000, pp. 100-104. doi:10.1007/s004670050021

[5] M. Oellerich, M. Shipkova, E. Schütz, *et al.*, "Pharmacokinetic and Metabolic Investigations of Mycophenolic Acid in Pediatric Patients after Renal Transplantation: Implications for Therapeutic Drug Monitoring," *Therapeutic Drug Monitoring*, Vol. 22, No. 4, 2000, pp. 20-26. doi:10.1097/00007691-200002000-00004

[6] L. T. Weber, T. Lamersdorf, M. Shipkova, *et al.*, "Area under Curve Concentration-Time Curve for Total, but Not for Free, Mycophenolic Acid Increases in the Stable Phase after Enal Transplantation: A Longitudinal Study in Pediatric Patients," *Therapeutic Drug Monitoring*, Vol. 21, No. 5, 1999, pp. 498-506. doi:10.1097/00007691-199910000-00002

[7] K. P. Braun, P. Glander, P. Hambach, *et al.*, "Pharmacokinetics and Pharmacodynamics of Mycophenolate Mofetil under Oral and under Intravenous Therapy," *Transplantation Proceedings*, Vol. 34, No. 5, 2002, pp. 1745-1747. doi:10.1016/S0041-1345(02)03051-8

[8] G. Filler, N. Lepage, B. Delisle, *et al.*, "Effect of Cyclosporine on Mycophenolic Acid Area under the Concentration-Time Curve in Pediatric Kidney Transplant Re-

cipients," *Therapeutic Drug Monitoring*, Vol. 23, No. 5, 2001, pp. 514-519. doi:10.1097/00007691-200110000-00003

[9] C. Mignat, "Clinically Significant Drug Interactions with New Immunosuppressive Agents," *Drug Safety*, Vol. 16, No. 4, 1997, pp. 267-278. doi:10.2165/00002018-199716040-00004

[10] D. Kuypers, K. Claes, P. Evenepoel, *et al*., "Long-Term Changes in Mycophenolic Acid Exposure in Combination with Tacrolimus and Corticosteroids Are Dose Dependent and Not Reflected by Trough Plasma Concentration: A Prospective Study in 100 De Novo Renal Allograft Recipients," *Journal of Clinical Pharmacology*, Vol. 43, No. 8, 2003, pp. 866-880. doi:10.1177/0091270003256151

[11] R. E. S. Bullingham, A. Nicholls and M. D. Hale, "Pharmacokinetics of Mycophenolate Mofetil: A Short Review," *Transplantation Proceedings*, Vol. 28, No. 2, 1996, pp. 925-929.

[12] R. E. S. Bullingham, A. Nicholls and B. R. Kamm, "Clinical Pharmacokinetics of Mycophenolate Mofetil," *Clinical Pharmacokinetics*, Vol. 34, No. 6, 1998, pp. 429-455. doi:10.2165/00003088-199834060-00002

[13] L. M. Shaw, A. Nawrocki, M. Korecka, *et al*., "Using Established Immunosuppressant Therapy Effectively: Lessons from the Measurement of Mycophenolic Acid Plasma Concentrations," *Therapeutic Drug Monitoring*, Vol. 26, No. 2, 2004, pp. 347-351. doi:10.1097/00007691-200408000-00002

[14] B. Krumme, K. Wollenberg, G. Kirste, *et al*., "Drug Monitoring of Mycophenolic Acid in the Early Period after Renal Transplantation," *Transplantation Proceedings*, Vol. 30, No. 5, 1998, pp. 1773-1774. doi:10.1016/S0041-1345(98)00425-4

[15] Pillans PI, Rigby RJ, Kubler P, *et al*., "A Retrospective Analysis of Mycophenolic Acid and Cyclosporine Concentrations with Acute Rejection in Renal Transplant Recipients," *Clinical Biochemistry*, Vol. 34, No. 1, 2001, pp. 77-81. doi:10.1016/S0009-9120(00)00196-X

[16] L. M. Shaw, M. Korecka, R. Venkataramanan, *et al*., "Mycophenolic Acid Pharmacodynamics and Pharmacokinetics Provide a Basis for Rational Monitoring Strategies," *American Journal of Transplantation*, Vol. 3, No. 5, 2003, pp. 534-542. doi:10.1034/j.1600-6143.2003.00079.x

[17] V. C. Cox and M. Ensom, "Mycophenolate Mofetil for Solid Organ Transplantation: Does the Evidence Support the Need for Clinical Pharmacokinetic Monitoring?" *Therapeutic Drug Monitoring*, Vol. 25, No. 2, 2003, pp. 137-157. doi:10.1097/00007691-200304000-00003

[18] L. M. Shaw, M. Korecka, D. DeNofrio, *et al*., "Pharmacokinetic, Pharmacodynamic, and Outcome Investigations as the Basis for Mycophenolic Acid Therapeutic Drug Monitoring in Renal and Heart Transplant Patients," *Clinical Biochemistry*, Vol. 34, No. 1, 2001, pp. 17-22. doi:10.1016/S0009-9120(00)00184-3

[19] A. G. Johnson, R. J. Rigby, P. J. Taylor, *et al*., "The Kinetics of Mycophenolic Acid and Its Glucuronide Metabolite in Adult Kidney Transplant Recipients," *Clinical Pharmacology & Therapeutics*, Vol. 66, No. 5, 1999, pp. 492-500. doi:10.1016/S0009-9236(99)70012-3

[20] K. Zucker, A. Rosen, A. Tsaroucha, *et al*., "Unexpected Augmentation of Mycophenolic Acid Pharmacokinetics in Renal Transplant Patients Receiving Tacrolimus and Mycophenolate Mofetil in Combination Therapy, and Analogous *in Vitro* Findings," *Transplant Immunology*, Vol. 5, No. 3, 1997, pp. 225-232. doi:10.1016/S0966-3274(97)80042-1

[21] P. J. Smak Gregoor, T. van Gelder, C. J. Hesse, *et al*., "Mycophenolic Acid Plasma Concentrations in Kidney Allograft Recipients with or without Cyclosporin: A Cross-Sectional Study," *Nephrology Dialysis Transplantation*, Vol. 14, No. 3, 1999, pp. 706-708. doi:10.1093/ndt/14.3.706

[22] L. Pou, M. Brunet, C. Cantarell, *et al*., "Mycophenolic Acid Plasma Concentrations: Influence of Comedication," *Therapeutic Drug Monitoring*, Vol. 23, No. 1, 2000, pp. 35-38. doi:10.1097/00007691-200102000-00007

[23] T. van Gelder, J. Klupp, M. J. Barten, *et al*., "Comparison of the Effects of Tacrolimus and Cyclosporin on the Pharmacokinetics of Mycophenolic Acid," *Therapeutic Drug Monitoring*, Vol. 23, No. 2, 2001, pp. 119-128. doi:10.1097/00007691-200104000-00005

[24] M. Glanemann, J. Klupp, J. M. Langrehr, *et al*., "Higher Immunosuppressive Efficacy of Mycophenolate Mofetil in Combination with FK 506 than in Combination with Cyclosporine A," *Transplantation Proceedings*, Vol. 32, No. 3, 2000, pp. 522-523. doi:10.1016/S0041-1345(00)00872-1

[25] D. Cattaneo, Perico N., F. Gaspari, *et al*., "Glucocorticoids Interfere with Mycophenolate Mofetil Bioavailability in Kidney Transplantation," *Kidney International*, Vol. 62, No. 3, 2002, pp. 1060-1067. doi:10.1046/j.1523-1755.2002.00531.x

[26] G. I. Hubner, R. Eismann and W. Sziegoleit, "Relationship between Mycophenolate Mofetil Side Effects and Mycophenolic Acid Plasma Trough Levels in Renal Transplant Patients," *Arzneimittelforschung*, Vol. 50, No. 10, 2000, pp. 936-940.

[27] I. Neumann, M. Haidinger, H. Jaeger, *et al*., "Pharmacokinetics of Mycophenolate Mofetil in Patients with Autoimmune Diseases Compared to Renal Transplant Recipients," *Journal of the American Society of Nephrology*, Vol. 14, No. 3, 2003, pp. 721-727. doi:10.1097/01.ASN.0000051598.12824.DA

[28] M. Brunet, J. Martorell, F. Oppenheimer, *et al*., "Pharmacokinetics and Pharmacodynamics of Mycophenolic Acid in Stable Renal Transplant Recipients Treated with Low Doses of Mycophenolat Mofetil," *Transplant International*, Vol. 13, No. S1, 2000, pp. S301-S305.

[29] P. Belitsky, G. A. Levy and A. Johnston, "Neoral Absorption Profiling: An Evolution in Effectiveness," *Transplantation Proceedings*, Vol. 32, No. 3A, 2000, pp. 45S-52S. doi:10.1016/S0041-1345(00)00863-0

[30] K. Mahalati, P. Belitsky, I. Sketris, *et al*., "Neoral Monitoring by Simplified Sparse Sampling Area under the Concentration-Time Curve," *Transplantation*, Vol. 68, No. 1, 1999, pp. 55-62. doi:10.1097/00007890-199907150-00011

2

The Effect of Exercise Therapy on Physical Function, Biochemistry and Dialysis Adequacy in Haemodialysis Patients: A Systematic Review and Meta-Analysis

Neil Smart[1*], James McFarlane[1], Veronique Cornelissen[2]
[1]Department of Exercise Science, University of New England, Armidale, Australia
[2]Department of Rehabilitation Sciences, University of Leuven, Leuven, Belgium
Email: *nsmart2@une.edu.au

ABSTRACT

Background: Patients undergoing dialysis have high mortality rates and a unique risk factor profile. Some improvements elicited by exercise training have been shown in dialysis populations, here we aimed to further explore the benefits of exercise. As well as changes in physical fitness we quantified cardiac function, depression, serum biochemistry, dialysis adequacy and energy intake following exercise training in people with chronic kidney disease (CKD) undertaking dialysis. **Methods:** A systematic literature search was completed in December 2012 identifying randomized, controlled trials of exercise training studies in haemodialysis (HD) patients. A subsequent meta-analysis was conducted. **Results:** Twenty four studies were included, totalling 879 patients. Exercise training produced significant improvements in physical fitness: peak VO_2 5.03 $mlO_2 \cdot kg^{-1} \cdot min^{-1}$ (95% CI 3.73, 6.33, $p < 0.0001$), Knee extensor strength 2.99 kg (95% CI 0.46, 5.52, $p = 0.02$) and 6 minute walk distance 60.7 metres (95% CI 18.9, 103, $p = 0.004$). Significant increases in energy intake MD 238 $Kcal \cdot day^{-1}$ (95% CI 94, 383, $p = 0.001$), serum Interleukin-6 MD −0.58 $pg \cdot ml^{-1}$ (95% CI −1.01, −0.15, $p = 0.008$) and C-reactive protein MD 0.92 mg/L^{-1} (95% CI 0.29, 1.56, $p = 0.004$), but not Albumin or BMI, were reported. Improved Beck Depression scores were reported MD −6.9 (95% CI −9.7, −4.1, $p < 0.00001$). Dialysis adequacy was reduced MD −0.23 (95% CI −0.29, −0.17, $p < 0.00001$), while serum potassium was higher MD 0.14 $mmol \cdot L^{-1}$ (95% CI 0.01, 0.27, $p = 0.04$). Moreover exercise training appeared safe, with no direct exercise- associated deaths in over 30,000 patient-hours. **Conclusions:** Our pooled analyses confirmed improvements in physical fitness following exercise training and suggested additional improvements in dialysis efficiency (kt/v), serum potassium, inflammation and depression in HD patients.

Keywords: Exercise Training; Haemodialysis; Meta-Analysis; Systematic Review

1. Introduction

Numerous trials have extolled the benefits of exercise training to chronic kidney disease (CKD) patients [1-3]. Common benefits often associated with exercise training are improved peak VO_2 [4], quality of life [5], cardiac function [6] and reduced sympatho-adrenal activity [7]. Reduced peak VO_2 and poor quality of life have been associated with increased mortality risk in HD patients [8]. Systematic reviews of exercise training have been completed previously but the common focus has been mainly on cardio-respiratory fitness and muscle strength [1,9,10].

The publication of several recent exercise training studies in HD patients prompted our group to conduct the first data pooling analyses to examine if exercise training can also improve dialysis adequacy, depression, body mass index, serum inflammatory markers, erythropoietin use and several biochemical markers vital to HD patient monitoring. Our analysis further sought to determine if any of these outcome measures, exercise adherence and safety can be optimized with a particular delivery method, e.g. program duration or modality of exercise training.

2. Methods

A systematic literature search was completed in December 2012 and subsequent meta-analysis undertaken.

2.1. Search Strategy

Potential studies were identified by a systematic search of Medline (Ovid) (1950-December 2012), Embase.com (1974-December 2012), Cochrane Central Register of Controlled Trials and CINAHL (1981-December 2012).

*Corresponding author.

The search strategy included a mix of MeSH and free text terms for the search terms chronic renal failure, chronic kidney disease, hemodialysis and exercise training, aerobic exercise, resistance exercise, physical activity, strength training and these were combined with a sensitive search strategy to identify randomized controlled trials. Reference list of papers found were scrutinized for new references. All identified papers were assessed independently by two reviewers (NS and JM) and a consensus reached. Searches of published papers were conducted up until December 3rd 2012.

2.2. Inclusions

Randomized, controlled trials of exercise training in adult (>18 years) chronic kidney disease patients receiving dialysis were included. Included studies reported the post-training mean and standard deviation (SD) or standard error (SE) in exercise and control group of at least one primary or secondary outcome measure (listed below). There were no language restrictions. Acute exercise response studies were not included.

2.3. Exclusions

Animal studies, review papers and non-randomized controlled trials were excluded. Studies that did not have an exercise intervention, desired outcome measures, participants who were not chronic kidney disease patients or not receiving dialysis in either treatment or control groups were also excluded. Authors were contacted to provide missing data or clarify if information was duplicated in multiple publications from the same authors. At the time of submission no additional data was forthcoming. Incomplete data or data from an already included study resulted in exclusion.

2.4. Data Synthesis

Data relating to chronic kidney disease patient characteristics and exercise training protocols were reviewed. Information was archived in a database and separated into studies that recruited patients undertaking dialysis. Where studies randomized patients to more than two groups only exercise training versus usual care (CKD versus control) data was analyzed. When reviewers suspected data had been duplicated between studies, only study data from the largest patient cohort was analysed.

Outcome measures were peak VO_2, 6 minute walk distance, knee extensor strength, cardiac function (left ventricular ejection %), left ventricular mass index, serum albumin and potassium, inflammatory markers (serum interleukin-6, C-reactive protein), quality of life (SF-36, Beck Depression score), daily energy intake, dialysis adequacy index (Kt/v) and body mass index. Data on exercise adherence and safety (number of adverse events were also collected. Measures of study quality were assessed by Jadad score which examined details of randomization, investigator blinding and study withdrawal [11].

2.5. Statistical Analysis

For continuous data, we took the approach of assuming randomization would adjust for baseline imbalance and used end-point data only as advised by the Cochrane Collaboration [12]. A random effects inverse variance was used with the effects measure of mean difference (MD). For dichotomous data Mantel-Haenszel fixed effects odds ratio was calculated. Heterogeneity was quantified using a Cochran Q test [13]. We conducted two sub-group analyses; first we compared home versus outpatient exercise training and second we compared those studies of 6 months or greater versus those less than 6 months. We used a 5% level of significance and 95% confidence interval, figures were produced by Review Manager version 5.0.

3. Results

3.1. Studies Included in the Review

Forty-nine randomized controlled trials were identified. Twenty five studies were excluded, leaving 24 full manuscripts. Included studies can be seen in **Table 1**. Assessment of study quality can be seen in **Table 2**. Reasons for study exclusion are seen in **Table 3**.

Twenty four studies yielding data on 879 HD patients, 493 were exercising participants and sedentary 386 controls. Generally exercise and control groups were well matched at baseline for age, gender, EPO use and peak VO_2. Data available from 24 studies of HD patients suggested mean time of receiving haemodialysis was 4.8 (exercise) and 4.5 years (control) and both exercise and control participants demonstrated a mean of two other co-morbid chronic diseases.

3.2. Peak VO_2

Nine studies (one study examined two types of exercise, hence 10 datasets in **Figure 1**) [4,6,7,14-19] measured peak VO_2 in 400 patients. Significantly greater post-training peak VO_2 values [+5.03 $mlO_2{\cdot}kg^{-1}{\cdot}min^{-1}$ (95% CI 3.73; 6.33, $p < 0.00001$)] were exhibited following exercise versus control (**Figure 1**). Mean post-intervention peak VO_2 for both exercise and control participants were 23.1 ± 2.6 and 18.1 ± 3.3 $mlO_2{\cdot}kg^{-1}{\cdot}min^{-1}$ respectively.

3.3. Effect of Exercise Training Duration

A further analysis was conducted to examine the effect of

Study or Subgroup	Exercise Mean	Exercise SD	Exercise Total	Control Mean	Control SD	Control Total	Weight	Mean Difference IV, Fixed, 95% CI
Deligannis 1999aiHomeEx	19	5.3	10	15.8	4.8	6	6.6%	3.20 [-1.85, 8.25]
Deligannis 1999aiID	23.7	7.7	16	15.8	4.8	6	5.8%	7.90 [2.52, 13.28]
Deligannis 1999b	24	7	30	16	6	30	15.5%	8.00 [4.70, 11.30]
Goldberg 1983	25	8	14	20	8	11	4.2%	5.00 [-1.32, 11.32]
Koufaki 2002	19.9	6.3	18	18.8	4.9	15	11.6%	1.10 [-2.72, 4.92]
Kouidi 1997	23.2	7.6	20	15.9	4.3	11	9.6%	7.30 [3.11, 11.49]
Kouidi 2009	21.4	6.8	30	16.5	4.5	29	19.7%	4.90 [1.97, 7.83]
Moros 2000	23.81	4.8	23	17.11	5.3	11	12.4%	6.70 [3.00, 10.40]
Painter 2002	22.1	8.9	10	19.9	6.7	14	4.0%	2.20 [-4.34, 8.74]
Van Vilsteren	28.02	8.8	53	26.25	10.8	43	10.6%	1.77 [-2.23, 5.77]
Total (95% CI)			**224**			**176**	**100.0%**	**5.03 [3.73, 6.33]**

Heterogeneity: Chi² = 13.95, df = 9 (P = 0.12); I² = 35%

Test for overall effect: Z = 7.57 (P < 0.00001)

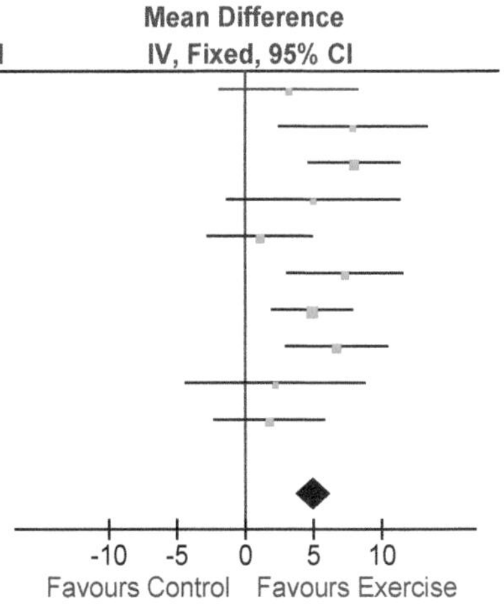

Figure 1. Comparison of peak VO_2 ($mlO_2 \cdot kg^{-1} \cdot min^{-1}$) following exercise training in HD patients.

Table 1. Summary characteristics of included studies.

Haemodialysis studies	N (ExT)	Training	Study duration, delivery method	Data extracted
Afshar, 2010 [30]	21 (7AT, 7RT)	AT, RT	2 months, ID	Cr, Kt/V, Hb, Albumin, CRP, Chol
Chen, 2010 [24]	50 (25)	RT	4 Months ID	Strength
Daniilidis 2004 [31]	34 (20)	AT	3 Months, ID	IL-6
Deligiannis, 1999 [14]	16 (10)	CT	6 months, ND, outpatient	Peak VO_2, Biochemistry, BP, LVMI, LVEF
Deligiannis, 1999 [14]	22 (16)	CT	6 months, ND, home	Peak VO_2, Biochemistry, BP, LVMI, LVEF
Deligiannis, 1999 [7]	60 (30)	CT	6 months, ND	Peak VO_2, HRV, Biochemistry
De Paul, 2002 [22]	38 (18)	CT	5 months, ND	6MWD, BP, Biochemistry
Dong, 2011 [27]	32 (15)	RT	6 months ID	BMI, Biochemistry, Kcals
Frey, 1999 [28]	11 (5)	AT	2 months, ID	Kcals, Kt/V, Albumin
Goldberg, 1983 [19]	25 (14)	AT	12 months, ND	Peak VO_2
Johansen, 2006 [33]	79 (40)	RT	3 months, ID	Muscle strength, Cr
Koh, 2010 [21]	70 (43)	AT	6 months, cycling, ID	SF-36, 6MWD, BP
Koufaki, 2002 [15]	18 (15)	AT	3 months, cycling, ID	Peak VO_2, Kcals, Hb, Albumin, BMI
Kouidi, 1997 [4]	31 (20)	AT	6 months, ND	Peak VO_2, BDI
Kouidi, 2009 [6]	59 (30)	CT	10 months, cycling ID	Peak VO_2, LVMI, LVEF, HRV, Hb
Kouidi, 2010 [5]	44 (24)	CT	12 months, ID	BDI (other data already used Kouidi 2009)
Makhlough, 2012 [32]	48 (25)	AT	2 months ID	Biochemistry
Moros-Garcia, 2000 [16]	34 (23)	AT	4 months, cycling ND	Peak VO_2
Oliveros, 2011 [23]	15 (9)	CT	4 months ND	Strength, SF-36, BDI, 6MWD, Kt/V
Painter, 2002 [17]	24 (10)	AT	5 months, cycling, ID	Peak VO_2, SF-36
Parsons, 2004 [37]	13 (6)	AT	2 months cycling, ID	SF-36
Reboredo, 2010 [29]	22 (11)	AT	3 months, ID	HRV, LVEF, KT/V, Biochemistry, LVMI
Van Vilsteren, 2005 [18]	96 (53)	CT	3 months, cycling ID	Peak VO_2, SF-36, LVMI
Willund, 2010 [26]	17 (8)	AT	4 months, ID cycling	BMI, IL-6, CRP, biochemistry, BP, LVMI

ExT: exercise training; RT: resistance training; AT: aerobic training; CT: combined training; ND: exercise on non-dialysis days; ID: exercise on dialysis days; HRV: heart rate variability; LVEF%: left ventricular ejection fraction; SF-36: short form 36 health questionnaire; BDI: beck depression inventory; Cr: serum creatinine; Hb: haemoglobin; Kt/V: dialysis adequacy index; CRP: C-reactive protein; Chol: total serum cholesterol; LVMI: left ventricular mass index; Kcals: daily energy intake (kilocalories); BP: blood pressure; 6MWD: six minute walk distance.

Table 2. Assessment of study quality—JADAD score.

Haemodialysis studies	Randomized	Blinding	Withdrawn	Jadad score
Ashfar, 2010 [30]	Yes	Unclear	Unclear	1
Chen, 2010 [24]	Yes	Yes	Yes	3
Daniilidis, 2004 [31]	Yes	Unclear	Yes	2
Deligiannis, 1999 [14]	Yes	Unclear	No	1
Deligiannis, 1999 [7]	Yes	Unclear	Unclear	1
De Paul, 2002 [22]	Yes	Yes	Yes	3
Dong, 2011 [27]	Yes	Unclear	Yes	2
Frey, 1999 [28]	Yes	Unclear	Yes	2
Goldberg ,1983 [19]	Yes	Unclear	Yes	2
Johansen, 2006 [33]	Yes	Yes	Yes	3
Koh, 2010 [21]	Yes	No	Yes	2
Koufaki, 2002 [15]	Yes	Unclear	Yes	2
Kouidi, 1997 [4]	Yes	Unclear	Yes	2
Kouidi, 2009 [6]	Yes	Yes	Yes	3
Kouidi, 2010 [5]	Yes	Yes	Yes	3
Makhlough, 2012 [32]	Yes	Yes	Yes	3
Moros-Garcia, 2000 [16]	Yes	Unclear	Yes	2
Oliveros, 2011 [23]	Yes	Unclear	Yes	2
Painter, 2002 [17]	Yes	Unclear	Yes	2
Parsons, 2004 [37]	Yes	Unclear	Yes	2
Reboredo, 2010 [29]	Yes	Yes	Yes	3
Van Vilsteren, 2005 [18]	Yes	Unclear	Yes	2
Willund, 2010 [26]	Yes	Yes	Yes	3

study duration on change in peak VO_2 in 9 studies. First, we removed the four studies that employed an exercise training program of less than 6 months from the analysis [15-18], mean change in peak VO_2 for the five studies of 6 months for longer was 32.1% ± 8.9%, while the four shorter duration studies yielded a significantly lower peak VO_2 change of 16.2% ± 5.3% (p = 0.002).

3.4. Effect of Exercise Modality and Delivery

Four studies of combined aerobic (AT) and strength (ST) training [6,7,14,18] appear to convey a weighted mean 28.6% ± 11.4% improvement in peak VO_2 compared to five isolated AT studies [4,15,16,17,19] which produced a weighted mean 22.2% ± 9.7% improvement in peak VO_2 (p = 0.37). None of the isolated resistance studies reported peak VO_2. Four studies [6,15,17,18] used inter-dialytic training (ID) and also reported weighted mean change in peak VO_2 was 17.8% ± 7.7% while the five studies [4,7,14,16,19] using exercise training on non-dialysis days showed 30.8% ± 9.6% improvement in peak VO_2 (p = 0.07). One study[20] directly compared exercise training induced improvements in peak VO_2 at 12 months with outpatient (ND) and (ID) training programs 38% versus 31% respectively (p = 0.07). Only two studies [14,21] examined home versus outpatient exercise with conflicting results. The former study [21] showed a greater improvement in six minute walk distance in the home group, while the latter study [20] reported a larger peak VO_2 improvement in the out-patient versus home exercise patients.

3.5. Walking Distance

Data from three studies [21-23] in 80 haemodialysis patients showed an improvement in six-minute walking

Table 3. Excluded randomized controlled trials.

Akiba 1995 [38]	No relevant outcome data
Balakrishnan, 2009 [39]	No relevant outcome data
Carney, 1987 [40]	No relevant outcome data
Castenada, 2001 [41]	Non-HD patients
Castenada, 2004 [42]	Non-HD patients
Chang, 2010 [43]	Relevant outcome data reported by physical activty levels
Cheema, 2007 [44]	Data could not be converted to post mean/standard deviation
Cheema, 2007 [45]	Data could not be converted to post mean/standard deviation
Cheema, 2011 [46]	Data could not be converted to post mean/standard deviation
Chen, 2010 [47]	Non-HD patients
Fitts, 1999 [48]	No relevant outcome data
Flesher, 2011 [49]	No relevant outcome data. Intervention included cooking classes
Goldberg, 1986 [50]	Duplicate Goldberg, 1983; Harter, 1985
Harter, 1985 [51]	Duplicate Goldberg, 1983; Goldberg, 1986
Headley, 2008 [52]	Acute exercise response, not training study
Konstantinou, 2002 [53]	Duplicate, control group data shared with Deligannis, 1999
Kouidi, 2004 [20]	No sedentary control group
Leehey, 2009 [54]	Non-HD patients
Matsumoto, 2007 [55]	Only baseline data reported
Molstead, 2004 [56]	Data reported as median and range
Mustata, 2011 [57]	Non-HD patients
Ouzouni, 2009 [58]	Possible duplicate with Kouidi, 2009 and Kouidi, 2010
Painter, 2002 [59]	Included transplant patients not receiving hemodialysis
Petraki, 2008 [35]	Possible duplicate with Kouidi, 2009
Segura-Orti, 2009 [60]	Possible duplicate with Kouidi, 2009

distance MD 60.7 metres (95% CI 18.9, 102.5 metres, $p = 0.004$) see **Figure 2**.

3.6. Muscle Strength

Three studies [23-25] reported knee extensor muscle strength in 95 HD patients, improvements were seen in exercising patients versus sedentary controls, MD 2.99 kg (95% CI 0.46, 5.52, $p = 0.02$), see **Figure 3**.

3.7. Erythropoietin (EPO) Use

As EPO use may have had significant impact on exercise training adaptations, particularly peak VO_2, relevant sub-analyses may have been informative, but this was not justified as thirteen of the HD studies did not provide details of patient EPO use during the studies. Three studies did however keep EPO use stable and the remaining eight studies targeted EPO use to haemoglobin levels, but only four of these 11 studies reported peak VO_2 rendering sub-analyses impractical.

3.8. Body Mass Index, Energy Intake, Serum Albumin and Inflammation

Three studies [15,26,27] reported post-training body mass index in 72 HD patients, BMI was not different between exercise and control participants MD 1.15 $kg{\cdot}m^{-2}$ (95% CI - 0.33, 2.63, $p = 0.13$), see **Figure 4**. Three studies [15,27,28] including 66 patients, employed dietary recall to estimate daily energy intake, exercise participants increased their intake by 4% from baseline. Meta-analysis, showed daily energy intake to be significantly higher in those who exercised versus controls MD

Study or Subgroup	Exercise Mean	Exercise SD	Exercise Total	Control Mean	Control SD	Control Total	Weight	Mean Difference IV, Fixed, 95% CI
Cheema 2007	513	35.3504	24	493	35.3504	25	81.7%	20.00 [0.20, 39.80]
De Paul 2002	464	94	20	430	80	18	10.5%	34.00 [-21.34, 89.34]
Koh 2010	526	97	15	452	144	16	4.3%	74.00 [-11.95, 159.95]
Oliveros 2011	630	85	5	506	75	6	3.5%	124.00 [28.33, 219.67]
Total (95% CI)			**64**			**65**	**100.0%**	**27.45 [9.55, 45.34]**

Heterogeneity: Chi² = 5.64, df = 3 (P = 0.13); I² = 47%
Test for overall effect: Z = 3.01 (P = 0.003)

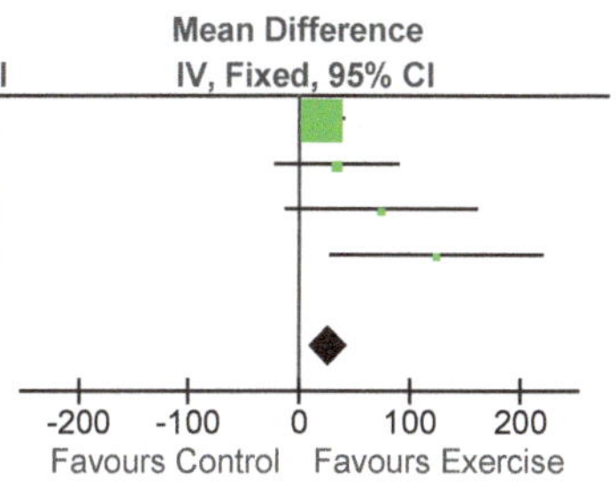

Figure 2. Comparison of six-minute walk distance (Metres) following exercise training in HD patients.

Study or Subgroup	Exercise Mean	Exercise SD	Exercise Total	Control Mean	Control SD	Control Total	Weight	Mean Difference IV, Fixed, 95% CI
Chen JL 2010	15.8	5	22	12.1	6.1	22	58.8%	3.70 [0.40, 7.00]
Johansen 2006	22.6	11.6	20	20	9.1	20	15.3%	2.60 [-3.86, 9.06]
Oliveros 2011	21	4	5	19.4	4.4	6	25.9%	1.60 [-3.37, 6.57]
Total (95% CI)			**47**			**48**	**100.0%**	**2.99 [0.46, 5.52]**

Heterogeneity: Chi² = 0.49, df = 2 (P = 0.78); I² = 0%
Test for overall effect: Z = 2.32 (P = 0.02)

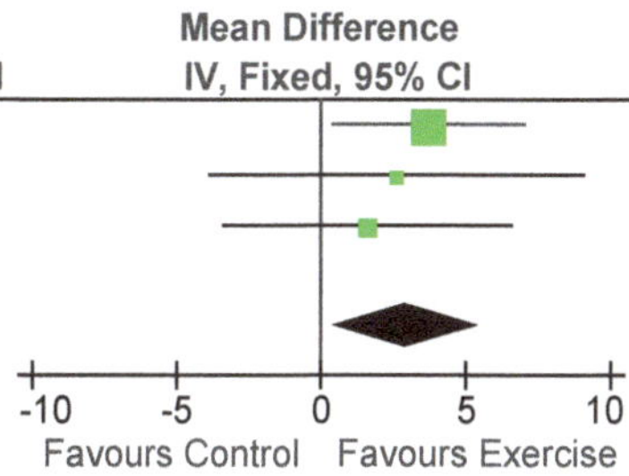

Figure 3. Comparison of knee-extensor strength (kg) following exercise training in HD patients.

Study or Subgroup	Exercise Mean	Exercise SD	Exercise Total	Sedentray Control Mean	Sedentray Control SD	Sedentray Control Total	Weight	Mean Difference IV, Fixed, 95% CI
Cheema 2007	27.3	0.5356	24	26.9	0.5356	25	96.1%	0.40 [0.10, 0.70]
Dong 2011	26.8	4.3	10	29.3	6.8	12	0.4%	-2.50 [-7.18, 2.18]
Koufaki 2002	25.7	3.3	18	24.7	3.5	15	1.6%	1.00 [-1.34, 3.34]
Wilund 2010	30.3	2.5	8	28.3	1.8	9	2.0%	2.00 [-0.09, 4.09]
Total (95% CI)			**60**			**61**	**100.0%**	**0.43 [0.14, 0.72]**

Heterogeneity: Chi² = 3.93, df = 3 (P = 0.27); I² = 24%
Test for overall effect: Z = 2.86 (P = 0.004)

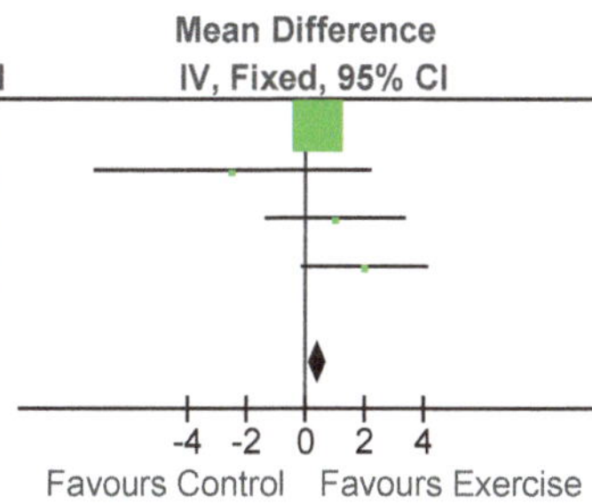

Figure 4. Comparison of BMI ($kg{\cdot}m^{-2}$) following exercise training in HD patients.

238 $Kcal{\cdot}day^{-1}$ (95% CI 94, 383, p = 0.001), see **Figure 5**. **Figure 6** shows a forest plot of 6 studies [15,26-30] reporting serum albumin in 126 HD patients. Albumin was significantly lower in exercising versus sedentary controls MD −0.07 $g{\cdot}L^{-1}$ (95% CI −0.16, −0.01, p = 0.08). Two studies [26,31] reported post-training serum levels of interleukin-6 (pg/ml) in 49 patients, IL-6 was significantly lower in exercising HD patients versus sedentary controls MD-0.58 $pg{\cdot}ml^{-1}$ (95% CI −1.01, −0.15, p = 0.008), see **Figure 7**. Two studies [26,30] reported post-training serum levels of C-reactive protein in 38 patients, CRP was significantly higher in exercising HD patients versus sedentary controls MD 0.92 mg/L^{-1} (95% CI 0.29, 1.56, p = 0.004), see **Figure 8**.

3.9. Cardiac Function

Following analysis of three studies [6,14,29] in 119 patients, a non-significant trend towards improved left ventricular ejection fraction was observed post-intervention in exercise training patients MD 2.8% (95% CI −1.4, 6.9%, p = 0.20).

3.10. Depression and Self-Reported Health (SF-36)

Three studies [4,5,23] reported Beck depression score (BDI) in 86 HD patients, BDI score was significantly lower (improved) in exercising patients versus sedentary controls MD −6.9 (95% CI −9.7, −4.1, p < 0.00001), see **Figure 9**. Neither the physical or mental components of SF-36 general health questionnaire were improved following exercise training.

3.11. Dialysis Related Biochemistry

Figure 10 shows four studies [23,28-30] reported dialysis adequacy index in 54 patients, Kt/V was significantly lower in exercising patients versus sedentary controls MD −0.25 (95% CI −0.34, −0.17, p < 0.00001). **Figure 11** shows 6 studies [4,6,7,14,26,32] reporting serum potassium in 253 patients, potassium was higher in exercising

Study or Subgroup	Exercise Mean	Exercise SD	Exercise Total	Control Mean	Control SD	Control Total	Weight	Mean Difference IV, Fixed, 95% CI
Dong 2011	1,977	530	10	2,379	1,026	12	4.7%	-402.00 [-1069.00, 265.00]
Frey 1999	2,027	549	5	1,392	325	6	7.0%	635.00 [88.02, 1181.98]
Koufaki 2002	2,680	306	18	2,439	121	15	88.3%	241.00 [86.95, 395.05]
Total (95% CI)			**33**			**33**	**100.0%**	**238.31 [93.56, 383.06]**

Heterogeneity: Chi^2 = 5.56, df = 2 (P = 0.06); I^2 = 64%
Test for overall effect: Z = 3.23 (P = 0.001)

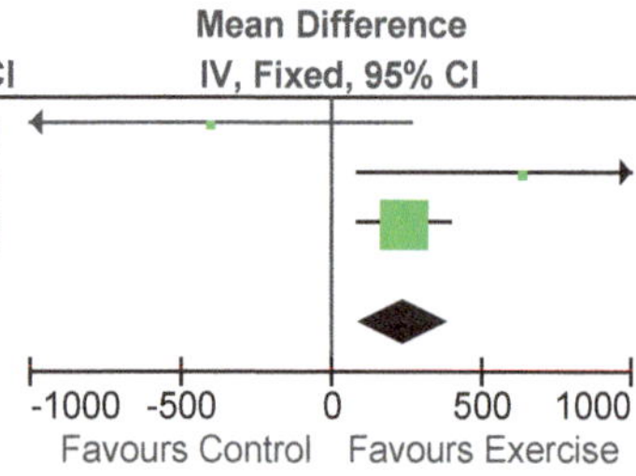

Figure 5. Comparison of daily energy intake (Kcals·day^{-1}) following exercise training in HD patients.

Study or Subgroup	Expercise Mean	Expercise SD	Expercise Total	Control Mean	Control SD	Control Total	Weight	Mean Difference IV, Fixed, 95% CI
Afshar 2010 Aerobic	4	0.4	7	4	0.3	4	3.9%	0.00 [-0.42, 0.42]
Afshar 2010 Resistance	4	0.3	7	4	0.3	3	4.1%	0.00 [-0.41, 0.41]
Cheema 2007	3.48	0.4106	24	3.34	0.4106	25	12.8%	0.14 [-0.09, 0.37]
Dong 2011	4.15	0.44	10	4.2	0.22	12	7.5%	-0.05 [-0.35, 0.25]
Frey 1999	4.4	0.5	5	3.7	0.7	6	1.3%	0.70 [-0.01, 1.41]
Koufaki 2002	3.52	0.7	18	4.05	0.36	15	4.9%	-0.53 [-0.90, -0.16]
Reboredo 2010	3.9	0.3	11	4.1	0.5	11	5.7%	-0.20 [-0.54, 0.14]
Wilund 2010	3.8	0.06	8	3.9	0.15	9	59.7%	-0.10 [-0.21, 0.01]
Total (95% CI)			**90**			**85**	**100.0%**	**-0.07 [-0.16, 0.01]**

Heterogeneity: Chi^2 = 14.69, df = 7 (P = 0.04); I^2 = 52%
Test for overall effect: Z = 1.75 (P = 0.08)

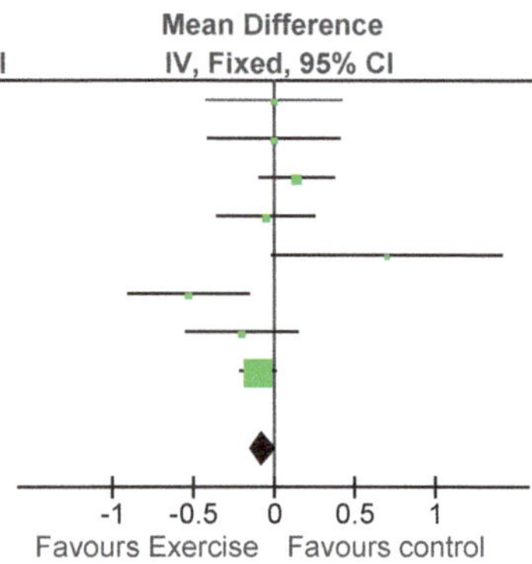

Figure 6. Comparison of serum albumin (g·L^{-1}) following exercise training in HD patients.

Study or Subgroup	Exercise Mean	Exercise SD	Exercise Total	Control Mean	Control SD	Control Total	Weight	Mean Difference IV, Fixed, 95% CI
Daniilidis 2004	6.23	1.04	18	6.61	0.98	14	37.1%	-0.38 [-1.08, 0.32]
Wilund 2010	1.8	0.66	8	2.5	0.44	9	62.9%	-0.70 [-1.24, -0.16]
Total (95% CI)			**26**			**23**	**100.0%**	**-0.58 [-1.01, -0.15]**

Heterogeneity: Chi^2 = 0.50, df = 1 (P = 0.48); I^2 = 0%
Test for overall effect: Z = 2.66 (P = 0.008)

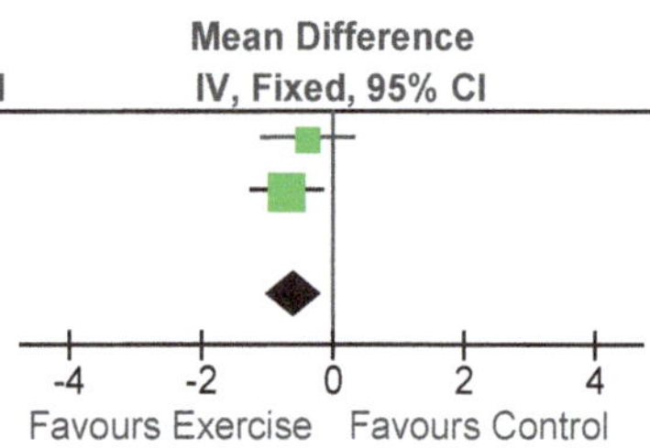

Figure 7. Comparison of serum interleukin-6 (pg·ml^{-1}) following exercise training in HD patients.

Study or Subgroup	Exercise Mean	Exercise SD	Exercise Total	Control Mean	Control SD	Control Total	Weight	Mean Difference IV, Fixed, 95% CI
Afshar 2010 Aerobic	0.88	0.59	7	4.14	3.87	4	2.7%	-3.26 [-7.08, 0.56]
Afshar 2010 Resistance	2.27	1.79	7	4.14	3.87	3	1.9%	-1.87 [-6.45, 2.71]
Wilund 2010	6	0.67	8	4.9	0.69	9	95.4%	1.10 [0.45, 1.75]
Total (95% CI)			**22**			**16**	**100.0%**	**0.92 [0.29, 1.56]**

Heterogeneity: Chi^2 = 6.33, df = 2 (P = 0.04); I^2 = 68%
Test for overall effect: Z = 2.87 (P = 0.004)

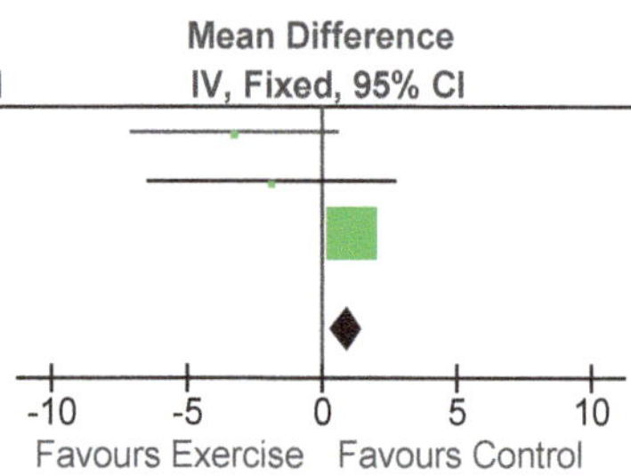

Figure 8. Comparison of C-reactive protein (mg·L^{-1}) following exercise training in HD patients.

patients versus sedentary controls MD 0.14 mmol·L^{-1} (95% CI 0.01, 0.27, p = 0.04).

3.12. Exercise Eligibility, Adherence and Safety

The following studies provided a complete CONSORT [6,18,21,22,24,27,29,33] statement. Two other studies [4, 15] provided partial data about eligibility, withdrawal and completion. Data from these studies showed that of 1421 patients approached for suitability for exercise training 551 or nearly 39% were ineligible due to various medical exclusion criteria. Exercise training appears safe with no deaths reported during exercise training in over 30,000 patients-hours of exercise.

3.13. Study Quality and Effect of Publication Bias

JADAD score [11] was used to assess study quality. We used a modified JADAD score on a scale 0 - 3, based

Study or Subgroup	Exercise Mean	Exercise SD	Exercise Total	Control Mean	Control SD	Control Total	Weight	Mean Difference IV, Fixed, 95% CI
Kouidi 1997	13.7	9.5	20	21.3	11.9	11	12.0%	-7.60 [-15.77, 0.57]
Kouidi 2010	14.61	4.15	24	22.1	6.24	20	78.4%	-7.49 [-10.69, -4.29]
Oliveros 2011	13.4	8	5	14.7	7.3	6	9.6%	-1.30 [-10.43, 7.83]
Total (95% CI)			**49**			**37**	**100.0%**	**-6.91 [-9.74, -4.08]**

Heterogeneity: Chi² = 1.61, df = 2 (P = 0.45); I² = 0%
Test for overall effect: Z = 4.78 (P < 0.00001)

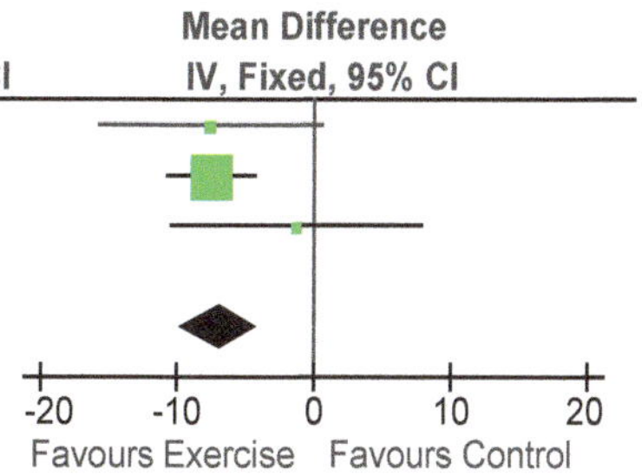

Figure 9. Comparison of Beck depression inventory following exercise training in HD patients.

Study or Subgroup	Expercise Mean	Expercise SD	Expercise Total	Control Mean	Control SD	Control Total	Weight	Mean Difference IV, Fixed, 95% CI
Afshar 2010 Aerobic	1	0.33	7	1.1	0.25	3	2.9%	-0.10 [-0.47, 0.27]
Cheema 2007	1.6	0.1785	24	1.8	0.1785	25	40.5%	-0.20 [-0.30, -0.10]
Frey 1999	1.8	0.3	5	1.7	0.1	6	5.4%	0.10 [-0.17, 0.37]
Oliveros 2011	1.2	0.08	5	1.5	0.07	6	50.2%	-0.30 [-0.39, -0.21]
Reboredo 2010	1.8	0.7	11	2	0.8	11	1.0%	-0.20 [-0.83, 0.43]
Total (95% CI)			**52**			**51**	**100.0%**	**-0.23 [-0.29, -0.17]**

Heterogeneity: Chi² = 8.69, df = 4 (P = 0.07); I² = 54%
Test for overall effect: Z = 7.13 (P < 0.00001)

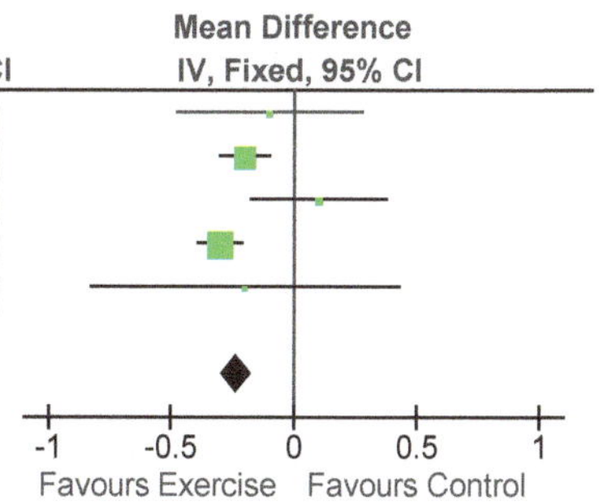

Figure 10. Comparison of dialysis adequacy index following exercise training in HD patients.

Study or Subgroup	Exercise Mean	Exercise SD	Exercise Total	Control Mean	Control SD	Control Total	Weight	Mean Difference IV, Fixed, 95% CI
Deligannis 1999aiHomeEx	5.5	0.7	10	5.4	0.4	6	5.9%	0.10 [-0.44, 0.64]
Deligannis 1999ailD	5.7	0.5	16	5.4	0.4	6	10.5%	0.30 [-0.10, 0.70]
Deligannis 1999b	5.8	0.5	30	5.7	0.7	30	18.0%	0.10 [-0.21, 0.41]
Kouidi 1997	5.6	0.5	20	5.5	0.7	11	7.8%	0.10 [-0.37, 0.57]
Kouidi 2009	5.6	0.6	30	5.3	0.4	29	25.4%	0.30 [0.04, 0.56]
Makhlough 2012	5.12	0.96	25	5.16	0.67	23	7.9%	-0.04 [-0.51, 0.43]
Wilund 2010	4.9	0.3	8	4.9	0.25	9	24.5%	0.00 [-0.26, 0.26]
Total (95% CI)			**139**			**114**	**100.0%**	**0.14 [0.01, 0.27]**

Heterogeneity: Chi² = 3.83, df = 6 (P = 0.70); I² = 0%
Test for overall effect: Z = 2.04 (P = 0.04)

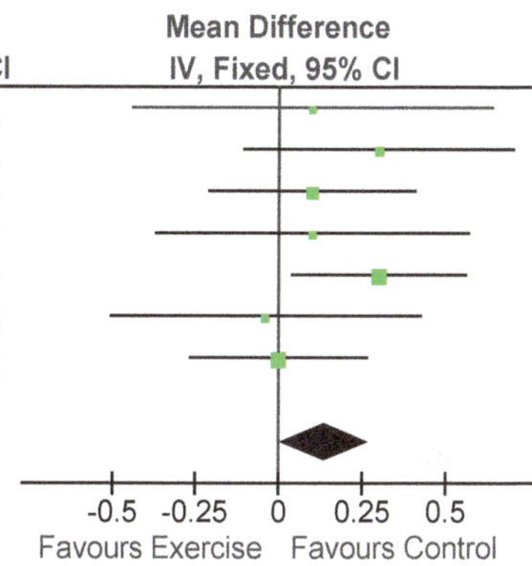

Figure 11. Comparison of serum potassium ($mmol \cdot L^{-1}$) following exercise training in HD patients.

upon investigator blinding, randomization of participants and reporting of participant withdrawals. Median JADAD was 2, three studies scored 1, 12 studies scored 2 and 13 studies scored 3. Funnel plots showed little evidence of publication bias.

3.14. Study Heterogeneity

Studies were extremely well matched for age, gender and baseline peak VO_2. Cochran Q tests revealed low (<50%) I^2 values for all but 3 analyses suggesting little heterogeneity between studies, these values indicate it was appropriate to pool data for all analyses except CRP, energy intake and dialysis adequacy.

4. Discussion

Our review includes previously unreported pooled analyses of changes in energy balance, dialysis adequacy, serum potassium, patient adherence recruitment and safety post-exercise training. Our work also provides a clinical update on pooled analyses undertaken following exercise training in studies of CKD patients published to date. Our work suggests that exercise training for patients undertaking HD is safe.

The mean baseline peak VO_2 value for HD patients is approximately 20 $mlO_2 \cdot kg^{-1} \cdot min^{-1}$, previous work has demonstrated that a peak VO_2 of 17.5 $mlO_2 \cdot kg^{-1} \cdot min^{-1}$ or less is associated with poor survival [8], so exercise training is likely to assist most those at risk of falling below this threshold. Data extracted demonstrates included patients showed reduced baseline peak VO_2 approximately 30% below age-adjusted norms. We observed that exercise training produces varied improvements in peak VO_2 depending on the type, increasing duration and intra-dialytic delivery of exercise. Our data suggest either combined aerobic and resistance exercise or isolated aerobic exercise, delivered on non-dialysis days, for at least 6 months is likely to offer the greatest magnitude of change in peak VO_2. Data on isolated resistance exercise in HD patients is limited currently. The magnitude of change in peak VO_2 in programs of 2 - 6 months duration concur with the 17% previously reported in HD patients [17,33], although only about a 12% improvement can be expected at 3 months. Larger increments (>30%) in post-training peak VO_2 have been observed in patients who complete combined aerobic and strength training for 6 months or more on non-dialysis days [7,14]. Moreover exercise training restores much of the deficit in age-adjusted peak VO_2 and meta-regression showed the extent of peak VO_2 restoration is positively correlated with increasing exercise training duration.

Our 6-minute walk data confirmed that the improvements in peak VO_2 were associated with improved physical function. One must remember though that such large improvements in peak VO_2 are facilitated because patients are often concurrently given erythropoietin (EPO) and optimizing oxygen carrying capacity of the blood will increase the potential to adapt to exercise training. The included studies had great variation in the criteria for managing EPO use.

Outcomes pertaining to muscle size and strength were available from three studies, these data suggest muscle size and strength can be improved via resistance training. The optimal exercise training program is therefore likely to retard muscle-wasting and improve muscle cross sectional area and strength, although there is an obvious need for a large, well-designed, randomized, controlled trial of resistance training in HD patients.

Three studies [15,27,28] reported exercising patients reported raised daily energy intakes by 238 $Kcal \cdot day^{-1}$ or 1666 $Kcal \cdot week^{-1}$. We estimate that exercise training energy expenditures from these studies are of the order of 1000 Kcal per week, providing a weekly energy surplus of about 670 Kcal. Despite this the four studies measuring change in BMI did not report a significant net gain. Data from heart failure studies suggest weight gain, especially body fat is beneficial [34], but this finding has yet to be established for HD patients even though intuittively poor nutrition is associated with muscle wasting, de-conditioning and the catabolic state. Serum levels of both interleukin-6 and C-reactive protein were both favourably attenuated following exercise training, suggesting that muscle mass can be preserved in HD patients and end stage cachexia delayed in those at risk.

Beck Depression score was impaired at baseline but did improve significantly. Baseline Beck depression data from this meta-analysis suggest values consistent with moderate to severe depression, which was significantly reduced post-training, in those who exercised [5], so exercise training may have benefit beyond the partial restoration of peak VO_2 deficits.

Dialysis Adequacy (kt/v) was lower in exercising versus control patients. Lower kt/v indicates that a smaller amount of fluid needs to be removed during dialysis and therefore there may be less strain on the cardiovascular system. Serum potassium was also higher in exercising patients which is likely to reduce fluid retention and this may be linked to changes observed in kt/v. The risk of hypotensive episodes during intra-dialytic exercise, due to fluid removal during dialysis, may preclude patients from achieving similar durations and activities of exercise that could be accomplished on non-dialysis days [35], however our analyses of this review suggest that adaptation to exercise may attenuate the risks associated with fluid removal.

To date no randomized, controlled, study of exercise training in patients with chronic renal failure has reported a death directly related to exercise in over 30,000 patient-hours of exercise. An analysis of exercise training study withdrawal suggests exercise patients are no more likely than control patients to drop out of a study. One may therefore postulate that exercise training for HD patients is safe and the derived benefits outweigh the risk of adverse events such as hypotensive or ischemic episodes.

Kidney Disease International recently recommended exercise training for people with chronic renal disease to guide specialist and allied health teams to incorporate exercise training into their clinical services [36]. Perhaps of most interest would be a long-term randomized, controlled trial of exercise training that examines the primary outcome measures of mortality, including cardiovascular mortality, hospitalization and cost-effectiveness in dialysis or preferably, pre-dialysis patients.

The limitations of this work were varying exercise program parameters; durations, type of delivery (intra-versus inter-dialytic), modalities (aerobic or resistance or combined), intensity. Moreover a wide range of outcome measures were employed, studies were generally small and strict eligibility criteria mean healthier patients were more likely to be selected. Despite these limitations included studies are exceptionally well matched in terms of age, gender and peak VO_2 at baseline for exercise and control group participants. Publication bias may affect the results although funnel plotting peak VO_2 changes suggest bias was minimal.

5. Conclusion

Our pooled analyses produced novel findings that exercise training may improve dialysis efficiency (kt/v), serum potassium, inflammation and depression in HD patients. Our analyses also confirm improvements in peak VO_2, muscle strength, walking distance and energy intake.

REFERENCES

[1] B. S. Cheema and M. A. Singh, "Exercise Training in Patients Receiving Maintenance Hemodialysis: A Systematic Review of Clinical Trials," *American Journal of Nephrology*, Vol. 25, No. 4, 2005, pp. 352-364. doi:10.1159/000087184

[2] E. J. Howden, R. G. Fassett, N. M. Isbel and J. S. Coombes, "Exercise Training in Chronic Kidney Disease Patients," *Sports Medicine*, Vol. 42, No. 6, 2012, pp. 473-488. doi:10.2165/11630800-000000000-00000

[3] K. L. Johansen and P. Painter, "Exercise in Individuals with CKD," *American Journal of Kidney Diseases*, Vol. 59, No. 1, 2012, pp. 126-134. doi:10.1053/j.ajkd.2011.10.008

[4] E. Kouidi, A. Iacovides, P. Iordanidis, S. Vassiliou, A. Deligiannis, C. Ierodiakonou and A. Tourkantonis, "Exercise Renal Rehabilitation Program: Psychosocial Effects," *Nephron Clinical Practice*, Vol. 77, No. 2, 1997, pp. 152-158.

[5] E. Kouidi, V. Karagiannis, D. Grekas, A. Iakovides, G. Kaprinis, A. Tourkantonis and A. Deligiannis, "Depression, Heart Rate Variability, and Exercise Training in Dialysis Patients," *European Journal Cardiovascular Prevention Rehabilitation*, Vol. 17, No. 2, 2010, pp. 160-167. doi:10.1097/HJR.0b013e32833188c4

[6] E. J. Kouidi, D. M. Grekas and A. P. Deligiannis, "Effects of Exercise Training on Noninvasive Cardiac Measures in Patients Undergoing Long-Term Hemodialysis: A Randomized Controlled Trial," *American Journal of Kidney Diseases*, Vol. 54, No. 3, 2009, pp. 511-521. doi:10.1053/j.ajkd.2009.03.009

[7] A. Deligiannis, E. Kouidi and A. Tourkantonis, "Effects of Physical Training on Heart Rate Variability in Patients on Hemodialysis," *American Journal of Cardiology*, Vol. 84, No. 2, 1999, pp. 197-202. doi:10.1016/S0002-9149(99)00234-9

[8] K. E. Sietsema, A. Amato, S. G. Adler and E. P. Brass, "Exercise Capacity as a Predictor of Survival among Ambulatory Patients with End-Stage Renal Disease," *Kidney International*, Vol. 65, No. 2, 2004, pp. 719-724. doi:10.1111/j.1523-1755.2004.00411.x

[9] N. Smart and M. Steele, "Exercise Training in Haemodialysis Patients: A Systematic Review and Meta-Analysis," *Nephrology* (*Carlton*), Vol. 16, No. 7, 2011, pp. 626-632.

[10] E. Segura-Orti, "Exercise in Haemodyalisis Patients: A Literature Systematic Review," *Nefrologia*, Vol. 30, No. 2, 2010, pp. 236-246.

[11] A. R. Jadad, R. A. Moore, D. Carroll, C. Jenkinson, D. J. Reynolds, D. J. Gavaghan and H. J. McQuay, "Assessing the Quality of Reports of Randomized Clinical Trials: Is Blinding Necessary?" *Controlled Clinical Trials*, Vol. 17, No. 1, 1996, pp. 1-12. doi:10.1016/0197-2456(95)00134-4

[12] P. Alderson and S. Green, "Cochrane Collaboration Open Learning Material for Reviewers," Version 1.1, 2002. http://www.cochrane-net.org/openlearning/PDF/Openlearning-full.pdf

[13] J. P. T. Higgins, S. G. Thompson, J. J. Deeks and D. G. Altman, "Measuring Inconsistency in Meta-Analysis," *British Medical Journal*, Vol. 327, No. 7414, 2003, pp. 557-560. doi:10.1136/bmj.327.7414.557

[14] A. Deligiannis, E. Kouidi, E. Tassoulas, P. Gigis, A. Tourkantonis and A. Coats, "Cardiac Effects of Exercise Rehabilitation in Hemodialysis Patients," *International Journal of Cardiology*, Vol. 70, No. 3, 1999, pp. 253-266. doi:10.1016/S0167-5273(99)00090-X

[15] P. Koufaki, T. H. Mercer and P. F. Naish, "Effects of Exercise Training on Aerobic and Functional Capacity of End-Stage Renal Disease Patients," *Clinical Physiology and Functional Imaging*, Vol. 22, No. 2, 2002, pp. 115-124. doi:10.1046/j.1365-2281.2002.00405.x

[16] G. Moros, R. Ros Mar, A. A. Villarroya, A. C. L. de Robles, M. Comin and S. Nerin Ballarriga, "Physical Exercise in Hemodialysis Patients," *Archivos de Medicina del Deporte*, Vol. 17, No. 77, 2000, pp. 235-244.

[17] P. Painter, G. Moore, L. Carlson, S. Paul, J. Myll, W. Phillips and W. Haskell, "Effects of Exercise Training plus Normalization of Hematocrit on Exercise Capacity and Health-Related Quality of Life," *American Journal of Kidney Diseases*, Vol. 39, No. 2, 2002, pp. 257-265. doi:10.1053/ajkd.2002.30544

[18] M. C. Van Vilsteren, M. H. de Greef and R. M. Huisman, "The Effects of a Low-to-Moderate Intensity Pre-Conditioning Exercise Programme Linked with Exercise Counselling for Sedentary Haemodialysis Patients in The Netherlands: Results of a Randomized Clinical Trial," *Nephrology Dialysis Transplantation*, Vol. 20, No. 1, 2005, pp. 141-146. doi:10.1093/ndt/gfh560

[19] A. P. Goldberg, E. M. Geltman, J. M. Hagberg, J. R. Gavin III, J. A. Delmez, R. M. Carney, A. Naumowicz, M. H. Oldfield and H. R. Harter, "Therapeutic Benefits of Exercise Training for Hemodialysis Patients," *Kidney International Supplements*, Vol. 16, 1983, pp. S303-S309.

[20] E. Kouidi, D. Grekas, A. Deligiannis and A. Tourkantonis, "Outcomes of Long-Term Exercise Training in Dialysis Patients: Comparison of Two Training Programs," *Clinical Nephrology*, Vol. 61, Suppl. 1, 2004, pp. S31-S38.

[21] K. P. Koh, R. G. Fassett, J. E. Sharman, J. S. Coombes and A. D. Williams, "Intradialytic versus Home-Based Exercise Training in Hemodialysis Patients: A Randomised Controlled Trial," *BMC Nephrology*, Vol. 10, 2009, p. 2.

[22] V. DePaul, J. Moreland, T. Eager and C. M. Clase, "The Effectiveness of Aerobic and Muscle Strength Training in Patients Receiving Hemodialysis and EPO: A Randomized Controlled Trial," *American Journal Kidney Diseases*, Vol. 40, No. 6, 2002, pp. 1219-1229. doi:10.1053/ajkd.2002.36887

[23] R. M. Oliveros, M. Avendano, D. Bunout, S. Hirsch, M. P. De La Maza, C. Pedreros and H. Muller, "A Pilot Study on Physical Training of Patients in Hemodialysis,"

Revista Médica de Chile, Vol. 139, No. 8, 2011, pp. 1046-1053.

[24] J. L. Chen, S. Godfrey, T. T. Ng, R. Moorthi, O. Liangos, R. Ruthazer, B. L. Jaber, A. S. Levey and C. Castaneda-Sceppa, "Effect of Intra-Dialytic, Low-Intensity Strength Training on Functional Capacity in Adult Haemodialysis Patients: A Randomized Pilot Trial," *Nephrology Dialysis Transplantation*, Vol. 25, No. 6, 2010, pp. 1936-1943. doi:10.1093/ndt/gfp739

[25] K. L. Johansen, P. L. Painter, G. K. Sakkas, P. Gordon, J. Doyle and T. Shubert, "Effects of Resistance Exercise Training and Nandrolone Decanoate on Body Composition and Muscle Function among Patients Who Receive Hemodialysis: A Randomized, Controlled Trial," *Journal of the American Society of Nephrology*, Vol. 17, No. 8, 2006, pp. 2307-2314. doi:10.1681/ASN.2006010034

[26] K. R. Wilund, E. J. Tomayko, P. T. Wu, H. Ryong Chung, S. Vallurupalli, B. Lakshminarayanan and B. Fernhall, "Intradialytic Exercise Training Reduces Oxidative Stress and Epicardial Fat: A Pilot Study," *Nephrology Dialysis Transplantation*, Vol. 25, No. 8, 2010, pp. 2695-2701. doi:10.1093/ndt/gfq106

[27] J. Dong, M. B. Sundell, L. B. Pupim, P. Wu, A. Shintani and T. A. Ikizler, "The Effect of Resistance Exercise to Augment Long-Term Benefits of Intradialytic Oral Nutritional Supplementation in Chronic Hemodialysis Patients," *Journal of Renal Nutrition*, Vol. 21, No. 2, 2011, pp. 149-159. doi:10.1053/j.jrn.2010.03.004

[28] S. Frey, A. R. Mir and M. Lucas, "Visceral Protein Status and Caloric Intake in Exercising versus Nonexercising Individuals with End-Stage Renal Disease," *Journal of Renal Nutrition*, Vol. 9, No. 2, 1999, pp. 71-77. doi:10.1016/S1051-2276(99)90003-1

[29] M. Reboredo Mde, V. Pinheiro Bdo, J. A. Neder, M. P. Avila, E. R. M. L. Araujo, A. F. de Mendonca, M. V. de Mello, A. C. Bainha, J. Dondici Filho and R. B. de Paula, "Effects of Aerobic Training during Hemodialysis on Heart Rate Variability and Left Ventricular Function in End-Stage Renal Disease Patients," *Jornal Brasileiro de Nefrologia*, Vol. 32, No. 4, 2010, pp. 367-373.

[30] R. Afshar, L. Shegarfy, N. Shavandi and S. Sanavi, "Effects of Aerobic Exercise and Resistance Training on Lipid Profiles and Inflammation Status in Patients on Maintenance Hemodialysis," *Indian Journal of Nephrology*, Vol. 20, No. 4, 2010, pp. 185-189. doi:10.4103/0971-4065.73442

[31] M. Daniilidis, E. Kouidi, E. Giagoudaki, A. Fleva, P. Nikolaides, A. Vasilaki, *et al.*, "The Immune Response in Hemodialysis Patients Following Physical Training," *Sport Sciences for Health*, Vol. 1, 2004, pp. 11-16. doi:10.1007/s11332-004-0003-y

[32] A. Makhlough, E. Ilali, R. Mohseni and S. Shahmohammadi, "Effect of Intradialytic Aerobic Exercise on Serum Electrolytes Levels in Hemodialysis Patients," *Iranian Journal of Kidney Diseases*, Vol. 6, No. 2, 2012, pp. 119-123. doi:10.1681/ASN.2007010009

[33] K. L. Johansen, "Exercise in the End-Stage Renal Disease Population," *Journal of the American Society of Nephrology*, Vol. 18, No. 6, 2007, pp. 1845-1854.

[34] S. D. Anker, W. Steinborn and S. Strassburg, "Cardiac Cachexia," *Annals of Medicine*, Vol. 36, No. 7, 2004, pp. 518-529. doi:10.1080/07853890410017467

[35] M. Petraki, E. Kouidi, D. Grekas and A. Deligiannis, "Effects of Exercise Training during Hemodialysis on Cardiac Baroreflex Sensitivity," *Clinical Nephrology*, Vol. 70, No. 3, 2008, pp. 210-219.

[36] "KDIGO 2012 Clinical Practice Guideline for the Evaluation and Management of Chronic Kidney Disease," *International Society of Nephrology*, Vol. 3, No. 1, 2013, pp. 1-163.

[37] T. L. Parsons, E. B. Toffelmire and C. E. King-Van Vlack, "The Effect of an Exercise Program during Hemodialysis on Dialysis Efficacy, Blood Pressure and Quality of Life in End-Stage Renal Disease (ESRD) Patients," *Clinical Nephrology*, Vol. 61, No. 4, 2004, pp. 261-274.

[38] T. Akiba, N. Matsui, S. Shinohara, H. Fujiwara, T. Nomura and F. Marumo, "Effects of Recombinant Human Erythropoietin and Exercise Training on Exercise Capacity in Hemodialysis Patients," *Artificial Organs*, Vol. 19, No. 12, 1995, pp. 1262-1268. doi:10.1111/j.1525-1594.1995.tb02297.x

[39] V. S. Balakrishnan, M. Rao, V. Menon, P. L. Gordon, M. Pilichowska, F. Castaneda and C. Castaneda-Sceppa, "Resistance Training Increases Muscle Mitochondrial Biogenesis in Patients with Chronic Kidney Disease," *Clinical Journal American Society Nephrology*, Vol. 5, No. 6, 2010, pp. 996-1002. doi:10.2215/CJN.09141209

[40] R. M. Carney, B. Templeton, B. A. Hong, H. R. Harter, J. M. Hagberg, K. B. Schechtman and A. P. Goldberg, "Exercise Training Reduces Depression and Increases the Performance of Pleasant Activities in Hemodialysis Patients," *Nephron Clinical Practice*, Vol. 47, No. 3, 1987, pp. 194-198.

[41] C. Castaneda, P. L. Gordon, K. L. Uhlin, A. S. Levey, J. J. Kehayias, J. T. Dwyer, R. A. Fielding, R. Roubenoff and M. F. Singh, "Resistance Training to Counteract the Catabolism of a Low-Protein Diet in Patients with Chronic Renal Insufficiency. A Randomized, Controlled Trial," *Annals of Internal Medicine*, Vol. 135, No. 11, 2001, pp. 965-976.

[42] C. Castaneda, P. L. Gordon, R. C. Parker, K. L. Uhlin, R. Roubenoff and A. S. Levey, "Resistance Training to Reduce the Malnutrition-Inflammation Complex Syndrome of Chronic Kidney Disease," *American Journal of Kidney Diseases*, Vol. 43, No. 4, 2004, pp. 607-616. doi:10.1053/j.ajkd.2003.12.025

[43] Y. Chang, S. Y. Cheng, M. Lin, F. Y. Gau and Y. F. Chao, "The Effectiveness of Intradialytic Leg Ergometry Exercise for Improving Sedentary Life Style and Fatigue among Patients with Chronic Kidney Disease: A Randomized Clinical Trial," *International Journal of Nursing Studies*, Vol. 47, No. 11, 2010, pp. 1383-1388. doi:10.1016/j.ijnurstu.2010.05.002

[44] B. Cheema, H. Abas, B. Smith, A. O'Sullivan, M. Chan, A. Patwardhan, J. Kelly, A. Gillin, G. Pang, B. Lloyd and M. F. Singh, "Progressive Exercise for Anabolism in Kidney Disease (PEAK): A Randomized, Controlled Trial of Resistance Training during Hemodialysis," *Journal of the American Society Nephrology*, Vol. 18, No. 5,

2007, pp. 1594-1601. doi:10.1681/ASN.2006121329

[45] B. Cheema, H. Abas, B. Smith, A. O'Sullivan, M. Chan, A. Patwardhan, J. Kelly, A. Gillin, G. Pang, B. Lloyd and M. Fiatarone Singh, "Randomized Controlled Trial of Intradialytic Resistance Training to Target Muscle Wasting in ESRD: The Progressive Exercise for Anabolism in Kidney Disease (PEAK) Study," *American Journal of Kidney Diseases*, Vol. 50, No. 4, 2007, pp. 574-584. doi:10.1053/j.ajkd.2007.07.005

[46] B. S. Cheema, H. Abas, B. C. Smith, A. J. O'Sullivan, M. Chan, A. Patwardhan, J. Kelly, A. Gillin, G. Pang, B. Lloyd, K. Berger, B. T. Baune and M. A. Fiatarone Singh, "Effect of Resistance Training during Hemodialysis on Circulating Cytokines: A Randomized Controlled Trial," *European Journal of Applied Physiology*, Vol. 111, No. 7, 2011, pp. 1437-1445. doi:10.1007/s00421-010-1763-5

[47] P. Y. Chen, Y. C. Huang, Y. H. Kao and J. Y. Chen, "Effects of an Exercise Program on Blood Biochemical Values and Exercise Stage of Chronic Kidney Disease Patients," *Journal of Nursing Research*, Vol. 18, No. 2, 2010, pp. 98-107. doi:10.1097/JNR.0b013e3181dda726

[48] S. S. Fitts, M. R. Guthrie and C. R. Blagg, "Exercise Coaching and Rehabilitation Counseling Improve Quality of Life for Predialysis and Dialysis Patients," *Nephron Clinical Practice*, Vol. 82, No. 2, 1999, pp. 115-121.

[49] M. Flesher, P. Woo, A. Chiu, A. Charlebois, D. E. Warburton and B. Leslie, "Self-Management and Biomedical Outcomes of a Cooking, and Exercise Program for Patients with Chronic Kidney Disease," *Journal of Renal Nutrition*, Vol. 21, No. 2, 2011, pp. 188-195. doi:10.1053/j.jrn.2010.03.009

[50] A. P. Goldberg, E. M. Geltman, J. R. Gavin III, R. M. Carney, J. M. Hagberg, J. A. Delmez, A. Naumovich, M. H. Oldfield and H. R. Harter, "Exercise Training Reduces Coronary Risk and Effectively Rehabilitates Hemodialysis Patients," *Nephron Clinical Practice*, Vol. 42, No. 4, 1986, pp. 311-316.

[51] H. R. Harter and A. P. Goldberg, "Endurance Exercise Training. An Effective Therapeutic Modality for Hemodialysis Patients," *Medical Clinics of North America*, Vol. 69, No. 1, 1985, pp. 159-175.

[52] S. A. Headley, M. J. Germain, C. M. Milch, M. P. Buchholz, M. A. Coughlin and L. S. Pescatello, "Immediate Blood Pressure-Lowering Effects of Aerobic Exercise among Patients with Chronic Kidney Disease," *Nephrology* (*Carlton*), Vol. 13, No. 7, 2008, pp. 601-606. doi:10.1111/j.1440-1797.2008.01030.x

[53] E. Konstantinidou, G. Koukouvou, E. Kouidi, A. Deligiannis and A. Tourkantonis, "Exercise Training in Patients with End-Stage Renal Disease on Hemodialysis: Comparison of Three Rehabilitation Programs," *Journal of Rehabilitation Medicine*, Vol. 34, No. 1, 2002, pp. 40-45. doi:10.1080/165019702317242695

[54] D. J. Leehey, I. Moinuddin, J. P. Bast, S. Qureshi, C. S. Jelinek, C. Cooper, L. C. Edwards, B. M. Smith and E. G. Collins, "Aerobic Exercise in Obese Diabetic Patients with Chronic Kidney Disease: A Randomized and Controlled Pilot Study," *Cardiovascular Diabetology*, Vol. 8, 2009, p. 62.

[55] Y. Matsumoto, A. Furuta, S. Furuta, M. Miyajima, T. Sugino, K. Nagata and S. Sawada, "The Impact of Pre-Dialytic Endurance Training on Nutritional Status and Quality of Life in Stable Hemodialysis Patients (Sawada Study)," *Renal Failure*, Vol. 29, No. 5, 2007, pp. 587-593. doi:10.1080/08860220701392157

[56] S. Molsted, I. Eidemak, H. T. Sorensen and J. H. Kristensen, "Five Months of Physical Exercise in Hemodialysis Patients: Effects on Aerobic Capacity, Physical Function and Self-Rated Health," *Nephron Clinical Practice*, Vol. 96, No. 3, 2004, pp. c76-c81. doi:10.1159/000076744

[57] S. Mustata, S. Groeneveld, W. Davidson, G. Ford, K. Kiland and B. Manns, "Effects of Exercise Training on Physical Impairment, Arterial Stiffness and Health-Related Quality of Life in Patients with Chronic Kidney Disease: A Pilot Study," *International Urology and Nephrology*, Vol. 43, No. 4, 2011, pp. 1133-1141. doi:10.1007/s11255-010-9823-7

[58] S. Ouzouni, E. Kouidi, A. Sioulis, D. Grekas and A. Deligiannis, "Effects of Intradialytic Exercise Training on Health-Related Quality of Life Indices in Haemodialysis Patients," *Clinical Rehabilitation*, Vol. 23, No. 1, 2009, pp. 53-63. doi:10.1177/0269215508096760

[59] P. L. Painter, L. Hector, K. Ray, L. Lynes, S. Dibble, S. M. Paul, S. L. Tomlanovich and N. L. Ascher, "A Randomized Trial of Exercise Training after Renal Transplantation," *Transplantation*, Vol. 74, No. 1, 2002, pp. 42-48. doi:10.1097/00007890-200207150-00008

[60] E. Segura-Orti, E. Kouidi and J. F. Lison, "Effect of Resistance Exercise during Hemodialysis on Physical Function and Quality of Life: Randomized Controlled Trial," *Clinical Nephrology*, Vol. 71, No. 5, 2009, pp. 527-537.

3

Protein Diet and Estimated Glomerular Filtration Rate

Supatra Lohsiriwat
Department of Physiology, Faculty of Medicine Siriraj Hospital, Mahidol University, Bangkok, Thailand
Email: supatra.loh@mahidol.ac.th

ABSTRACT

Chronic kidney disease (CKD) is a common health problem worldwide. CKD staging or classification, together with patients' prognosis and treatment plan depend on the patients' kidney function which is assessed by measurement of glomerular filtration rate (GFR). Estimated GFR can be obtained using serum or plasma creatinine as a main variable in equations or formulae such as Cockcroft-Gault equation, MDRD equation (Modification of Diet in Renal Disease), the Schwartz and Counahan-Barratt formulae. These equations, though widely accepted, still have to be adjusted or validated among different groups of patients according to the variation in some factors such as race, diet, and genetic heterogenicity. Diet, especially the high protein load, can affect GFR representing the renal functional reserve. A high protein diet can cause an increase in GFR that lasts for many hours. Long-term consumption of vegetarian diet which is low in protein and contains only protein from plant sources can cause a low baseline GFR while the renal functional reserve is still preserved. This paper aims to remind of the role of protein diet effect on GFR measurement especially when assessing the renal function in vegetarians or individuals on long-term low-protein intake.

Keywords: Protein Diet; Glomerular Filtration Rate; eGFR; Vegetarian

1. Introduction

Chronic kidney disease (CKD) is becoming an increasing health problem in many countries, its prevalence and staging were studied and reported from all over the globe including United States [1], Australia [2], European countries [3], the Republic of China [4], and Japan [5]. In Thailand, the National Health Examination Survey 2004 found that the prevalence of CKD (compiling only those of stage 3, 4 and 5) in Thai adults was 8.45% [6].

These reports show that CKD is becoming a more serious problem worldwide as the patients with end stage renal disease (ESRD) need dialysis and/or transplantation which need complicate health care and also a high cost of health service. CKD stages were most often classified based on Kidney Disease Outcome Quality Initiatives (K/DOQI) which classified CKD patients into 5 stages according to their glomerular filtration rate (GFR) [7]. So the measurement of GFR should be reliable and accurate.

Intake of cooked meat has a significant effect on serum creatinine concentration and GFR. Misclassification of CKD is possible if measurements are made after high protein diet [8], and in individuals with exceptional dietary intake such as vegetarian [9].

2. GFR Measurement: Clearance Technique

GFR provides the best index of overall kidney function especially glomerular function. GFR is not measured directly but can be assessed by clearance technique using creatinine, inulin, radionuclide-labeled markers, radiocontrast markers or other substances that are freely filtered but not transported in the renal tubules. Clearance (C) of a substance is the rate at which an indicator substance is removed from plasma per unit concentration, specifying a volume from which all of the substance is removed per unit time. Clearance can be calculated from the formula $C = UV/P$, where C is clearance in ml/min, U means the urine concentration of the substance in mg/mL, V means the urine volume in one minute and P means plasma concentration of the substance in mg/mL [10,11].

3. Estimated GFR (eGFR)

Clearance method needs accurate urine collection which is not easily accomplished, time consuming and can be cumbersome leading to inadequate compliance and unreliability. In 1976 Cockcroft and Gault proposed the prediction of creatinine clearance from serum creatinine (S_{cr})

[12]. The principle has been accepted, modified, and called estimated GFR.

Cockcroft-Gault equation predicts clearance of creatinine (Ccr) as Ccr = (140 − age) × (weight)/(72 × Scr) (multiply by 0.85 if female).

Other equations to estimate GFR from serum creatinine have come out and been widely used as well. Levey *et al.* [13] in 1999 presented a new prediction equation called the MDRD equation (Modification of Diet in Renal Disease) claimed to be more accurate especially in the black.

$eGFR = 170 \times [S_{cr}\ (mg/dL)]^{-0.999} \times [age]^{-0.176} \times [0.762$ if patient is female$] \times [1.18$ if patient is black$]$.

Among children, the Schwartz [14] and Counahan-Barratt [15] formulae provide clinical useful estimates of GFR.

Manjunath *et al.* in 2001 stated that measurement of creatinine clearance using timed (e.g., 24-hour) urine collections does not improve the estimate of GFR over that provided by prediction equations. Anyhow, they indicated that a 24-hour urine sample provides useful information for GFR estimation in individuals with exceptional dietary intake (vegetarian diet, use of creatine supplements) or muscle mass (amputation, malnutrition, muscle wasting) [16].

4. Variation of Serum Creatinine

Creatinine has a molecular weight of 113 D. It is a break down product of creatine and phosphocreatine in muscle, and is usually produced at a rather constant rate in the body. Creatinine generation is proportional to muscle mass. The liver plays important role in formation of creatinine through methylation of guanidine aminoacetic acid [17].

Creatinine is freely filtered by the renal glomeruli. There is no renal tubular reabsorption of the substance, while approximately 3% of creatinine in the urine is secreted from the renal tubules. With a decrease in GFR, blood concentration of creatinine rises, presenting a reciprocal relationship between GFR and serum creatinine concentration.

In CKD patients with reduced glomerular and nephron function, serum creatinine rises and renal tubular secretion of creatinine is in relatively higher proportion.

Elevated level of serum creatinine usually indicates reduced GFR, but normal level does not exclude possibility of reduced GFR especially when renal damage is not immense. Renal clearance representing GFR is a more accurate method to measure kidney function.

Serum creatinine level can be affected by numerous factors. It is slightly increased just after ingestion of high meat diet, vigorous exercise, or due to some drugs that block tubular secretion of creatinine especially in CKD patients who already have high concentration of creatinine in the blood. Serum creatinine level is lower in individuals with muscle wasting, malnutrition, dietary protein restriction, and advanced liver disease. So in CKD patients with severe malnutrition and severe muscle wasting, serum creatinine might not be as high as in those with more muscle mass though their kidney functions are in the same level.

5. Protein Diet and GFR, Renal Functional Reserve

Intake of cooked meat has a significant effect on serum creatinine concentration and GFR [18,19]. Proteins of different sources, for example animal protein vs vegetable protein, do not affect GFR at the same magnitude [20,21],

The capacity of the kidney to increase its renal blood flow and GFR after a dietary protein load is called renal functional reserve [22]. The increase in GFR after high protein diet can be due both to an increase in the serum creatinine concentration and the known postprandial increase of true GFR [8,22]. Healthy vegetarians are known to have a statistically reduced baseline GFR [18] but the ability to increase the GFR after high protein diet is still maintained [23], unlike in patients with a reduced number of nephrons whose renal functional reserve may be diminished or absent [22].

Protein diet from animal source produced more increment in postprandial GFR compared to that from vegetable source [21]. Kontessis *et al.* in 1995 reported that, after a high protein diet of animal source, plasma concentrations of valine, lysine, and IGF-I were higher than after a vegetable protein diet, while the plasma levels of growth hormone and glucagon did not differ significantly. The plasma valine was strongly correlated to the GFR [20].

6. The Classification of Chronic Kidney Disease in Vegetarian

Since the classification of chronic kidney disease is based on baseline GFR [7], and strict and long-term healthy vegetarians are known to have a statistically reduced baseline GFR [18], therefore physicians need to bear this in mind when dealing with diagnosis and classification of chronic kidney disease in vegetarians. Barai et al. reported that basal GFR in 109 healthy Indian subjects consuming vegetarian diet for 10 days was 82.4 ± 12.7 mL/min/1.73sq.m. which was significantly lower than the normal value of 120 - 130 mL/min/1.73sq.m. in western population [24]. They suggested that the conventional cutoff value of 60 mL/min/1.73sq.m. for defining chronic kidney disease might not be appropriate in India. Preiss *et al.* in 2007 concluded in their report that misclassification of chronic kidney disease is possible if measurement of serum creatinine and GFR estimation are made after meat-containing meals [8]. Wiseman et al. measured GFR (as 51Cr-EDTA clearance) in vegans and lactovegetarians in comparison to omnivorous control subjects matched for age [25]. They found lower GFR in vegans and lactovegetarians but higher mean urinary albumin excretion rate in the omnivores.

In Thailand, it is our Thai tradition to consume rice meals with more carbohydrate and local vegetables, with less meat than the western style, especially in the rural area. The effect of meat on baseline serum creatinine and GFR estimation may play some minor part when dealing with diagnosis and classification of chronic kidney disease.

7. Conclusion

Vegetarians and individuals consuming long-term low-protein diet exhibit low baseline GFR though their renal functional reserve is still preserved. To assess renal function or survey of the prevalence of CKD using single measurement of baseline GFR, these low protein consumers may be mistaken as patients with early stages of CKD.

REFERENCES

[1] J. Coresh, B. Astor, T. Greene, G. Eknoyan and A. Levey, "Prevalence of Chronic Kidney Disease and Decreased Kidney Function in the Adult US Population: Third National Health and Nutrition Examination Survey," *American Journal of Kidney Diseases*, Vol. 41, No. 1, 2003, pp. 1-12. doi:10.1053/ajkd.2003.50007

[2] R. C. Atkins, K. R. Polkinghorne, E. M. Briganti, J. E. Shaw, P. Z. Zimmet and S. J. Chadban, "Prevalence of Albuminuria in Australia. The Ausdiab Kidney Study," *Kidney International*, Vol. 66, 2004, pp. S22-S24. doi:10.1111/j.1523-1755.2004.09206.x

[3] B. Rutkowski and E. Krol, "Epidemiology of Chronic Kidney Disease in Central and Eastern Europe," *Blood Purification*, Vol. 26, 2008, pp. 381-385. doi:10.1159/000137275

[4] C. P. Wen, T. Y. Cheng, M. K. Tsai, *et al.*, "All-Cause Mortality Attributable to Chronic Kidney Disease: A Prospective Cohort Study Based on 462,293 Adults in Taiwan," *Lancet*, Vol. 371, No. 9631, 2008, pp. 2173-2182. doi:10.1016/S0140-6736(08)60952-6

[5] T. Konta, Z. Hao, H. Abiko, *et al.*, "Prevalence and Risk Factor Analysis of Microalbuminuria in Japanese General Population: The Takahata Study," *Kidney International*, Vol. 70, 2006, pp. 751-756. doi:10.1038/sj.ki.5001504

[6] L. Ong-Ajyooth, K. Vareesangthip, P. Khonputsa and W. Aekplakorn, "Prevalence of Chronic Kidney Disease in Thai Adults: A National Health Survey," *BMC Nephrology*, Vol. 10, 2009, p. 35. doi:10.1186/1471-2369-10-35

[7] "National Kidney Foundation. K/DOQI Clinical Practice Guidelines for Chronic Kidney Disease: Evaluation, Classification, and Stratification," *American Journal of Kidney Diseases*, Vol. 39, No. 5, 2002, pp. S1-266. doi:10.1016/S0272-6386(02)70054-1

[8] D. J. Preiss, I. M. Godber, E. J. Lamb, R. N. Dalton and I. R. Gunn, "The Influence of a Cooked-Meat Meal on Estimated Glomerular Filtration Rate," *Annals of Clinical Biochemistry*, Vol. 44, No. 1, 2007, pp. 35-42. doi:10.1258/000456307779595995

[9] G. Manjunath, M. J. Sarnak and A. S. Levey, "Estimating the Glomerular Filtration Rate. Dos and Don'ts for Assessing Kidney Function," *Postgraduate Medicine*, Vol. 110, No. 6, 2001, pp. 55-62.

[10] P. B. Rehberg, "Studies on Kidney Function I. The Rate of Filtration and Reabsorption in the Human Kidney," *Biochemical Journal*, Vol. 20, 1926, p. 447.

[11] J. M. Hayman Jr., J. A. Halsted and L. E. Seyler, "A Comparison of the Creatinine and Urea Clearance Tests of Kidney Function," *JCI*, Vol. 12, No. 5, 1933, pp. 861-875. doi:10.1172/JCI100545

[12] D. W. Cockcroft and M. H. Gault, "Prediction of Creatinine Clearance from Serum Creatinine," *Nephron*, Vol. 16, No. 1, 1976, pp. 31-41. doi:10.1159/000180580

[13] A. S. Levey, J. P. Bosch, J. B. Lewis, T. Greene, N. Rogers and D. Roth, "A More Accurate Method to Estimate Glomerular Filtration Rate from Serum Creatinine: A New Prediction Equation. Modification of Diet in Renal Disease Study Group," *Annals of Internal Medicine*, Vol. 130, No. 6, 1999, pp. 461-470. doi:10.7326/0003-4819-130-6-199903160-00002

[14] G. L. Schwartz and B. Gauthier, "A Simple Estimate of Glomerular Filtration Rate in Adolescent Boys," *The Journal of Pediatrics*, Vol. 106, No. 3, 1985, pp. 522-526. doi:10.1016/S0022-3476(85)80697-1

[15] R. Counahan, C. Chantler, S. Ghazali, B. Kirkwood, F. Rose and T. M. Barrett, "Estimation of Glomerular Filtration Rate from Plasma Creatinine Concentration in Children," *Archives of Disease in Childhood*, Vol. 51, No. 11, 1976, pp. 875-878. doi:10.1136/adc.51.11.875

[16] G. Manjunath, M. J. Sarnak and A. S. Levey, "Estimating the Glomerular Filtration Rate. Dos and Don'ts for Assessing Kidney Function," *Postgraduate Medicine*, Vol. 110, No. 6, 2001, pp. 55-62.

[17] M. H. Rosner and K. Bolton, "Core Curriculum in Nephrology. Renal Function Test," *American Journal of Kidney Diseases*, Vol. 47, No. 1, 2006, pp. 174-183. doi:10.1053/j.ajkd.2005.08.038

[18] R. Hirschberg, H. Rottka, D. von Herrath, A. Pauls and K. Schaefer, "Effect of an Acute Protein Load on the Creatinine Clearance in Healthy Vegetarian," *Klinische Wochenschrift*, Vol. 63, No. 5, 1985, pp. 217-220. doi:10.1007/BF01731172

[19] S. Lohsiriwat and M. Sriponyaskul, "Effect of High-Protein Diet on the Glomerular Filtration Rate in the Adult and the Elderly," *Siriraj Medical Journal*, Vol. 51, 1999, pp. 21-26.

[20] P. A. Kontessis, I. Bossinakou, L. Sarika, E. Iliopoulou, A. Papantiniou, R. Trevisan, D. Roussi, K. Stipsanelli, S. Grigorakis and A. Souvatzoglou, "Renal, Metabolic, and Hormonal Responses to Proteins of Different Origin in Normotensive, Nonproteinuric Type I Diabetic Patients," *Diabetic Care*, Vol. 18, No. 9, 1995, p. 1233. doi:10.2337/diacare.18.9.1233

[21] S. Lohsiriwat and S. Thophol, "Effects of Vegetable and Animal Protein Meals on Glomerular Filtration Rate," *The Nephrology Society of Thailand*, Vol. 6, 2000, pp. 217-223.

[22] J. P. Bosch, A. Saccaggi, A. Lauer, C. Ronco, M. Belledonne and S. Glabman, "Renal Functional Reserve in Humans. Effect of Protein Intake on Glomerular Filtration Rate," *The American Journal of Medicine*, Vol. 75, No. 6, 1983, pp. 943-950. doi:10.1016/0002-9343(83)90873-2

[23] S. Lohsiriwat and A. Buageaw, "Renal Functional Reserve in Lacto-Vegetarian Adolescents," *Siriraj Medical Journal*, Vol. 54, 2002, pp. 217-223.

[24] S. Barai, S. Gambhir, N. Prasad, R. K. Sharma, M. Ora, A. Kumar, A. Gupta, D. S. Parasar and B. Suneetha, "Levels of GFR and Protein-Induced Hyperfiltration in Kidney Donors: A Single Center Experience in India," *American Journal of Kidney Diseases*, Vol. 51, No. 3, 2008, pp. 407-414. doi:10.1053/j.ajkd.2007.11.008

[25] M. J. Wiseman, R. Hunt, A. Goodwin, J. L. Gross, H. Keen and G. C. Viberti, "Dietary Composition and Renal Function in Healthy Subjects," *Nephron*, Vol. 46, No. 1, 1987, pp. 37-42. doi:10.1159/000184293

4

Body Fluid Changes, Cardiovascular Deconditioning and Metabolic Impairment Are Reversed 24 Hours after a 5-Day Dry Immersion

Mickael Coupé[1,2], Elena Tomilovskaya[3], Françoise Larcher[4], Bertrand Diquet[5], Liudmila Kh. Pastushkova[2,3], Inesa B. Kozlovskaya[3], Irina M. Larina[2,3], Guillemette Gauquelin-Koch[6], Vladimir A. Kulchitsky[7], Marc-Antoine Custaud[1,2], Nastassia M. Navasiolava[1,2]

[1]CNRS UMR 6214, INSERM U1083, Angers University, Angers, France
[2]Associated French-Russian Laboratory CaDyWEC, Angers, France & Moscow, Russia
[3]Institute of Biomedical Problems RAS SSC, Moscow, Russia
[4]Biochemistry Laboratory, Angers University Hospital, Angers, France
[5]Pharmacokinetics Laboratory, Angers University Hospital, Angers, France
[6]French Space Agency (CNES), Paris, France
[7]Institute of Physiology, National Academy of Sciences, Minsk, Belarus
Email: nastassia.navasiolava@etud.univ-angers.fr

ABSTRACT

Dry immersion is an effective and useful model for research in physiology and physiopathology. The focus of this study was to provide integrative insight into renal, endocrine, circulatory, autonomic and metabolic effects of dry immersion. We assessed if the principal changes were restored within 24 h of recovery, and determined which changes were mainly associated with immersion-induced orthostatic intolerance. Five-day dry immersion without countermeasures, and with *ad libitum* water intake, standardized diet and a permitted short daily rise was performed in a relatively large sample for this experiment type (14 healthy young men). Reduction of total body water derived mostly from extracellular compartment, and stabilized rapidly at the new operating point. Decrease in plasma volume was estimated at 20% - 25%. Five-day immersion was sufficient to impair metabolism with a decrease in glucose tolerance and hypercholesterolemia, but was not associated with pronounced autonomic changes. Five-day immersion induced marked cardiovascular impairment. Immediately after immersion, over half of the subjects were unable to accomplish the 20-min 70° tilt; during tilt, heart rate and total peripheral resistance were increased, and stroke volume was decreased. However, 24 hours of normal physical activity appeared sufficient to reverse orthostatic tolerance and all signs of cardiovascular impairment, and to restitute plasma volume and extracellular fluid volume. Similarly, metabolic impairment was restored. In our study, the major factor responsible for orthostatic intolerance appeared to be hypovolemia. The absence of pronounced autonomic dysfunction might be explained by relatively short duration of dry immersion and daily short-time orthostatic stimulation.

Keywords: Physical Inactivity; Modeled Weightlessness; Water-Electrolyte Balance; Body Fluid Compartments; Orthostatic Intolerance

1. Introduction

Water immersion has been demonstrated as an efficient and useful model for renal, neuro-hormonal and body fluid physiology [1-3]. Since antiquity, it is known that immersion induces diuresis, indeed the Latin word "urinator" means wisely "diver". However, the water immersion method is generally limited to several hours because of skin maceration. This method has been modified to separate the subject from water using elastic tissue (dry immersion, DI), which allows for longer immersion periods and increased comfort for the subjects [4] (**Figure 1**). Using longer duration, it becomes possible to study the effects of a new body fluid steady state on major bodily functions.

DI allows for studying of acute expansion of central volume (first hours), maintained hypovolemic state (continuation of DI for days), and acute diminution of central volume (immediate recovery). DI rapidly induces hypovolemia and cardiovascular deconditioning, observed as orthostatic hypotension, increased heart rate and reduced exercise capacity. DI has also been recognized as a

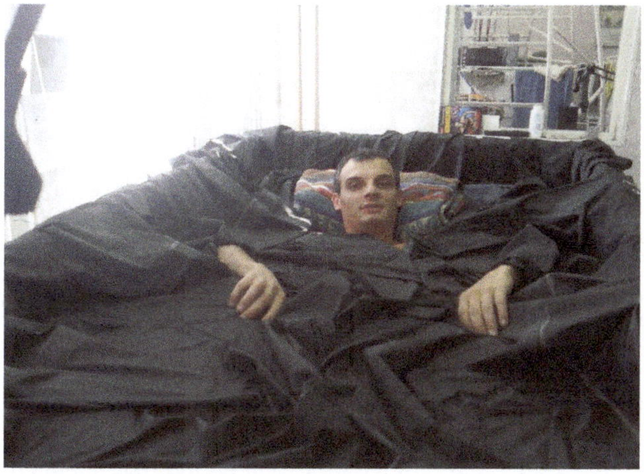

Figure 1. Dry immersion method. The subject is separated from water with waterproof tissue.

valuable model for physical inactivity [5], due to acute limitation of voluntary muscular activity, reduction of gravitational stress on muscles, and deep atonia [4].

The DI model was first developed by Russian physicians and scientists to mimic the space environment. This method, however, might be directly useful in some common disease. DI appeared effective in treatment of refractory edema of different etiologies (cardiovascular diseases, renal pathologies, liver cirrhosis, and burns). In patients with edema, the 1.5 - 3 fold increase in diuresis observed after 4 - 6 hours of DI persisted for 2 days [6, 7]. In patients with treatment-resistant hypertensive crisis, 1.5 hours of DI induced a rapid and prolonged blood pressure reduction and sedation [8]. Together this indicates the interest of DI model for physiology and physiopathology studies.

In DI studies, the volunteers' number rarely exceeds 6 - 8 subjects. We had the unique opportunity to study the effects of DI in a relatively large population (n = 14) for this specific protocol. Our first aim was to provide a comprehensive analysis of body fluid, autonomic, cardiovascular and metabolic changes induced by a 5-day DI. We further examined whether the 24-hour recovery period was sufficient to restore the principal changes induced by DI. Finally, we determined the main changes associated with orthostatic intolerance induced by DI.

2. Methods

2.1. Subjects

The study included a group of 14 healthy non-smoking Russian men (age 22 ± 1 y, height 174 ± 1 cm, weight 67.9 ± 1.5 kg; mean ± SE). All volunteers provided written informed consent, in compliance with the Helsinki Declaration. The experimental protocol was approved by the Committee of Biomedicine Ethics of the Russian Academy of Sciences. The subjects were randomly divided into 2 groups (group R0, n = 7, and group R+1, n = 7), according to the day of orthostatic test in the recovery period.

2.2. General Protocol

The protocol used in this study is schematized in **Figure 2**. DI was performed for 5 days (120 hours) at the Dry Immersion Facility of the Institute of Biomedical Problems (Moscow, Russia). For baseline and recovery measurements and sampling, ambulatory periods of 3 and 4 days preceded and followed DI, respectively (B-3 to B-1, and R0 to R+3). The subjects were immersed one after another. Thermoneutral water temperature (32° - 33.5°) was continuously maintained; air temperature was maintained at 24°C - 25°C, and air humidity was 40% - 50%.

The present study was one of 16 studies conducted during this DI protocol. Some experiments required extraction from bath; in this case, the subjects remained supine on a lifting platform. Total out-of-bath supine time for the 120 h of immersion was 4.11 ± 0.15 h (mean ± SE). In addition, once a day (in the evening) the subjects were allowed to leave the bath for personal hygiene procedures (defecation and shower in a sitting position) and weighing (in a standing position). Total out-of-bath sitting/standing time for the 120 hours of immersion was 1.43 ± 0.07 h (mean ± SE). Otherwise, the subjects remained in a supine position during DI for all activities and were continuously observed by video monitoring. Blood pressure and heart rate (using a sphygmomanometer) were measured daily at 8 a.m. The onset and end of the immersion were both at 10 a.m., so morning measurements on day 1 were performed before immersion, and on day R0—still under immersion. Before, during and after DI, water intake was *ad libitum* (measured), and diet was standardized. Daily caloric intake was ~2880 ± 60 kcal. Dietary sodium was set to 2.8 mmol/kg/day, calcium—to ~1100 mg/day, and protein intake to 1.15 g/kg/day.

2.3. Bio-Impedance Measurements

Bio-impedance measurements by multifrequency impedance device Hydra ECF/ICF 4200 (Xitron Technologies, San Diego, USA) were performed out of the bath in the evening (at 5 p.m.) at baseline (B-2 or B-1), day 1 (7 hours after beginning DI), day 3, day 5, R0 (7 hours after the end of DI) and R+1. Each measurement was repeated 3 times, and mean values were calculated. We estimated extracellular fluid (ECF), intracellular fluid (ICF) and total body water. Whole body wrist-ankle measurement approach was used. The subject was in supine position for at least 10 minutes prior to the start of measurements, without contact with metal or water. The arms were

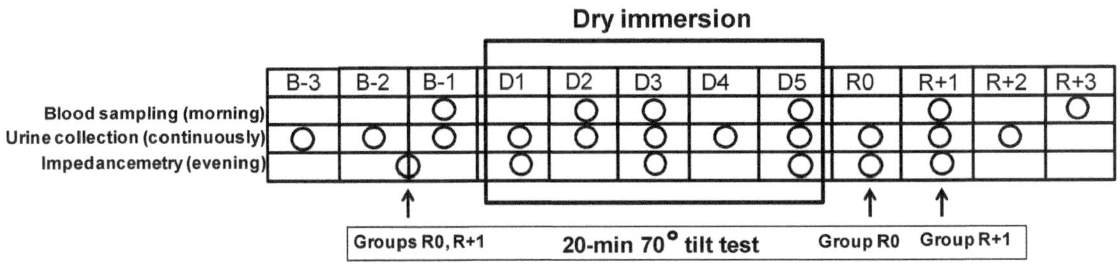

Figure 2. Schematic outlining of the experimental protocol. B-3, B-2 and B-1, baseline days prior to immersion; D1-D5, days of dry immersion; R0 - R+3, recovery days; circles, days of sampling or measurement; arrows, days of tilt-test.

abducted from the body and legs were separated. Four gum-based electrodes measuring 5 cm^2 were used: two current injection electrodes on the hand and foot on the dorsal surfaces proximal to the metacarpal-phalangeal and metatarsal-phalangeal joints, respectively, and two voltage detector electrodes on the mid-line between the prominent ends of the radius and ulna of the wrist and mid-line between the medial and lateral malleoli of the ankle.

Both before and after immersion, the subjects were weighed prior to measurements. During immersion, body weight data from the evening of the previous day were used for calculations.

2.4. Tilt Test

The head-up tilt test was performed in a quiet room with an ambient air temperature of 24°C - 25°C, in the morning, before immersion (day B-2 or B-1) and immediately after completing the 5-day DI (first rising, group R0) or on the second day of recovery (group R+1). The subject was placed on a tilt-table in a supine position, and allowed to rest for at least 30 min; the data were then recorded from this resting supine position for 10 minutes. Afterwards, the subject was tilted 70° head-up. Subjects were instructed to stand with feet shoulder-width apart, keeping as still as possible to avoid muscle pump activity. Subjects remained in the 70° head-up tilt (HUT) position with continuous monitoring for 20 min, until presyncope, or until the subject's request to stop.

Standard ECG was recorded continuously, and beat-to-beat R-R intervals and heart rate (HR) were extracted from the signal. Blood pressure was measured continuously on the third finger using a non-invasive finger cuff device (Finapres, Ohmeda, Englewood, Colorado). The finger cuff was maintained at heart level in both supine and standing positions. Additionally, arm blood pressure was measured by Dinamap (Carescape V100, GE Healthcare, Finland) at baseline, and at 5th, 10th and 15th minutes of the HUT. Skin blood flow at the calf level was estimated using Laser-Doppler flowmetry as previously described [9]. Calf skin temperature was controlled by monitoring using a thermocouple connected to an electronic thermometer (BAT-12, Physitemp Instruments, Clifton, New Jersey).

The stable 5 min of data for each period (basal and end tilt) were averaged and used for analysis. In case of orthostatic intolerance, the 5 minutes prior to intolerance were chosen for analysis [10]. For the single subject who developed orthostatic intolerance at the third minute of tilt, the 2 min mark prior to intolerance was analyzed. Cardiac output (CO), stroke volume (SV), and total peripheral resistance (TPR) were estimated by an analysis of blood pressure waveform.

Analysis of orthostatic responses, power spectrum analysis of heart rate variability, and analysis of the spontaneous baroreflex sensitivity was performed as previously described [10]. Skin vascular resistance (SVR) was calculated by dividing mean blood pressure by skin blood flow. In the tilted position, heart-Laser-Doppler probe distance (hydrostatic component of blood pressure) was taken into account to correct blood pressure at the probe level and calculate SVR.

2.5. Sample Collection and Analyses

2.5.1. Blood Sampling and Estimation of Plasma Volume Dynamics

Blood sampling was performed with participants in the supine position in the morning before breakfast on baseline (B-1), day 2, day 3, day 5, and the second and fourth recovery days (R+1 and R+3).

Fasting glucose (using Accu Check Performa glucometer), hemoglobin (using HemoCue hemoglobin analyzer) and hematocrit (using microhematocrit method) were determined immediately after blood collection. Percentage changes in plasma volume were calculated indirectly using:

- Hb and Hct count (Dill and Costill formula):

$$DPV (\%) = 100 \times [HbB\,(1 - 0.01Hcti)]/[Hbi\,(1 - 0.01HctB)] - 100;$$

- Only Hct count (van Beaumont formula):

$$DPV (\%) = [100/(100 - HctB)] \times [100 \times (HctB - Hcti)/Hcti)]$$

- Plasma protein count [11]:

DPV (%) = 100 × [Prot B/Prot i] − 100;

where HctB, HbB and Prot B are hematocrit, hemoglobin and proteins concentrations at baseline, respectively, and Hcti, Hbi and Prot i are the corresponding values on day 2, day 3, day 5 and R+1.

Plasma and serum samples were analyzed for renin, aldosterone, brain natriuretic peptide (BNP), electrolytes (Na^+, K^+, Cl^-, Ca^{2+}), osmolality, proteins, urea and creatinine concentrations, high-sensitivity CRP, insulin, leptin, triglycerides, total cholesterol, and HDL-cholesterol. LDL-cholesterol was calculated using the Friedewald formula. Homeostasis model assessment-insulin resistance index (HOMA-IR) was calculated as fasting insulin concentration (μU/ml) × fasting glucose concentration (mmol/L)/22.5.

2.5.2. Urine Sampling

Urine pools were collected over 24 hours for 3 days prior to immersion (B-3, B-2 and B-1), 5 days of immersion (day 1-day 5) and 3 recovery days (R0, R+1 and R+2). Urine volume was measured and the aliquots were stored at −80°C. The partial water balance, defined as the difference between consumed water (including drinking water, tea, juice, soup) and urine volume, was calculated. Urine samples were analyzed for electrolytes (Na^+, K^+, Cl^-), osmolality, creatinine, urea and urinary free cortisol (UFC), urinary catecholamines (epinephrine, norepinephrine, metanephrine, normetanephrine, dopamine). Creatinine, free water and osmolal clearances were calculated for days B-2, day 1, day 2, day 4, R0 and R+2 using the 24-h urine samples from these days and the morning blood samples from the next days (*i.e.* B-1, day 2, day 3, day 5, R+1, R+3).

2.5.3. Biochemical Analyses

Active renin analysis was performed using a chemiluminescence immunoassay on the Liaison analyzer (DiaSorin). BNP was measured using a chemiluminescence immunoassay on the "Architect i2000" analyser (Abbott). Plasma aldosterone was determined by a competition radioimmunoassay using a commercially available RIA kit (Immunotech, Beckman Coulter). Urinary free cortisol was detected by liquid chromatography-tandem mass spectrometry (LC-MS/MS) with an Applied Biosystems/MDS Sciex Api 3000 triple quad mass spectrometer equipped with turbolon spray source. Plasma and urine osmolality were measured by freezing-point depression in comparison to pure water. Urinary catecholamines were determined by high-pressure liquid chromatography.

All the other variables from blood and urine samples were evaluated using the Architect c16000 automated clinical chemistry analyzer (Abbot).

Minimal detectable level for plasma aldosterone and BNP was 10 ng/L, for serum hs-CRP −0.1 mg/L, for urinary epinephrine −2 μg/L, and for urinary metanephrine −0.1 μg/L. Results that were less than the minimal detectable level were taken for half minimal value.

2.6. Data Analysis

All values are presented as mean ± SE. The effects of DI were tested with ANOVA for repeated measures. Statistically significant differences were further analyzed by post-hoc pairwise comparisons (Least Significant Difference). Differences were considered to be statistically significant at $p < 0.05$. Analyses were performed using SPSS 15.0 for Windows.

3. Results

3.1. General Data

Overall, the five-day DI was well tolerated by the study group; all the subjects, however, had a moderate backache at the beginning, which disappeared by the third to fourth day of immersion.

3.2. Body Fluids and Kidney Regulation

3.2.1. Body Fluids

Plasma volume changes determined by Hb and Hct count, and by Hct count alone, were similar. Plasma volume decreased by 17% - 18% within the first 24 hours of immersion, and remained at reduced level until the end of immersion. Plasma protein count also revealed plasma volume reduction under immersion, but less pronounced, at approximately 7% - 8%. On the second recovery day, plasma volume as determined by all 3 methods did not differ from baseline (**Figure 3**). *Water intake* varied throughout the experiment without significance. *Daily diuresis* was increased by approximately 90% on day 1, and remained elevated throughout the immersion. *Partial water balance* at day 1 was approximately 1 L less than at baseline, and remained negative throughout the immersion. On the first recovery day, we observed a compensatory decrease in diuresis and increase in water balance (**Table 1**). *Free water clearance* did not significantly change throughout the protocol. *Osmolal clearance* was decreased during immersion (significantly on day 4; p = 0.09 on day 1 and day 2) (**Table S1**). The dynamics of fluid compartments are shown in **Figure 4**. *Extracellular fluid* decreased with the onset of immersion (by 5.1% ± 1.3%), with the maximal decrease of 7.8% ± 1.4% on day 3. In absolute values, the extracellular volume lost on day 3 was approximately 1.4 ± 0.3 L. *Total body water* also decreased to approximately 1.6 L on day 3, and remained decreased on day 5. In recovery, and already within 7 hours after the end of DI, the extracellular fluid and total body water did not significantly

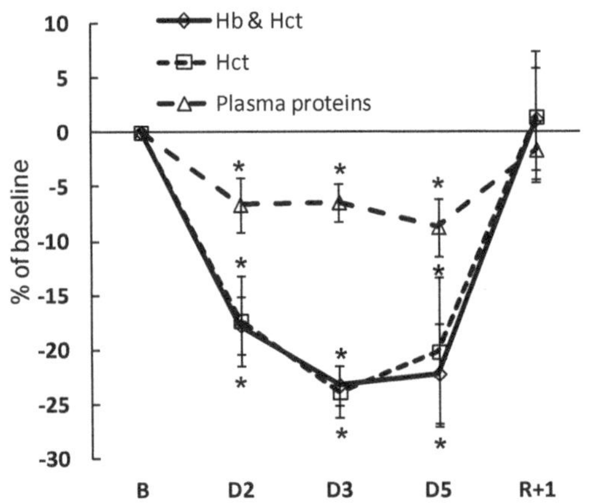

Figure 3. Variations in plasma volume in percentage of baseline, calculated indirectly by hemoglobin and hematocrit count (Hb and Hct), hematocrit count alone (Hct), and plasma proteins count. B: baseline; D: dry immersion; R: recovery. Values are means ± SE; *p < 0.05 vs baseline.

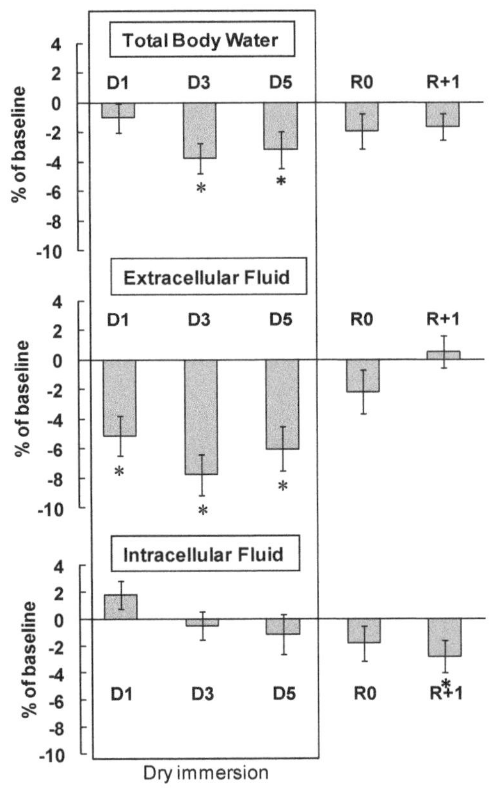

Figure 4. Variations of fluid compartments. D: dry immersion; R: recovery. Values are means ± SE; *p < 0.05 vs baseline.

differ from baseline levels. *Intracellular fluid* showed non-significant variations during DI and was decreased by approximately 3% at R+1.

3.2.2. Blood and Urine Biochemistry

Blood levels of Na^+, K^+, Cl^-, Ca^{2+}, proteins, urea, creatinine and osmolality remained within normal values at all measurements. DI was accompanied by a significant increase in blood K^+, Ca^{2+} and protein content. Blood urea was slightly decreased at the beginning of DI, and slightly increased 24 hours after the end of DI (**Table 2**).

Urinary sodium loss increased at the beginning of DI (with a two-fold increase on day 1), followed by decrease in recovery (with a 3-fold decrease on R0). The dynamics of urinary Cl^- excretion showed similar trends. Urinary potassium excretion was not significantly changed. The urinary Na^+/K^+ ratio increased significantly only on day 1 and did not differ from the baseline during the rest of immersion. The end of immersion was accompanied by a decrease in the Na^+/K^+ ratio (**Table 1**).

Urinary osmolality was reduced during immersion, with a significant reduction on day 3, and tendency to reduction—with p = 0.07 to 0.09—on days 1, 2 and 4, with no significant difference compared to baseline in recovery (**Table 1**). Urinary urea and urinary creatinine did not change significantly (**Table 1**). Urea clearance increased on day 1 and decreased on R0. Creatinine clearance did not change throughout the DI (**Table S1**).

3.3. Cardiovascular System at Rest

3.3.1. Morning Heart Rate and Blood Pressure

Heart rate and blood pressure remained within normal limits. Heart rate was slightly reduced at the beginning of DI, and systolic blood pressure was slightly lower at the end of DI (**Table S2**).

3.3.2. Cardiovascular Hormones Regulating Volemia

Twenty-four hours after the onset of DI, plasma renin decreased two-fold and plasma BNP increased four-fold. Plasma aldosterone was not significantly changed. Twenty-four hours after the end of DI, we observed a two-fold increase in renin and 3-fold increase in aldosterone. On the fourth recovery day, renin and aldosterone were not modified, and BNP was significantly increased (**Figure 5**).

3.4. Cardiovascular Variables during Tilt Test

3.4.1. Tolerance

Before DI, only one subject (assigned to group R0) out of 14 was unable to complete the 20-min HUT. After DI, on day R0, 4 out of 7 subjects were non-finishers. On day R+1, all subjects finished the test.

3.4.2. Hemodynamic Responses to Tilt Test: Supine and Upright Position

The hemodynamic responses to the tilt test are presented in **Table 3**. Measurements on R0 compared to pre-immersion, performed in the supine position, showed a

Table 1. Urine biochemistry, diuresis, water intake and partial water balance before, during and following dry immersion.

	B-3	B-2	B-1	DI 1	DI 2	DI 3	DI 4	DI 5	R0	R+1	R+2
K^+, mmol/24h	35 ± 6	35 ± 5	39 ± 6	40 ± 2	41 ± 4	45 ± 6	47 ± 5	55 ± 6	38 ± 4	42 ± 3	51 ± 4
Na^+, mmol/24h	132 ± 12	120 ± 15	123 ± 21	211 ± 17*	163 ± 17*	131 ± 13	137 ± 15	157 ± 14	46 ± 4*	70 ± 8	113 ± 19
Na^+/K^+ ratio	3.8 ± 0.4	3.8 ± 0.4	3.4 ± 0.6	5.6 ± 0.7*	4.0 ± 0.3	3.2 ± 0.3	3.0 ± 0.2	3.0 ± 0.2	1.5 ± 0.2*	1.8 ± 0.3*	2.1 ± 0.3
Cl^-, mmol/24h	132 ± 13	108 ± 13	121 ± 21	181 ± 13*	160 ± 18*	128 ± 12	130 ± 15	147 ± 14	54 ± 4*	61 ± 7*	111 ± 17
Creatinine, mmol/24h	9.1 ± 1.2	8.7 ± 1.0	8.9 ± 1.4	9.1 ± 0.6	9.3 ± 1.0	9.5 ± 1.2	8.5 ± 0.8	10.8 ± 1.2	7.4 ± 0.7	7.8 ± 0.6	8.2 ± 0.9
Urea, mmol/24h	209 ± 25	208 ± 29	203 ± 30	231 ± 20	205 ± 23	231 ± 24	223 ± 18	275 ± 21	171 ± 20	210 ± 13	252 ± 30
Osmolality, mOS/kg	496 ± 56	497 ± 42	487 ± 56	360 ± 27	375 ± 22	348 ± 40*	377 ± 40	386 ± 52	534 ± 43	502 ± 59	537 ± 29
UFC (µg/24h)	33 ± 7	20 ± 4	28 ± 4	46 ± 13	46 ± 8*	40 ± 5	44 ± 8*	35 ± 6	22 ± 4	20 ± 2	36 ± 6
Epinephrine, µg/24h	5.02 ± 0.75	6.34 ± 1.04	6.79 ± 0.95	6.46 ± 0.91	6.65 ± 1.09	7.33 ± 0.83	6.06 ± 0.65	7.37 ± 1.01	6.26 ± 0.93	5.34 ± 0.62	6.75 ± 0.9
Norepinephrine, µg/24h	25 ± 5	22 ± 2	24 ± 3	30 ± 4	27 ± 3	32 ± 3*	28 ± 4	29 ± 4	29 ± 4	28 ± 3	28 ± 4
Metanephrine, µmol/24h	0.44 ± 0.07	0.51 ± 0.05	0.53 ± 0.06	0.6 ± 0.06	0.59 ± 0.08	0.62 ± 0.05	0.5 ± 0.07	0.59 ± 0.07	0.41 ± 0.03*	0.4 ± 0.02*	0.56 ± 0.07
Normetanephrine, µmol/24h	0.93 ± 0.24	0.85 ± 0.11	0.88 ± 0.14	1.04 ± 0.1	0.88 ± 0.1	0.98 ± 0.08	0.92 ± 0.12	0.97 ± 0.12	0.88 ± 0.13	0.94 ± 0.11	1.1 ± 0.13
Dopamine, µg/24h	250 ± 39	173 ± 18	221 ± 30	311 ± 32	247 ± 19	254 ± 31	236 ± 32	229 ± 31	174 ± 27	180 ± 30	223 ± 41
Diuresis, l/24h	1.37 ± 0.22	1.13 ± 0.1	1.23 ± 0.15	2.31 ± 0.21*	1.94 ± 0.19*	2.24 ± 0.34*	1.99 ± 0.2*	2.26 ± 0.31*	0.91 ± 0.11*	1.06 ± 0.1	1.23 ± 0.13
Water intake, l/24h	1.91 ± 0.17	1.54 ± 0.19	1.50 ± 0.19	1.50 ± 0.12	1.47 ± 0.16	2.0 ± 0.22	1.86 ± 0.2	2.14 ± 0.24	1.95 ± 0.17	1.64 ± 0.19	1.34 ± 0.16
Partial water balance, ml/24h	770 ± 210	420 ± 190	320 ± 110	−780 ± 170*	−520 ± 110*	−230 ± 180*	−210 ± 150*	−230 ± 160*	1030 ± 180*	590 ± 160	200 ± 85

B: baseline; DI: dry immersion; R: recovery; UFC: urinary free cortisol; values are means ± SE, *$p < 0.05$ vs B-1.

Table 2. Blood biochemistry before, during and following dry immersion.

	B-1	DI 2	DI 3	DI 5	R+1	R+3
Na^+, mmol/l	136 ± 2	138 ± 2	139 ± 3	137 ± 2	135 ± 2	136 ± 2
K^+, mmol/l	3.6 ± 0.1	4.0 ± 0.1*	4.1 ± 0.1*	4.0 ± 0.1*	3.7 ± 0.1	3.7 ± 0.1
Cl^-, mmol/l	103 ± 2	104 ± 1	105 ± 2	102 ± 1	102 ± 1	103 ± 2
Ca^{2+}, mmol/l	2.14 ± 0.05	2.22 ± 0.04*	2.23 ± 0.05*	2.27 ± 0.05*	2.18 ± 0.04	2.08 ± 0.05
Proteins, g/l	65 ± 2	70 ± 2*	70 ± 2*	72 ± 2*	67 ± 2	64 ± 2
Urea, mmol/l	4.5 ± 0.3	3.6 ± 0.2*	4.1 ± 0.2	4.5 ± 0.3	5.4 ± 0.3*	5.2 ± 0.4
Creatinine, µmol/l	74 ± 2	72 ± 2	75 ± 3	76 ± 2	77 ± 3	72 ± 2
Osmolality, mOS/kg	288 ± 7	283 ± 3	283 ± 4	290 ± 4	284 ± 3	284 ± 6
hs-CRP, mg/l	0.35 ± 0.08	0.43 ± 0.12	0.52 ± 0.14	0.4 ± 0.09	0.47 ± 0.09	0.72 ± 0.22
Fasting glucose, mmol/l	4.97 ± 0.11	4.96 ± 0.08	4.99 ± 0.08	4.82 ± 0.08	4.86 ± 0.11	4.66 ± 0.09
Fasting insulin, µU/ml	5.73 ± 0.54	7.24 ± 0.49*	7.19 ± 0.44	8.2 ± 0.63*	6.16 ± 0.61	5.31 ± 0.79
HOMA-IR	1.27 ± 0.13	1.59 ± 0.11*	1.59 ± 0.09	1.76 ± 0.15*	1.35 ± 0.16	1.11 ± 0.17
Leptin, ng/ml	2.23 ± 0.31	2.49 ± 0.28*	2.73 ± 0.38*	2.66 ± 0.33	2.05 ± 0.22	2.75 ± 0.55
Total cholesterol, mmol/l	3.71 ± 0.18	4.14 ± 0.18*	4.31 ± 0.23*	4.52 ± 0.31*	3.61 ± 0.2	3.53 ± 0.17
HDL cholesterol, mmol/l	1.23 ± 0.08	1.32 ± 0.08*	1.28 ± 0.07	1.32 ± 0.1*	1.12 ± 0.08	1.15 ± 0.07
LDL cholesterol, mmol/l	2.11 ± 0.17	2.41 ± 0.16*	2.59 ± 0.21*	2.76 ± 0.27*	2.04 ± 0.16	2.03 ± 0.14
Triglycerides, mmol/l	0.81 ± 0.11	0.86 ± 0.12	0.96 ± 0.06	0.97 ± 0.07	0.97 ± 0.09	0.76 ± 0.07

B: baseline; DI: dry immersion; R: recovery; values are means ± SE, *$p < 0.05$ vs baseline.

Table 3. Hemodynamic and autonomic responses to tilt test.

	Group R0, n = 7					Group R+1, n = 7				
	B	n	R0	n	P value, B vs R0	B	n	R+1	n	p value, B vs R+1
					Supine					
HR, bpm	70.3 ± 6.5	7	83.1 ± 6.4*	7	0.017	61.9 ± 1.6	7	60.1 ± 2.8‡	7	0.457
SBP, mmHg	112.7 ± 2.5	7	124.0 ± 4.2*	7	0.034	113.6 ± 4.2	7	114.7 ± 4.9	7	0.750
DBP, mmHg	56.7 ± 3.6	7	69.3 ± 4.1	7	0.058	57.0 ± 4.3	7	55.7 ± 3.2‡	7	0.555
SV, ml	86.9 ± 5.9	7	64.7 ± 2.3*	7	0.01	86.0 ± 3.3	7	93.3 ± 5.0‡	7	0.102
CO, l/min	6.04 ± 0.64	7	5.28 ± 0.33	7	0.148	5.31 ± 0.26	7	5.63 ± 0.45	7	0.233
TPR, AU	0.876 ± 0.077	7	1.173 ± 0.138	7	0.061	0.894 ± 0.057	7	0.909 ± 0.091	7	0.871
SVR, AU	8.6 ± 1.1	7	19.8 ± 4.3	7	0.063	11.7 ± 1.9	7	10.2 ± 2.0	7	0.555
LF RRi normalized	0.63 ± 0.08	7	0.75 ± 0.03	5	0.115	0.62 ± 0.04	7	0.60 ± 0.06	7	0.852
LF/HF RRi	2.65 ± 0.81	7	3.28 ± 0.43	5	0.983	1.80 ± 0.29	7	1.97 ± 0.60	7	0.786
SBRs, ms/mmHg	17.1 ± 2.2	7	13.4 ± 2.4	7	0.207	18.2 ± 2.2	6	16.8 ± 1.7	6	0.496
					End tilt					
HR, bpm	97.9 ± 7.1†	7	127.4 ± 6.2*†	7	0.001	92.6 ± 4.3†	7	95.5 ± 3.7‡†	7	0.477
SBP, mmHg	114.4 ± 2.5	7	116.4 ± 3.2	7	0.586	118.9 ± 3.9	7	119.0 ± 4.9	7	0.975
DBP, mmHg	60.0 ± 2.9	7	70.6 ± 2.1*	7	0.019	70.7 ± 4.3†	7	70.9 ± 3.6†	7	0.970
SV, ml	45.8 ± 4.0†	7	31.8 ± 1.7*†	6	0.024	54.4 ± 5.8†	7	54.5 ± 2.3‡†	7	0.988
CO, l/min	4.30 ± 0.13†	7	4.12 ± 0.30	6	0.867	4.98 ± 0.49	7	5.18 ± 0.29‡	7	0.693
TPR, AU	1.498 ± 0.099†	7	1.692 ± 0.176†	6	0.469	1.087 ± 0.083	6	1.139 ± 0.051‡†	6	0.603
SVR, AU	36.1 ± 5.8†	7	37.2 ± 5.5	6	0.567	45.5 ± 7.9†	6	40.3 ± 11.7†	7	0.966
LF RRi normalized	0.80 ± 0.06	7	0.81 ± 0.04†	4	0.182	0.80 ± 0.03†	7	0.82 ± 0.03†	7	0.562
LF/HF RRi	6.63 ± 1.66†	7	4.97 ± 0.76†	4	0.099	4.61 ± 0.70†	7	5.75 ± 1.01†	7	0.394
SBRs, ms/mmHg	6.0 ± 0.8†	7	4.3 ± 0.5†	6	0.072	6.1 ± 0.9†	7	5.2 ± 0.4†	7	0.227

B: baseline; R: recovery; n: subjects number; HR: heart rate; SBP: systolic blood pressure; DBP: diastolic blood pressure; SV: stroke volume; CO: cardiac output; TPR: total peripheral resistance; SVR: skin vascular resistance; LF: low frequency band; HF: high frequency band; RRi: R-R interval; LF/HF: sympathetic index; SBRs: spontaneous baroreflex sensitivity; values are mean ± SE; *$p \leq 0.05$ vs before; †$p \leq 0.05$ vs supine; ‡$p \leq 0.05$ vs group.

significant increase in HR and SBP, and a tendency towards increase for DBP ($p = 0.058$), TPR ($p = 0.06$) and SVR (more than 2-fold increase, $p = 0.063$). SV was decreased, and CO remained unchanged. Measurements taken in the upright position showed increased HR and DBP and decreased SV after immersion, whereas SBP, TPR, SVR and CO remained unchanged.

On R+1, all measured hemodynamic variables did not show significant difference from pre-immersion levels, in both supine and upright positions.

SVR in the upright position was significantly higher than in the supine position for all measurements except those taken on R0.

3.5. Autonomic Nervous System

3.5.1. Catecholamines and Their Metabolites

Urinary epinephrine and normetanephrine were not significantly changed throughout the experiment. Urinary metanephrine decreased during recovery. Urinary norepinephrine showed a tendency towards increase during the first half of immersion (day 1, $p = 0.076$; day 2, $p = 0.072$; day 3, $p < 0.05$). Urinary dopamine also tended to increase during the first half of immersion (day 1, p =

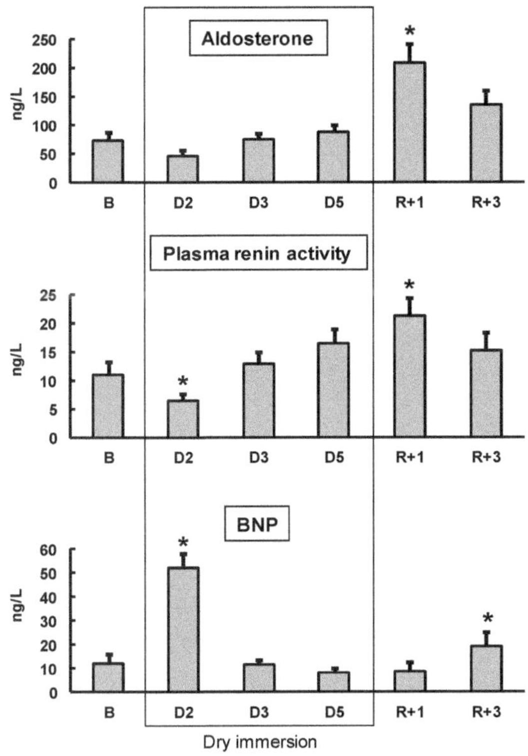

Figure 5. Blood aldosterone, renin and brain natriuretic peptide (BNP) before, during and following dry immersion. B: baseline; D: dry immersion; R: recovery. Values are means ± SE; *p < 0.05 vs baseline.

0.08; day 2, p = 0.09), with tendency to decrease on R0 (p = 0.07) (**Table 1**).

3.5.2. Cardiac Autonomic Neural Control

There was no significant difference in heart rate variability spectrum (LF, LF/HF) before and after DI (both R0 and R+1) (**Table 3**). Spontaneous baroreflex slope in upright position tended towards decrease on R0, but not on R+1 (**Table 3**).

3.6. Metabolism

3.6.1. Weight Changes

Body weight during immersion decreased by approximately 700 - 800 g. This decrease was significant on day 2 and day 3, with day 4 and day 5 showing a tendency towards decrease (p = 0.06). During recovery, there was no significant variation in body weight.

3.6.2. Blood Variables Relevant to Metabolism

All studied blood variables relevant to metabolism were within normal limits. Insulin, estimated insulin resistance (HOMA-IR), leptin and both LDL- and HDL-cholesterol fractions increased during DI. On the second recovery day, these variables did not differ from baseline. Fasting glucose and triglyceride levels were not significantly altered during DI (**Table 2**).

3.6.3. UFC and hs-CRP

Urinary free cortisol was slightly increased during immersion (significantly on day 2 and day 4), and unmodified in recovery (**Table 1**).

hs-CRP was unmodified (**Table 2**).

4. Discussion

Our results showed that during a 5-day DI, the decrease in total body water (3% - 4%) comes mostly from extracellular compartment (decrease 6% - 8%), and shows rapid stabilization at the new level. Five days of DI are sufficient to impair metabolism with decrease in glucose tolerance and hypercholesterolemia, but are not associated with pronounced autonomic changes. The 5-day DI induces marked cardiovascular impairment with altered orthostatic tolerance at first rising, which is quickly reversed (within 24 hours upon resuming normal activities).

4.1. Regulation of Body Fluids: Excretion and Redistribution

Extracellular osmolality, approximated by blood osmolality, remained stable under DI, suggesting no important changes regarding the intracellular volume. The main changes detected in response to the DI involved extracellular fluid, namely intravascular and interstitial volume.

4.1.1. Intravascular Volume: Water Loss by Neuroendocrine Regulation

Fundamental studies of body fluid regulation during short-term water immersion were performed by Gauer-Henry and Epstein [2]. Water-electrolyte changes in immersion are triggered by congestion of the central vascular regions: hydrostatic compression lowers the peripheral vascular capacity and shifts Starling balance towards increased absorption of interstitial fluid (hemodilution), leading to central hypervolemia. Twenty-four hours after the onset of DI, hormonal regulation was still in process (confirmed by a 2-fold renin decrease and 4-fold BNP increase), but after 48 hours of immersion, the major redistributions were over and hormonal concentrations remained at pre-immersion levels until the end of DI. The increase in BNP on the fourth recovery day may be not directly related to body fluid regulation, but rather reflect increased heart load after a period of enhanced physical inactivity during DI. Previously, we observed a similar increase in NT-proBNP, a proxy measure of BNP, on the fourth recovery day after 7-day DI [12]. The absence of BNP increase in first 24 hours of recovery may reflect the necessity to retain water and compensate for hypovolemia, which is prioritized over the need to "unload" the deconditioned heart.

4.1.2. Interstitial Volume: Water Redistribution by Protein Transfer

Plasma volume reduction calculated using plasma proteins consisted of as little as 1/3 of that calculated using Hct or Hb and Hct. This difference might be explained by the partial transfer of albumins (which make up approximately 60% of total protein pool) to interstitial fluid. During immersion, with compression of superficial tissues and continuous transcapillary "autotransfusion" [13], enhanced loss of interstitial fluid occurs. To limit tissue dehydration, plasma albumins might shift to interstitial fluid and increase its oncotic pressure. The partial transfer of proteins from plasma to interstitial fluid prevents the further decrease in interstitial fluid volume, which ensures the limitation of liquid loss and its adequate redistribution between intra-and extravascular departments [14]. Plasma proteins can be deposited in extravascular fluid compartments, and, if necessary, quickly return to restore the plasma protein loss. This was demonstrated by experiments with dry immersion and head-down bed rest, in which the plasma protein pool was restored during recovery at a rate exceeding the possibility of its synthesis *de novo* [15].

4.2. Hemodynamics

Five days of DI induced marked impairment of the cardiovascular system with tachycardia and stroke volume diminution both during resting and orthostatic challenge. The increase in HR, TPR and skin vasoconstriction, observed during first rising, might help to maintain blood pressure in conditions of decreased blood volume. The over two-fold increase in supine SVR together with the lack of further increase in SVR when upright immediately after DI might reflect the tension of systems maintaining cerebral blood perfusion.

4.3. Autonomic Nervous System

Dry immersion conditions might, on one hand, increase sympathetic activity due to hypovolemia and stress, and on the other hand, decrease it due to physical inactivity. Most DI studies suggest that DI conditions increase sympathetic activation [4]. However, we did not observe pronounced autonomic changes. Heart rate variability remained unmodified, though baroreflex sensitivity was somewhat weakened. The concentrations of urinary cathecolamines and theirs metabolites were not seriously altered.

4.4. Metabolism

The metabolic effects of DI are mainly related to the enforced physical inactivity. DI rapidly impaired glucose metabolism and lipid profile, inducing a decrease in insulin sensitivity and dyslipidemia. The same changes were observed in bed rest experiments [16-18]. It is important to note that physical inactivity for even a short-time is sufficient to impair metabolism ([18], this study). The increase in UFC during DI may be related to increased diuresis, as UFC and cortisone excretion depends on urine volume [19]. It also might reflect stress induced by new environment and the efforts of the organism to preserve homeostasis. Unmodified hs-CRP suggests the absence of a pronounced inflammatory state in DI.

4.5. Hypovolemia as Major Reason for DI-Induced Cardiovascular Deconditioning

A number of mechanisms may contribute to cardiovascular deconditioning induced by DI: circulatory blood volume loss [20,21], impaired baroreflex sensitivity [22, 23], autonomic dysfunction [22,24], increased venous compliance [21] enforced by decreased muscle tone [25], macrovascular [26] and microvascular [27] impairment promoted by physical inactivity and prolonged decrease of shear stress forces [28], myocardial impairment, hormonal changes, vestibular changes, or metabolic changes. Hypovolemia appears to be the major contributor for the observed rapid cardiovascular impairment in DI. The importance of hypovolemia is shown by inverse relationships between microgravity-induced plasma volume reduction and orthostatic tolerance [29]. Coyle *et al.* [30] showed that the decline in SV and $\dot{V}O_2$ max and the increase in HR and TPR during upright exercise following a few weeks of inactivity (only sedentary daily routines and no training) in men who had been training intensely for several years, was largely due to a decline in blood volume. When blood volume was expanded by dextran solution, the reduction of cardiovascular function after a few weeks of detraining was minimal. It is interesting to compare our study, in which plasma volume was normalized spontaneously, with studies in which plasma volume was restored after a prescription. Plasma volume normalization with salt tablets and water after a 12-day head down bed rest (HDBR) prevented orthostatic hypotension and changes in supine hemodynamics and endocrine variables, but was not effective to prevent tachycardia and epinephrine hyperresponsiveness to upright tilt [31]. Plasma volume restoration with fludrocortisone (a synthetic mineralocorticoid) after a 7-day HDBR significantly limited orthostatic intolerance (only one out of 7 subjects remained intolerant), and prevented changes in the baroreflex sensitivity [32]. However, while use of thigh cuffs during a 7-day HDBR significantly (but not completely) limited the decrease in plasma volume and the baroreflex sensitivity, it was unable to prevent orthostatic intolerance [33].

In summary, our results suggest that dry immersion induces remarkable changes at renal, endocrine, circulatory and metabolic levels, with pronounced orthostatic intolerance related mainly to hypovolemia. These changes are characterized by both a very rapid onset and very rapid restoration within return to normal activities.

4.6. Perspectives

DI is very original and efficient tool for physiological and physiopathological studies, especially in renal and body-fluid domain. In healthcare context, pronounced diuretic, sedative and muscle tone-decreasing effects of DI make it therapeutically promising. DI had already been tested in nephrology and cardiology for treatment of hypertension and edemas, in pediatrics for rehabilitation of preterm infants, and in neurology for muscle spasm relief. It may appear an efficient, easy and low-cost method of non-drug treatment. But to consider larger clinical implementation of DI, it is essential to dispose comprehensive detailed information concerning its effects. Our study on healthy volunteers aimed to contribute to this general knowledge. This work should be continued to further elucidate the mechanisms and potential applications of DI.

5. Acknowledgements

The authors thank all the volunteers for their enthusiastic participation in this study.

This study was supported by CNES, CNRS, the regional council "Région des Pays de la Loire" (DC-VACE project), RFFI, and the European FEDER program (Televasc program).

REFERENCES

[1] M. Epstein, "Cardiovascular and Renal Effects of Head-Out Water Immersion in Man: Application of the Model in the Assessment of Volume Homeostasis," *Circulation Research*, Vol. 39, No. 5, 1976, pp. 619-628. doi:10.1161/01.RES.39.5.619

[2] M. Epstein, "Renal, Endocrine and Hemodynamic Effects of Water Immersion in Humans," In: M. J. Fregly and C. M. Blatteis, Eds., *Handbook of Physiology, Environmental Physiology*, Oxford University Press, Oxford, 1996, pp. 845-853.

[3] J. E. Greenleaf, "Physiological Responses to Prolonged Bed Rest and Fluid Immersion in Humans," *Journal of Applied Physiology*, Vol. 57, No. 3, 1984, pp. 619-633.

[4] N. M. Navasiolava, M. A. Custaud, E. S. Tomilovskaya, I. M. Larina, T. Mano, G. Gauquelin-Koch, C. Gharib and I. B. Kozlovskaya, "Long-Term Dry Immersion: Review and Prospects," *European Journal of Applied Physiology*, Vol. 111, No. 7, 2011, pp. 1235-1260. doi:10.1007/s00421-010-1750-x

[5] M. E. Widlansky, "The Danger of Sedenterism: Endothelium at Risk," *Heart and Circulatory Physiology: American Journal of Physiology*, Vol. 299, No. 2, 2010, pp. 243-244. doi:10.1152/ajpheart.00505.2010

[6] M. A. Iunusov, V. N. Orlov and T. V. Vinokhodova, "Effect of the Model of 'Dry' Immersion on the Indicators of Water-Electrolyte Metabolism and Aldosterone and Cortisol in the Plasma of Persons with Different Levels of Body Water," *Kosmicheskaia Biologiia i Aviakosmicheskaia Meditsina*, Vol. 19, No. 4, 1985, pp. 42-45.

[7] S. G. Ivanov and E. E. Bogomazov, "'Dry' Immersion and Prospects of Its Use in Clinical Practice," *Kosmicheskaia Biologiia i Aviakosmicheskaia Meditsina*, Vol. 22, No. 5, 1988, pp. 4-6.

[8] S. G. Ivanov and L. I. Markova, "Use of a 'Dry' Immersion Method in the Treatment of Hypertensive Crisis," *Kosmicheskaia Biologiia i Aviakosmicheskaia Meditsina*, Vol. 24, No. 1, 1990, pp. 40-42.

[9] N. M. Navasiolava, V. de Germain, T. Levrard, I. M. Larina, I. B. Kozlovskaya, B. Diquet, A. Le Bouil, M. A. Custaud and J. O. Fortrat, "Skin Vascular Resistance in the Standing Position Increases Significantly after 7 Days of Dry Immersion," *Autonomic Neuroscience*, Vol. 160, No. 1-2, 2011, pp. 64-68. doi:10.1016/j.autneu.2010.10.003

[10] M. Coupé, M. Yuan, C. Demiot, Y. Q. Bai, S. Z. Jiang, Y. Z. Li, P. Arbeille, G. Gauquelin-Koch, T. Levrard, M. A. Custaud and Y. H. Li, "Low-Magnitude Whole Body Vibration with Resistive Exercise as a Countermeasure against Cardiovascular Deconditioning after 60 Days of Head-Down Bed Rest," *American Journal of Physiology—Regulatory, Integrative and Comparative Physiology*, Vol. 301, No. 6, 2011, pp. 1748-1754. doi:10.1152/ajpregu.00234.2011

[11] V. P. Krotov, T. E. Burkovskaia, M. A. Dotsenko, Iu. V. Gordeev, A. M. Nosovskiĭ and N. A. Chel'naia, "Blood Plasma Volume Dynamics in Monkeys during Immersion," *Aviakosmicheskaia i Ekologicheskaia Meditsina*, Vol. 38, No. 3, 2004, pp. 30-36.

[12] N. M. Navasiolava, A. Pajot, Y. Gallois, L. Kh. Pastushkova, V. A. Kulchitsky, G. Gauquelin-Koch, I. B. Kozlovskaya, M. Heer, O. Hand, I. M. Larina and M. A. Custaud, "NT-ProBNP Levels, Water and Sodium Homeostasis in Healthy Men: Effects of 7 Days of Dry Immersion," *European Journal of Applied Physiology*, Vol. 111, No. 9, 2011, pp. 2229-2237. doi:10.1007/s00421-011-1858-7

[13] J. A. Krasney, "Head-Out Water Immersion: Animal Studies," In: M. J. Fregly and C. M. Blatteis, Eds., *Handbook of Physiology, Environmental Physiology*, Oxford University Press, Oxford, 1996, pp. 855-887.

[14] K. I. Gogolev, E. A. Aleksandrova and E. B. Shul'zhenko, "Comparative Assessment of Changes during Antiorthostatic Hypokinesia and Immersion in Man," *Human Physiology*, Vol. 6, No. 6, 1980, pp. 392-396.

[15] A. M. Chaĭka and I. S. Balakhovskiĭ, "Changes in Plasma and Extracellular Fluid Volumes and Plasma Protein Mass under Conditions of Head-Down Tilt Hypokinesia

and Immersion," *Kosmicheskaia Biologiia i Aviakosmicheskaia Meditsina*, Vol. 16, No. 6, 1982, pp. 22-28.

[16] A. Bergouignan, I. Momken, D. A. Schoeller, S. Normand, A. Zahariev, B. Lescure, C. Simon and S. Blanc, "Regulation of Energy Balance during Long-Term Physical Inactivity Induced by Bed Rest with and without Exercise Training," *Journal of Clinical Endocrinology & Metabolism*, Vol. 95, No. 3, 2010, pp. 1045-1053. doi:10.1210/jc.2009-1005

[17] S. Blanc, S. Normand, C. Pachiaudi, J. O. Fortrat, M. Laville and C. Gharib, "Fuel Homeostasis during Physical Inactivity Induced by Bed Rest," *Journal of Clinical Endocrinology & Metabolism*, Vol. 85, No. 6, 2000, pp. 2223-2233. doi:10.1210/jc.85.6.2223

[18] N. M. Hamburg, C. J. McMackin, A. L. Huang, S. M. Shenouda, M. E. Widlansky, E. Schulz, N. Gokce, N. B. Ruderman, J. F. Keaney Jr. and J. A. Vita, "Physical Inactivity Rapidly Induces Insulin Resistance and Microvascular Dysfunction in Healthy Volunteers," *Arteriosclerosis, Thrombosis, and Vascular Biology*, Vol. 27, No. 12, 2007, pp. 2650-2656. doi:10.1161/ATVBAHA.107.153288

[19] M. Fenske, "Urinary Free Cortisol and Cortisone Excretion in Healthy Individuals: Influence of Water Loading," *Steroids*, Vol. 71, No. 11-12, 2006, pp. 1014-1018. doi:10.1016/j.steroids.2006.08.004

[20] J. C. Buckey Jr., L. D. Lane, B. D. Levine, D. E. Watenpaugh, S. J. Wright, W. E. Moore, F. A. Gaffney and C. G. Blomqvist, "Orthostatic Intolerance after Spaceflight," *Journal of Applied Physiology*, Vol. 81, No. 1, 1996, pp. 7-18.

[21] V. A. Convertino, "Exercise and Adaptation to Microgravity Environment," In: M. J. Fregly and C. M. Blatteis, Eds., *Handbook of Physiology, Environmental Physiology*, Oxford University Press, Oxford, 1996, pp. 815-843.

[22] V. A. Convertino, "Mechanisms of Microgravity Induced Orthostatic Intolerance: Implications for Effective Countermeasures," *Journal of Gravitational Physiology*, Vol. 9, No. 2, 2002, pp. 1-13.

[23] K. A. Engelke, D. F. Doerr, C. G. Crandall and V. A. Convertino, "Application of Acute Maximal Exercise to Protect Orthostatic Tolerance after Simulated Microgravity," *American Journal of Physiology*, Vol. 271, No. 4, 1996, pp. R837-R847.

[24] T. Mano, "Autonomic Neural Functions in Space," *Current Pharmaceutical Biotechnology*, Vol. 6, No. 4, 2005, pp. 319-324. doi:10.2174/1389201054553743

[25] A. I. Grigor'ev, I. B. Kozlovskaia and B. S. Shenkman, "The Role of Support Afferents in Organization of the Tonic Muscle System," *Rossiĭskii Fiziologicheskiĭ Zhurnal Imeni I.M. Sechenova*, Vol. 90, No. 5, 2004, pp. 508-521.

[26] L. F. Zhang, "Vascular Adaptation to Microgravity: What Have We Learned?" *Journal of Applied Physiology*, Vol. 91, No. 6, 2001, pp. 2415-2430.

[27] M. Coupe, J. O. Fortrat, I. M. Larina, G. Gauquelin-Koch, C. Gharib and M. A. Custaud, "Cardiovascular Deconditioning: From Autonomic Nervous System to Microvascular Dysfunctions," *Respiratory Physiology & Neurobiology*, Vol. 169, No. 1, 2009, pp. 10-12. doi:10.1016/j.resp.2009.04.009

[28] P. C. de Groot, M. W. Bleeker and M. T. Hopman, "Magnitude and Time Course of Arterial Vascular Adaptations to Inactivity in Humans," *Exercise and Sport Sciences Reviews*, Vol. 34, No. 2, 2006, pp. 65-71. doi:10.1249/00003677-200604000-00005

[29] V. A. Convertino, "Clinical Aspects of the Control of Plasma Volume at Microgravity and during Return to one Gravity," *Medicine & Science in Sports & Exercise*, Vol. 28, No. 10, 1996, pp. 45-52. doi:10.1097/00005768-199610000-00033

[30] E. F. Coyle, M. K. Hemmert and A. R. Coggan, "Effects of Detraining on Cardiovascular Responses to Exercise: Role of Blood Volume," *Journal of Applied Physiology*, Vol. 60, No. 1, 1986, pp. 95-99.

[31] W. W. Waters, S. H. Platts, B. M. Mitchell, P. A. Whitson and J. V. Meck, "Plasma Volume Restoration with Salt Tablets and Water after Bed Rest Prevents Orthostatic Hypotension and Changes in Supine Hemodynamic and Endocrine Variables," *Heart and Circulatory Physiology*: *American Journal of Physiology*, Vol. 288, No. 2, 2005, pp. 839-847. doi:10.1152/ajpheart.00220.2004

[32] J. Vernikos and V. A. Convertino, "Advantages and Disadvantages of Fludrocortisone or Saline Load in Preventing Post-Spaceflight Orthostatic Hypotension," *Acta Astronaut*, Vol. 33, 1994, pp. 259-266. doi:10.1016/0094-5765(94)90133-3

[33] M. A. Custaud, C. Millet, J. Frutoso, A. Maillet, G. Gauquelin, C. Gharib and J. O. Fortrat, "No Effect of Venoconstrictive Thigh Cuffs on Orthostatic Hypotension Induced by Head-Down Bed Rest," *Acta Physiologica Scandinavica*, Vol. 170, No. 2, 2000, pp. 77-85. doi:10.1046/j.1365-201x.2000.00763.x

Supplementary Data

Table S1. Variations from baseline for creatinine, free water, osmolal and urea clearances (Δ = valueday − valuebaseline).

	DI 1	DI 2	DI 4	R0	R+2
ΔCCr, ml/min	5.6 ± 7.0	8.9 ± 10.7	−2.9 ± 13.9	−18.9 ± 8.4	4.9 ± 5.8
ΔCH_2O, ml/min	0.42 ± 0.2	0.61 ± 0.3	0.43 ± 0.22	0.45 ± 0.2	0.11 ± 0.22
ΔCosm, ml/min	−0.32 ± 0.14	−0.23 ± 0.09	−0.41 ± 0.14*	0.08 ± 0.19	0.15 ± 0.11
ΔCurea, ml/min	13.9 ± 1.9*	6.8 ± 3.8	5.9 ± 5.3	−9.6 ± 2.6*	5.4 ± 3.3

CCr: creatinine clearance; CH_2O: free water clearance; Cosm: osmolal clearance; Curea: urea clearance; B: baseline; DI: dry immersion; R: recovery; values are means ± SE, *$p < 0.05$ vs baseline.

Table S2. Morning blood pressure and heart rate before, during and after dry immersion.

	B-2	B-1	DI 1	DI 2	DI 3	DI 4	DI 5	R0	R+1	R+2
SBP, mmHg	124 ± 3	123 ± 3	121 ± 3	116 ± 2	121 ± 2	123 ± 3	113 ± 2*	121 ±3	123 ± 2	118 ± 2
DBP, mmHg	72 ± 2	69 ± 2	71 ± 2	68 ± 1	73 ± 2	68 ± 2	70 ± 2	71 ± 1	68 ± 2	64 ± 2
HR, bpm	64 ± 4	65 ± 4	67 ± 4	57 ± 2*	56 ± 3*	61 ± 3	58 ± 2	57 ± 2	69 ± 3	71 ± 2

B: baseline; DI: dry immersion; R: recovery; SBP: systolic blood pressure; DBP: diastolic blood pressure; HR: heart rate; values are means ± SE. *$p < 0.05$ vs B-1.

5

Cyclosporine-Associated Nephrotoxicity

Maria Delia Colombo[1,2*], Renata Perego[2], Gilberto Bellia[1]
[1]Novartis Farma S.p.A., Origgio (VA), Italy
[2]Department of Dermatology, Marchesi Hospital, Inzago (MI), Italy
Email: *delia.colombo@novartis.com

ABSTRACT

Cyclosporine (CsA) has revolutionized transplant medicine and is currently one of the most important immunosuppressive agents for a wide range of organ transplantations and of autoimmune and inflammatory diseases, such as rheumatoid arthritis, uveitis, psoriasis, and atopic dermatitis. Renal impairment represents the main limitation to CsA long-term continuous therapy. However, it has been shown that nephrotoxicity is associated with longer treatment duration, larger cumulative doses and higher daily dose of CsA. With low dose regimens (<5 mg/kg/day), stable serum creatinine levels have been observed up to 15 - 20 years after kidney transplantation. Intermittent therapy may offer a good therapeutic strategy to limit long-term renal dysfunction, given the fact that renal structural changes are dose- and time-dependent. The best predictor of permanent renal damage is a persistent increase in serum creatinine level one month after treatment withdrawal. In patients with autoimmune diseases, the percentage increase in serum creatinine above baseline value during CsA therapy has been shown to predict CsA-induced nephropathy. Before CsA therapy initiation, patients should undergo a thorough baseline evaluation including laboratory assessments, in particular electrolytes, serum creatinine, and urea levels. Furthermore, patients should be evaluated for factors that might increase the risk of nephrotoxicity, such as obesity, older age, hypertension, concomitant use of nephrotoxic drugs, and pre-existing renal conditions. In the present paper, CsA-induced nephropathy will be reviewed in terms of pathophysiology, pathologic and clinical findings, and strategies for prevention and management.

Keywords: Cyclosporine; Nephrotoxicity; Immunosuppression; Transplant; Creatinine

1. Introduction

Since its discovery in Sandoz laboratories in 1972, cyclosporine (CsA) has revolutionized transplant medicine. CsA is currently one of the most important immunosuppressive agents for a wide range of organ transplantations, including kidney, liver, heart, lung, pancreas, and intestine [1]. CsA has been found to have many immunologic properties that make it an attractive agent for immunosuppression: it is found to inhibit both *in vitro* cell-mediated lysis as well as lymphocyte sensitization by allogeneic target cells [2]. Clinically, as summarized by Hariharan *et al.* in 2000, who reviewed 93,000 transplants from 1988 and 1996, CsA obtained one-year graft survival rates in 94% and 88% in living related and deceased donor allografts respectively [3]. More recent data from the United Network for Organ Sharing (UNOS) from 1998 to 2007 show one-year adjusted survival rates of 96.6% and 91.6% in living related and deceased donor allografts respectively. In its 40 years of life, CsA was shown to be also an effective treatment option in autoimmune and inflammatory diseases, such as rheumatoid arthritis, uveitis, psoriasis, and atopic dermatitis [4-8].

The fact CsA was nephrotoxic was discovered early after its initial use, when Calne *et al.* found a significant and unexpected nephrotoxicity that had not been observed in animal experiments in their first attempt to use CsA following transplantation using a dose of 25 mg/kg [9]. Currently, it is well known that renal damage may be an important side effect of CsA therapy, but it is also known that most persistent renal dysfunction is related to prolonged therapy, or doses of greater than 5 mg/kg/day, both of which can result in structural renal changes. Furthermore, it has been reported that nephrotoxicity is also related to individual susceptibility [10]. In the present paper, CsA-induced nephropathy will be reviewed in terms of pathophysiology, pathologic and clinical findings, and strategies for prevention and management.

*Corresponding author.

2. Risk Factors for CsA Nephrotoxicity

2.1. Systemic Levels of CsA

The main issue after renal transplantation is to maintain a reasonable balance between efficacy against rejection and toxicity, especially nephrotoxicity. Klintmalm *et al.* were the first to demonstrate a relationship between CsA doses, plasma levels, and renal allograft interstitial fibrosis [11,12]. This association between CsA nephrotoxicity and higher CsA doses (>5 mg/kg/day) was then confirmed by others [13]. After these findings, it became evident that CsA has a relatively narrow therapeutic window and great care has to be given to keep dosage within preset target ranges [14].

However, maintaining CsA concentrations within preset target ranges proved to be difficult due to its high inter-and intraindividual pharmacokinetic variability [15], which was especially observed with the first CsA formulation, Sandimmun. This variability appeared to be largely due to significant inter- and intraindividual variability in the expression and function of the metabolizing cytochrome P450 3A isoenzymes, mainly CYP3A4 and CYP3A5, and of the multidrug efflux transporter P- glycoprotein. This was partly attributed to interactions with other drugs, which cause either inhibition or stimulation of expression or activity of these enzymes and transporter. After development of a new CsA emulsion, Neoral, better absorption, less inter- and intraindividual variability, earlier stabilization of pharmacokinetics, and dose linearity in CsA exposure were observed compared with the old formulation [16-18]. However, it has been suggested that during chronic treatment of transplant recipeents, therapeutic drug monitoring of CsA may be useful and in fact, it is now adopted in clinical practice [19].

2.2. Local Renal Exposure to CsA

It has been demonstrated that levels of CsA in the renal tissue are much higher than in blood [20,21]. In addition to the degree of renal CsA exposure, there is also evidence that the susceptibility to CsA nephrotoxicity is determined by local renal factors, independent of local CsA levels. These factors include both the age of the recipient and of the transplanted kidney, the latter being independently associated with chronic histologic damage [22]. Second, local renal P-glycoprotein not only could play a role in renal accumulation of CsA, but could also be important for tubular epithelial cell detoxification and protection against apoptotic stress. Third, the use of nonsteroidal anti-inflammatory drugs (NSAIDs) has been shown to increase renal susceptibility to acute CsA nephrotoxicity, with decreases in renal plasma flow and GFR [23-26]. Finally, genetic polymorphisms in genes involved in the pathogenesis of CsA nephrotoxicity have been associated with the risk for chronic nephrotoxicity [27-37].

Given the above evidences, it could be anticipated that younger patients with native kidneys or recipients of transplanted kidneys from younger donors could be less susceptible to CsA nephrotoxicity. Moreover, great attention should be paid to drug interactions: **Table 1** lists the drugs that may increase the risk of CsA-associated nephrotoxicity. Finally, determination of a patient's or donor's genotype of drug-metabolizing genes or of molecules involved in CsA nephrotoxicity, like TGF-β, could provide a reasonable tool to determine which patients are most susceptible for CsA nephrotoxicity.

2.3. CsA-Independent Risk of Chronic Renal Failure Following Transplantation

Ojo *et al.* conducted a population-based cohort analysis to evaluate the incidence of chronic renal failure and the risk factors for it in 69,321 patients undergone non renal transplantation in the United States between 1990 and 2000 [38]. The 5-year risk varied depending on the type of organ transplanted, ranging from 7% among heart-lung recipients to 21% in recipients of intestine transplants. Other risk factors were increasing age, female sex, hypertension, diabetes mellitus, pre-transplantation heaptitis B infection, and postoperative acute renal failure. These data show that after transplantation of non-renal organs patients are at higher risk of chronic renal failure, independently from the post-transplantation immunosuppressive therapy.

3. Pathophysiology of CsA Nephrotoxicity

The etiology of chronic CsA nephrotoxicity has been studied extensively. A combination of CsA-induced hemodynamic changes and direct toxic effects of CsA on tubular epithelial cells is thought to play a role [19]. Renal dysfunction can be functional or structural. Functional impairment, which may begin soon after commencing

Table 1. Drugs that may increase the risk of CsA-associated nephrotoxicity [115].

Aminoglycosides
Melfalan
Diclofenac
Amphotericin B
Ketoconazole
Trimetoprim (with or without sulphametoxazole)
Fluoroquinilones
Acyclovir
Cidofovir
Foscarnet
Cimetidine, ranitidine
Tacrolimus
Colquicine
NSAIDs
Analgesics
Contrast media
Fibrates

treatment, can be subdivided into vascular dysfunction and tubular dysfunction. Vascular dysfunction is caused by vasoconstriction of the afferent glomerular arterioles, leading to increased vascular resistance. This results in decreased renal glomerular filtration rate (GFR) and renal blood flow with decreased clearance of creatinine. Tubular dysfunction is characterized by decreased magnesium reabsorption, decreased uric acid excretion, decreased potassium and hydrogen ion secretion, and distal tubular acidosis. Hypomagnesemia, decreased bicarbonate concentration, hyperuricemia, and hyperkalemia may also result. There is no loss of urinary concentrating power, as is the case with other nephrotoxins.

3.1. Acute Nephrotoxicity

Vasoconstriction of the afferent arterioles was first suggested by Murray *et al.* in 1985, which was proposed to be due to activation of the renal sympathetic nervous system, since a concomitant stimulation of plasma renin activity was demonstrated [39]. These authors also noted a reduction in the rate of decline of renal blood flow in denervated rats. Barros *et al.* also demonstrated an increase in vascular resistance in both afferent and efferent arterioles with a reduction in renal plasma flow and glomerular filtration rate (GFR), an effect that was attenuated by the administration of the angiotensin-converting enzyme (ACE) inhibitor captopril and the calcium channel blocker verapamil [40]. In addition to its activation of the renin-angiotensin system (RAS), CsA has been shown to increase the vasoconstrictor factors endothelin and tromboxane. It also demonstrated to reduce vasodilator factors, prostacyclin, prostaglandin E2 and nitric oxide (NO) [41,42]. Activation of the RAS by CsA occurs by two mechanisms, a direct effect on juxtaglomerular cells [43] and indirectly through arterial vasoconstriction and reduced renal plasma flow. Another pathogenic mechanism was that observed by Hoecherl *et al.* who demonstrated a marked reduction of COX-2 expression and of the down- stream production of arachidonic acid metabolites, and a consequent vasoconstriction [44].

The role of the innate immune system has also been implicated in the nephrotoxicity of CsA. Injured tubular epithelial cells may activate toll-like receptors (TLR) and TNF-alfa which, in turn, stimulate secretion of chemokines that initiate phagocytic activity and immune activation [45]. This mechanism may provide a link between innate immunity and the direct effects of CsA on renal tubular cells.

3.2. Chronic Nephrotoxicity

Chronic nephrotoxicity is the main drawback of current CsA immunosuppressive regimens [46]. Myers *et al.* in 1984 were the first demonstrating that high doses of CsA not only induce reversible alterations in renal vascular resistance, but may also be associated with irreversible damage of the renal architecture [46]. In cardiac transplant recipients surviving more than 12 months and treated with CsA at very high doses (up to 17 mg/kg/day), which are no longer used even in transplant recipients, they observed significant reduction in GFR, renal plasma flow, and renal blood flow. Biopsies of five CsA-treated patients showed tubulointerstitial injury and focal glomerular sclerosis, which seemed to correlate in intensity with the degree of renal impairment47. Further evidence of chronic nephrotoxicity related to high dose (>5 mg/kg/die), long-term CsA use (>2 years) was the finding of impaired renal function in heart, liver, and lung transplant recipients as well as in patients with autoimmune diseases [47-49].

More recently, other authors reported much more encouraging results following long-term use of CsA in kidney transplant recipients. Sandrini *et al.* reported on renal function in 638 cadaveric kidney transplant patients treated with CsA for up to 15 years. At 15 years, patient and graft survival rates were 82.7% and 56.1% respecttively, renal function remained stable in 266 patients (46.6%) with preserved serum creatinine values observed even after a 15-year treatment period [50]. Kandaswamy *et al* studied the impact of continuing CsA-based immunosuppression in the second decade after kidney transplantation in a total of 1263 patients [10]. They observed that not all transplanted patients on CsA developed progressive renal changes, but conversely in a subset or patients on long term CsA, serum creatinine levels were stable up to 20 years post-transplantation. The authors' conclusions were that identifying recipients' predisposetion to CsA toxicity and individualizing immunosuppressive therapy might be important in order to improve long-term kidney function. They also noted that reducetion in CsA exposure over time might preserve renal function.

4. Pathologic Findings

The hallmark finding in CsA nephrotoxicity is arteriolar hyalinosis, characterized by nodular hyaline deposits in the tunica media of afferent arterioles. Another common finding is interstitial or so-called striped fibrosis. This is hypothesized to be secondary to the above mentioned vasoconstriction effects of CsA with subsequent arterial narrowing. The subsequent tissue ischemia/hypoxia leads to a reperfusion type injury, with the formation of reactive oxygen species and free radicals, leading to cellular injury and apoptosis [19,51].

Activation of the RAS is also implied in the pathogenesis of CsA nephrotoxicity, not only for its vasoconstrictive effects but also due to the action of angiotensin

II, which has been shown to possibly induce fibrosis [19, 52,53].

Nankivell *et al* in 2004 gave one of the most important contributions to the documentation of the long-term nephrotoxic effects of CsA and the associated pathologic findings [54]. These authors examined serial kidney biopsies, performed at the time of organ implantation, at weeks 1, 2 and 4, at months 3, 6 and 12, and then yearly for 10 years. In total 888 biopsies were obtained in 99 patients. At 10 years these authors observed lesions consistent with chronic CsA toxicity in 100% of patients, but it has to be taken into account that immunosuppression protocols in those years were complex, with transplanted patients usually receiving triple therapy, including CsA, prednisone and azathioprine, so that renal damage cannot be attributed to CsA alone [55].

Table 2 summarizes the histological lesions associated with CsA acute and chronic use. However, the differential diagnosis between CsA-related nephrotoxicity and other injury phenomena is very difficult, especially in kidney transplantation. The calcineurin inhibitors nephrotoxicity score proposed by Kambham *et al.* in 2007 [56] represents a first step in the standardization of the composite histological changes induced by CsA, but further validation studies are necessary. In non-renal organ transplantation the picture may be clearer and the study of CsA nephrotoxicity in native kidneys seems to be less troublesome [38,57].

5. CsA-Induced Nephropathy in Patients with Autoimmune Diseases

Feutren *et al.* in 1992 [4] studied the incidence of and the risk factors for CsA-induced nephropathy in patients with various autoimmune diseases. They retrospectively analyzed clinical and renal biopsy data from 192 patients (152 with insulin-dependent diabetes mellitus, 23 with posterior uveitis, 11 with psoriasis, 5 with Sjoegren, 1 with polychondritis), including 63 children of ≤15 years of age. The duration of CsA therapy ranged from 4 to 39 months and in most patients CsA doses were higher than currently recommended (8.2 ± 2.8 mg/kg/day) and were increased during the first months of therapy. Renal biopsies were performed in all patients and CsA-induced nephropathy was defined as the presence of moderate or more severe alterations of the tubulointerstitial space, the glomerular arterioles or both. Forty-one of the 192 patients had evidence of CsA-induced nephropathy: 25 had diabetes, 14 had uveitis, and 1 each had polychondritis and Sjoegren's syndrome. Interstitial fibrosis with tubular atrophy were the predominant morphologic lesions in CsA-induced nephropathy. The percent increase in serum creatinine above baseline values was the best predictor of nephropathy. The impairment of renal function did not seem to be a direct consequence of the morphologic alterations, since it was reversible in most patients after a reduction in the dose or discontinuation of CsA therapy, even when morphologic lesions were present. The dose of CsA, the type of underlying disease, and the patient's age were additional risk factors for nephropathy. The incidence of nephropathy was lower in children than in adults, probably because the clearance of CsA is greater in children [58]. In the authors' opinion, the results of this study suggest that CsA-induced nephropathy may not be the result of long-term and cumulative toxic effects on arterioles and tubules, but rather a consequence of a brief insult brought about by the administration of excessive doses of CsA (≥ 10 mg/kg/day), which were rather frequent in early nineties. This analysis suggests that in patients with autoimmune and inflammatory disease and normal renal function, the likelihood of the development of CsA-induced nephropathy can be minimized by using doses ≤ 5 mg/kg/day and avoiding increases in serum creatinine concentrations greater than 30% above the patient's baseline value by appropriate dose.

Table 2. Histological lesions associated with cyclosporine use (modified from Naesens *et al.* [19]).

Acute CsA nephrotoxicity	• Acute arteriolopathy = renal dysfunction without histological alterations • Tubular vacuolization • Thrombotic microangiopathy
Chronic CsA nephrotoxicity	• Interstitial fibrosis and tubular atrophy • Medial arteriolar hyalinosis • Glomerular capsular fibrosis • Global glomerulosclerosis • Focal segmental glomerulosclerosis • Juxtaglomerular apparatus hyperplasia • Tubular microcalcification

Several studies have been conducted specifically in psoriasis patients treated with CsA. Nine studies evaluated changes in renal structure, assessed in kidney biopsy specimens, together with the variation in GFR, in patients with psoriasis treated with CsA [59,67]. Different grading and scoring systems were used to evaluate CsA nephrotoxicity, making it difficult to combine the results. Biopsy studies included a total of 104 patients receiving CsA for a period ranging from 1 to 10 years at doses commonly ranging between 1.9 and 5 mg/kg/day, with some patients receiving up to 7.5 mg/kg/day. These studies showed slight to moderate interstitial fibrosis after 1 year of CsA in some subjects, and after 3 to 4 years, interstitial fibrosis was moderate to severe [59,61-64]. The frequency of glomerular sclerosis in biopsies increased from 12.5% at 3 years to 26% at 10 years [60,66]. Tubular atrophy has also been described. Renal arteriolar abnormalities, consisting of either necrosis of smooth-muscle cells and nodular protein deposits in the wall of afferent glomerular arterioles or arteriolar intima hyalinosis may also be seen [68]. The percentage of increase in serum creatinine above 30% of baseline was found to be a predictor of structural kidney changes. Moreover, the severity of recurrent acute nephrotoxicity was shown to correlate with chronic histological changes ($r = 0.8$, $p = 0.0003$) [64]. Increases in serum creatinine were reversible 1 month to 10 years [65,66,69] after stopping CsA therapy. It seems that structural kidney damage can be expected in patients in whom serum creatinine does not decrease after cessation of CsA therapy. Young *et al.* [62] showed that older patients may be more vulnerable to CsA-induced renal injury and that CsA-associated hypertension was associated with a greater degree of progressive renal interstitial fibrosis on serial biopsies. Other six studies described the incidence of increases in serum creatinine by more than 30% above the baseline value in psoriasis patients [4,70-74]. Overall, more than 50% of the patients had a significant increase in serum creatinine (>30% of baseline) if treatment was prolonged for ≥2 years. Comparing the incidence of in- creases in serum creatinine >30% in patients receiving continuous or intermittent CsA treatment no significant difference was found (OR 1.35, $p = 0.66$). In conclusion, in psoriasis patients nephrotoxicity was associated with longer use, larger cumulative dose, higher daily dose and the occurrence of acute increases in serum creatinine. Slight to moderate interstitial fibrosis was observed in patients treated for at least 1 - 2 years, while glomerular sclerosis or severe interstitial fibrosis were seen in some cases after 3 years or more. The functional signification and the reversibility of the structural changes have not been fully characterized in the available studies.

Regarding rheumatoid arthritis (RA), following the estimation of potential risk factors for the development of CsA-induced nephropathy in autoimmune diseases4, dosing recommendations for the use of CsA in RA were established, stating that the starting dose should be 2.5 - 3.5 mg/kg/day, the maximum daily dose should not exceed 5 mg/kg/day and that the dose should be reduced whenever serum creatinine increases by ≥ 30% [75,76]. The 1994 International Consensus Report on the treatment of RA by CsA concluded that CsA-induced nephropathy can be avoided when these rules are observed. Subsequently, data from the Kidney Biopsy Registry on 60 first and 14 second renal biopsies performed in RA patients treated with CsA for up to 87 months were reviewed by Rodriguez *et al.* in order to describe the biopsy findings in all evaluable RA patients, collect information about the long-term follow-up of renal function and discuss the risk factors for the development of nephrotoxicity [5]. Of the 22 patients who started CsA at dosages <4 mg/kg/day and did not exceed 5 mg/kg/day, none developed CsA-associated nephropathy. Continuous assessment of renal function did not show any evidence of deterioration over time in patients maintained on long-term, low-dose CsA.

A single-center prospective cohort study was conducted to assess the long-term renal tolerance of a low-dose CsA treatment in patients affected by sight-threatening posterior idiopathic uveitis, having healthy kidneys before CsA therapy [6]. Forty-one patients were included in the study undergoing a mean CsA treatment duration of 44.9 ± 3.6 months and receiving no other nephrotoxic drugs. Mean CsA daily dosage was gradually tapered from 4.3 ± 1.6 mg/kg/day to 1.8 ± 0.9 mg/kg/day over 5 years. Renal effects were evaluated by creatinine clearance, GFR and effective renal plasma flow; additionally 11 patients underwent kidney biopsies before and after 2 years of CsA treatment. The authors suggest that in order to obtain the expected benefits to patients with uveitis, CsA should be used at the lowest effective dose, possibly ≤ 3 mg/kg/day, so that CsA-associated nephrotoxicity might be prevented.

A large cohort of 285 recently diagnosed type 1 diabetic patients having received CsA for a mean of 20 months was monitored for 13 years and compared with a parallel group of 100 similar patients treated with insulin alone. The CsA-treated patients showed a transient increase in creatininemia during the first 18 months of treatment, associated with a transient increase in renal vascular resistance, both of which disappeared later, with values remaining then normal [77]. The authors conclude that low-dose CsA combined with tight and careful monitoring should not result in long-term renal dysfunction.

6. Prevention of CsA Nephrotoxicity

Despite the above mentioned evidences of CsA-associated renal toxicity, the exclusion of CsA from the immunosuppressive regimens following organ transplantation does not allow to preserve the allograft function, due to the inadequate rejection prophylaxis obtained with other immunosuppressive regimens [78-81]. Therefore, different strategies aimed at prevent- ing renal damage during long-term CsA treatment have been developed. For example, the week-end therapy was evaluated in the PREWENT study, which assessed the impact on efficacy and safety of a two consecutive days a week regimen in psoriasis patients, no difference in the incidence of adverse effects was observed between placebo and CsA [82].

6.1. CsA Minimization

There is increasing interest in CsA minimization protocols, in which the doses of CsA are adjusted to lower target levels, both in de novo immunosuppressive protocols both from time of transplantation and for rescue therapy after detection of renal histologic damage or dysfunction [80]. These CsA-sparing regimens appear to be relatively safe [79-81]. By minimizing CsA levels, nephrotoxicity might be partially avoided, but it has become clear that the increased risk of allograft rejection could annihilate these positive effects. It will be important to develop and apply new tools for clinical immunologic monitoring in order to avoid that minimization strategies will result in under-immunosuppression with the risk of chronic rejection.

6.2. Calcium Antagonists

Because vasoconstriction of the afferent arterioles appears to play a pivotal role in acute and chronic CsA nephrotoxicity, many authors have studied the preventive effects of vasodilatory agents. The calcium antagonist nitrendipine and later lacidipine were shown to prevent the fall in renal plasma flow and GFR associated with CsA administration [83-85]. In a randomized trial in renal transplant recipients, patients treated with the combination of CsA and nifedipine had better renal function with the same degree of blood pressure control [86]. A similar effect was shown by lacidipine in another randomized trial [87].

Likewise, in heart transplantation, treatment with nifedipine normalized BP and improved renal function [88]. More recently, another randomized trial with amlodipine confirmed these positive effects of calcium antagonists on CsA nephrotoxicity again in heart transplant recipients [89]. In contrast, a long-term follow-up study did not find a protective effect of calcium channel blockers in preventing CsA nephrotoxicity [90], but it has to be pointed out that the type of calcium antagonist is not specified in this study.

6.3. RAS Inhibition

Given the pivotal role of RAS activation in the pathogenesis of CsA nephrotoxicity, it can be expected that RAS inhibition will be useful in preventing its development. In human studies, ACE inhibitors showed to reduce CsA nephrotoxicity [91] and to improve the cardiovascular alterations observed in renal transplant recipients [92]. On the other hand, results with the angiotensin-receptor blocker (ARB) losartan are currently contradictory [93,94] and it is therefore not clear whether combination with ARB could effectively slow the progression of CsA-associated renal toxicity. Similarly inconsistent are the results of the comparison between nifedipine and lisinopril [95,96].

6.4. Other Pharmacological Approaches

Vasodilatory prostanoids, like misoprostol, did not prevent CsA nephrotoxicity both in transplant recipients and in rheumatoid arthritis patients [97,98]. Despite promising results in rats, the nitric oxide donor L-arginine showed no effect on CsA nephrotoxicity prevention in humans [99].

Other therapeutic approaches are promising, such as anti-TGF-β antibodies [100,101], antioxidants [102-105], statins [106] and magnesium supplementation [107,108], but no human studies are yet available with these agents.

7. Management of CsA Nephrotoxicity

A protocol for the management of nephrotoxicity associated with long term CsA administration has been proposed by Griffith *et al.* in their international consensus statement on CsA in psoriasis clinical practice [7]. Based on the observation that CsA nephropathy is strictly related to drug dose (>5 mg/kg/day) and treatment duration [60,70,109], these authors propose that the risk of renal toxicity during CsA treatment is reduced by the use of intermittent, short courses of the drug. The drug-free days should allow renal recovery and restoration of normal renal function [109]. Renal safety during short course CsA therapy has been shown in studies where only a minority of patients (4%, 17% and 10% - 27%) [72,110-112] experienced an elevation in serum creatinine, which was typically transient and commonly returned to baseline within 4 weeks following dose reduction or treatment cessation [72].

According to Griffiths *et al.* [7], the chance of developing renal impairment during CsA therapy should be minimized by screening patients at baseline for any risk factors of renal toxicity: hypertension, advanced age, pre-existing renal conditions, and abnormalities in absorption of CsA. Concomitant medications and weight may represent additional risk factors [4]. Most importantly, the dose of CsA should only exceptionally exceed 5 mg/kg/day and the duration should be only as long as is necessary to achieve clearance or near-clearance of the disease. Further management guidelines for monitoring renal safety during CsA therapy proposed by Griffiths *et al* are summarized in **Figure 1**.

8. Conclusions

Renal impairment represents the main limitation to CsA long-term continuous therapy. However, it has been shown that nephrotoxicity is associated with longer treatment duration, larger cumulative doses and higher daily dose of CsA. Its prevalence with doses ≤5 mg/kg/day is low. Renal structural changes including slight to moderate interstitial fibrosis were mainly observed in patients treated for ≥2 years consecutively with high dosages, significant lesions such as glomerular sclerosis or severe interstitial fibrosis seen after 3 years or more.

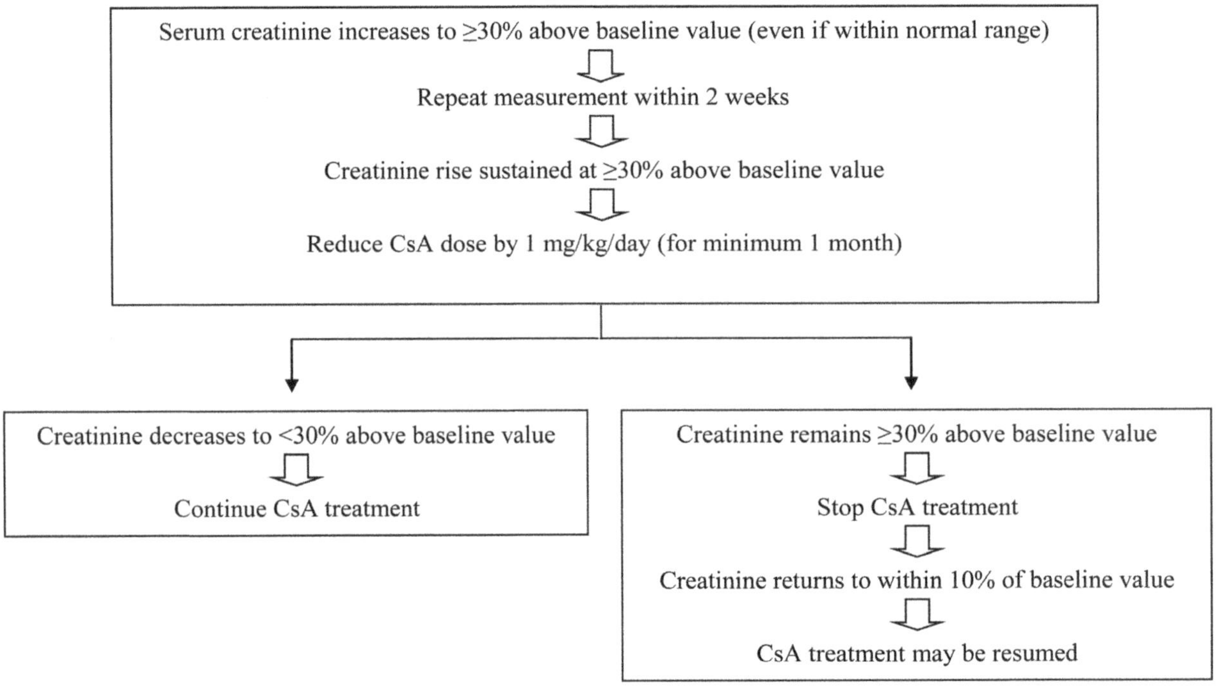

Figure 1. Management of renal toxicity during CsA therapy proposed by Griffiths *et al.* [7].

With low dose regimens, stable serum creatinine levels have been observed up to 15 - 20 years after kidney transplantation [10,50]. Intermittent therapy may offer a good therapeutic strategy to limit long-term renal dysfunction, given the fact that renal structural changes are dose- and time-dependent. Besides, the conventional CsA dose must be adapted to the ideal and not the real weight in obese patients to limit the risk of nephrotoxicity.

The best predictor of permanent renal damage is a persistent increase in serum creatinine level one month after treatment withdrawal. The percentage increase in serum creatinine above baseline value during CsA therapy has been shown to predict CsA-induced nephropathy in patients with autoimmune diseases [4]. Thus, patients must be examined and have serum creatinine levels measured monthly, in order to monitor increases >30% of baseline value, which may precede histological lesions and should prompt dose reduction.

Initiation of CsA therapy requires a thorough baseline evaluation including laboratory assessments with full blood counts, electrolytes, serum creatinine, urea, liver enzymes, cholesterol and triglycerides [113]. Furthermore, patients should be evaluated for factors that might increase the risk of nephrotoxicity. These risk factors include obesity [66], older age [60], hypertension, concomitant use of nephrotoxic drugs [114], and pre-existing renal conditions.

In general, if CsA is administered at a dose of 5 mg/kg/day or less and patients' serum creatinine levels are carefully monitored to ensure that they do not increase to more than 30% above baseline, renal side effects will be fully reversible after discontinuation of the drug.

In summary, CsA has with no doubt revolutionized transplant medication and has proven to be effective in autoimmune and inflammatory diseases. Despite the discovery of acute and chronic nephrotoxicity, its use continues to be a mainstay in immunosuppression, and CsA remains irreplaceable despite the enormous efforts otherwise. Available data indicate that low-dose CsA regimens (2.5 - 5 mg/kg/die) would provide an interesting balance between efficacy and toxicity.

REFERENCES

[1] D. Tedesco and L. Haragsim, "Cyclosporine: A Review," *Journal of Transplantation*, 2012, Article ID 230386, 2012, 7 pages.

[2] J. F. Borel, "Comparative Study of *in Vitro* and *in Vivo* Drug Effects on Cell Mediated Cytotoxicity," *Immunology*, Vol. 31, No. 4, 1976, pp. 631-641.

[3] S. Hariharan, C. P. Johnson, B. A. Bresnahan, S. E. Taranto, M. J. McIntosh and D. Stablein, "Improved Graft Survival after Renal Transplantation in the United States 1988-1996," *The New England Journal of Medicine*, Vol. 342, 2000, pp. 605-612. doi:10.1056/NEJM200003023420901

[4] G. Feutren and M. J. Mihatsch, "Risk Factors for Cyclosporine-Induced Nephropathy in Patients with Autoimmune Diseases," *The New England Journal of Medicine*,

Vol. 326, 1992, pp. 1654-1660. doi:10.1056/NEJM199206183262502

[5] F. Rodriguez, J. C. Krayenbuehl, W. B. Harrison, O. Forre, B. A. C. Dijkmans, P. Tugwell, *et al.*, "Renal Biopsy Findings and Follow Up of Renal Function in Rheumatoid Arthritis Patients Treated with Cyclosporine A. An Update from the International Kidney Biopsy Register," *Arthritis & Rheumatism*, Vol. 39, No. 9, 1996, pp. 1491-1498. doi:10.1002/art.1780390908

[6] C. Isnard Bagnis, S. Tezenas du Montcel, H. Beaufils, C. Jouanneau, C. Jaudon, P. Macsud, *et al.*, "Long-Term Renal Effects of Low-Dose Cyclosporine in Uveitis-Treated Patients: Follow-Up Study," *Journal of the American Society of Nephrology*, Vol. 13, No. 12, 2002, pp. 2962-2968. doi:10.1097/01.ASN.0000034945.61533.26

[7] C. E. M. Griffiths, L. Dubertret, C. N. Ellis, A. Y. Finlay, A. F. Finzi, V. C. Ho, *et al.*, "Cyclosporin in Psoriasis Clinical Practice: An International Consensus Statement," *British Journal of Dermatology*, Vol. 150, No. 67, 2004, pp. 11-23. doi:10.1111/j.0366-077X.2004.05949.x

[8] J. I. Harper, J. Berth-Jones, R. D. Camp, M. J. Dillon, A. Y. Finlay, C. A. Holden, *et al.*, "Cyclosporin for Atopic Dermatitis in Children," *Dermatology*, Vol. 203, No. 1, 2001, pp. 3-6. doi:10.1159/000051694

[9] R. Y. Calne, S. Thiru and D. J. G. White, "Cyclosporin A in Patients Receiving Renal Allografts from Cadaver Donors," *Lancet*, Vol. 2, No. 8104, 1978, pp. 1323-1327.

[10] R. Kandaswamy, A. Humar, V. Casingal, K. J. Gillingham, H. Ibrahim and A. J. Matas, "Stable Kidney Function in the Second Decade after Kidney Transplantation While on Cyclosporine-Based Immunosuppression," *Transplantation*, Vol. 83, No. 6, 2007, pp. 722-726 doi:10.1097/01.tp.0000256179.14038.e2

[11] G. Klintmalm, S. O. Bohman, B. Sundelin and H. Wiczek, "Interstitial Fibrosis in Renal Allografts after 12 to 46 Months of Cyclosporine Treatment: Beneficial Effects of Low Doses in Early Post-Transplantation Period," *Lancet*, Vol. 2, No. 8409, 1984, pp. 950-954 doi:10.1016/S0140-6736(84)91166-8

[12] G. Klintmalm, J. Sawe, O. Ringden, B. C. Von Bahr and A. Magnusson, "Cyclosporine Plasma Levels in Renal Transplant Patients. Association with Renal Toxicity and Allograft Rejection," *Transplantation*, Vol. 39, No. 2, 1985, pp. 132-137. doi:10.1097/00007890-198502000-00005

[13] F. C. Henny, C. H. Kleinbloesem, A. J. Moolenaar, L. C. Paul, D. D. Breimaer and L. A. van Es, "Pharmacokinetics and Nephrotoxicity of Cyclosporine in Renal Transplant Recipients," *Transplantation*, Vol. 40, No. 3, 1985, pp. 261-265. doi:10.1097/00007890-198509000-00008

[14] R. J. Ptachcinski, G. J. Burckart and R. Venkataramanan, "Cyclopsorine Concentration Determinations for Monitoring and Pharmacokinetic Studies," *The Journal of Clinical Pharmacology*, Vol. 26, No. 5, 1986, pp. 358-366. doi:10.1002/j.1552-4604.1986.tb03538.x

[15] A. Fahr, "Cyclosporine Clinical Pharmacokinetics," *Clinical Pharmacokinetics*, Vol. 24, No. 6, 1993, pp. 472-495. doi:10.2165/00003088-199324060-00004

[16] D. W. Holt, E. A. Mueller, J. M. Kovarik, J. B. van Bree, F. Richard and K. Kutz, "Sandimmun Neoral Pharmacokinetics: Impact of the New Oral Formulation," *Transplant Proceeding*, Vol. 27, No. 1, 1995, pp. 1434-1437.

[17] M. A. Masri, A. Barbari, A. Stephan, G. Kamel, G. Frem, F. Younan, *et al.*, "Cyclosporine Pharmacokinetics in Stable Renal Transplant Patients: Effect of Formulation Sandimmun versus Consupren versus Neoral," *Transplant Proceeding*, Vol. 28, No. 3, 1996, pp. 1318-1320.

[18] H. Humbert, "Variability of the Bioavailability of Cyclosporine: Benefit of the Neoral Formulation," *Therapie*, Vol. 52, No. 4, 1997, pp. 353-357.

[19] M. Naesens, D. R. J. Kuypers and M. Sarwal, "Calcineurin Inhibitors Nephrotoxicity," *Clinical Journal of the American Society of Nephrology*, Vol. 4, No. 2, 2009, pp. 481-508.

[20] P. F. Halloran, L. M. Helms, L. Kung and J. Noujaim, "The Temporal Profile of Calcineurin Inhibition by Cyclosporine *in Vivo*," *Transplantation*, Vol. 68, No. 9, 1999, pp. 1356-1361.doi:10.1097/00007890-199911150-00023

[21] K. Iwasaki, T. Shiraga, H. Matsuda, Y. Teramura, A. Kawamura, T. Hata, *et al.*, "Absorption, Distribution, Metabolism and Excretion of Tacrolimus (FK506) in the Rat," *Drug Metabolism and Pharmacokinetics*, Vol. 13, No. 3, 1998, pp. 259-265. doi:10.2133/dmpk.13.259

[22] M. Kubo, Y. Kiyohara, I. Kato, Y. Tanizaki, R. Katafuchi, H. Hirakata, *et al.*, "Risk Factors for Renal Glomerular and Vascular Changes in an Autopsy-Based Population Survey: The Hisayama Study," *Kidney International*, Vol. 63, 2003, pp. 1508-1515. doi:10.1046/j.1523-1755.2003.00886.x

[23] N. D. Sturrock, C. C. Lang and A. D. Struthers, "Indomethacin and Cyclosporine Together Produce Marked Renal Vasoconstriction in Humans," *Journal of Hypertension*, Vol. 12, No. 8, 1994, pp. 919-924. doi:10.1097/00004872-199408000-00009

[24] R. D. Altman, G. O. Perez and G. N. Sfakianakis, "Interaction of Cyclosporine A and Nonsteroidal Anti-Inflammatory Drugs on Renal Function in Patients with Rheumatoid Arthritis," *The American Journal of Medicine*, Vol. 93, No. 4, 1992, pp. 396-402. doi:10.1016/0002-9343(92)90169-C

[25] J. M. Kovarik, P. Kurki, E. Mueller, M. Guerret, E. Markert, R. Alten, *et al.*, "Diclofenac Combined with Cyclosporine in Treatment Refractory Rheumatoid Arthritis: Longitudinal Safety Assessment and Evidence of a Pharmacokinetic/Dynamic Interaction," *Journal of Rheumatology*, Vol. 23, No. 12, 1996, pp. 2033-2038.

[26] R. M. Soubhia, G. E. Mendes, F. Z. Mendonca, M. A. Baptista, J. P. Cipullo and E. A. Burdmann, "Tacrolimus and Nonsteroidal Anti-Inflammatory Drugs: An Association to Be Avoided," *American Journal of Nephrology*, Vol. 25, 2005, pp. 327-334. doi:10.1159/000086569

[27] C. C. Baan, A. H. Balk, C. T. Holweg, I. C. van Riemsdijk, L. P. Maat, P. J. Vantrimpont, *et al.*, "Renal Failure after Clinical Heart Transplantation Is Associated with the TGF-beta 1 Codon 10 Gene Polymorphism," *Journal of Heart Lung Transplant*, Vol. 19, No. 9, 2000, pp. 866-872. doi:10.1016/S1053-2498(00)00155-8

[28] J. van de Wetering, C. H. Weimar, A. H. Balk, J. I.

Roodnat, C. T. Holweg, C. C. Baan, *et al.*, "The Impact of Transforming Growth Factor-Beta1 Gene Polymorphism on End-Stage Renal Failure after Heart Transplantation," *Transplantation*, Vol. 82, No. 12, 2006, pp. 1744-1748. doi:10.1097/01.tp.0000250360.78553.5e

[29] S. Di Filippo, A. Zeevi, K. K. McDade, G. J. Boyle, S. A. Miller, S. K. Gandhi and S. A. Webber, "Impact of TGFbeta1 Gene Polymorphisms on Late Renal Function in Pediatric Heart Transplantation," *Human Immunology*, Vol. 66, No. 2, 2005, pp. 133-139. doi:10.1016/j.humimm.2004.09.018

[30] J. R. Jonsson, C. Hong, D. M. Purdie, C. Hawley, N. Isbel, M. Butler, *et al.*, "Role of Cytokine Gene Polymorphisms in Acute Rejection and Renal Impairment after Liver Transplantation," *Liver Transplant*, Vol. 7, No. 3, 2001, pp. 255-263. doi:10.1053/jlts.2001.22450

[31] J. Mytilineos, G. Laux and G. Opelz, "Relevance of IL10, TGF-beta1, TNFalpha, and IL4Ralpha Gene Polymorphisms in Kidney Transplantation: A Collaborative Transplant Study Report," *American Journal of Transplantation*, Vol. 4, No. 10, 2004, pp. 1684-1690. doi:10.1111/j.1600-6143.2004.00561.x

[32] B. Rigat, C. Hubert, F. Henc-Gelas, F. Cambien, P. Corvol and F. Soubrier, "An Insertion/Deletion Polymorphism in the Angiotensin I-Converting Enzyme Gene Accounting for Half the Variance of Serum Enzyme Levels," *Journal of Clinical Investigation*, Vol. 86, No. 4, 1990, pp. 1343-1346. doi:10.1172/JCI114844

[33] J. Beige, S. Scherer, A. Weber, S. Engeli, G. Offermann, G. Opelz, A. Distle and A. M. Sharma, "Angiotensin-Converting Enzyme Genotype and Renal Allograft Survival," *Journal of the American Society of Nephrology*, Vol. 8, No. 8, 1997, pp. 1319-1323.

[34] J. Broekroelofs, C. A. Stegeman, G. Navis, A. M. Tegzess, Z. D. De and P. E. De Jong, "Risk Factors for Long-Term Renal Survival after Renal Transplantation: A Role for Angiotensin-Converting Enzyme (Insertion/Deletion) Polymorphism?" *Journal of the American Society of Nephrology*, Vol. 9, No. 11, 1998, pp. 2075-2081.

[35] S. Barocci, F. Ginevri, U. Valente, F. Torre, R. Gusmano and A. Nocera, "Correlation between Angiotensin-Converting Enzyme Gene Insertion/Deletion Polymorphism and Kidney Graft Long-Term Outcome in Pediatric Recipients: A Single-Center Analysis," *Transplantation*, Vol. 67, No. 4, 1999, pp. 534-538. doi:10.1097/00007890-199902270-00008

[36] M. B. Juckett, E. P. Cohen, C. A. Keever-Taylor, Y. Zheng, C. A. Lawton, J. E. Moulder and J. Klein, "Loss of Renal Function Following Bone Marrow Transplantation: An Analysis of Angiotensin Converting Enzyme D/I Polymorphism and Other Clinical Risk Factors," *Bone Marrow Transplant*, Vol. 27, No. 4, 2001, pp. 451-456. doi:10.1038/sj.bmt.1702797

[37] R. Abdi, T. B. Tran, R. Zee, B. M. Brenner and E. L. Milford, "Angiotensin Gene Polymorphism as a Determinant of Post-Transplantation Renal Dysfunction and Hypertension," *Transplantation*, Vol. 72, No. 4, 2001, pp. 726-729. doi:10.1097/00007890-200108270-00028

[38] A. O. Ojo, P. J. Held, F. K. Port, R. A. Wolfe, A. B. Leichtman, E. W. Young, *et al.*, "Chronic Renal Failure after Transplantation of Non-Renal Organ," *New England Journal of Medicine*, Vol. 349, 2003, pp. 931-940. doi:10.1056/NEJMoa021744

[39] B. M. Murray, M. S. Paller and T. F. Ferris, "Effect of Cyclosporine Administration on Renal Hemodynamics in Conscious Rats," *Kidney International*, Vol. 28, 1985, pp. 767-774. doi:10.1038/ki.1985.196

[40] E. J. G. Barros, M. A. Boim and H. Ajzen, "Glomerular Hemodynamics and Hormonal Participation on Cyclosporine Nephrotoxicity," *Kidney International*, Vol. 32, 1987, pp. 19-25. doi:10.1038/ki.1987.166

[41] S. C. Textor, J. C. Burnett, J. C. Romero Jr., V. J. Canzanello, S. J. Taler, R. Wiesner, *et al.*, "Urinary Endothelin and Renal Vasoconstriction with Cyclosporine or FK506 after Liver Transplantation," *Kidney International*, Vol. 47, 1995, pp. 1426-1433. doi:10.1038/ki.1995.200

[42] S. Hortelano, M. Castilla, A. M. Torres, A. Tejedor and L. Bosc′a, "Potentiation by Nitric Oxide of Cyclosporin A and FK506-Induced Apoptosis in Renal Proximal Tubule Cells," *Journal of the American Society of Nephrology*, Vol. 11, No. 12, 2000, pp. 2315-2323.

[43] A. Kurtz, R. Della Bruna and K. Kuhn, "Cyclosporine A Enhances Renin Secretion and Production in Isolated Juxtaglomerular Cells," *Kidney International*, Vol. 33, 1988, pp. 947-953. doi:10.1038/ki.1988.92

[44] K. Hoecherl, F. Dreher, H. Vitzthum, J. Koehler and A. Kurtz, "Cyclosporin A Suppresses Cyclooxygenase-2 Expression in the Rat Kidney," *Journal of the American Society of Nephrology*, Vol. 13, No. 10, 2002, pp. 2427-2436. doi:10.1097/01.ASN.0000031702.86799.B9

[45] S. W. Lim, C. Li, K. O. Ahn, *et al.*, "Cyclosporine-Induced Renal Injury Induces Toll-Like Receptor and Maturation of Dendritic Cells," *Transplantation*, Vol. 80, No. 5, 2005, pp. 691-699. doi:10.1097/01.tp.0000173594.69089.a0

[46] W. M. Bennet, A. De Mattos, M. M. Meyer, T. Andoh and J. M. Barry, "Chronic Cyclosporine Nephropathy: The Achilles' Heel of Immunosuppressive Therapy," *Kidney International*, Vol. 50, 1996, pp. 1089-1100. doi:10.1038/ki.1996.415

[47] B. D. Myers, J. Ross and L. Newton, "Cyclosporine-Associated Chronic Nephropathy," *New England Journal of Medicine*, Vol. 311, No. 11, 1984, pp. 699-705.

[48] M. E. Falkenhain, F. G. Cosio and D. D. Sedmak, "Progressive Histologic Injury in Kidneys from Heart and Liver Transplant Recipients Receiving Cyclosporine," *Transplantation*, Vol. 62, No. 3, 1996, pp. 364-370. doi:10.1097/00007890-199608150-00011

[49] J. S. Zaltzman, Y. Pei, J. Maurer, A. Patterson and D. C. Cattran, "Cyclosporine Nephrotoxicity in Lung Transplant Recipients," *Transplantation*, Vol. 54, No. 5, 1992, pp. 875-878. doi:10.1097/00007890-199211000-00021

[50] S. Sandrini, G. Setti, N. Bossini, R. Zubani, S. Cassamali, P. Maiorca, *et al.*, "Experience with Cyclosporine," *Transplant Proceedings*, Vol. 36, Suppl. 2S, 2004, pp. 152S-157S. doi:10.1016/j.transproceed.2003.12.036

[51] D. Diederich, J. Skopec, A. Diederich and F.-X. Dai, "Cyclosporine Produces Endothelial Dysfunction by Increased Production of Superoxide," *Hypertension*, Vol. 23, 1994, pp. 957-961. doi:10.1161/01.HYP.23.6.957

[52] R. Christiane and W. Gunter, "Renin-Angiotensin-Aldosterone System and Progression of Renal Disease," *Journal of the American Society of Nephrology*, Vol. 17, No. 11, 2006, pp. 2985-2991. doi:10.1681/ASN.2006040356

[53] G. Wolf, "Renal Injury Due to Renin-Angiotensin-Aldosterone System Activation of the Transforming Growth Factor-β Pathway," *Kidney International*, Vol. 70, No. 11, 2006, pp. 1914-1919.

[54] B. J. Nankivell, R. J. Borrows, C. L. S. Fung, P. J. O'Connell, J. R. Chapman and R. D. M. Allen, "Calcineurin Inhibitor Nephrotoxicity: Longitudinal Assessment by Protocol Histology," *Transplantation*, Vol. 78, No. 4, 2004, pp. 557-565. doi:10.1097/01.TP.0000128636.70499.6E

[55] E. M. Johnson, D. M. Canafax, K. J. Gillingham, A. Humar, K. Pandian, S. R. Kerr, *et al.*, "Effect of Early Cyclosporine Levels on Kidney Allograft Rejection," *Clinical Transplantation*, Vol. 11, No. 6, 1997, pp. 552-557.

[56] N. Kambham, S. Nagarajan, S. Shah, L. Li, O. Salvatierra and M. M. Sarwal, "A Novel, Semiquantitative, Clinically Correlated Calcineurin Inhibitor Toxicity Score for Renal Allograft Biopsies," *Clinical Journal of the American Society of Nephrology*, Vol. 2, No. 1, 2007, pp. 135-142. doi:10.2215/CJN.01320406

[57] A. Greenberg, J. W. Egel, M. E. Thompson, R. L. Hardesty, B. P. Griffith, H. T. Bahnson, *et al.*, "Early and Late Forms of Cyclosporine Nephrotoxicity: Studies in Cardiac Transplant Recipients," *American Journal of Kidney Diseases*, Vol. 9, No. 1, 1987, pp. 12-22.

[58] P. F. Hoyer, G. Offner, K. Wonigeit, J. Brodehl and R. Pichelmayr, "Dosage of Cyclosporin A in Children with Renal Transplant," *Clinical Nephrology*, Vol. 22, No. 2, 1984, pp. 68-71.

[59] H. Zachariae, K. Kragballe, H. E. Hansen, N. Marcussen and S. Olsen, "Renal Biopsy Findings in Long-Term Cyclosporin Treatment of Psoriasis," *The British Journal of Dermatology*, Vol. 136, No. 4, 1997, pp. 531-535.

[60] N. J. Lowe, J. M. Wieder, A. Rosenbach, K. Johnson, R. Kunkel, C. Bainbridge, *et al.*, "Long-Term Low-Dose Cyclosporine Therapy for Severe Psoriasis: Effects on Renal Function and Structure," *Journal of the American Academy of Dermatology*, Vol. 35, No. 5, 1996, pp. 710-719. doi:10.1016/S0190-9622(96)90726-4

[61] J. M. Messana, K. J. Johnson and M. J. Mihatsch, "Renal Structure and Function Effects after Low Dose Cyclosporine in Psoriasis Patients: A Preliminary Report," *Clinical Nephrology*, Vol. 43, No. 3, 1995, pp. 150-153.

[62] E. W. Young, C. N. Ellis, J. M. Messana, K. J. Johnson, A. B. Leichtman, M. J. Mihatsch, *et al.*, "A Prospective Study of Renal Structure and Function in Psoriasis Patients Treated with Cyclosporine," *Kidney International*, Vol. 46, 1994, pp. 1216-1222. doi:10.1038/ki.1994.387

[63] E. Svarstad, S. Helland, T. Morken, L. Bostad, A. Myking, B. M. Iversen and J. Ofstad, "Renal Effects of Maintenance Low-Dose Cyclosporin A Treatment in Psoriasis," *Nephrology, Dialysis, Transplantation*, Vol. 9, No. 10, 1994, pp. 1462-1467.

[64] Y. Pei, J. W. Scholey, A. Katz, R. Schachter, G. F. Murphy and D. Cattran, "Chronic Nephrotoxicity in Psoriatic Patients Treated with Low-Dose Cyclosporine," *American Journal of Kidney Diseases*, Vol. 23, No. 4, 1994, pp. 528-536.

[65] A. V. Powles, T. Cook, B. Hulme, B. S. Baker, H. M. Lewis, E. Thomas, *et al.*, "Renal Function and Biopsy Findings after 5 Years' Treatment with Low-Dose Cyclosporin for Psoriasis," *The British Journal of Dermatology*, Vol. 128, No. 2, 1993, pp. 159-165. doi:10.1111/j.1365-2133.1993.tb15145.x

[66] A. V. Powles, C. M. Hardman, W. M. Porter, T. Cook, B. Hulme and L. Fry, "Renal Function after 10 Years' Treatment with Cyclosporin for Psoriasis," *The British Journal of Dermatology*, Vol. 138, No. 3, 1998, pp. 443-439. doi:10.1046/j.1365-2133.1998.02122.x

[67] H. Zachariae, H. E. Hansen, K. Kragballe and S. Olsen, "Morphologic Renal Changes during Cyclosporine Treatment of Psoriasis. Studies on Pretreatment and Post-Treatment Kidney Biopsy Specimens," *Journal of the American Academy of Dermatology*, Vol. 26, No. 3, 1992, pp. 415-419.

[68] M. J. Mihatsch, G. Thiel and B. Ryffel, "Morphology of Cyclosporine Nephropathy," *Progress in Allergy*, Vol. 38, 1986, pp. 447-465.

[69] U. Mrowietz, L. Faerber, H. H. Henneicke-von Zepelin, H. Bachmann, D. Welzel and E. Christophers, "Long-Term Maintenance Therapy with Cyclosporine and Post-Treatment Survey in Severe Psoriasis: Results of a Multicenter Study. German Multicenter Study," *Journal of the American Academy of Dermatology*, Vol. 33, No. 3, 1995, pp. 470-475.

[70] C. Laburte, R. Grossman, J. Abi-Rached, K. H. Abeywickrama and L. Dubertret, "Efficacy and Safety of Oral Cyclosporin A (CyA; Sandimmun) for Long-Term Treatment of Chronic Severe Plaque Psoriasis," *British Journal of Dermatology*, Vol. 130, No. 3, 1994, pp. 366-375. doi:10.1111/j.1365-2133.1994.tb02935.x

[71] J. Shupack, E. Abel, E. Bauer, M. Brown, L. Drake, R. Freinkel, *et al.*, "Cyclosporine as Maintenance Therapy in Patients with Severe Psoriasis," *Journal of the American Academy of Dermatology*, Vol. 36, No. 3, 1997, pp. 423-432.

[72] V. C. Ho, C. E. Griffiths, G. Albrecht, F. Vanaclocha, G. León-Dorantes, N. Atakan, *et al.*, "Intermittent Short Courses of Cyclosporin (Neoral^R) for Psoriasis Unresponsive to Topical Therapy: A 1-Year Multicentre, Randomized Study. The PISCES Study Group," *British Journal of Dermatology*, Vol. 141, No. 2, 1999, pp. 283-291. doi:10.1046/j.1365-2133.1999.02977.x

[73] P. Gisondi, M. Del Giglio, V. Di Francesco, *et al.*, "Weight Loss Improves the Response of Obese Patients with Moderate-to-Severe Chronic Plaque Psoriasis to Low-Dose Cyclosporine Therapy: A Randomized, Controlled, Investigator-Blinded Clinical Trial," *The American Journal of Clinical Nutrition*, Vol. 88, No. 5, 2008,

pp. 1242-1247.

[74] J. F. Honeyman, L. Sànchez and P. Valdés, "Low-Dose Cyclosporine A Improves Severe Disabling Psoriasis in Latin America. Latin American Multicenter Study," *International Journal of Dermatology*, Vol. 34, No. 8, 1995, pp. 583-588. doi:10.1111/j.1365-4362.1995.tb02961.x

[75] G. S. Panayi and P. Tugwell, "An International Consensus Report: The Use of Cyclosporin A in Rheumatoid Arthritis," *British Journal of Rheumatology*, Vol. 32, Suppl. 1, 1993, pp. 1-3.

[76] G. S. Panayi and P. Tugwell, "The Use of Cyclosporin A in Rheumatoid Arthritis: Conclusions of an International Review," *British Journal of Rheumatology*, Vol. 33, No. 10, 1994, pp. 967-969. doi:10.1093/rheumatology/33.10.967

[77] R. Assan, F. Blanchet, G. Feutren, J. Timsit, E. Larger, C. Boitard, *et al.*, "Normal Renal Function 8 to 13 Years after Cyclosporin A Therapy in 285 Diabetic Patients," *Diabetes/Metabolism Research and Reviews*, Vol. 18, No. 6, 2002, pp. 464-472. doi:10.1002/dmrr.325

[78] H. Ekberg, H. Tedesco-Silva, A. Demirbas, S. Vitko, B. Nashan, A. Gurkan, *et al.*, "Reduced Exposure to Calcineurin Inhibitors in Renal Transplantation," *New England Journal of Medicine*, Vol. 357, 2007, pp. 2562-2575. doi:10.1056/NEJMoa067411

[79] H. Ekberg, J. Grinyo, B. Nashan, Y. Vanrenterghem, F. Vincenti, A. Voulgari, *et al.*, "Cyclosporine Sparing with Mycophenolate Mofetil, Daclizumab and Corticosteroids in Renal Allograft Recipients: The CAESAR Study," *American Journal of Transplantation*, Vol. 7, No. 3, 2007, pp. 560-570. doi:10.1111/j.1600-6143.2006.01645.x

[80] T. R. Srinivas and H. U. Meier-Kriesche, "Minimizing Immunosuppression, an Alternative Approach to Reducing Side Effects: Objectives and Interim Result," *Clinical Journal of the American Society Nephrology*, Vol. 3, Suppl. 2, 2008, pp. S101-S116. doi:10.2215/CJN.03510807

[81] S. M. Flechner, J. Kobashigawa and G. Klintmalm, "Calcineurin Inhibitor-Sparing Regimens in Solid Organ Transplantation: Focus on Improving Renal Function and Nephrotoxicity," *Clinical Transplantation*, Vol. 22, No. 1, 2008, pp. 1-15.

[82] D. Colombo, N. Cassano, G. Altomare, A. Giannetti and G. A. Vena, "Psoriasis Relapse Evaluation with Week-End Cyclosporine A Treatment: Results of a Randomized, Double-Blind, Multicenter Study," *International Journal of Immunopathology and Pharmacology*, Vol. 23, No. 4, 2010, pp. 1143-1152.

[83] P. Ruggenenti, N. Perico, L. Mosconi, F. Gaspari, A. Benigni, C. S. Amuchastegui, *et al.*, "Calcium Channel Blockers Protect Transplant Patients from Cyclosporine-Induced Daily Renal Hypoperfusion," *Kidney International*, Vol. 43, 1993, pp. 706-711. doi:10.1038/ki.1993.101

[84] K. H. Rahn, M. Barenbrock, F. Fritschka, A. Heinecke, J. Lippert, K. Schroeder, *et al.*, "Effect of Nitrendipine on Renal Function in Renal-Transplant Patients Treated with Cyclosporin: A Randomised Trial," *The Lancet*, Vol. 354, No. 9188, 1999, pp. 1415-1420. doi:10.1016/S0140-6736(99)08421-4

[85] B. J. Nankivell, J. R. Chapman, G. Bonovas and S. Gruenewals, "Oral Cyclosporine But Not Tacrolimus Reduces Renal Transplant Blood Flow," *Transplantation*, Vol. 77, No. 9, 2004, pp. 1457-1459. doi:10.1097/01.TP.0000121196.71904.E0

[86] J. M. Morales, E. Rodriguez-Paternina, A. Araque, A. Andres, E. Hernandez, L. M. Ruilope and J. L. Rodicio, "Long-Term Protective Effect of a Calcium Antagonist on Renal Function in Hypertensive Renal Transplant Patients on Cyclosporine Therapy: A 5-Year Prospective Randomized Study," *Transplant Proceedings*, Vol. 26, No. 5, 1994, pp. 2598-2599.

[87] D. R. Kuypers, H. H. Neumayer, L. Fritsche, K. Budde, J. Rodicio, Y. Vanrenterghem (Lacidipine Study Group), "Calcium Channel Blockade and Preservation of Renal Graft Function in Cyclosporine-Treated Recipients: A Prospective Randomized Placebo-Controlled 2-Year Study," *Transplantation*, Vol. 78, No. 8, 2004, pp. 1204-1211. doi:10.1097/01.TP.0000137793.23371.42

[88] L. Legault, R. I. Ogilvie, C. J. Cardella and F. H. Leenen, "Calcium Antagonists in Heart Transplant Recipients: Effects on Cardiac and Renal Function and Cyclosporine Pharmacokinetics," *The Canadian Journal of Cardiology*, Vol. 9, No. 5, 1993, pp. 398-404.

[89] F. H. Leenen, E. Coletta and R. A. Davies, "Prevention of Renal Dysfunction and Hypertension by Amlodipine after Heart Transplant," *American Journal of Cardiology*, Vol. 100, No. 3, 2007, pp. 531-535. doi:10.1016/j.amjcard.2007.03.058

[90] B. Lindelow, C. H. Bergh, H. Herlitz and F. Waagstein, "Predictors and Evolution of Renal Function during 9 Years Following Heart Transplantation," *Journal of the American Society of Nephrology*, Vol. 11, No. 5, 2000, pp. 951-957.

[91] T. P. Hannedouche, S. Natov, C. Boitard, B. Lacour and J. P. Grunfeld, "Angiotensin Converting Enzyme Inhibition and Chronic Cyclosporine-Induced Renal Dysfunction in Type 1 Diabetes," *Nephrology Dialysis Transplantation*, Vol. 11, No. 4, 1996, pp. 673-678. doi:10.1093/oxfordjournals.ndt.a027358

[92] M. Hausberg, M. Kosch, H. Hohage, B. Suwelack, M. Barenbrock, K. Kisters and K. H. Rahn, "Antihypertensive Treatment in Renal Transplant Patients—Is There a Role for ACE Inhibitors?" *Annals of Transplantation*, Vol. 6, No. 4, 2001, pp. 31-37.

[93] J. M. Campistol, P. Inigo, W. Jimenez, S. Lario, P. H. Clesca, F. Oppenheimer and F. Rivera, "Losartan Decreases Plasma Levels of TGF-Beta1 in Transplant Patients with Chronic Allograft Nephropathy," *Kidney International*, Vol. 56, 1999, pp. 714-719. doi:10.1046/j.1523-1755.1999.00597.x

[94] P. Inigo, J. M. Campistol, S. Lario, C. Piera, B. Campos, M. Bescos, *et al.*, "Effects of Losartan and Amlodipine on Intrarenal Hemodynamics and TGF-Beta(1) Plasma Levels in a Crossover Trial in Renal Transplant Recipients," *Journal of the American Society of Nephrology*, Vol. 12, No. 4, 2001, pp. 822-827.

[95] G. Mourad, J. Ribstein and A. Mimran, "Converting-

Enzyme Inhibitor Versus Calcium Antagonist in Cyclosporine-Treated Renal Transplants," *Kidney International*, Vol. 43, 1993, pp. 419-425. doi:10.1038/ki.1993.61

[96] K. Midtvedt, A. Hartmann, A. Foss, P. Fauchald, K. P. Nordal, K. Rootwelt and H. Holdaas, "Sustained Improvement of Renal Graft Function for Two Years in Hypertensive Renal Transplant Recipients Treated with Nifedipine as Compared to Lisinopril," *Transplantation*, Vol. 72, No. 11, 2001, pp. 1787-1792. doi:10.1097/00007890-200112150-00013

[97] M. Moran, M. F. Mozes, M. Maddux, S. Veremis, C. Bartkus, B. Ketel, *et al.*, "Prevention of Acute Graft Rejection by the Prostaglandin E1 Analogue Misoprostol in Renal-Transplant Recipients Treated with Cyclosporine and Prednisone," *New England Journal of Medicine*, Vol. 322, 1990, pp. 1183-1188. doi:10.1056/NEJM199004263221703

[98] M. Boers, W. G. Bensen, D. Ludwin, C. H. Goldsmith and P. Tugwell, "Cyclosporine Nephrotoxicity in Rheumatoid Arthritis: No Effect of Short Term Misoprostol Treatment," *The Journal of Rheumatology*, Vol. 19, No. 4, 1992, pp. 534-537.

[99] X. Z. Zhang, G. Ardissino, L. Ghio, A. S. Tirelli, V. Dacco, D, Colombo, *et al.*, "L-Arginine Supplementation in Young Renal Allograft Recipients with Chronic Transplant Dysfunction," *Clinical Nephrology*, Vol. 55, No. 6, 2001, pp. 453-439.

[100] H. Ling, X. Li, S. Jha, W. Wan, L. Karetskaya, B. Pratt and S. Ledbetter, "Therapeutic Role of TGF-Beta-Neutralizing Antibody in Mouse Cyclosporin A Nephropathy: Morphologic Improvement Associated with Functional Preservation," *Journal of the American Society of Nephrology*, Vol. 14, No. 2, 2003, 377-388. doi:10.1097/01.ASN.0000042168.43665.9B

[101] M. Islam, J. F. Burke Jr., T. A. McGowan, Y. Zhu, S. R. Dunn, P. McCue, *et al.*, "Effect of Anti-Transforming Growth Factor-Beta Antibodies in Cyclosporine-Induced Renal Dysfunction," *Kidney International*, Vol. 59, 2001, pp. 498-506. doi:10.1046/j.1523-1755.2001.059002498.x

[102] M. Tariq, C. Morais, S. Sobki, M. Al Sulaiman and A. Al Khader, "N-Acetylcysteine Attenuates Cyclosporin-Induced Nephrotoxicity in Rats," *Nephrology Dialysis Transplantation*, Vol. 14, No. 4, 1999, pp. 923-929. doi:10.1093/ndt/14.4.923

[103] P. Barany, P. Stenvinkel, A. Ottosson-Seeberger, A. Alvestrand, J. Morrow, J. J. Roberts and A. K. Salahudeen, "Effect of 6 Weeks of Vitamin E Administration on Renal Haemodynamic Alterations Following a Single Dose of Neoral in Healthy Volunteers," *Nephrology Dialysis Transplantation*, Vol. 16, No. 3, 2001, pp. 580-584. doi:10.1093/ndt/16.3.580

[104] J. K. Jenkins, H. Huang, K. Ndebele and A. K. Salahudeen, "Vitamin E Inhibits Renal mRNA Expression of COX II, HO I, TGF-Beta, and Osteopontin in the Rat Model of Cyclosporine Nephrotoxicity," *Transplantation*, Vol. 71, No. 2, 2001, pp. 331-334. doi:10.1097/00007890-200101270-00028

[105] C. Lessio, S. F. de Assuncao, M. A. Gloria, A. B. Di Tommaso, M. M. Gori, G. S. Di Marco, *et al.*, "Cyclosporine A and NAC on the Inducible Nitric Oxide Synthase Expression and Nitric Oxide Synthesis in Rat Renal Artery Cultured Cells," *Kidney International*, Vol. 68, 2005, pp. 2508-2516. doi:10.1111/j.1523-1755.2005.00726.x

[106] C. Li, B. K. Sun, S. W. Lim, J. C. Song, S. W. Kang, Y. S. Kim, *et al.*, "Combined Effects of Losartan and Pravastatin on Interstitial Inflammation and Fibrosis in Chronic Cyclosporine-Induced Nephropathy," *Transplantation*, Vol. 79, No. 11, 2005, pp. 1522-1529.

[107] A. K. Pere, L. Lindgren, P. Tuomainen, L. Krogerus, P. Rauhala, J. Laakso, *et al.*, "Dietary Potassium and Magnesium Supplementation in Cyclosporine-Induced Hypertension and Nephrotoxicity," *Kidney International*, Vol. 58, 2000, pp. 2462-2472. doi:10.1046/j.1523-1755.2000.00429.x

[108] T. Asai, T. Nakatani, S. Tamada, N. Kuwabara, S. Yamanaka, K. Tashiro, *et al.*, "Activation of Transcription Factors AP-1 and NF-kappaB in Chronic Cyclosporine A Nephrotoxicity: Role in Beneficial Effects of Magnesium Supplementation," *Transplantation*, Vol. 75, No. 7, 2003, pp. 1040-1044. doi:10.1097/01.TP.0000057242.96219.AF

[109] M. J. Mihatsch, D. Belghiti and S. O. Bohman, "Kidney Biopsies in Control of Cyclosporine A Treated Psoriatic Patients," *British Journal of Dermatology*, Vol. 122, Suppl. 22, 1990, pp. 95-100. doi:10.1111/j.1365-2133.1990.tb02887.x

[110] L. Faerber, M. Braeutigam, G. Weidinger, U. Mrowietz, E. Christophers, H. J. Schulze, *et al.*, "Cyclosporine in Severe Psoriasis: Results of a Meta-Analysis," *American Journal of Clinical Dermatology*, Vol. 2, No. 1, 2001, pp. 41-47. doi:10.2165/00128071-200102010-00007

[111] J. Berth-Jones, C. A. Henderson, C. S. Munro, S. Rogers, R. J. Chalmers, M. J. Boffa, *et al.*, "Treatment of Psoriasis with Intermittent Short-Course Cyclosporine (Neoral®). A Multicentre Study," *British Journal of Dermatology*, Vol. 136, No. 4, 1997, pp. 527-530.

[112] V. C. Y. Ho, C. E. M. Griffiths, J. Berth-Jones, K. A. Papp, F. Vanaclocha, E. Dauden, *et al.*, "Intermittent Short Courses of Cyclosporine Microemulsion for the Long-Term Management of Psoriasis: A 2-Year Cohort Study," *Journal of the American Academy of Dermatology*, Vol. 44, No. 4, 2001, pp. 643-651. doi:10.1067/mjd.2001.112400

[113] D. Pathirana, A. D. Ormerod, P. Saiag, C. Smith, P. I. Spuls, A. Nast, *et al.*, "European S3-Guidelines on the Systemic Treatment of Psoriasis Vulgaris," *Journal of the European Academy of Dermatology and Venereology*, Vol. 23, No. 2, 2009, pp. 1-70. doi:10.1111/j.1468-3083.2009.03389.x

[114] G. Feutren, K. Abeywickrama, D. Friend and B. Von Graffenried, "Renal Function and Blood Pressure in Psoriatic Patients Treated with Cyclosporine A," *British Journal of Dermatology*, Vol. 122, No. 36, 1990, pp. 57-69. doi:10.1111/j.1365-2133.1990.tb02883.x

[115] H. I. Katz, "Potential Drug Interactions with Cyclosporine," *International Journal of Dermatology*, Vol. 36, No. 1, 1997, pp. 18-24. doi:10.1046/j.1365-4362.36.s1.5.x

6

Surface Treated Catheters for Vascular Access—Useful?

Rolf Bambauer[1*], Ralf Schiel[2], Carolin Bambauer[3], Reinhard Latza[4]
[1]Institute for Blood Purification, Homburg, Germany
[2]Inselklinik Heringsdorf GmbH, Seeheilbad Heringsdorf, Germany
[3]Main Hospital Darmstadt, Darmstadt, Germany
[4]Laboratorium of Medicine, St. Ingbert, Germany
Email: *rolf.bambauer@t-online.de

ABSTRACT

Background: Catheter-related infections (CRI), thrombosis, and stenosis are among the most frequent complications associated with catheters which are inserted in vessels as vascular access. These problems are usually related to the handling of the staff, the catheter materials, and the surface properties of the catheter. To mitigate such complications surface treatment process of the outer surface, such as ion beam assisted deposition is investigated in a retrospective study from 1992 to 2007, to prove if the surface treatment of the catheters is a sufficient solution. Methods: This study (1992-2007) evaluated silver coated and non-coated implanted large-bore catheters used for extracorporeal detoxification. In 159 patients, 54 patients received a silver coated catheter (Spi-Argent, Spire Corporation, Bedford, MA, USA) and 105 patients, an untreated catheter served as controls. The catheters were inserted into the internal jugular or subclavian veins. After removal, the catheters were cultured for bacterial colonization using standard microbiologic assays. They were also examined using a scanning electron microscope (SEM). Results: The silver coated catheters showed a tendency towards longer *in situ* time. The microbiologic examinations of the catheter tips were in both catheter types high positive, but not significant. Conclusion: The silver coated catheters showed no significant reduction in infection rate by evaluation of all collected data in this retrospective study. There was no association between both catheters in significantly reducing patient discomfort. Other surface treatments which include the outer and inner surface are necessary. New developed catheter materials such as the microdomain structured inner and outer surface, as an example, are considered more biocompatible because they mimic the structure of natural biological surface.

Keywords: Surface Treated Large Bore Catheters; Hemodialysis; Apheresis; Ion Been Assisted Deposition (IBAD); Microdomain-Structered Surface (PUR-SMA Coated Catheter)

1. Introduction

Since the first introduction of large-bore catheters for acute hemodialysis in 1961 by Shaldon *et al.* [1], many problems with handling, materials, and contamination of these catheters have arisen. Nevertheless, vascular catheters have become essential tools for management of hospitalized or chronically ill patients requiring intensive medical treatments [2]. The increased insertion of such devices has been accompanied by a corresponding increase in complications, such as bloodstream infection and thrombosis [3]. Infections are particular concern, because they can appear at any time, even years after implantation, and are not material dependent. They are usually attributed to microbial colonization of the skin or handling of the catheters by attending staff. Complication rates due to venous catheter-relates infection are reported to range from 34 to 40 percent [4,5]. Despite recent technical innovations in hemodialysis, problems related to temporary or permanent vascular access have found no satisfactory solutions. Temporary vascular access is particularly problematic.

Catheterization of the femoral vessels produces more complications than the catheterization of the superior vena cava (SVC). Cannulation of the SVC versus the subclavian vein is difficult to implement and involves a high complication rate [6]. Using the infraclavicular catheterization technique is often difficult to push the large-bore catheter under the clavicle. Because of the anatomical position of the subclavian vein, perforation is more likely with a rigid, large-bore catheter, apart from the danger of causing a pneumothorax or a hematorax [7-10].

*Corresponding author.

Therefore, Bambauer *et al.* have introduced the insertion of large-bore catheters in the superior vena cava rather than in the internal jugular or the subclavian veins [11,12]. Dialysis catheters are used for vascular access in 65% of incident hemodialysis (HD) patients, and in 25% of the prevalent HD populations [13]. Today, the first choice of vascular access is the vena cava superior over the internal jugular vein.

Catheter-related bacteremia is a major cause of morbidity among hemodialysis patients. Treatment with systemic antibiotics alone without removal of the catheter fails to definitely eradicate the infection in most patients [14]. Catheter-related bacteremia must be managed by either catheter removal with delayed placement of a new catheter or management of the infected catheter with a new catheter over a guide-wire and additional systemic antibiotic therapy. These catheter-related complications are contributing factors to increasing cost of medical care. They are responsible for patient readmissions and longer hospital stays as well as patient discomfort, morbidity, and occasional mortality.

The source of catheter-related bacteremia is in most patients a bacterial biofilm that forms in the catheter lumen or on the outer surface. This biofilm, most consisting of *staphylococcus aureus*, cannot be destroyed or eliminated by a systemic antibiotic therapy because of antimicrobial resistance [15]. Bacteriae could most of the time colonize rough surfaces [16]. The combination of rough surfaces and protein deposits should be an ideal situation for the colonization of bacteria. The bacteria could produce and become covered with a slime layer, in which case antibiotic drugs have no influence on the bacteria. The bacteria under the slime layer use the organic substances of the catheter material for their metabolism. The toxins of the bacteria can penetrate the slime layer and enter the patient blood provoking a catheter infection [16]. Biofilm is a microbial derived sessile community characterized by cells that are irreversibly attached to a substratum or interface to each other, embedded in a matrix of extracellular polymeric substances that have produced [17]. Such a biofilm can be the origin of fibrin sheath formations leading to catheter dysfunction due to blood reducing and to blood disturbances. The therapy must be to remove the catheter immediately, or exchange it over a guide-wire with a new catheter and additional systemic antibiotic therapy.

Biocompatibility of synthetic materials is another major problem. The interaction of blood with a synthetic surface causes coagulation and activation of the complement system. This can lead to the adsorption of various proteins and the formation of a layer of protein on the synthetic surface. Thrombocytes, other cells and bacteria adhere to this layer of protein so that thrombi may form which can lead to blood flow disturbances and catheter dysfunction [18].

To influence catheter-related bacteremia different new developments are available today, such as new catheter materials, coating of the catheter surface with antibiotic-heparin, or silver and silicone, cuffs on the outer surface, catheter for tunnelling, installation of an antibiotic-anticoagulant lock into the catheter lumen after the HD, etc. [14,19,20]. The first results with available catheters which coated on the outer surface with silver or silicone were encouraged [18,21].

In a retrospective study from 1992 to 2007, outer surface treated catheters with silver versus untreated catheter in 159 patients, who needed a large-bore catheter, were investigated. The results of a preliminary study from 2001, which showed 75% decline in the infection rate with the surface treated catheters cannot be confirmed with the present study. One reason may be that on the surface treated catheters only the outer surface was coated with silver and the possibility of contamination by the handling during the extracorporeal treatments.

Therefore, new materials and surface treatment technologies are needed to save health care costs for hemodialysis catheters, to reduce infection rates and thrombus formations and to help improve the patients' outcome. The handling of the catheter by the attending staff must be improved and done after the guidelines of different medical communities [22]. In this study, the authors try to give an overview of the surface treated catheters and show a new technique of microdomain-structured surface catheters (PUR-SMA coated catheters, (Gambro, Germany) as an example if these technologies are useful in reducing catheter-related infections and thrombogenicities.

2. Catheter and Material

All available single-, double-, or triple-lumen catheters have some deficiencies depending on the material. Not all catheters are radiopaque. No problem is experienced with the polyurethane catheters after the incorporation of contrast media; however, the latter material may affect catheter durability when using Teflon. This problem was overcome by making a thicker catheter wall, but this caused endothelial irritation and early thrombus formation [23]. Catheters providing radio contrast are not absolutely necessary however, because their position can be controlled more simply and gently with an intra-atrial electrocardiogram (ia-ECG) lead [24]. The three most important criteria of any catheter material are a good tolerance, a low thrombogenicity, and a low infection rate.

Rarely do the material properties perfectly match every requirement in a given application and biomaterials are no exception. Therefore, it often becomes necessary to strike a compromise so that a material has acceptable properties. For example, in a product such a hemodialysis catheter, which demands both good flexibility and low surface friction, the best candidate may be a slippery, less flexible material rather than a more supple one with unacceptable high friction [25].

The importance of surface-engineered biomaterials has been recognized by major medical device companies, because surface modification processes can reduces the rate of infection, thrombogenicity, and other catheter-related complications without adversely affecting the basic design function of catheters.

Although the field of surface-engineered biomaterials is still essentially in its infancy, the range of services currently offered by surface treated vendors is varied and continually expanding. Surface modification processes can reduces the rate of infection, thrombogenicity, and other catheter-related complications without adversely affecting the basic design function of catheters. Examples include conventional coating process such as depending and spraying: vacuum-deposition techniques (e.g., sputtering), and surface modification approaches such as diffusion (e.g., nitriding, carburizing), laser and plasma processes, chemical plating, grafting or bonding, and bombardment with energetic particles (as in plasma immersion or ion implantation). Of the available techniques, those based on ionised particle bombardment have been particularly successful in biomaterial surface modification, primarily because they combine versartility and low-temperatures processing with superior control, reliability, and reproducibility [25,26].

The ion beam-based technology used for the treatment of catheters covered herein is ion beam-assisted deposition (IBAD: Spi-Argent®, Spire corporation, Bedford, MA, USA) [21,25,27]. The process is typically performed at low temperature under high vacuum. The affected layer in the typical films deposited by the IBAD process, is in the order of 1 μm or less vacuum- compatible catheter materials may, therefore, be treated without adversely affecting bulk mechanical properties. The IBAD is line-of-directly: however, parts with complicated geometries may be manipulated for uniform coverage of all surfaces [26].

Silver has been indicated as a good prospect for an infection-resistant coating material for catheters. The problem previously preventing the use of silver on catheters has been the inability to deposit adherent films of silver on flexible polymeric substances. The IBAD process permits the formation of silver coatings at a relatively low temperature with extremely good adhesion that prevents delamination of the film during extended exposure to bodily fluids. The IBAD silver-deposited film has a low coefficient of friction, is highly uniform, and has a cytotoxicity test and the USP Systemic Injection Test. Excellent results were obtained in both tests [25,26, 28,29].

Another possibility shows the new developed catheter material, the microdomain structured surface (PUR-SMA coated catheter, Gambro Germany) [23]. Microdomain surfaces are considered the most biocompatible because the mimic the structure of natural biological surfaces. Microdomain structures are used to match the multiple requirements for improved catheter surfaces, that is reduced thrombogenicity and improved antimicrobial properties. An SMA-modified polyurethane coating consists of hydrophobic and hydrophilic microdomain in range below 50 nmm. Up to 50 percent of the molecule is presented to the surface and creates microdomain structured surfaces. If the domains are below a critical dimension of approximately 100 nmm, theoretical considerations indicate that interaction with proteins, blood cells, or even bacteria will be unstable and therefore not occur as frequently as on non-microdomain structured surfaces.

3. Patients

In the retrospective study of a single center from 1992 to 2007, all catheter data of all included patients were collected from the patients´s charts. The inclusion criteria were patients >18 years of age who required a large-bore catheter (in-/outpatient), were free of bacteremia and provided informed consent. The exclusion criteria were a pregnant or lactating female, a hypersensitivity of silver and a bacteremia at the time of catheter insertion. An IRB approval was in 1992 not necessary [30]. After the patients had given their consent to this study, the physician chose the catheter which he inserted after a randomization of one surface treated catheter, and than two untreated catheters, and so on.

In the study a total of 159 patients (age 66.5 ± 13.2 years, female n = 94 (59%)) are involved. Large-bore, single-lumen catheters were inserted percutaneously in the internal jugular or subclavian veins. The percutaneously catheterization was necessary in renal failure because of acute kidney injury (AKI) for hemodialysis due to cardio-vascular disease, postoperative AKI etc., and in end-stage renal disease (ESRD) because of clotting fistula, septicaemia, abscess and catheter thrombosis and faults in the catheter material (n = 138 (86.8%)). Further indications of catheterization were access problems in patients with familial hypercholesterolemia (n = 12 (7.5%)) under LDL-apheresis treatment, different indications for plasmapheresis (n = 7 (4.4%)) and in 2 patients with carcinoma (n =2) (1.3%)).

In 54 patients (34%) a catheter with silver coating on the outer surface (Spi-Argent®, Spire, Bedford, MA, USA) was inserted and 105 patients (66%) received untreated catheters after a randomization of one treated and two untreated catheters. Patients with untreated catheters were younger (62.2 ± 16.2 versus 68.8 ± 10.7, p = 0.003) but there were no differences between the groups regarding gender distribution, diagnosis, or extracorporeal detoxification methods. Catheterization must always be done under aseptic conditions (wearing sterile gown each time, sterile gloves, mask etc). The patient should be correctly positioned, according to the vascular access point to be used and should be given adequate local anesthetic.

The catheters were placed by nephrologists after the Seldinger technique and/or under fluoroscopic guidance. Before percutaneous insertion each patient skin was disinfected using a consistent method, and a sterile skin smear was taken for microbiologic examination, and than the catheter was inserted. Before fixing the catheter with a suture, its position (particularly the catheter tip) should be checked with a normal radiological control and/or with an ia ECG [24]. Before and after the extracorporeal detoxification procedures, the staff worked under sterile conditions with disinfection and sterile gloves etc. In long-term catheters, a blood smear was taken every 4 weeks or earlier if an inflammation was seen on the insertion side of the catheter to screen for bacteria. Catheters were removed either when other vascular access routes became available or when serious infections developed, or if the catheter was not longer necessary.

Before catheter removal, a skin smear was taken. The catheters were then removed under sterile conditions, and the tip was examined bacteriologically. The remainder of the catheter was rinsed in physiological saline solution and fixed in a solution of phosphate buffer containing glutaraldehyde and formaldehyde for histological investigation.

4. Statistical Analysis

Statistical analysis was performed using the Statistical Package for Social Sciences (SPSS 13.0). All continuous data are presented as mean ± standard deviation (SD) or if the data showed no normal distribution, as median and range. Dichtomous data were presented as a number (n) or in percent (%). Univariante, unadjusted analysis were performed with the independent samples t-test, chi-square test, Fisher´s exact test for frequencies at or below 5 and the Wilcoxon´s rank sum test. Pearson's correlation coefficient was calculated and multivaria's analysis was used to evaluate the presence of associated variables. Significance was defined at the 0.05 level.

5. Results

The median in situ period untreated and silver coated catheters were 138.9 (range, 1 - 1,845) and 115.0 (range, 4 - 1,348) days respectively ($p = 0.653$). Calculating the in situ times after classification for different age groups, it will be overt, that in patients older than 45 years in situ times were significantly longer ($p < 0.01$). Comparing the in situ times of untreated catheters after classification for *in situ* times, there was a tendency towards longer in situ times for the silver coated catheters. In the median catheters were used for 44 (range, 1 - 670) treatment sessions. Untreated catheters were used for 51 (range, 1 - 625) treatments, silver coated catheters for 39 (range, 1 - 670, $p = 0.849$) treatment sessions [30].

Performing microbiologic examinations of the catheter tips some differences were overt. Of the untreated catheter tips 55 % cultured positive for bacteria. Of the cultures in patients with surface treated catheters 52 % were positive, not significantly lower. Although untreated catheters showed a lower infection rate with *Staphylococcus aureus*, in treated catheters the infection rate with *Staphylococcus epidermidis*, *pseudomonas*, and others such as saphrophytes was not significantly lower (**Table 1**). A catheter thrombosis rate was not proved in the removed catheters.

Performing multivariante analysis there was a strong association between catheters' in situ period ($R\text{-square} = 0.96$), the number of treatment sessions ($\beta = 0.97$, $p < 0.001$) and patients' age ($\beta = 0.095$, $p = 0.002$). There was no association between the in situ time and silver coated/untreated catheters, results of the bacteriological examination, and patients diagnosis outcome. Catheter malfunction or fibrin sheath formation as an outcome of both groups was not investigated.

The decrease of the infection rate in surface treated catheter in the preliminary study from 2001 cannot be seen in this presented study from 1992 to 2007. An explanation could be that all and more available data are now evaluated. The untreated catheters showed a higher positive culture for bacteria of 55% versus 52% to the surface treated catheters, but without significance. The procedure for both studies was the same.

The PUR-SMA coating prevents contact of blood components with barium sulphate, possibly leading to leaching as particles or dissolved in the surrounding media. The advantage of the PUR-SMA surface treatment is the coating of the inner and the outer surface in contrast to the ion beam-based surface treatment technologies in which can be treated only the outer surface of the catheters. The preliminary results with these PUR-SMA coated catheters showed a good biocompatibility without any blood deposits and a low thrombogenicity and coagulation activity. The microbiological results were low and of those from the Spi-Argent® catheters [30].

6. Discussion

Catheter-related infections are the most dangerous complications of large-bore catheter aside from accidential puncture of an artery. In addition to colonization, biocompatibility of a catheter material is an important con-

Table 1. Microbiological examinations of 105 untreated and 54 surface treated catheters.

Microorganism	Untreated (n)	%	Treated (n)	%	p-value
Negative	47	45	26	48	n.s
S. aureus	31	29	21	38	n.s
S.epidermidis	7	7	1	2	n.s.
Pseudomonas	1	1	0	0	n.s.
Enterobacter	1	1	1	2	n.s.
Others	18	17	5	10	n.s.

tributing factor to a successful clinical outcome, particularly in catheters that remain in situ for several weeks or months. Although improved since the use of centrally placed catheters, the incidence of catheter clotting was previously very high.

Infection rates range from 5% to 30 % and the most bacteria found is the *Staphylococcus aureus*. These rates do not depend on the route of vascular access [31]. Catheter-related *Staphylococcus aureus* bacteremiae are one of the main causes of morbidity and preventable cause of death in hemodialysis. Patients on dialysis are at a high risk of *Staphylococcus aureus* bacteremia and they have a four times higher mortality from central venous catheter-related *Staphylococcus aureus* bacteremia than other patients [15,32,33].

Recent data have suggested that methicillin-resistant *S. aureus* (MSRA) and vancomycin intermediate *S. aureus* (VISA) organisms may have increased [34]. One of the proposed mechanisms of vancomycin resistance is the bacterial cell wall thickening following vancomycin exposure [35]. Vancomycin´s activity may be decreased due to the thickness of the bacterial cell, the results are MSRA and VISA [36].

To reduce infection rates and thrombogenicity, coated catheters and cuffs were investigated [37-40]. The clinical results of our preliminary investigations showed a significantly reduced infection rate in treated versus untreated catheters, a reduction of more than 75% [18]. With the silver surface treatment, a very smooth metallic surface was obtained which was responsible for a lower thrombogenicity rate. The activation of coagulation factors at the catheter surfaces, and the catheter thrombosis rate was not investigated. Silver ions are bactericidal, therefore, no bacteria growth is possible on the treated catheter surface. The positive association between the in situ time of the catheters and the patients' age may be because of an alteration of the immune system in elderly patients, especially in hemodialysis patients.

But in our retrospective study of all silver coated catheters no significantly reduction in infection rate, improvement, or life expectancy of silver coated versus untreated catheters, which were inserted during 1992 and 2007, was observed. One reason can be that with the IBAD technology only the outer surface is coated with silver. The postulated penetration of silver ions from the outer to the inner surface cannot be shown with these results. The only outer surface treated surface catheters with silver have no advantage in point of view of reducing infection rate and improvement of patients versus the untreated catheters. The handling of the catheters under sterile conditions before, during and after the extracorporeal treatments probably cannot prevent the contamination with bacteria, especially the untreated inner side.

Based on these results, new materials must be developed, which should have better biocompatibility to reduce side effects so that they can be left in situ for a long time, because the part of dialysis patients with vascular problems is increasing in the last decade, and now about 30 % of all hemodialysis patients [41], because the age of HD patients is permanent growing up. As the requirement for more and more artificial organs and/or organ replacement increases, especially in elderly patients, there will be a definite need for new materials with better biocompatibility and for suitable technologies to solve these infection, thrombosis and medical problems to reduce the costs and get better improvement of patients. A disadvantage of drugs such as antibiotics in the catheter surfaces or administration to patient or disinfection substances is that they can develop resistance by mutation or other mechanisms. Therefore the need of new surgical techniques and materials are necessary [42].

More new materials must be developed, which should have better biocompatibility to reduce side effects so that they can be left in situ for a long time, because the part of dialysis patients with vascular problems is increasing in the last decade. As the requirement for more and more artificial organs and/or organ replacement increases, there will a definite need for new materials with better biocompatibility and for suitable technologies to solve these infection, thrombosis and medical problems to reduce the costs and get a better improvement of patients. But it appears impossible to create a surface with an absolute "zero" adherence due to thermal-dynamical reasons and due to the fact that a modified material surface is *in vivo* rapidly covered by plasma and connective tissue proteins.

Therefore other concepts of the prevention of implant-associated infections must involve the impregnation of the devices the inner and outer surface with antibiotics, antimicrobial substances and/or metals [43,44]. Another point is to understand the processes leading to the development of catheter-related bacteremia in order to can offer effective preventive and therapeutic possibilities [45] such as new polymer-antibiotic systems in inhibiting bacterial biofilm formation and in reducing neutrophil activation after surface contact on different biomaterials, thus reducing the risk for biomaterial-mediated inflammatory reactions [46-48], or the development of new biofilm to serve in a communication system termed quorum sensing [49], or molecules that inhibit quorum sensing signal generation among organism could block microbial biofilm formation [50].

These catheters related complications are contributing factors to the increasing cost of medical care. They are responsible for patient readmissions and longer hospital stays as well as patients discomfort, morbidity, and occasional mortality. Feldman *et al.* calculated in 1996 the costs of the morbidity due to catheter infections will soon exceed $ 1 billion per year [51]. Therefore he demanded to reduce vascular access-related morbidity, that strategies must be developed not only to prevent and detect appropriately early synthetic vascular access dysfunction, but to better identify the patients in a whom radial arterio-venous fistula is a viable clinical option. The representative health care cost savings for hemodialysis catheters, given specific infection rates and potential infection rate reductions achieved by treated catheters [23].

The cost analysis was calculated using the literature and the available costs of different companies which distribute these catheters [52]. Potential health care cost reductions that could be achieved through the use of surface treated-catheters by an annual usage of 125,971 hemodialysis catheter devices and an infection rate of 5% - 20%, savings per year of $ 17.7 million, reduction about 40% [52]. Besides a high number of patients who die to CRI, the costs of these infections are increasingly steady. After Schwebel *et al.* the costs are $ 2118/intensive care unit day, and after Pronovost *et al.* $ 45,000 per each infection [53,54]. Tacconelli *et al.* estimated in 2009 the costs associated with CRI in four European countries (France, Germany, Italy, and UK) between € 35.9 and € 163.9 million per year [55].

Due to these tremendous high costs it must be possible of scientists, physicians, bioengineers and others to develop new techniques and new materials to reduce these high costs and to increase the improvement of patients.

But besides the high costs due catheter-related infections, the patients′ longer hospital stays, and patients discomfort, mortality, and occasionally mortality are the most important problems which must be resolved. To reduce these complications it is necessary that the handling of the catheters must be done first after the numerous recommendation and guidelines available in the literature [22,56,57].

Surface treatment of catheter is necessary, but of the inner and the outer surface. Therefore new technology must be developed for the surface treatment with antibitotics, antimicrobial substances and/or metal. New material and new-polymer-antibiotic systems are demanded. The developed of new biofilm to serve in a communication system termed quorum sensing [49], or molecules which inhibit quorum sensing signal generation among organism could block microbial biofilm formation [50]. This reqirement shows perhaps the new developed catheter material, the microdomain-structured surface [PUR-SMA-coated catheters, Gambro, Germany) [18]. Microdomain surfaces are considered the most biocompatible because they mimic the structure of natural biological surfaces. Microdomain structures are used to match the multiple requirements for improved catheter surfaces, that is reduced thromgenecity and improved antimicrobial properties. First results with these catheters are very encouraged.

Most important is the improvement of the handling of the catheters by the attending staff which is recommended in numerous available guidelines to reduce the tremendous high costs to treat the CRI and the discomfort and morbidity of the patients.

7. Conclusion

The results showed that catheters which were surface treated only on the outside had no advantages versus untreated catheters. In a retrospective study from 1992 to 2007, outer surface treated catheters with silver versus untreated catheters in 159 patients, who needed a large bore catheter, were investigated. There was no association between the *in situ* time and silver coated/uncoated catheters, resulting in the bacteriological examination, and patients' diagnosis or outcome. Reasons may be that on the surface treated catheters only the outer surface was coated with silver and the possibility of contamination by the handling during the extracorporeal treatments. Therefore, new materials and surface treatment on both surfaces, the inner and outer surface, are needed to save the tremendous high health costs for hemodialysis catheters, to reduce infection rates, and thrombus formations and to improve the patients' outcome.

REFERENCES

[1] L. Beloqui, S, Shaldon, L, Chiandussi and B. Higgs, "Haemodialysis by Percutaneous Catheterization of the Femoral Artery and Vein with Reginal Heparinisation," *Lancet*, Vol. 11, 1961, p. 857.

[2] D. G. Maki, "Infection Due to Infusion Therapy," In: I. V. Bennett and P. S. Brachman, Eds., *Hospitals Infections*, Little Brown and Co., Boston, 1992, pp. 849-859.

[3] J. S. Groegor, A. B. Lucas and H. A. T. Thaler, "Infectious Morbidity Associated with Long-Term Use of Venous Access Devices in Patients with Cancer," *Annals of Internal Medicine*, Vol. 119, No. 12, 1993, pp. 1168-1174. doi:10.7326/0003-4819-119-12-199312150-00003

[4] R. Bambauer, P. Mestres and K. J. Pirrung, "Frequency, Therapy, and Prevention of Infections Associated with Large-Bore Catheter," *ASAIO Journal*, Vol. 38, No. 2, 1992, pp. 96-101.

[5] R. Bambauer, R. Inninger and K. J. Pirrung, "Complications and Side Effects Associated with Large-Bore Catheters in the Suclavian and Internal Veins," *Artificial Organs*, Vol. 18, No. 4, 1994, pp. 318-321. doi:10.1111/j.1525-1594.1994.tb02204.x

[6] C. M. Kjellstrand, G. G. Merino, S. M. Mauer, *et al.*, "Complications of Percutaneous Femoral Vein Catheterization for Hemodialysis," *Clinical Nephrology*, Vol. 4, No. 1, 1975, pp. 37-40.

[7] A. Schwarzbeck, W. D. Brittinger, G. E. von Henning, *et al.*, "Cannulation of Subclavian Vein for Hemodialysis Using Seldinger Technique," *Transactions of American Society for Artificial Internal Organs*, Vol. 27, No. 1, 1978, pp. 24-31.

[8] A. De Cubber, C. De Wolf, N. Lameire, *et al.*, "Single Needle Hemodialysis with Double Headpump via the Subclavian Vein," *Dialysis & Transplantation*, Vol. 7, No. 11, 1978, pp. 1261-1263.

[9] P. R. Uldall, P. R. Dyck and F. Woods, "A Subclavian Cannula for Temporary Vascular Access for Hemodialysis or Plasmapheresis," *Dialysis & Transplantation*, Vol. 8, No. 9, 1979, pp. 963-968.

[10] C. T. Flynn and R. McGowan, "Subclavian Vein Catheter and Clockwork Pump," *Dialysis & Transplantation*, Vol. 9, No. 5, 1980, pp. 556-616.

[11] R. Bambauer and G. A. Jutzler, "Jugularis-Interna Punktion zur Shaldon-Katheterisierung. Ein neuer Zugang für Akute Hämodialysen," *Nieren-Hochdruckh*, Vol. 9, No. 3, 1980, pp. 109-116

[12] R. Bambauer and G. A. Jutzler, "Transcutaneous Insertion of the Shaldon Catheter through the Internal Jugular Vein as Access for Acute Hemodialysis," *Dialysis & Transplantation*, Vol. 11, No. 9, 1982, pp. 766-771.

[13] D. Philibert, M. Agharazii, E. Audy, *et al.*, "Clinical Experience with a Chronic Hemodialysis Catheter with Symmetrical Tip Configuration (Palindrone TM)," *JASN*, Vol. 16, 2005.

[14] M. Allon, "Dialysis Catheter-Related Bacteremia Treatment and Prophylaxis," *American Journal of Kidney Diseases*, Vol. 44, No. 5, 2004, pp. 779-791.

[15] J. Nielsen, H. J. J. Kolosk and F. Espersen, "*Staphylococcus aureus* Bacteremia among Patients Undergoing Dialysis: Focus Dialysis Catheter-Related Cases," *Nephrology Dialysis Transplantation*, Vol. 13, No. 1, 1988, pp. 139-145. doi:10.1093/ndt/13.1.139

[16] R. Locci, G. Peters and G. Pulverer, "Microbiological Colonization of Prosthetic Devices. Microtopological Characteristics of Intravenous Catheters as Detected by Scanning Electron Microscopy," *Zentralblatt für Bakteriologie, Mikrobiologie und Hygiene*, Vol. 173, No. 2, 1981, pp. 285-292.

[17] J. W. Costerton, L. Montanaro and C. R. Arciola, "Biofilm in Implant Infections: Its Production and Regulation," *International Journal of Artificial Organs*, Vol. 28, No. 9, 2005, pp. 1065-1068.

[18] R. Bambauer, R. Schiel, S. Bambauer and P. Sioshansi, "Large Bore Catheters with Surface Treatments versus Untreated Catheters for Blood Access," *The Journal of Vasclar Access*, Vol. 2, No. 3, 2001, pp. 97-105.

[19] J. D. Maya, D. Carlton, E. Estrada, *et al.*, "Treatment of Dialysis Catheter-Related *Staphylococcus aureus* Bacteremia with an Antibiotic Lock: A Quality Improvement Report," *American Journal of Kidney Diseases*, Vol. 50, No. 2, 2007, pp. 289-295. doi:10.1053/j.ajkd.2007.04.014

[20] G. K. Dogra, H. Herson, B. Hutchison, *et al.*, "Prevention of Tunnelled Hemodialysis Catheter-Related Infections Using Catheter Restricted Filling with Gentamycin and Citrate: A Randomized Controlled Study," *Journal of the American Society of Nephrology*, Vol. 13, No. 8, 2002, pp. 2133-2139. doi:10.1097/01.ASN.0000022890.29656.22

[21] R. Bambauer, R. Schiel, P. Mestres and P. Sioshansi, "Scanning Electron Microscopic Investigation of Catheters for Blood Access," *International Journal of Artificial Organs*, Vol. 18, No. 5, 1995, pp. 326-331.

[22] R. Hollenbeck, V. Mickley, J. Brunkwall, *et al.*, "Gefäßzugang zur Hämodialyse" *Der Nephrologe*, Vol. 4, No. 2, 2009, pp. 158-176. doi:10.1007/s11560-009-0281-0

[23] R. Bambauer, R. Schiel, S. Bambauer and P. Sioshansi, "Long-Term Catheters for Apheresis and Dialysis with Surface Treatment with Infection Resistance and Low Thrombogenicity," *Therapeutic Apheresis and Dialysis*, Vol. 7, No. 2, 2003, pp. 225-231. doi:10.1046/j.1526-0968.2003.00042.x

[24] R. Bambauer and G. A. Jutzler, "Lagekontrolle Großlumiger Zentraler Venenkatheter Mittels Intrakardialer Elektrographie," *Intensivmed*, Vol. 17, No. 6, 1980, pp. 12-17.

[25] P. Sioshansi and E. J. Tobin, "Surface Treatment of Biomaterials by Ion-Beam Processes," *Medical Plastics and Biomaterials*, Vol. 2, 1995, pp. 50-59.

[26] P. Sioshansi, "New Process for Surface Treatment of Catheters," *Artificial Organs*, Vol. 18, No. 4, 1994, pp. 226-271. doi:10.1111/j.1525-1594.1994.tb02193.x

[27] R. Bambauer, P. Mestres, R. Schiel, *et al.*, "New Surface Treatment Technologies for Catheters Used for Extracorporeal Detoxication Methods," *Dialysis & Transplantation*, Vol. 24, No. 5, 1995, pp. 228-237.

[28] P. Sioshansi, "Ion Implantation of Cobalt Chronicum Prosthetic Components to Reduce Polyethylene Wear," *Orthopedics Today*, Vol. 11, No. 1, 1991, pp. 24-25.

[29] D. Schierholz, A. Rump and W. Pulverer, "Klinische und Präklinische Effizienz Antimikrobieller Katheter," *Anaesthesiol Intensivmed Notfallmed Schmerzther*, Vol. 32, No. 5, 1997, pp. 289-305. doi:10.1055/s-2007-995058

[30] R. Bambauer, R. Schiel, C. Bambauer and R. Latza, "Surface-Treted versus Untreated Large-Bore Catheters as Vascular Access in Hemodialysis and Apheresis," *International Journal of Nephrology*, Vol. 2012, 2012, Article ID: 956136, 8 pages. http://www.Hindawi.com/journals/ijn(2012/956136/

[31] R. Vanholder, N. Hoenich, S. Ringoir, *et al.*, "Morbidity and Mortality of Central Venous Catheter Hemodialysis, a Review of 10 Years' Experience," *Nephron*, Vol. 47, No. 4, 1987, pp. 247-279. doi:10.1159/000184523

[32] G. Jean, B. Charra, C. Chazot, *et al.*, "Risk Factor Analysis for Long-Term Tunnelled Dialysis Catheter-Related Bacteremias," *Nephron*, Vol. 91, No. 2, 2002, pp. 399-405. doi:10.1159/000064279

[33] S. H. Kim, K. I. Song, J. W. Chang, *et al.*, "Prevention of Uncuffed Hemodialysis Catheter-Related Bacteremia Using an Antibiotic Lock Technique: A Prospective, Randomised Clinical Trial," *Kidney International*, Vol. 69, No. 1, 2006, pp. 161-164. doi:10.1038/sj.ki.5000012

[34] E. A. King, D. McCoy, S. Desai, *et al.*, "Vancomycin Resistant Enterococcal Bacteraemia and Daptomycin: Are Higher Doses Necessary?" *Journal of Antimicrobial Chemotherapy*, Vol. 66, No. 9, 2011, pp. 2112-2118. doi:10.1093/jac/dkr255

[35] I. Cui, A. Iwamoto and I. O. Lian, "Novel Mechanism of Antibiotic Resistance Originating in Vancomycin-Intermediate *Staphylococcus aureus*," *Antimicrobial Agents and Chemotherapy*, Vol. 50, No. 2, 2006, pp. 428-438. doi:10.1128/AAC.50.2.428-438.2006

[36] I. Cui, F. Tominage, H. M. Nenh, *et al.*, "Correlation between Reduced Daptomycin Suscetibility and Vancomycin Resistance in Vancomycin-Intermediate *Staphylococcus aureus*," *Antimicrobial Agents and Chemotherapy*, Vol. 50, No. 3, 2006, pp. 1079-1082. doi:10.1128/AAC.50.3.1079-1082.2006

[37] D. G. Maki, J. K. Garman, J. M. Shapiro, *et al.*, "An Attachable Silver-Impregnated Cuff for Prevention of Infection with Central Venous Catheters: A Prospective Randomized Multicenter Trial," *The American Journal of Medicine*, Vol. 85, No. 3, 1988, pp. 307-314. doi:10.1016/0002-9343(88)90579-7

[38] K. S. Tweden, J. D. Cameron, A. J. Razzouk, *et al.*, "Silver Modification of Polyethylene Terphthalate Textile for Antimicrobial," *ASAIO Journal*, Vol. 43, No. 2, 1997, pp. M475-M481. doi:10.1097/00002480-199703000-00088

[39] A. Oloffs, C. Gosse-Siestrup, S. Bisson, *et al.*, "Biocompatibility of Silver Coated Polyurethane Catheters and Silver Coated Dacron Material," *Biomaterials*, Vol. 15, No. 10, 1994, pp. 753-758. doi:10.1016/0142-9612(94)90028-0

[40] R. Bambauer, P. Mestres, R. Schiel, *et al.*, "Surface Treated Large-Bore Catheters with Silver Based Coating Versus Untreated Catheters for Extracorporeal Detoxication Methods," *ASAIO Journal*, Vol. 44, No. 4, 1998, pp. 3003-3008. doi:10.1097/00002480-199807000-00013

[41] K. S. Rabindranath, T. Bansal, J. Adams, *et al.*, "Systematic Review of Antimicrobials for Prevention of Hemodialysis Catheter-Related Infections," *Nephrology Dialysis Transplantation*, Vol. 24, No. 12, 2009, pp. 3763-3774. doi:10.1093/ndt/gfp327

[42] A. A. Hampton and R. J. Sheretz, "Vascular Access Infections in Hospitalised Patients," The *Surgical Clinics of North America*, Vol. 68, No. 1, 1988, pp. 57-71.

[43] C. Von Eif, W. Kohnen, K, Becker, *et al.*, "Modern Strategies in the Prevention of Implant-Associated Infections," *The International Journal of Artificial Organs*, Vol. 28, No. 11, 2005, pp. 1146-1156.

[44] J. F. Timsit, O. Mimoz, B. Mourviller, *et al.*, "Randomized Controlled Trial of Chlorhexidine Dressing and Highly Adhesive Dressing for Preventing Catheter-Related Infections in Critically Ill Adults," *American Journal of Respiratory and Critical Care Medicine*, Vol. 186, No. 12, 2012, pp. 1272-1278. doi:10.1164/rccm.201206-1038OC

[45] L. Troidle and F. O. Finkelstein, "Catheter-Related Bacteremia in Hemodialysis Patients: The Role of the Central Venous Catheter in Prevention and Therapy," *The International Journal of Artificial Organs*, Vol. 31, No. 9, 2008, pp. 827-833.

[46] S. Cicalini, F. Palmieri and N. Petrosillo, "Clinical Review: New Technologies for Prevention of Intravascular Catheter-Related Infections," *Critical Care*, Vol. 8, 2004, pp. 157-162. doi:10.1186/cc2380

[47] G. Donelli, I. Francolini, A. Piozzi, *et al.*, "New Polymer-Antibiotic Systems to Inhibit Bacterial Biofilm Formation: A Suitable Approach to Prevent Central Venous Catheter-Associated Infections," *Journal of Chemotherapy*, Vol. 14, No. 5, 2002, pp. 501-507.

[48] S. Schmitt, G. Haase, E. Csomor, *et al.*, "Inhibitor of Complement, Compstatin, Prevents Polymer-Mediated Mac-1 Up-Regulation of Human Neutrophils Independent of Biomaterial Type Tested," *Journal of Biomedical Materials Research*, Vol. 66A, No. 3, 2003, pp. 491-499. doi:10.1002/jbm.a.10031

[49] M. R. Parsek, D. L. Val, B. L. Hanzelka, *et al.*, "Acyl Homoserine-Lactone Quorum-Sensing Signal Generation," *Proceedings of the National Academy of Sciences of the United States of America*, Vol. 96, No. 8, 1999, pp. 4360-4365. doi:10.1073/pnas.96.8.4360

[50] D. G. Davies, M. R. Parsek, J. P. Pearson, *et al.*, "The Involvement of Cell-to-Cell Signals in the Development of a Bacterial Biofilm," *Science*, Vol. 280, No. 5361, 1998, pp. 295-298. doi:10.1126/science.280.5361.295

[51] H. J. Feldmann, S. Kobrina and A. Wasserstein, "Hemodialysis Vascular Morbidity," *Journal of the American Society of Nephrology*, Vol. 7, No. 4, 1996, 523- 535.

[52] S. Bambauer, "Cost Reduction Benefits of Applying an Antimicrobial Surface Treatment to Catheters," Personnel Communication, 1996.

[53] C. Schwebel, J. C. Lucet, A. Vesin, *et al.*, "Economic Evaluation of Chlorhexidine-Impregnated Sponges for Preventing Catheter-Related Infection in Critically Ill Adults in the Dressing Study," *Critical Care Medicine*, Vol. 40, No. 1, 2012, pp. 11-17. doi:10.1097/CCM.0b013e31822f0604

[54] P. J. Pronovost, C. A. Goeschel, E. Colantuoni, *et al.*, "Sustaining Reductions in Catheter-Related Bloodstream Infections in Michigan Intensive Care Units: Observa-

tional Study," *British Medical Journal*, Vol. 340, 2010, p. c309. doi:10.1136/bmj.c309

[55] E. Toccanelli, G. Smith, A. Hiske, *et al*., "Epidemiology, Medical Outcomes and Costs of Catheter-Related Bloodstream Infections in Intensive Care Units of Four European Countries: Literature- and Registry-Based Estimates," *Journal of Hospital Infection*, Vol. 72, No. 2, 2009, pp. 97-103. doi:10.1016/j.jhin.2008.12.012

[56] N. P. O'Grady, M. Alexander, L. A. Burns, *et al*., "Guidelines for the Preventions of Intravascular Catheter-Related Infections," *Clinical Infectious Diseases*, Vol. 52, No. 9, 2011, pp. e162-e193.

[57] T. Nagai, S. Kohsaka, T. Anzai, *et al*., "Low Incidence of Catheter-Related Complications in Patients with Advanced Pulmonary Arterial Hypertension Undergoing Continuous Epoprostenol Infusions," *Chest*, Vol. 141, No. 1, 2012, pp. 272-273.doi:10.1378/chest.11-1893

7

Does Current Nephrology Fellowship Training Affect Utilization of Peritoneal Dialysis in the United States?*

Nand K. Wadhwa[1], Catherine R. Messina[2], Nasser M. Hebah[3]
[1]Division of Nephrology, Stony Brook School of Medicine, Stony Brook, New York, USA
[2]Department of Preventive Medicine, Stony Brook School of Medicine, Stony Brook, New York, USA
[3]Corporate Home Dialysis, Dialysis Clinic Inc., Nashville, USA.
Email: nand.wadhwa@stonybrookmedicine.edu

ABSTRACT

Background: The 2010 US Renal Data System annual report revealed that peritoneal dialysis is used by only 7% of end-stage renal disease patients on chronic dialysis vs. hemodialysis which is used by 93% of such patients, despite documented benefits of peritoneal dialysis over hemodialysis in these cases. **Purpose:** We examined whether education of nephrology fellows contributed to underutilization of peritoneal dialysis in the US. **Methods:** Self-report questionnaires were administered electronically to nephrology fellowship training program directors, October 2010-March 2011 (55% response). **Results:** Median number of training faculty and patients/fellow were significantly lower for peritoneal-dialysis vs. hemodialysis training. Hours of didactic teaching for fellows over their 2-year training period were significantly lower for peritoneal dialysis vs. hemodialysis. Peritoneal dialysis training was 20% of total training vs. 80% for hemodialysis. Most program directors (87%) believed lack of trained faculty in peritoneal dialysis and insufficient peritoneal dialysis patient population contributed to inadequate fellows' peritoneal dialysis training. **Conclusions:** Findings suggest that current nephrology fellowship training in peritoneal dialysis is inadequate and contributes to its underutilization.

Keywords: Peritoneal Dialysis; Hemodialysis; Utilization; Nephrology Fellowship Training

1. Introduction

Renal replacement therapy for patients with end-stage renal disease (ESRD) includes kidney transplantation and chronic dialysis. Most ESRD patients are treated with in-center hemodialysis (HD) and home peritoneal dialysis (PD) for prolonged periods because of limited availability of organ donors for kidney transplantation. As of December 31, 2010, among chronic dialysis patients, approximately 383,992 (93%) patients were receiving HD while 29,733 (7%) were on PD [1]. The incident HD population reached 103,874 patients in 2010. New PD patients peaked at 9408 in 1995, and have since fallen to 7586 [1]. This decline continues despite the cost effectiveness of PD therapy as compared to in-center HD, improving patient outcomes, advances in PD therapy including a decrease in peritonitis rate, new solutions such as icodextrin and the new generation of automated cycling machines allowing appropriate dialysis clearances [1-5]. PD underutilization has occurred despite the fact that nephrologists in the United States report that about 35% of ESRD patients should be maintained on PD therapy [6]. Not only are PD and HD associated with similar survival in incident dialysis patients starting therapy electively as outpatients [7], but also PD offers survival benefits in almost 67% of incident ESRD patients who are non-diabetics and younger diabetics with no additional comorbidity [8].

PD underutilization is related in part to inadequate training of nephrologists in PD [9]. A recent (2010) survey of self-perceived competency among US nephrologists after completion of nephrology fellowship training revealed that only 56% felt well trained and competent in the care of chronic PD patients vs. 80% who felt well trained and competent in the care of chronic in-center HD patients—although 92% ranked care of chronic PD patients as an area that is "somewhat or very important" [10]. Related to nephrologist concerns about lack of competence or comfort with PD, is inadequate exposure to PD patients during their training. Although US neph-

*Authors and Affiliations: The authors do not have any conflicts of interest or financial relationships to disclose.

rologists spent >35% of their time providing care for ESRD patients [11], Mehrotra *et al.* [12] reported a decnade ago that 29% of fellows in US training programs were exposed to <5 PD patients and 14% of these fellows spent <5% of their training time caring for PD patients.

Lack of exposure to PD during training influences nephrologist's referral patterns (*i.e.*, preferences for treatment modality) throughout their career and may influence patients' treatment choice [13] and therefore affect patient outcomes. While some have suggested that choice of dialysis modality selection is driven by patient preference [14,15]. Wuerth *et al.* reported that 83% of interviewed patients indicated that their physician influenced their ESRD treatment choice [16]. Of note is Stack's finding that patients who were autonomous in the ESRD treatment decision-making process were more likely to receive PD rather than HD compared to patients whose medical team were more actively involved in treatment modality decision making [17].

In 2002, Mehrotra *et al.* [12] described the status of dialysis training in the US in terms of the availability of resources and allocation of time for training fellows. We undertook this study to update Mehrotra *et al.*'s 2002 [12] observations and examine the current status of nephrology fellowship training in hemodialysis and peritoneal dialysis in the US.

2. Materials and Methods

The project protocol was approved by the Stony Brook University institutional review board. Self-report questionnaires were administered electronically via Survey Monkey, during October 2010-March 2011, to US Nephrology fellowship program directors. The names and email addresses of all US adult Nephrology fellowship program directors were obtained from the American Society of Nephrology listserv (directors of pediatric nephrology programs were excluded). Questionnaire responses were obtained anonymously. Questionnaires were re-administered to Program Directors approximately 4 weeks after the initial administration to encourage replies from those who had not already done so. This was repeated two more times. No incentives were offered.

The questionnaire was developed by the first author and reviewed by the second and third authors. Questionnaire items obtained information on training program characteristics (e.g., number of clinical nephrology faculty; number of nephrology fellows) and training activities relating to HD and PD (e.g., number of adult patients on HD and PD; percent of fellows time managing HD and PD; didactic lectures in HD and PD; type of training (block rotation or continuity care) and estimate of time spent on HD and PD; etc). Program directors described their perceptions of the adequacy of PD training at their institution and in the US, and noted barriers to the utilization of PD in the US The questionnaire took approximately 15 minutes to complete, and was pretested on a small group of physicians prior to distribution.

Study data were downloaded from Survey Monkey directly into an SPSS-formatted file and the statistical program SPSS (IBM SPSS, version 19) was used for all data analyses. Descriptive statistics (frequencies, proportions, medians, and ranges) are provided for all study data. The Wilcoxon signed rank test was used for comparisons of median values.

3. Results

3.1. Response Rate and Distribution of Respondent Training Programs

Questionnaires were administered to directors of 143 nephrology fellowship programs. Directors of 78 programs completed the questionnaires to yield an overall response rate of 54.5%. Our response rate is comparable to the response rate of 47.3% attained by a prior survey of members of the National Kidney Foundation regarding opinions and attitudes about dialysis modality selection conducted in 1997 [6]. Response rates varied by US Census Region [18]: 45% (n = 35) of responding US Program directors were located in the northeast; 13% (n = 10) were located in the west; 26% (n = 20) were located in the south; and 17% (n = 13) were in the mid-west [NOTE: denominator = 78 responding program directors]. When examined by the regional location of nephrology programs listed on the American Society of Nephrology listserv (*i.e.*, denominator represents total programs in the specific region): 69% (n = 35) of programs located in the northeast, 55% (n = 10) of those located in the west; 48% (n = 20) of those located in the south; and 42% (n = 13) of those located in the mid-west, were represented.

3.2. Training Resources and Program Characteristics

Self-reported HD and PD training resources are presented in **Table 1**. The median faculty/fellow ratio was significantly lower for PD compared to HD as was the median patients / fellow ratio (all p's < 0.001).

94% (n = 67/71) and 93% (n = 66/71) of program directors indicated that their fellows receive didactic teaching lectures during their tenure in HD and/or PD, respectively. However, the median number of teaching lecture hours reported was significantly lower for PD (6 hours (2 - 30 hours)) compared to HD (10 hours (range = 2 - 30 hours)), p < 0.001 [data not shown].

98.7% of the responding program directors (n = 77/78)

Table 1. Program director (n = 78 respondents) reports of hemodialysis and peritoneal dialysis training resources for nephrology fellows.

Training resource	Total	Hemodialysis (median, range)	Peritoneal dialysis (median, range)
Number of full and/or part time faculty	11 (1 - 28)	6 (0 - 24)	1 (0 - 14)
Faculty/fellow ratio	1.8 (0.1 - 5.0)	1.2* (0.3 - 4.0)	0.5* (0.1 - 2.5)
Number of adult patients on HD and PD		200 (40 - 700)	30 (1 - 20)
Patients/fellow ratio		37.5* (5.5 - 200)	5.0* (0.2 - 17.1)

*p < 0.001 for Hemodialysis vs. Peritoneal dialysis comparison; Wilcoxon Signed Ranks Test.

provide chronic dialysis training for their fellows. With regard to training characteristics of their outpatient chronic dialysis programs, 38% (n = 29/77) of responding program directors indicated that they only provide continuity care; 29% (n = 22/77) responded that they only provide block of time rotation; and 34% (n = 26/77) indicated that they provide both continuity care and block of time rotation [data not shown]. As shown in **Table 2**, among programs providing continuity care or block rotation and continuity care, the smaller proportion assigning dialysis patients to fellows were for PD rather than HD. Similarly, the smaller proportion of total dialysis training time among programs offering block rotation, continuity care, or both was devoted to PD rather than HD.

3.3. Perceived Adequacy of PD Training in the US

87% (n = 60/75) of responding program directors believe that PD training in the US is inadequate. When asked to describe the reason for this belief, the primary reasons noted by these program directors included: insufficient numbers of PD patients/lack of exposure to PD patients (71%); and lack of available training in PD/faculty not comfortable with PD (20%) [data not shown].

3.4. Estimations of Adequate PD Training

Figures 1(a) and **(b)** present program directors estimations of what is needed for adequate PD training. Overall, 76% (n = 52/68) of program directors felt that >5% of total training time is adequate for PD training. Of these, the most frequent percent total training time noted was 5% - 10% (35%; 24/68) followed by 10% - 20% (25%; 17/68). In general, 81% (n = 56/69) of program directors felt that assigning >5 chronic PD patients/fellow is adequate for PD training over the fellows' two year training period. The most frequently cited number of chronic PD patients/fellow was 5 - 10 (52%; 36/69). Among those program directors who felt that assigning >5 chronic PD patients/fellow is adequate for PD training over the fellows' two year training period, approximately 50% (n = 29/56) indicated having 30 or more patients on PD within their programs, with patient/fellow ratios ranging from 6.00 to 17.00 (data not shown).

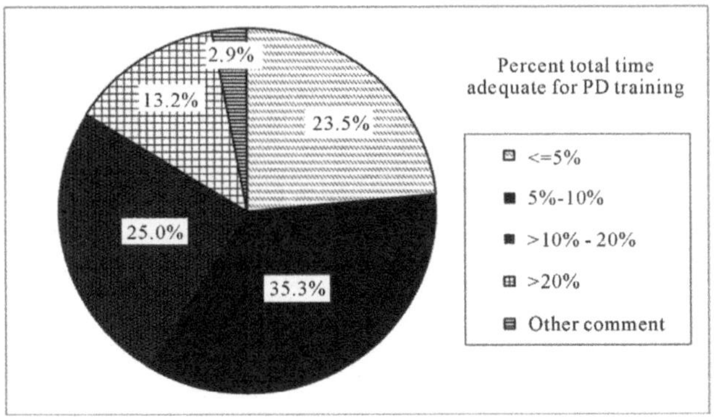

(a)

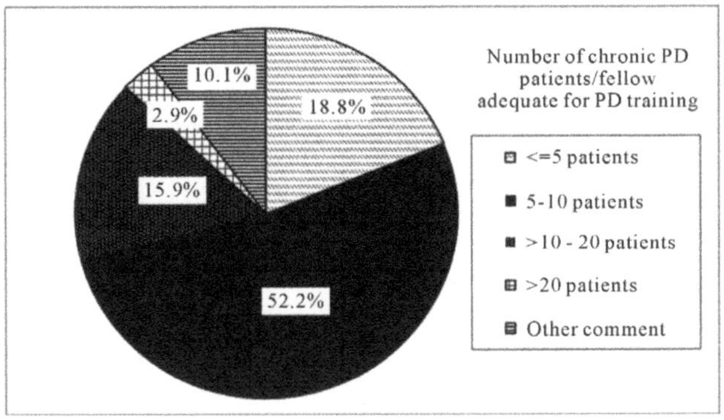

(b)

Figure 1. Percent total training time and number of patients/fellow program directors believe is adequate for PD training. (a) Percent total training time program directors believe is adequate for PD training. Note: %'s represent the proportion of responding program directors indicating a specific amount for training time. Other comments = "hard to quantify what proportion of time translates into competency", etc.; (b) Number of patients/fellow program directors believe is adequate for PD training. Note: %'s represent the proportion of responding program directors indicating a specific number of patients. Other comments = "not a set number"; "exposure to complications more important", etc.

3.5. Factors Which Limit Utilization of PD in the US

As seen in **Table 3**, program directors most often cited limited physician training in PD (88%) as a physician/nurse related factor which limits utilization of PD in the US Greater than 50% of respondents also cited poor

Table 2. Program directors' estimates of training in hemodiaysis and peritoneal dialysis (n = 77 respondents).

	Block rotation	Continuity care	Block rotation and continuity care		
	% (n) of programs where fellows are assigned dialysis patients	% of training during 2 years tenure (median (range))	% (n) of programs where fellows are assigned dialysis patients	% (n) of programs where fellows are assigned dialysis patients	% of training during 2 years tenure (median (range))
Hemodialysis	0	80 (34 - 95)	27.6 (8)	26.9 (7)	80 (0 - 100)
Peritoneal dialysis	5 (1)	20 (5 - 66)	10.3 (3)	7.7 (2)	20 (0 - 100)
Both	95 (21)	----	62.1 (18)	65.4 (17)	----

Table 3. Program director beliefs regarding factors which limit utilization of peritoneal dialysis therapy in the US (n = 69 respondents).

Factors which can potentially limit utilization of PD	Program directors of dialysis training: % respondents* (n)
Physician/nurse related factors:	
Limited physician training in PD	88.4 (61)
Poor personal experience with PD	59.4 (41)
Problems with hospital support for PD	53.6 (37)
Lack of nursing expertise to support PD program	49.3 (34)
Lower physician reimbursement for PD	20.3 (14)
None of these are barriers	13.0 (9)
Dialysis provider related factors:	
Lack of PD experienced and dedicated management	75.4 (52)
Lack of PD infrastructure, dedicated resources, and support	66.7 (46)
Proliferation of in-center HD units	55.1 (38)
None of these are barriers	7.2 (5)
Patient related factors:	
Lack of patient education on PD	78.3 (54)
Other patient related barrier	20.03 (14)
Patient education is not a barrier	17.4 (12)
Therapy related factors:	
Concerns about PD clinical outcomes (relative to HD outcomes)	43.5 (30)
Concerns about relative mortality rates with PD	31.9 (22)
None of these are barriers	49.3 (34)

*Respondents could indicate more than one factor.

personal experience with PD and approximately 50% cited problems with hospital and nursing support as limiting factors.

With regard to dialysis provider related factors, lack of PD experience and dedicated management was cited most often (75%) followed by lack of PD infrastructure, dedicated resources, and support (67%) and proliferation of in-center HD units (55%). Among the patient related factors limiting utilization of PD, 78% of program directors cited lack of patient education on PD. However, less than half of program directors (43%) cited concerns about PD clinical outcomes (relative to HD outcomes) as a therapy related factor limiting utilization of PD.

4. Discussion

Mehrota *et al.*'s 2002 national survey of nephrology training program directors described disparities in resources available for PD vs. HD training [12]. Approximately 10 years later, we found that the large majority of responding Program Directors in our national sample still believe that PD training in the US is inadequate. The primary reasons given relate to inadequacy of training in PD and include insufficient numbers of PD patients for adequate exposure to PD, and faculty who are not comfortable with PD. These findings are also consistent with another prior study which found that only 56% of nephrologists felt well trained and competent in the care of chronic PD patients while approximately 80% of respondents reported that they were well trained and felt competent after leaving fellowship in the care of chronic HD patients [10]. Level of physician perceived comfort and competence in the care of PD patients impacts both provider and patient decisions about choice of therapy [13] and consequently influences the rate of utilization of PD.

Related to adequacy of training, our survey of program directors suggest that the availability of training resources (faculty and patients) and allocation of didactic and training time for fellows in providing care to ESRD patients receiving dialysis are significantly lower for PD than HD in the US. The main limiting factors indicated by program directors were insufficiently trained faculty in PD and/or insufficient PD patient population to ensure appropriate training for fellows in providing care for patients undergoing PD. In addition, our findings suggest that the availability of training resources for PD has declined in the US since Mehrotra *et al.* reported on this in 2002 [12]. We found that median number of full/part-time faculty members were significantly lower for PD than for HD. Faculty numbers for PD have dropped from a median of 4 reported 10 years ago [12], to a median of 1 noted in our recent survey. Similarly, the median faculty/fellow ratio for PD training decreased from 1 [12] to 0.5, as evidenced by our data. The patients/fellow ratio has declined from a median of 6.7 [12], to 5.0 (our data). In contrast, we found that median numbers of faculty members, faculty/fellow ratio and patients/fellow ratio for HD training have remained similar to those noted 10 years earlier by Mehrotra *et al.* [12]. We found that among programs providing continuity care or block rotation and continuity care (continuity care is the preferred experience [19]), the smaller proportion assigned dialysis patients to fellows for PD rather than HD. Similarly, the smaller proportion of total dialysis training time among programs offering block rotation, continuity care, or both was devoted to PD rather than HD. This has not changed in comparison to the previous report [12].

A decline in the number of ESRD patients on PD has worsened this resource for nephrology fellowship training. Responding program directors most often cited limited physician training in PD as a physician/nurse related factor which limits utilization of PD in the US and greater than half also cited poor personal experience with PD. This sets up an adverse cycle since new ESRD patients' treatment choices are often influenced by their physicians [13,16]. We found that among patient related factors limiting utilization of PD, the majority of program directors cited lack of patient education on PD compared to less than half who cited concerns about PD clinical outcomes (relative to HD outcomes) as a therapy related factor limiting utilization of PD. Our data suggest that program directors perceive training and education as greater impediments to utilization of PD, than clinical factors.

What is needed for adequate PD training is debatable. 76% of program directors felt that allocating >5% of total training time is adequate for PD training and in general, 81% felt that assigning >5 chronic PD patients/fellow was also adequate for PD training over the fellows' two year training period). This may reflect program directors' beliefs that these are the number of patients needed for a fellow to attain competency. However, our questionnaire did not explicitly address the competency of PD training. Future surveys should specifically ask about training resources and experiences needed to attain competency in this area and should focus on evaluating and achieving competency in PD among fellows [20].

Study limitations include the response rate of 55%. However, given the voluntary nature of the survey, this response rate is comparable to that achieved in the other studies [6,12]. Furthermore, response rates varied regionally with representation greatest in the northeast. There is some evidence that the likelihood of PD placement is greatest in the northeast [17], although others have found that PD use did not differ in urban vs. rural settings [21], it is not surprising that directors of nephrology fellowship programs located in the northeast might more frequently to respond to a survey about PD utilization. Nonetheless, despite the over-representation of programs located in areas of highest PD use, our findings still suggest underutilization of PD related to inadequate training in PD.

Another limitation relates to the accuracy of self-report data obtained from this present survey, particularly descriptions of the distribution of time spent by fellows on PD vs. HD activities. This was estimated by responding program directors and not based on actual documentation of individual fellows' time. Nonetheless, we believe that their estimates of training practices and activities are adequate and reliable because most program directors are closely involved in outlining or designing the structure of dialysis training. In addition, estimates of time spent by fellows on PD vs. HD activities given by our responding program directors were similar to estimates provided by nephrology training program fellows in a prior study [19].

In conclusion, our survey of the program directors supports the contention that current nephrology fellowship training in PD in the US remains inadequate, despite documented advantages of PD over HD for treatment of ESRD among chronic dialysis patients. The adequacy of PD training resources needs appraisal by the nephrology community and competency in PD training needs to be defined and evaluated [19,20]. Minimum standards of PD training for each nephrology fellow should to be established similar to that of nephrology transplant training as mandated by the American College of Graduate Medical Education. Targeting current faculty for PD-directed educational efforts can also do much to enhance PD utilization and improve ESRD patient outcomes. Current faculty involved in training programs need to be trained or retrained in PD so that they feel comfortable in training fellows in PD and providing care to PD patients.

5. Acknowledgements

This project was supported by a grant from Dialysis Clinics Inc., to Nand Wadhwa MD, FACP, FRCP. The sponsor did not have a role in any of the following: study design; collection, analysis, and interpretation of data; writing this report; and the decision to submit this report for publication

REFERENCES

[1] US Renal Data System, "USRDS 2012 Annual Data Re-

port," Department of Health and Human Services, National Institutes of Health, Bethesda, 2012.

[2] P. K. Li, C. C. Szeto, B. Piraino, *et al.*, "Peritoneal Dialysis-Related Infections Recommendations: 2010 Update," *Peritoneal Dialysis International*, Vol. 30, No. 4, 2010, pp. 393-423. doi:10.3747/pdi.2010.00049

[3] J. E. Frampton and G. L. Plosker, "Icodextrin: A Review of Its Use in Peritoneal Dialysis," *Drugs*, Vol. 63, No. 19, 2003, pp. 2079-2105. doi:10.2165/00003495-200363190-00011

[4] P. H. Juergensen, A. L. Murphy, K. A. Pherson, A. S. Kliger and F. O. Finkelstein, "Tidal Peritoneal Dialysis: Comparison of Different Tidal Regimens and Automated Peritoneal Dialysis," *Kidney International*, Vol. 57, 2001, pp. 2603-2607. doi:10.1046/j.1523-1755.2000.00120.x

[5] R. Mehrotra, D. Kermah, L. Fried, *et al.*, "Chronic Peritoneal Dialysis in the United States: Declining Utilization Despite Improving Outcomes," *Journal of the American Society of Nephrology*, Vol. 18, No. 10, 2007, pp. 2781-2788. doi:10.1681/ASN.2006101130

[6] D. C. Mendelssohn, S. R. Mullaney, B. Jung, P. G. Blake and R. L. Mehta, "What Do American Nephrologists Think about Dialysis Modality Selection?" *American Journal of Kidney Diseases*, Vol. 37, No. 1, 2001, pp. 22-29.

[7] R. R. Quinn, J. E. Hux, M. J. Oliver, P. C. Austin, M. Tonelli and A. Laupacis, "Selection Bias Explains Apparent Differential Mortality between Dialysis Modalities," *Journal of the American Society of Nephrology*, Vol. 22, No. 8, 2011, pp. 1534-1542. doi:10.1681/ASN.2010121232

[8] R. Mehrotra, Y. Chiu, Kalantar-Zadeh, J. Bargman and E. Vonesh, "Similar Outcome with Hemodialysis and Peritoneal Dialysis in Patients with End-Stage Renal Disease," *Archives of Internal Medicine*, Vol. 171, No. 2, 2007, pp. 110-118. doi:10.1001/archinternmed.2010.352

[9] M. A. Perazella, "Nephrology Fellowship Training in the 21st Century: Where Do We Stand?" *Clinical Journal of the American Society of Nephrology*, Vol. 5, No. 3, 2010, pp. 387-389. doi:10.2215/CJN.00070110

[10] J. S. Berns, "A Survey-Based Evaluation of Self-Perceived Competency after Nephrology Fellowship Training," *Clinical Journal of the American Society of Nephrology*, Vol. 5, No. 3, 2010, pp. 490-496. doi:10.2215/CJN.08461109

[11] W. Mitch and W. M. McClellan, "Patterns of Patient Care Reported by Nephrologists: Implications for Nephrology Training," *American Journal of Kidney Diseases*, Vol. 32, No. 4, 1998, pp. 551-556. doi:10.1016/S0272-6386(98)70016-2

[12] R. Mehotra, P. Blake, N. Berman and K. Nolph, "An Analysis of Dialysis Training in the United States and Canada," *American Journal of Kidney Diseases*, Vol. 40, No. 1, 2002, pp. 152-160. doi:10.1053/ajkd.2002.33924

[13] E. Grapsa, "Is the Underutilzation of Peritoneal Dialysis in Relation to Hemodialysis as Renal Replacement Therapy, Justifiable Worldwide," *Hippkratia*, Vol. 15, Suppl. 1, 2011, pp. 13-15.

[14] P. G. Blake and F. O. Finkelstein, "Why Is the Proportion of Patients Doing Peritoneal Dialysis Declining in North America?" *Peritoneal Dialysis International*, Vol. 21, No. 2, 2001, pp. 107-114.

[15] L. Troidle, A. Kliger and F. Finkelstein, "Barriers to Utilization of Chronic Peritoneal Dialysis in Network #1, New England," *Peritoneal Dialysis International*, Vol. 26, 2006, pp. 452-457.

[16] D. Wuerth, S. Finkelstein, O. Schwetz, H. Carey, A. Kliger and F. Finkelstein, "Patients' Descriptions of Specific Factors Leading to Modality Selection of Chronic Peritoneal Dialysis or Hemodialysis," *Peritoneal Dialysis International*, Vol. 22, No. 2, 2002, pp. 184-190.

[17] A. G. Stack, "Determinants of Modality Selection among Incident Dialysis Patients: Results from a National Study," *Journal of the American Society of Nephrology*, Vol. 13, No. 5, 2002, pp. 1279-1287.

[18] US Census Bureau, "Census Bureau Regions and Divisions with State FIPS Codes," 2011. http:///www.census.gov/geo/www/us_regdiv.pdf

[19] A. R. Nissenson, R. Agarwal, M. Allon, A. K. Cheung, W. Clark, T. Depner, *et al.*, "Improving Outcomes in CKD and ESRD Patients: Carrying the Torch from Training to Practice," *Seminars in Dialysis*, Vol. 17, No. 5, 2004, pp. 380-397. doi:10.1111/j.0894-0959.2004.17350.x

[20] M. G. Parker, "Nephrology Training in the 21st Century: Toward Outcomes-Based Education," *American Journal of Kidney Diseases*, Vol. 56, No. 1, 2010, pp. 132-142.

[21] N. G. Kutner, R. Zhang, Y. Huang and H. Wasse, "Patient Awareness and Initiation of Peritoneal Dialysis," *Archives of Internal Medicine*, Vol. 171, No. 2, 2011, pp. 119-124. doi:10.1001/archinternmed.2010.361

8

Idiopathic Hypereosinophilic Syndrome Presenting as IgA Nephropathy with Nephrotic Range Proteinuria

Tajamul H. Shah, Ajaz N. Koul, Sonaullah Shah, Umar H. Khan, Parvaiz A. Koul, Fayaz A. Sofi, Mufti S., Rafi Ahmed Jan*

Intrenal & Pulmonary Medicine, Sheri Kashmir Institute of Medicine, Srinagar, India

Email: *rafiahmedjan@gmail.com

ABSTRACT

Idiopathic hypereosinophilic syndrome (IHES) is a disorder characterized by increased eosinophil count (eosinophilia) along with organ dysfunction secondary to organ infiltration of eosinophils and release of inflammatory markers [1-4], with no obvious cause for eosinophilia. The onset of symptoms is insidious in most of the cases and eosinophilia is detected incidentally. However, in others, the initial manifestations are severe and life-threatening due to the rapid evolution of cardiac or neurologic complications [5]. Renal involvement is rarely reported [6] in IHES. Herein we reported a case of IHES with predominant renal involvement as nephrotic syndrome with focal necrotizing IgA nephropathy.

Keywords: Idiopathic Hypereosinophilic Syndrome; Eosinophilia; Renal Involvement; Nephrotic Syndrome

1. Case Report

A 50-year old male presented with a 3-week history of a non-productive cough, associated with intermittent low grade fever, periorbital puffiness and lower extremity edema. Patient denied any history of breathlessness, chest-pain, hemoptysis, orthopnea, paroxysmal nocturnal dyspnea, drop in urine output, skin rash or arthritis. His past history was insignificant and he denied any history of drug intake.

Hisexamination revealed mild pallor, with periorbitalpuffiness, lower extremity pitting edema and mild splenomegaly. He had hemoglobin of 11 g/dL with a total leucocyte count of 9.2×10^9/cumm and an ESR of 23 mmhr. His differential count included 46% polymorphs 11% lymphocytes and 41% eosinophils with AEC count of 3800 which repeatedly was high and ranged from 3800 to 5500. A peripheral blood film showed features of normochromic normocytic anaemia with no abnormal cells. His serum creatinine was 1.7 mg/dL with a creatinine clearance of 44 ml/min. Liver functions showed hypoporoteinemia with hypoalbuminemia. He had an active urinary sedimentand urine which showed presence of eosinophils on wright's staining. 24 hours urinary protein was 5.04 g/24hours which was reproduced twice. Repeated stool examination for the presence of ova/parasite was negative.

Radiograph of the chest was normal. High resolution computerized tomography of the chest did not reveal any abnormality. His electrocardiograph and echocardiography were normal. Ultrasonography of abdomen was normal as well.

Patient was investigated further to look for eosinophilic infiltration of other organ systems in view of persistant hypereosinophilia.

Patient was subjected to bronchoscopy to obtain bronchoalveolar lavage for eosinophils which revealed 62% eosinophils. Bone marrow aspiration and biopsy revealed 56% eosinophils with no dysplasia and blasts. p-ANCA andc-ANCA were within normal limits. Serum tryptase levels were within normal limits.

Patient was subjected to percutaneous renal biopsy to look for the etiology of nephrotic range proteinuria. Renal biopsy revealed, marked interstitial edema and patchy inflammation including aggregates of eosinophils admixed with mononuclear cells and occasional neutrophils. An eosinophilic infiltrate was also seen in medulla with eosinophillic tubulitis and patchy destruction of tubular basement membrane. Direct immunofluorescence showed

*Corresponding author.

deposition of IgA, IgG, IgM and C_3 predominantly in mesangium with final impression of foal necrotizing IgA nephropathy (**Figure 1**).

A diagnosis of Idiopathic hypereosinophilia with renal involvement in the form of focal necrotizing IgA nephropathy presenting as nephrotic syndrome was made.

Patient was started on 1 mg/kg/day of prednisolone. Repeat eosinophil count after 2 weeks of steroids was within normal limits and protein was undetectable in urine after 4 weeks of steroid therapy.

2. Discussion

IHES is a group of disorders characterized by sustained overproduction of eosinophil's in which eosinophillic infiltration and mediator release cause damage to organ. Renal involvement in IHES is reported rarely [6,7], limited mostly to the case reports. Renal involvement could be the first manifestation of HES [8]. The first case of renal involvement in IHES was reported in 1979 by Lanfranchi *et al.* [9]. They observed glomerular sclerosis and eosinophilicintersititial infiltrate on renal histology.

Renal involvement can present as renal dysfunction [5,6] or proteinuria [10], which can range from sub-nephrotic to nephrotic range [11]. Our case presented with renal dysfunction with serum creatinine of 1.7 and creatinine clearance of 44 ml/min. He also had nephrotic range proteinuria which was reproduced twice.

There is not much literature on renal histological pattern in IHES [12]. Various histological patterns reported by various authors include Ischemic lesions secondary to intrarenal thrombus formation [13], crescentic glomerulonephritis [14], mesangial expansion [15], proliferative glomerulonephritis [13], immuno-tactoid glomerulopath [11], glomerular sclerosis [6], interstitial nephritis with

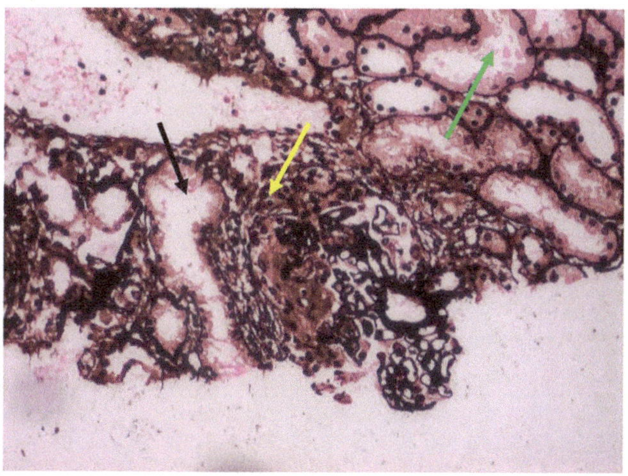

Figure 1. Microscopic view of kidney biopsy (H & E) Eosinophilic infiltration (yellow arrow), tubular epithelial shedding (black arrow) and tubular casts (green arrow).

eosinophilic infil-tratcs [8,10] and membranous nephropathy [11]. Findings on immunofluorescence of renal biopsy in patients with IHES vary with deposition of immune complex and complement in some cases and lack of their deposition in others.

In our case the histological features were suggestive of eosinophilic interstitial infiltrate and focal necrotizing IgA nephropathy. There was deposition of immunoglobulin'sand compliment.

This is probably the first case reported in literature till date of renal involvement in patient with IHES.

Renal involvement with peripheral eosinophilia can occur in a number of conditions like drugs [16], myeloproliferative disorders [17], parasitic manifestation [18], cholesterol embolization [19] or necrotizing vasculitis. No such cause was obvious from history and investigations in our case.

Treatment is indicated in all symptomatic patients or those with evidence of organ dysfunction.

Steroids are the initial therapy of choice [20] for patients with organ involvement who do NOT have the FIP1L1-PDGFRA fusion or another imatinib-sensitive tyrosine kinase mutation. In the large series, partial or complete remission was achieved in 85 percent at one month (4 weeks).

Other drugs include hydoxyurea, or Anti-IL-5 [20-22], either adding to steroids or as steroid sparing.

We managed our patient with oral prednisolone 60 mg/day (1 mg/kg/day). Patient was reevaluated at 2 weeks of steroid therapy for eosinophil count and proteinuria. At 2 weeks AEC was within normal limits but proteinuria persisted although decreased. At 4 weeks AEC was within normal limits and proteinuria had settled.

REFERENCES

[1] P. F. Weller and G. J. Bubley, "The Idiopathic Hypereosinophilic Syndrome," *Blood*, Vol. 83, No. 10, 1994, p. 2759.

[2] F. Roufosse, E. Cogan and M. Goldman, "Recent Advances in Pathogenesis and Management of Hypereosinophilic Syndromes," *Allergy*, Vol. 59, No. 7, 2004, pp. 673-689. doi:10.1111/j.1398-9995.2004.00465.x

[3] A. D. Klion, B. S. Bochner, G. J. Gleich, *et al.*, "Approaches to the Treatment of Hypereosinophilic Syndromes: A Workshop Summary Report," *Journal of Allergy and Clinical Immunology*, Vol. 117, No. 6, 2006, pp. 1292-1302. doi:10.1016/j.jaci.2006.02.042

[4] J. Sheikh and P. F. Weller, "Clinical Overview of Hypereosinophilic Syndromes," *Immunology and Allergy Clinics of North America*, Vol. 27, No. 3, 2007, pp. 333-355. doi:10.1016/j.iac.2007.07.007

[5] V. Ambarus and A. Cosovanu, "The Evolutionary Cha-racteristics of the Hypereosinophilic Syndrome," *Re-*

vista Medico-Chirurgicala a Societatii de Medici si Naturalisti din Lasi'S, Vol. 102, No. 1-2, 1998, pp. 69-75.

[6] J. L. Motellon, C. Bernis, A. Garcia-Sanchez, E. Gruss and J. A. Traver, "Renal Involvement in the Hyper-Eosinophilic Syndrome," *Nephrology Dialysis Transplantation*, Vol. 10, No. 3, 1995, pp. 401-403.

[7] A. S. Fauci, J. B. Harley, W. C. Roberts, V. J. Ferrans, H. R. Gralmick and B. H. Bhorson, "The Idiopathic Hypereosinophilic Syndrome: Clinical, Pathophy-Siologic and Therapeutic Considerations," *Annals of Internal Medicine*, Vol. 97, No. 1, 1982, pp. 78-92. doi:10.7326/0003-4819-97-1-78

[8] I. Navarro, J. Torras, M. Gomà, J. M. Cruzado and J. M. Grinyó, "Renal Involvement as the First Manifestation of Hypereosinophilic Syndrome," *Clinical Kidney Journal*, Vol. 2, No. 5, 2009, pp. 379-381.

[9] C. J. Spry, J. Davies, P. C. Tai, E. G. Oslen, C. M. Oakley and J. F. Goodwin, "Clinical Features of Fifteen Patients with the Hypereosinophilic Syndrome," *Journal of Nuclear Medicine*, Vol. 205, No. 52, 1983, pp. 1-2.

[10] F. Bulucu, C. Can, V. Inal, Y. Baykal and S. Erikci, "Renal Involvement in a Patient with Idiopathic Hypereosinophilic Syndrome," *Clinical Nephrology*, Vol. 57, No. 2, 2002, pp. 171-172.

[11] M. Frigui, M. B. Hmida, M. Jallouli, M. Kechaou, F. Frikha and Z. Bahloul, "Membranousglomerulopathy Associated with Idiopathic Hypereosinophilic Syndrome," *Saudi Journal of Kidney Diseases and Transplantation*, Vol. 21, No. 2, 2010, pp. 320-322.

[12] Y. J. Choi, J. D. Lee, K. H. Yang, B. K. Kim, B. K. Bang and S. I. Shim, "Immunotactoidglomerulopathy Associated with Idiopathic Hypereosinophilic Syndrome," *American Journal of Nephrology*, Vol. 18, 1998, pp. 337-343. doi:10.1159/000013362

[13] M. J. Chusid, D. C. Dale, B. C. West and S. M. Wolff, "The Hypereosinophilic Syndrome: Analysis of Fourteen Cases with Review of the Literature," *Medicine*, Vol. 54, No. 1, 1975, p. 27.

[14] P. Richardson, G. Dickinson, S. Nash, L. Hoffman, R. Steingard and M. Germain, "Crescentic Glome-Rulonephritis and Eosinophilic Interstitial Infiltrates in a Patient with Hypereosinophilic Syndrome," *Postgraduate Medical Journal*, Vol. 71, 1995, pp. 175-178. doi:10.1136/pgmj.71.833.175

[15] C. P. Guidicelli, F. Didelot, C. Duvic, J. Desrame, M. Herody and G. Nedelec, "Eosinophilia and Renal Pathology," *Medicine Tropicale*, Vol. 58, Suppl. 4, 1998, pp. 477- 481.

[16] U. Schnetzke, T. Bossert, *et al.*, "Drug-Induced Lymphadenopathy with Eosinophilia and Renal Failure Mimicking Lymphoma Disease: Dramatic Onset of DRESS Syndrome Associated with Antibiotic Treatment," *Annals of Hematology*, Vol. 90, No. 11, 2011, pp. 1353-1355.

[17] R Talwar, S. C. Dash, *et al.*, "A Case of Chronic Myeloid Leukemia Complicated with Minimal Change Nephrotic Syndrome," *Acta Haematologica*, Vol. 109, No. 2, 2003, pp. 101-103.

[18] M. L. F. van Velthuysen and S. Florquin, "Glomerulopathy Associated with Parasitic Infections," *Clinical Microbiological Review*, Vol. 13, No. 1, 2000, pp. 55-66.

[19] B. S. Kasinath and E. J. Lewis, "Eosinophilia as a Clue to the Diagnosis of Atheroembolic Renal Disease," *Archives of Internal Medicine*, Vol. 147, No. 8, 1987, pp. 1384-1385.

[20] P. U. Ogbogu, B. S. Bochner, J. H. Butterfield, *et al.*, "Hypereosinophilic Syndrome: A Multicenter, Retrospective Analysis of Clinical Characteristics and Response to Therapy," *Journal of Allergy and Clinical Immunology*, Vol. 124, No. 6, 2009, pp. 1319-1325. doi:10.1016/j.jaci.2009.09.022

[21] A. B. Kay and A. D. Lion, "Anti-IL-5 Therapy for Asthma and Hypereosinophilicsyndrome," *Immunology and Allergy Clinics of North America*, Vol. 24, No. 4, 2004, pp. 645-666. doi:10.1016/j.iac.2004.06.007

[22] M. E. Rothenber, *et al.*, "Treatment of Patients with the Hypereosinophilic Syndrome with Mepolizumab," *New England Journal of Medicine*, Vol. 358, 2008, pp. 1215-1228. doi:10.1056/NEJMoa070812

Alarming Presentation of a Seemingly Common Condition in a Patient with Renal Impairment

Mohammad Budruddin[1*], Muhammad Yasir Khalil[2], Issa Al Salmi[2], Ramaiah Shilpa[2]
[1]Nephrology Department, Tawam Hospital, Al Ain, UAE
[2]Nephrology Department, Royal Hospital, Muscat, Oman
Email: [*]drbudruddin@gmail.com

ABSTRACT

We received a 23-year-old male, working in the Army for 18 months, with advanced renal impairment, haemoptysis and hyperkalemia. An impression of the pulmonary renal syndrome was made and he was managed aggressively with haemodialysis, plasma exchange and pulsing with methyl prednisolone. His condition improved, but the renal functions did not. The vasculitic workup including Extractable Nuclear Antigen (ENA) and Anti-Neutrophil Cytoplasmic Antibody (ANCA) which were sent on admission came out to be negative. As he apparently responded to the initial management protocol, he was subjected to renal biopsy which did not reveal any vasculitis but was consistent for end-stage renal disease. Subsequently he was subjected to lung biopsy which also was not supportive for vasculitis. However, we concluded that the initial pointers for Wegener's granulomatosis were misleading. The haemoptysis entirely subsided as the congestion improved. He was maintained on Haemodialysis three times per week schedule and discharged to the peripheral health care facility.

Keywords: Haemoptysis; Renal Impairment; Pulmonary Renal Syndrome; Haemodialysis; ENA; ANCA; Vasculitis; Pulmonary Oedema

1. Introduction

Pulmonary oedema is not an unusual presentation in patients with end-stage renal disease. This may be associated with haemoptysis. Radiological imaging of the chest may at times be very confusing, mimicking alveolar haemorrhage. We had a young patient who presented acute onset advanced renal failure with haemoptysis. In the course of his management, we concluded that his haemoptysis was secondary to pulmonary oedema and not pulmonary renal syndrome.

2. Case Summary

Mr. IRS, a 23-year-old Omani male was referred from a peripheral Hospital with advanced renal failure and haemoptysis. He was not know to have any medical problems in the past and was not on any medications before this presentation. Neither was he ever told in any health care facility to be having renal impairment. He presented with the advanced renal failure with serum creatinine more than 2000 mmol/l and urea 84 mmol/l. He was in severe respiratory distress (tachypnoeic RR of 35/m, desaturating to 78% on room air) and developed massive frank haemoptysis immediately after admission. The chest X-ray **Figure 1** on admission and urgent high resolution CT (HRCT) **Figure 2** done after two sessions of Haemodialysis with good ultrafiltration showed extensive alveolar haemorrhage with perivascular nodules. This concurred with our initial impression of pulmonary renal syndrome (Wegener's granolomatosis). Further CT of the sinuses did show the polypoidal thickening of the mucous membrane of the right frontal sinus. The complements level done were normal.

His condition was critical with severe drop in Hb to 4 gm/dl. He was started on emergent aggressive treatment for Wegner's granulomatosis with 7 sessions of plasma exchange and methylprednisolone 1 gm pulse daily for three days. His haemoptysis subsided after the forth session of plasma exchange and his general condition also improved with improvement in the pulmonary congestion and uremia following several sessions of haemodialysis and ultrafiltrations.

[*]Corresponding author.

The vasculitic workup subsequently came out to be negative for Extactable Neuclear antigens (ENA), Anti-Neutrophil Cytoplasmic Antibody but equivocal for Anti-glomerular basement membrane antibody (Anti GBM). Serology for HBV, HCV and HIV were negative. Repeat radiology showed improvement in the alveolar shadows. Ultrasound estimation of kidney size was normal with increased ecogenicity. The urine analysis was bland (no active sediments) showed <2 RBC, <2 WBC, of 25 mg/L Protien.

After stabilizing he was subjected to renal biopsy in order to get the tissue diagnosis. The histopathology did not show any evidence of vasculitis, tubulointerstitial compartment showed marked sclerosis of the interstitium and scattered moderate inflammatory cells, tubular atrophy with dilatation. The features were consistent with the end stage renal disease (**Figure 3**)

Even the lung tissue biopsy done did not reveal any granuloma, pneumonic changes and evidence of vasculitis. However there were findings of scanty recent and old intra-alveolar haemorrhage (5% of the tissue sample) (**Figure 4**)

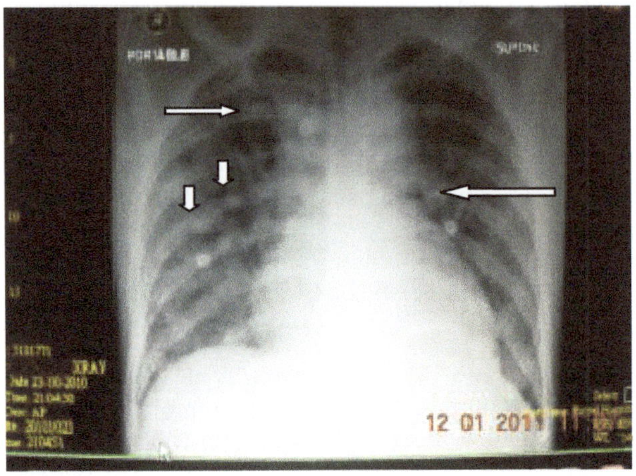

Figure 1. Chest X-ray showing nodular opacities (indicated by small and big arrows).

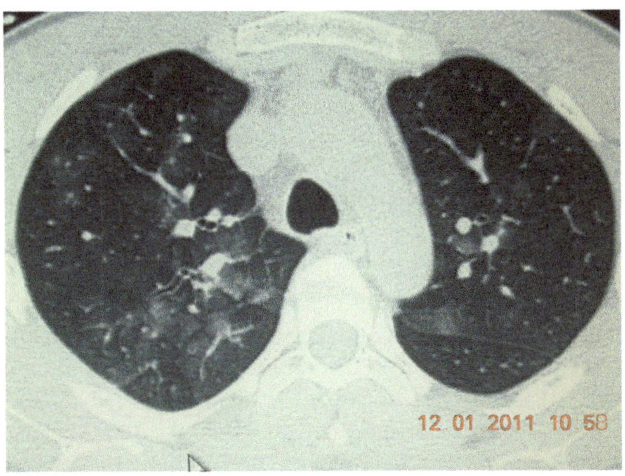

Figure 2. CT scan of the chest showing ground glass appearance.

Semi-permanent vascular access (Right Internal Jugular vein tunneled catheter) was inserted for him and he was put on maintenance haemodialysis three times per week and radiocephalic fistula was also created for him. He was discharged to the peripheral health care facility with dialysis facility, in a stable condition with a plan for living related renal transplantation from his brother in the future.

3. Discussion

The presentation with pulmonary oedema is very common in patients on maintenance haemodialysis. These end stage renal disease patients irrespective of etiology are at times polyuric before being started on dialysis. However after initiating on haemodialysis they tend to decrease their urine output. Little excess of fluid intake inter dialytic period leads to pulmonary congestion and at times frank pulmonary oedema. This is exacerbated by the concurrent presence of poorly functioning heart.

In our patient the scenario was a bit perplexing as he presented for the first time with very advanced renal failure and pulmonary congestion. However his urine

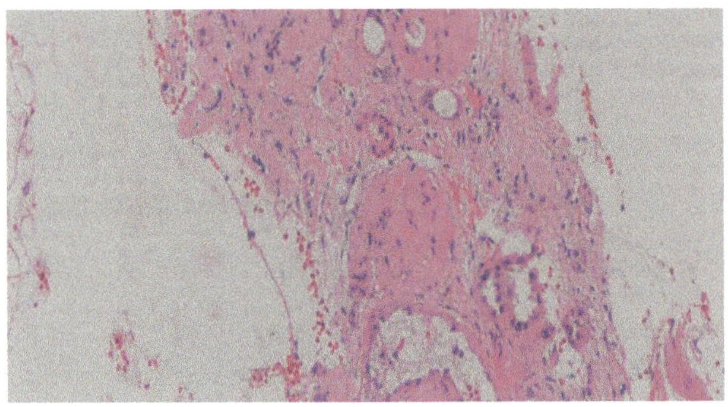

Figure 3. Haematoxylin Eosin stain section shows a core of kidney tissue with two globally hyalinised glomeruli, (black arrow heads) marked tubulointerstitial sclerosis and mild chronic inflammation.

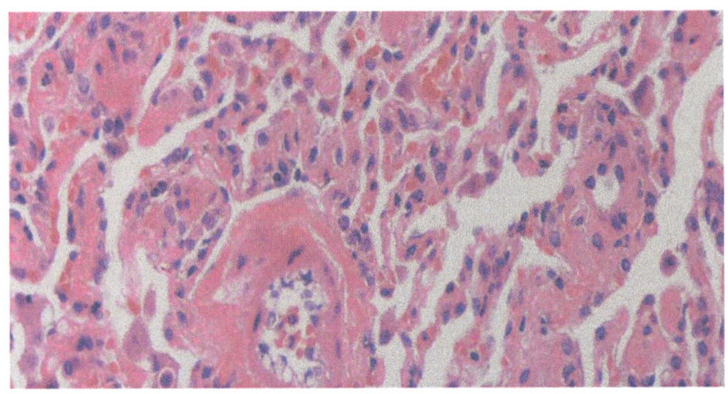

Figure 4. Section showing the lung tissue with mild thickening of the alveolar septa and congestion. No vasculitis or granuloma seen.

output was nearly 1500 ml in 24 Hours. The clinical presence of frank haemoptysis with first time documentation of grossly deranged renal functions and CT finding of alveolar haemorrhage was quite suggestive of pulmonary renal syndrome (Wegener's Granulomatosis/Good pastures syndrome).

Pulmonary oedema can at times present with haemoptysis but again it usually does not show alveolar haemorrhages.

However going through the literature we realized that radiological findings of pulmonary oedema can present in several forms [1].

a) Postobstructive pulmonary edema.

b) Pulmonary edema with chronic pulmonary embolism.

c) Pulmonary edema with veno-occlusive.

d) Stage 1 near drowning pulmonary edema manifests as Kerley lines, peribronchial cuffing, and patchy, perihilar alveolar areas of airspace consolidation;

e) stage 2 and 3 lesions are radiologically nonspecific.

f) Pulmonary edema following administration of cytokines.

g) High-altitude pulmonary edema.

(h) Neurogenic pulmonary edema manifests as bilateral, rather homogeneous airspace consolidations that predominate at the apices in about 50% of cases.

i) Reperfusion pulmonary edema.

j) Postreduction pulmonary edema manifests as mild airspace consolidation involving the ipsilateral lung.

k) Pulmonary edema due to air embolism initially demonstrates interstitial edema followed by bilateral, peripheral alveolar areas of increased opacity that predominate at the lung bases.

The typical alveolar shadows seen in our patients CT is one of the forms.

Further it is well known that those patients with obstructive airway disease who develop congestive heart failure have much higher pulmonary extravascular volume. Left ventricular failure due to hypoxia leads to left atrial hypertension, which could be the patho-physiologic basis of interstitial pulmonary oedema [2].

Histological studies in uremic lungs have proven the presence of proteinaceous oedema fluid though many have even shown intra-alveolar haemorrhage [3]. Evaluation of the oedema fluid by direct endotracheal aspiration have even shown high content of protein which could suggest increased pulmonary vascular permeability to plasma proteins in renal failure [4]. Though a common feature of pulmonary oedema is increased permeability of the basement membrane to water and low molecular weight solutes, this may be attributable to the hemodynamic factors playing role in the alveolar interstitium and basement membrane [5].

4. Conclusion

Patients with pulmonary edema may present not only blood tinged frothy sputum but may even present massive haemoptysis, which may be life threatening and mimicking serious medical conditions, clinically and radiologically. Keeping this in mind one must deal cautiously with patients presenting pulmonary haemorrhage (haemoptysis) and advanced renal failure.

REFERENCES

[1] T. Gluecker, P. Capasso, P. Schnyder, F. Gudinchet, M.-D. Schaller, J.-P. Revelly and R. Chiolero, "Clinical and Radiologic Features of Pulmonary Edema," *Radio Graphics*, Vol. 19, No. 6, 1999, pp. 1507-1531. http://dx.doi.org/10.1148/radiographics.19.6.g99no211507

[2] R. M. McCredie, "Pulmonary Oedema in Lung Disease," *British Heart Journal*, Vol. 32, No. 1, 1970, pp. 66-70. http://dx.doi.org/10.1136/hrt.32.1.66

[3] L. Doniach, "Uremic Oedema of the Lungs," *The American Journal of Roentgenology, Radium Therapy and Nuclear Medicine*, Vol. 58, No. 5, 1947, pp. 620-628.

[4] E. C. Rackow, I. A. Fein, C. Sprung, R. S. Grodman, "Uremic Pulmonary Oedema," *American Journal of Medicine*, Vol. 64, No. 6, 1978, pp. 1084-1088.

[5] D. G. Gibson, "Hemodynamic Factors in the Development of Acute Pulmonary Oedema in Renal Failure," *The Lancet*, Vol. 288, No. 7475, 1966, pp. 1217-1220. http://dx.doi.org/10.1016/S0140-6736(66)92302-6

10

Study of Dialyzer Membrane (Polyflux 210H) and Effects of Different Parameters on Dialysis Performance

Md Shihamul Islam*, **Jerzy Szpunar**
Department of Mechanical Engineering, University of Saskatchewan, Saskatoon, Canada
Email: *msi875@mail.usask.ca

ABSTRACT

Problems frequently encountered in kidney malfunction include abnormal fluid levels in the body, increased acid levels, abnormal levels of Urea, Glucose, Endothelin, $\beta 2$-Microglobulin and Complement Factor D. Parameters characterizing the structure of dialyzers are very important because they decide overall clearance of toxin molecules and at the same time should allow retaining useful molecules in the blood. In this paper, a cross sectional image of the dialyzer membrane with details of the porosity is presented. A multilayered membrane model with different porosity for each layer, describes the actual structure of Polyflux 210H membrane. This model is developed using Finite Element Software—COMSOL Multiphysics 4.3. A blood flow with substances like—Urea, Glucose, Endothelin, $\beta 2$-Microglobulin, Complement Factor D and Albumin is introduced. For a certain blood flow rate, the toxins diffuse through the membrane and on the other side of the membrane a dialysate flow removes the toxins. Here, different parameters, such as flow rate of blood and dialysate, length and radius of the fiber are changed to simulate how these changes affect toxin clearance and the removal of useful molecules.

Keywords: Simulation, Dialysis; Axisymmetric Model; 3-Layered Membrane; Effective Diffusivity; Parameters; COMSOL Multiphysics 4.3

1. Introduction

A substantial amount of research has been performed regarding homogeneous dialyzer membranes. These homogeneous dialyzer membranes are mostly made of cellulose. These membranes have a uniform pore structure from the inner to the outer side of the membrane. The surface of such membranes was not very biocompatible, because exposed hydroxyl groups would activate complement in the blood passing by the membrane. Therefore, these days dialyzer membranes are made from synthetic materials, using polymers such as polyarylethersulfone, polyamide, polyvinylpyrrolidone, polycarbonate and polyacrylonitrile. These synthetic membranes activate complement to a lesser degree than cellulose membranes [1]. They have a structure which is known as asymmetric. This actually means that the shape of a pore gradually changes from inner to outer surface of the membrane. Synthetic membranes can be made in either low- or high-flux configuration, but most are high-flux. Polyflux 210H is an example of such high flux asymmetric polymer membrane. Sakai *et al.* [2] studied and captured the images of inner and outer surface images of such an asymmetric membrane. They calculated the surface porosity based on those photomicrographs. These give an idea of the surface porosity. But to what extend that porosity continues from one surface to another is not sure. Taking cross sectional image of the membrane and calculating the porosity from that image allow a better description of it. Experimental studies [3,4] have been done to determine whether increasing the dialysate or blood flow rate leads to better clearance or not. But these studies did not consider the structure of the membrane. Also these studies were limited to clearance of Urea only. A reasonable concern for doctors, in these days, is whether the necessary elements like Albumin are diffused through the membrane during the dialysis or not. Most of the experimental studies are done with dialyzers which are commercially available. So they actually give a comparison between different dialyzers. But which parameters of dialysis process are really important to have a better overall clearance of toxin molecules and at the same time retain useful molecules is not clear. Also

*Corresponding author.

how the change of those parameters will affect the clearance is important and will be investigated in this work.

2. Polyflux 210H Dialyzer Membrane

In one dialyzer of Polyflux 210H, there are approximately 12,000 fibers. These fibers are made of Polyamix which is a blend of Polyarylethersulfone, Polyvinylpyrrolidone and Polyamide [5]. Polyflux 210H fiber has a porous structure. A single fiber has a length of 270 mm.

The fibers used in this research were fixed using a mixture of 2.5% glutaraldehyde and 2% paraformaldehyde in a 0.1 M phosphate buffer. A series of mixtures of pure ethanol and distilled water in different ratios were used to dehydrate the fibers. To investigate the internal surface of the fibers, some fibers were placed on a carbon double sided adhesive scanning electron microscopy (SEM) tape glued from the other side to an SEM stub. The SEM stub with the fibers glued to its surface was transferred for viewing under the stereoscopic optical microscope. The fiber walls were dissected longitudinally using a surgical scalpel. Then a 250 Å layer of gold (purity 99.991%) is applied to render the surfaces of the capillaries conductive for observation under the Scanning Electron Microscope (SEM) and the Field Emission Scanning Electron Microscope (FESEM). The SEM used here is a Joel-6010LV and the FESEM is a SU6600 Hitachi.

At first the longitudinal image (**Figure 1**) of the fiber is taken from the outside.

A cross section of the fiber is showed in **Figure 2**.

Then images of the outer and inner side of the membrane are taken to get an idea of the pore size and porosity. The outer surface has a range of pore size which varies between 0.45 μm to 20.40 μm (**Figure 3**).

But for the inner surface the range is between 34 nm and 45 nm (**Figure 4**). Then to get a better idea of the porosity changes, cross sectional images of the membrane are taken. This gives a clear idea of the porosity changes across the thickness.

In **Figure 5**, a dialyzer membrane having a total thickness of 45 μm is divided into three different layers to calculate the porosity for each of the layer. The first layer (thickness of 8 μm) has a porosity of around 0.1, second layer (thickness of 12 μm) has a porosity of around 0.27 and third layer (thickness of 25 μm) has a porosity of around 0.4. Several photomicrographs from each of the layers are taken to calculate the porosity and then an average value of porosity is introduced for each layer.

3. Method of Developing Model

The configuration of a modern hollow fiber dialysis assembly can be seen in **Figure 6**. The blood flows through the fibers while the dialysate flows over the capillaries in a counter-current manner similar to a shell and tube heat exchanger. In this application the flow is laminar.

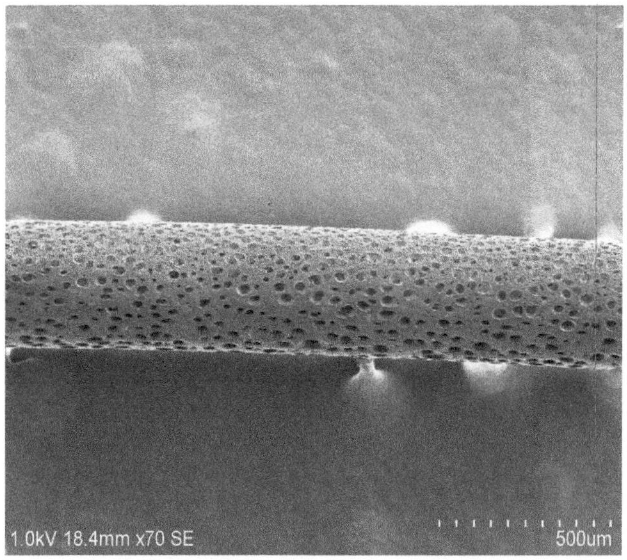

Figure 1. Longitudinal image of a fiber.

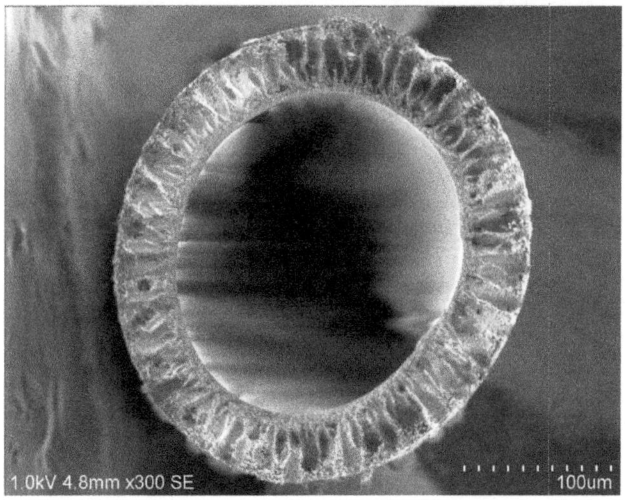

Figure 2. Cross section of the fiber.

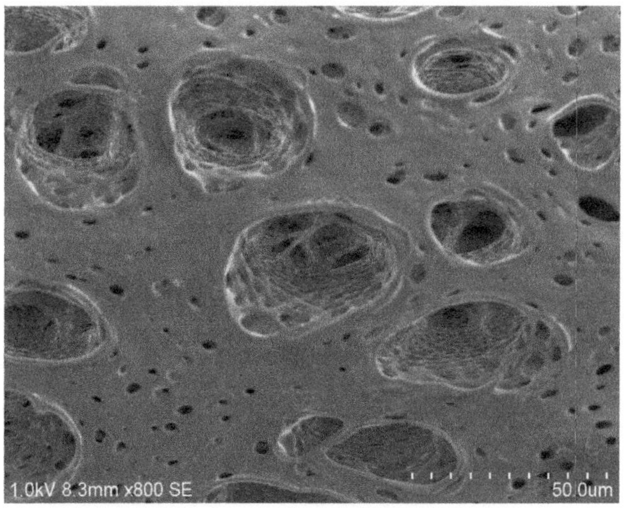

Figure 3. Outer surface of the dialyzer membrane.

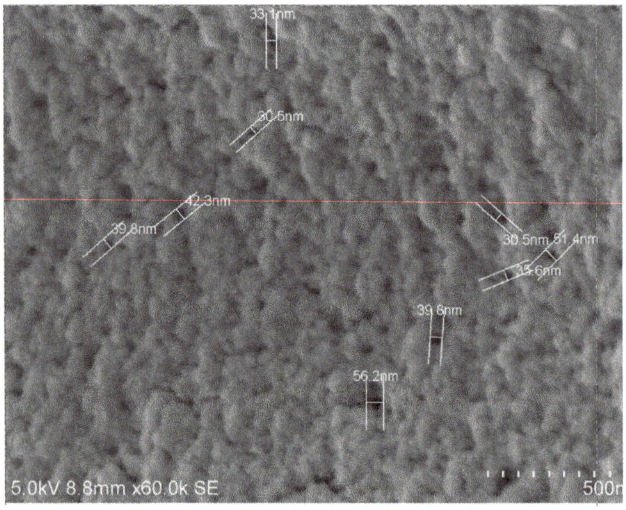

Figure 4. Inner surface of the dialyzer membrane.

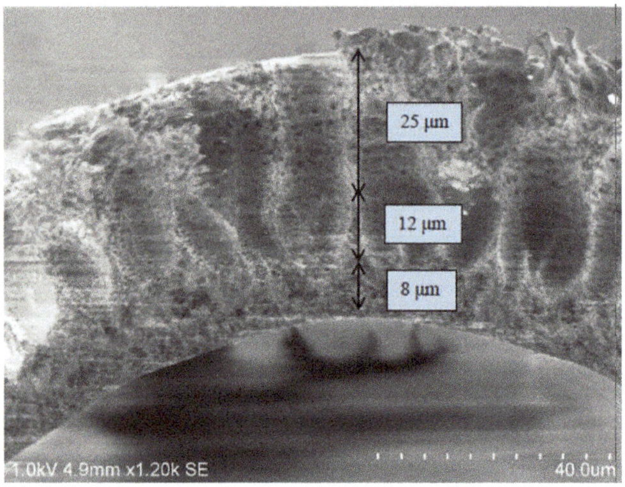

Figure 5. Cross section of the membrane.

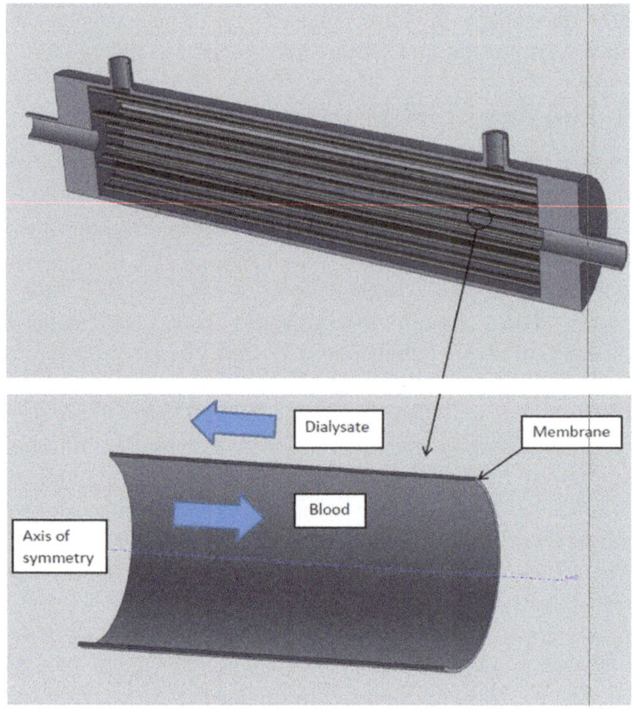

Figure 6. Diagram of dialysis hollow-fiber dialyzer.

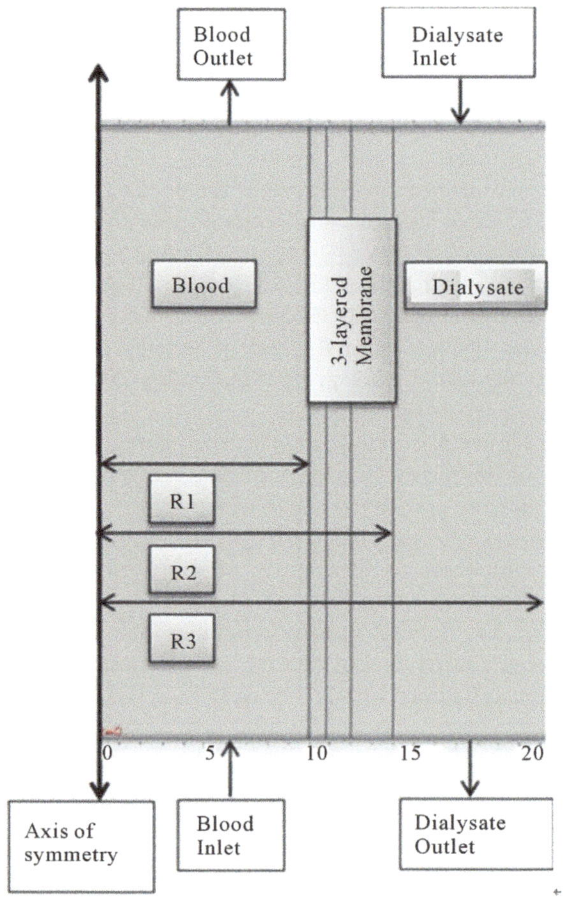

Figure 7. Model Geometry with R1, R2, R3.

Figure 7 shows the three sections of the axisymmetrical domain: the domain on the left represents the blood flow in the fiber, the small domain in the middle with three layers represents the membrane, and the domain on the right represents the outer dialysate flow in the shell.

4. Equations

The following simplified PDE (Partial Differential Equation) describes the convective and diffusion processes in the blood and the dialysate [6].

$$\nabla \cdot (-D_i \nabla c_i + c_i u) = 0 \qquad (1)$$

where c_i denotes the concentration of the toxin (mol/m^3) in the respective phase, D denotes the diffusion coefficient (m^2/s) in the liquid phases and u denotes the velocity (m/s) in the respective liquid phase.

For different toxins the diffusion coefficient is different and it can be calculated from [7]

$$D = 1.62 \times 10^{-4} (MW)^{-0.552} \quad (2)$$

where MW is the molecular weight of the respective toxin.

Both the blood and dialysate flow is considered fully developed laminar flow. For an inlet velocity of blood along the axial direction [8],

$$v_B = \left(\frac{2Q_B}{\pi R_1^2 n}\right)\left[1 - \left(\frac{r}{R_1}\right)^2\right] \quad (3)$$

where Q_B is the volume flow rate of blood, R_1 is the inner radius of the hollow fiber, r is the radial coordinate and n is the number of fibers in a dialyzer which is 12,000 for Polyflux 210H dialyzer.

For the phenomenon of diffusion through the membrane, the following equation has been used-

$$\nabla \cdot (-D_{e,i} \nabla c_i) = 0 \quad (4)$$

where c_i denotes the concentration of the molecules (mol/m^3) in the respective phase, D denotes the diffusion coefficient (m^2/s) of the molecules and D_e denotes the effective diffusion coefficient of the molecules in the porous media.

The term effective diffusivity is defined [9] as

$$D_e = Df(q) S_D A_k \quad (5)$$

$$q = \frac{r_s}{r_p} \quad (6)$$

$$f(q) = \frac{1 - 2.1050q + 2.0865q^3 - 1.7068q^5 + 0.72603q^6}{1 - 0.75857q^5} \quad (7)$$

$$S_D = (1-q)^2 \quad (8)$$

Where D is the diffusion coefficient of molecule, $f(q)$ the friction coefficient, S_D the steric hindrance factor at the pore inlet in diffusion, A_k the membrane porosity, q is the ratio of solute radius r_s to pore radius r_p. Here, the porosity values of the three layers of the membrane are used for A_k.

The six molecules that are considered in this paper are listed in **Table 1** with their molecular weight [10], diameter [11] and diffusion coefficient.

5. COMSOL Multiphysics 4.3

COMSOL Multiphysics 4.3 is used for developing and simulating the model of Polyflux 210H dialyzer. COMSOL Multiphysics is a finite element analysis, solver and simulation software / FEA Software package for various physics and engineering applications, especially coupled phenomena or multiphysics.

After developing the model with necessary inlet, outlet and boundary conditions, simulations are done for changes of different parameters. A post processing result is showed in **Figure 8**.

Table 1. Six molecules with their molecular weight, diameter and diffusion coefficient.

Molecule	Molecular weight (Da)	Diameter (nm)	Diffusion coefficient (x 10^{-8} cm^2/s)
Urea	60	0.48	1690.35
Glucose	180	1.0	921.73
Endothelin	4282.8	2.60	160.25
β2-Microglobulin	11800	3.88	91.59
Complement Factor D	24000	5.12	61.89
Albumin	66000	7.8	35.41

6. Validation

At first, the clearance rate of Urea at different blood flow rate is compared with the experimental results provided by the manufacturer [5].

From **Figure 9**, it can be concluded that the clearance rate of Urea at different blood flow rate is in good agreement with the data provided by the Polyflux 210H manufacturer.

7. Results

7.1. Effects of Blood Flow Rate on Clearance Rate

For the blood flow rate of Q_B = 300, 400 and 500 ml/min and dialysate flow rate of Q_D = 500ml/min, the clearance rate for six molecules is calculated.

As it can be seen from **Figure 10**, with the increasing blood flow rate, the clearance rate of both Urea and Glucose increase rapidly. Specially, for Urea, when the blood flow rate increases from 300 to 500 ml/min, the clearance rate almost gets doubled. And from **Figure 11**, it is evident that the clearance rate of Albumin remains almost constant.

7.2. Effects of Dialysate Flow Rate on Clearance Rate

The blood flow rate, Q_B= 400 ml/min is kept constant and the dialysate flow rate, Q_D is gradually increased.

From **Figures 12** and **13**, it can be said that at a constant blood flow rate, the increasing dialysate flow rate ensures further clearance of Urea and Glucose.

7.3. Effects of Length of the Dialyzer Fiber on Clearance Rate

The length of the dialyzer fiber is varied from 270 to 540 mm when Q_B = 300 ml/min and Q_D = 500 ml/min.

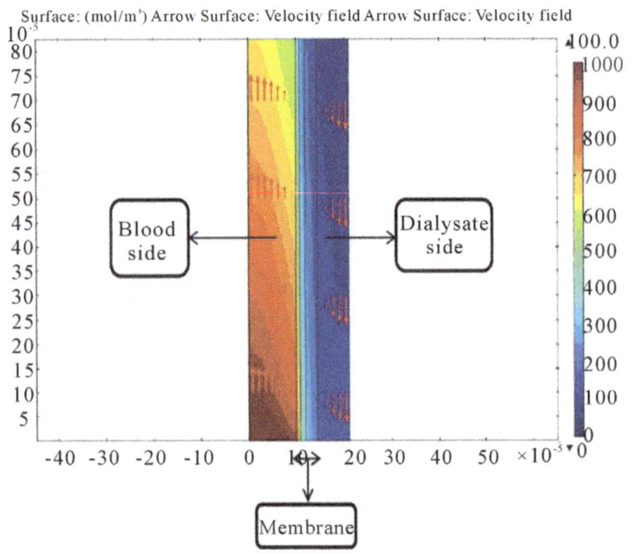

Figure 8. Concentration of Urea at both blood and dialysate side along the membrane (axisymmetric).

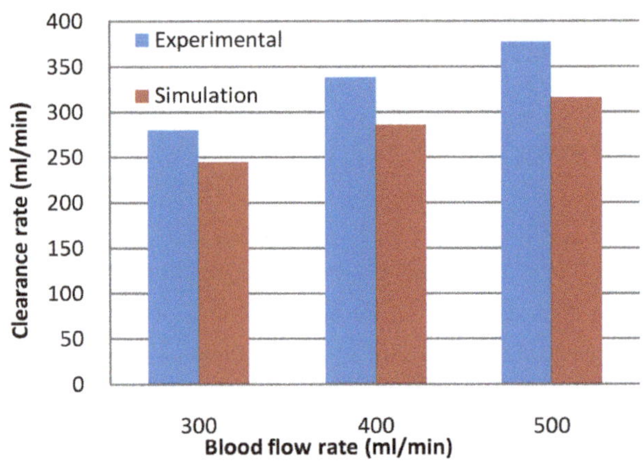

Figure 9. Clearance of Urea for both experimental and simulation cases at blood flow rate, QB = 300, 400 and 500 ml/min whereas dialysate flow rate, QD = 500 ml/min.

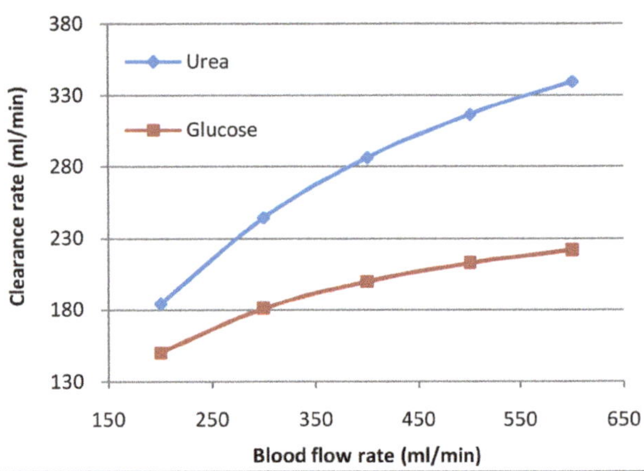

Figure 10. Clearance rate of Urea and Glucose at different blood flow rates when QD = 500 ml/min.

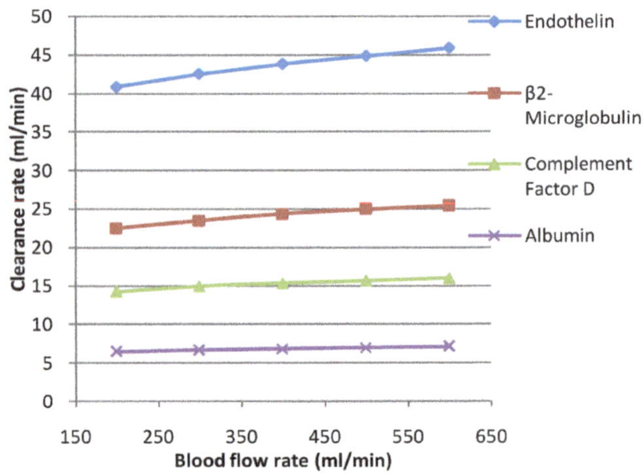

Figure 11. Clearance rate of Endothelin, *β*2-Microglobulin, Complement Factor D and Albumin at different blood flow rates when QD = 500 ml/min.

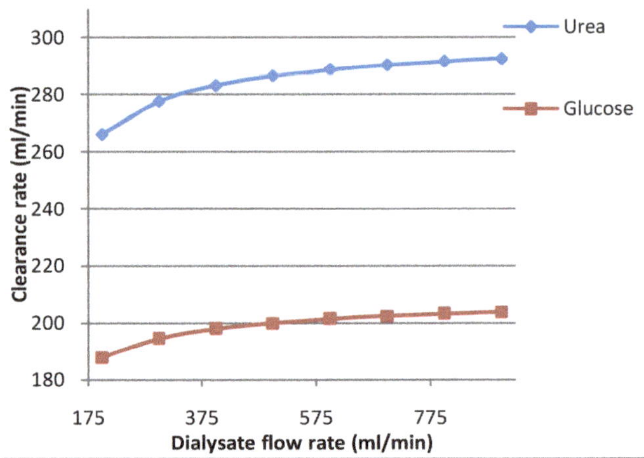

Figure 12. Clearance of Urea and Glucose at different Dialysate flow rates when QB = 400ml/min.

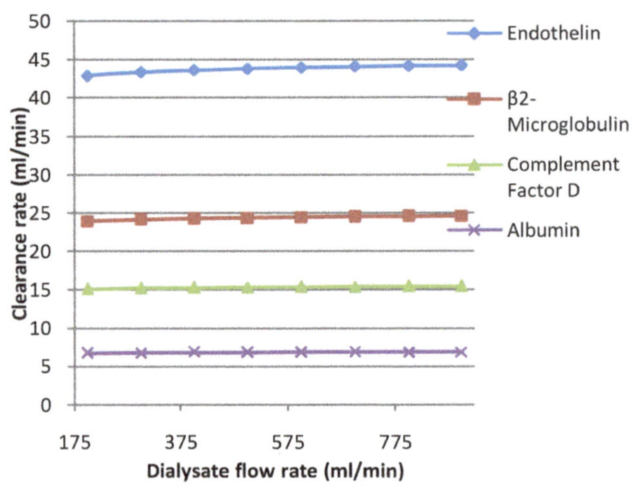

Figure 13. Clearance of Endothelin, *β*2-Microglobulin, Complement Factor D and Albumin at different Dialysate flow rates when QB = 400 ml/min.

From **Figure 14**, it can be seen that if the length of the dialyzer fiber is increased, the clearance rate of Glucose increases more rapidly than the clearance rate of Urea. For Endothelin and *β*2-Microglobulin (**Figure 15**) the clearance rate increases twice compared to the initial condition. Meanwhile, the clearance rate of Albumin does not change that much.

7.4. Effects of Radius of the Dialyzer Fiber on Clearance Rate

The radius of the dialyzer fiber is increased from 0.1 mm to 0.2 mm when Q_B = 300 ml/min and Q_D = 500 ml/min.

From **Figures 16** and **17** it is evident that the effect of increasing radius of dialyzer fiber is similar to that of increasing the length of the dialyzer fiber. However, if a case is considered where the clearance rate of Albumin is similar for length of 450 mm with a radius of 0.1 mm and radius of 0.17 mm with a length of 270 mm dialyzer fiber.

From **Table 2**, it is evident that for the same level of clearance rate of Albumin (or loss of Albumin), the dialyzer fiber with relatively higher length and lower radius shows better clearance of Urea, Glucose, Endothelin, *β*2-Microglobulin and Complement Factor D than the dialyzer fiber with relatively higher radius and lower length.

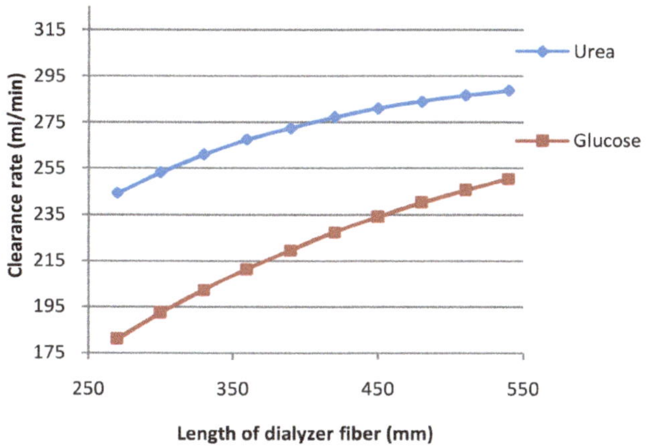

Figure 14. Clearance rate of Urea and Glucose at QB = 300ml/min and QD = 500 ml/min.

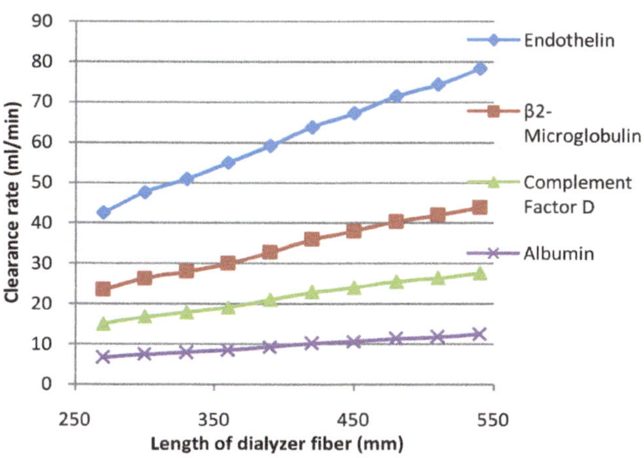

Figure 15. Clearance of Endothelin, *β*2-Microglobulin, Complement Factor D and Albumin at QB = 300 ml/min and QD = 500 ml/min.

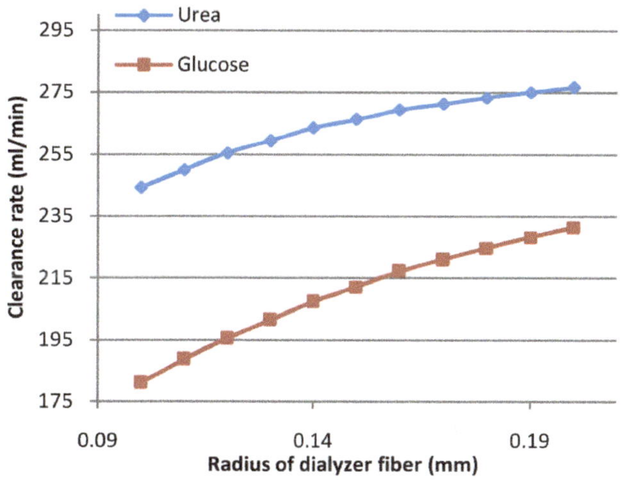

Figure 16. Clearance rate of Urea and Glucose at QB = 300 ml/min and QD = 500 ml/min.

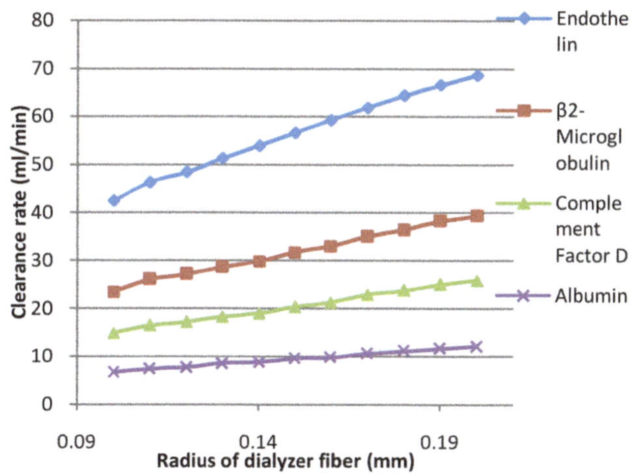

Figure 17. Clearance of Endothelin, *β*2-Microglobulin, Complement Factor D and Albumin at QB = 300 ml/min and QD = 500 ml/min.

Table 2. Clearance rate of different molecules for two dialyzer fibers consisting length = 450 mm, radius = 0.1 mm and length = 270 mm, radius = 0.17 mm.

	Length = 450 mm, Radius = 0.1 mm	Length = 270 mm, Radius = 0.17 mm
Urea	281.1	271.3
Glucose	234.1	221
Endothelin	67.21	61.8
*β*2-Microglobulin	37.97	35.05
Complement Factor D	24.04	22.92
Albumin	10.67	10.7

8. Conclusion

The clearance rate of Urea at different blood flow rate is in good agreement with the data provided by the Polyflux 210H manufacturer which ensures that the equations used to represent the phenomenon of dialysis process are reasonable. The clearance rate of small molecules—Urea and Glucose, increases rapidly with increasing blood flow rate while the clearance rate of Albumin is almost constant. Also increasing dialysate flow rate ensures further clearance of Urea and Glucose. Increasing the length or radius of the dialyzer fiber ensures better clearance of Glucose and middle molecules, such as Endothelin and $\beta 2$-Microglobulin. Moreover, increasing the length of the dialyzer fiber shows better clearance than increasing the radius of the dialyzer fiber, in the case of same amount of Albumin loss.

REFERENCES

[1] R. M. Hakim, P. J. Held, D. C. Stannard, R. A. Wolfe, F. K. Port, J. T. Daugirdas and L. Agodoa, "Effect of the Dialysis Membrane on Mortality of Chronic Hemodialysis Patients," *Kidney International*, Vol. 50, 1996, pp. 566-570. doi:10.1038/ki.1996.350

[2] M. Hayama, F. Kohori and K. Sakai, "AFM Observation of Small Surface Pores of Hollow-Fiber Dialysis Membrane Using Highly Sharpened Probe," *Journal of Membrane Science*, Vol. 197, No. 1-2, 2002, pp. 243-249. doi:10.1016/S0376-7388(01)00627-5

[3] S. R. Borzou, M. Gholyaf, M. Zandiha, R. Amini, M. T. Goodarzi and B. Torkaman, "The Effect of Increasing Blood Flow Rate on Dialysis Adequacy in Hemodialysis Patients," *Saudi Journal of Kidney Diseases and Transplantation*, Vol. 20, No. 4, 2009, pp. 639-642.

[4] A. T. Azar, "Increasing Dialysate Flow Rate Increases Dialyzer Urea Clearance and Dialysis Efficiency: An *in Vivo* Study," *Saudi Journal of Kidney Diseases and Transplantation*, Vol. 20, No. 6, 2009, pp. 1023-1029.

[5] Gambro, "Polyflux™ H–Gambro," 2013. www.gambro.com/PageFiles/7431/HCEN2489_5%20Polyflux_H.pdf?epslanguage=en

[6] T. Stocker, "Introduction to Climate Modelling," Springer, Verlag Berlin Heidelberg, 2011, p. 57. doi:10.1007/978-3-642-00773-6

[7] B. N. Preston, W. D. Comper, A. E. Hughes, I. Snook and W. V. Megen, "Diffusion of Dextran at Intermediate Concentrations," *Journal of the Chemical Society, Faraday Transactions* 1, Vol. 78, 1982, pp. 1209-1221. doi:10.1039/f19827801209

[8] R. B. Bird, W. E. Stewart and E. N. Lightfoot, "Transport Phenomena," John Wiley & Sons, Hoboken, 1960. pp. 42-46.

[9] K. Yamamoto, M. Hayama, M. Matsuda, T. Yahushiji, M. Fukuda, T. Miyasaka and K. Sakai, "Evaluation of Asymmetrical Structure Dialysis Membrane by Tortuous Capillary Pore Diffusion Model," *Journal of Membrane Science*, Vol. 287, 2007, pp. 88-93. doi:10.1016/j.memsci.2006.10.018

[10] R. Ouseph, C. A. Hutchison and R. A. Ward, "Differences in Solute Removal by Two High-Flux Membranes of Nominally Similar Synthetic Polymers," *Nephrology Dialysis Transplantation*, Vol. 23, No. 5, 2008, pp. 1704-1712. doi:10.1093/ndt/gfm916

[11] A. Hedayat, J. Szpunar, N. A. P. Kiran Kumar, R. Peace, H. Elmoselhi and A. Shoker, "Morphological Characterization of the Polyflux 210H Hemodialysis Filter Pores," *International Journal of Nephrology*, 2012. doi:10.1155/2012/304135

Intensive Antihypertensive Treatment with Angiotensin Receptor Blocker Combined with Hydrocholorthiazide Reduces Urinary Angiotensinogen in Patients with Type 2 Diabetes Mellitus*

Satoru Kuriyama, Naoki Sugano, Kohki Takane, Akimitsu Kobayashi, Yasushi Otsuka, Tatsuo Hosoya

Division of Kidney & Hypertension, Department of Internal Medicine, School of Medicine, Jikei University, Tokyo, Japan

Email: kuriyamas218@yahoo.ac.jp

ABSTRACT

Purpose: Local activation of rennin-angiotensin system (RAS) is involved in the progression of chronic kidney disease (CKD). One of the RAS components, angiotensinogen (AGT) has been known to be a potential surrogate biomarker for the renal RAS activity. Measuring the daily urinary excretion of AGT (U-AGT), the present study addressed whether the intensive blood pressure (BP) lowering with combined antihypertensive agents could improve such an abnormality in diabetic CKD patients. **Methods:** Uncontrolled hypertensive patients with type 2 diabetes with mild to moderate nephropathy previously receiving angiotensin receptor blockers (ARB) in an optimal dose alone were recruited for a better blood pressure (BP) control. Urinary specimens were subjected to a quantitative measurement of a daily urinary protein (U-prot) and U-AGT. After the baseline measurement, intensive antihypertensive therapy was attempted by switching the ARB dose to a fixed combination formula of candesartan 8 mg plus hydrochlorthiazide (HCTZ) 6.25 mg and the patients were followed up for 24 weeks. Comparison of parameters was then made between the values at the baseline and the end of the study. **Results:** At baseline, there was a significant positive correlation between U-AGT and U-prot, and between U-AGT and serum creatinine (Cr) concentration. In addition, U-AGT was inversely correlated with estimated glomerular filtration rate (e-GFR). Switching the antihypertensive regime from ARB alone to the combined ARB/HCTZ significantly reduced BP, U-AGT and U-prot. The magnitude of the reduction in U-prot was positively correlated with that in U-AGT. A stepwise regression analysis showed that HbA1c, e-GFR and the reduction in U-prot in response to the intensive antihypertensive therapy were positively correlated with the reduction in U-AGT. **Conclusion:** U-AGT is increased and positively correlated with U-prot in patients with type 2 diabetic nephropathy. Intensive antihypertensive treatment with ARB combined with HCTZ reduces both U-AGT and U-prot, presumably via an amelioration of an accelerated renal RAS activity. These data also suggest that U-AGT can be used as a potential therapeutic surrogate biomarker for the activated renal RAS in patients with diabetic nephropathy.

Keywords: Hypertension; Angiotensinogen; Proteinuria; Renin-Angiotensin System; ARB; Diabetic Nephropathy

1. Introduction

The role of the rennin-angiotensin system (RAS) in the pathophysiology of chronic renal disease (CKD) has been highlighted in relation to the local RAS activity in the kidney. Experimental studies revealed that intrarenal angiotensin II (AII) is regulated by a mechanism independent of circulating AII, and that elevated levels of intrarenal AII may link to renal functional derangement and tissue injury, leading to the progression of CKD [1,2]. Of importance is that the source of renal AII is not only derived from the systemic circulation but also from the locally formed AII substrate, angiotensinogen (AGT) [3-8]. Animal studies suggest that AGT levels in the renal tissues reflect the activity of intrarenal RAS [1-6,8]. In human, Yamamoto *et al.* showed that urinary AGT levels were elevated in patients with CKD [9]. In addition, similar results have recently demonstrated that urinary AGT levels in renal tissues are increased in human

*Conflict of interest: No conflict of interest is declared.

IgA glomerulonephritis [10,11]. These studies indicated that urinary AGT is mainly derived from the renal tissues, and that it can be used as a potential surrogate biomarker for the local RAS activity in CKD.

A plethora of reports have proven that the effective antihypertensive interventions are undoubtedly associated with a decline in urinary protein excretion, contributing to renoprotection. However, it is also obvious that treatment with RAS inhibitor, either ACEIs or ARBs, is successful in mitigating CKD in a BP independent manner [12-14]. However, reports on whether BP lowering unequivocally induces reduction in urinary AGT are still scant. Reviewing the literatures, Bakris *et al.* have shown that in order to achieve lower BP of less than 130/80 mmHg, more than two drugs are needed in most patients [15]. Indeed, many guidelines for the management of hypertension have recommended that combination of multiple antihypertensive agents with different pharmacological mode of action is more efficacious than a single agent alone in terms of renal protection [16]. The combination of an AII receptor blocker (ARB) and hydrochlorothiazide (HCTZ) has been widely recognized as a preferable prescription, because combining ARB with HCTZ exerts a complementary antihypertensive effect by suppressing RAS with the former and body fluid system with the latter, which provides a greater reduction in BP than either agent alone. A fixed combination formulation of ARB plus HCTZ may be more advantageous because of a better adherence to therapy and less side effects [17].

With the above-mentioned background taken into consideration, the present study made an attempt to investigate 1) whether abnormality exists in urinary AGT excretion in patients with type 2 diabetic nephropathy, and 2) whether the intensive antihypertensive treatment consisting of ARB plus HCTZ can improve such abnormality.

2. Patients & Methods

2.1. Patients

Enrolled in the present study were patients with type 2 diabetic nephropathy (DN) (average age: 66.4 +/− 9.7, male/female: 20/15) who agreed to participate in the collection of 24 hour urine collection for the evaluation of a daily urinary protein (U-prot) and angiotensinogen excretion (U-AGT). Patients whoes semi-quantitative measurement of urinary test was positive for proteinuria at least once were included in the study. The basic clinical characteristics of the patients enrolled are shown in **Table 1**. BP at the entry was 148 +/− 9 mmHg in systolic and 88 +/− 5 mmHg in diastolic. The diagnosis of diabetes mellitus was made based upon clinical and laboratory findings. Patients all satisfied the American Diabetes Association (ADA) diagnostic criteria of diabetes mellitus [18].

Table 1. Patient characteristics.

Age (y)	66.4 ± 9.7
Male/Female	M/F = 20/15
BMI (kg/m^2)	23.8 ± 2.8
SBP/DBP (mmHg)	148 ± 9/88 ± 5
Serum Cr (mg/dL)	2.3 ± 1.5
Hb (mg/dL)	12.2 ± 1.8
HbA1c (%)	6.1 ± 1.2
K (mEq/l)	4.6 ± 0.4
Ccr (ml/min/1.73m^2)	50.6 ± 37.4
e-GFR (ml/min/1.73m^2)	33.0 ± 20.9
U-prot (g/day)	1.5 ± 1.3
U-AGT (μg/g·Cr)	331 ± 351
U-AGT (μg/day)	386 ± 389
ARB use (%)	100
Insulin use (%)	63

2.2. Treatment Plans

The inclusion criteria were outpatients whose BP was more than 130/80mmHg despite previous antihypertensive agents (ARB alone) prescribed for more than 3 months prior to the study entry. Such ARBs had been prescribed in the optimal dose of each including candesartan 8 mg in 12 cases, losartan 50 mg in 8, ormesartan 40 mg in 8, valsartan 80 mg in 7 cases. At the entry, ARBs were switched to a single formulation tablet of candesratan 8 mg plus hydrochrolothiazide (HCTZ) 6.25 mg (Ecard HD®). These strategies were based upon an assumption that the combination therapies might exert more intense reduction in U-prot and U-AGT than ARB alone. Addition of HCTZ to ARB has been widely recommended to effectively reduce U-prot. Due to an ethical reason, drugs which are known to affect renal outcomes such as statins, anti-platelet agents, erythrocyte stimulating agents, remained unchanged throughout the study period. Dietary interventions were also kept unchanged.

The institution received prior ethics committee and or institutional review board approval (# 193), and the trial was conducted in accordance with the principles of Good Clinical Practice and the ethical principles of the concurrent Declaration of Helsinki which also protected the privacy of the patients. All patients gave written informed consent before study enrollment. Clinical trial Number by UMIN was 000001950.

2.3. Measurement of Urinary Parameters

Blood samples were obtained between 10 - 12 AM at the sitting position after more than 30 minutes rest. One day before the blood tests, 24 hours urine collection was made and samples were subjected to the quantitative measurement of a daily excretion on urinary protein and AGT. AGT was measured by a sandwich EIA method based on the theory reported elsewhere (19). The measuring plate is commercially available as a Human Total Angiotensinogen Assay Kit-IBL (Takasaki, Japan). The detection limit of this assay is estimated to be 0.30 ng/ml.

2.4. Statistical Analyses

Student t-test, the Chi-square test, and the Stepwise regression analysis were carried out with JMP 9.0 software. The computer used for the analysis was a Dynabook Satellite 2590X (Toshiba, Tokyo, Japan). Because of their skewed distribution, logarithmic transformation of AGT values was performed as the geometric means with 95% confidence intervals in some parts of the statistical analyses. Data were presented as mean +/− SD, unless otherwise indicated. A p-value of less than 0.05 was considered statistically significant.

3. Results

Figure 1 shows the effect of switching the previous treatment with ARB alone to the intensive therapy with ARB plus HCTZ on BP, U-prot (a total daily urinary excretion) and U-AGT (a total daily urinary excretion of AGT). After introducing the intensive antihypertensive therapy (so-called "treatment"), both systolic (from 148 +/− 9 to 132 +/− 5 mmHg, $p < 0.001$) and diastolic BP (from 88 +/− 5 to 82 +/− 4mmHg, $p < 0.001$) were reduced significantly. Similarly, both U-prot (from 1.5 +/− 1.3 to 1.2 +/− 0.8 g/day, $p < 0.001$) and U-AGT (from 386 +/− 389 to 208 +/− 204 μg/day, $p < 0.001$) were reduced in the majority of patients in the 24 weeks treatment period.

Figure 2 shows the relationship between pre-treatment U-AGT and U-prot. There was a close correlation between the two parameters (**Figure 1**, right). When logarithmic transformation was considered, such a correlation appeared to be more apparent (**Figure 1**, left).

Figure 3 show the relationship between pre-treatment AGT and serum Cr concentration or e-GFR. There was a significant positive correlation between serum Cr concentration and pre-treatment U-AGT, and in exchange negative correlation between serum Cr concentration and e-GFR.

Figure 4 shows relationship between the reduction ratio of a daily urinary protein excretion (ΔU-prot) and that of a daily urinary excretion of AGT (ΔU-AGT), in response the intensive antihypertensive treatment. The former was significantly positively correlated with the latter.

Figure 5 shows relationship between the total amount of the reduced daily urinary excretion (U-prot, plotted in the X-axis) and the ratio of the reduction in a daily urinary excretion of AGT (ΔU-AGT, plotted in the Y-axis). Similar to **Figure 2**, the former was significantly positively correlated with the latter.

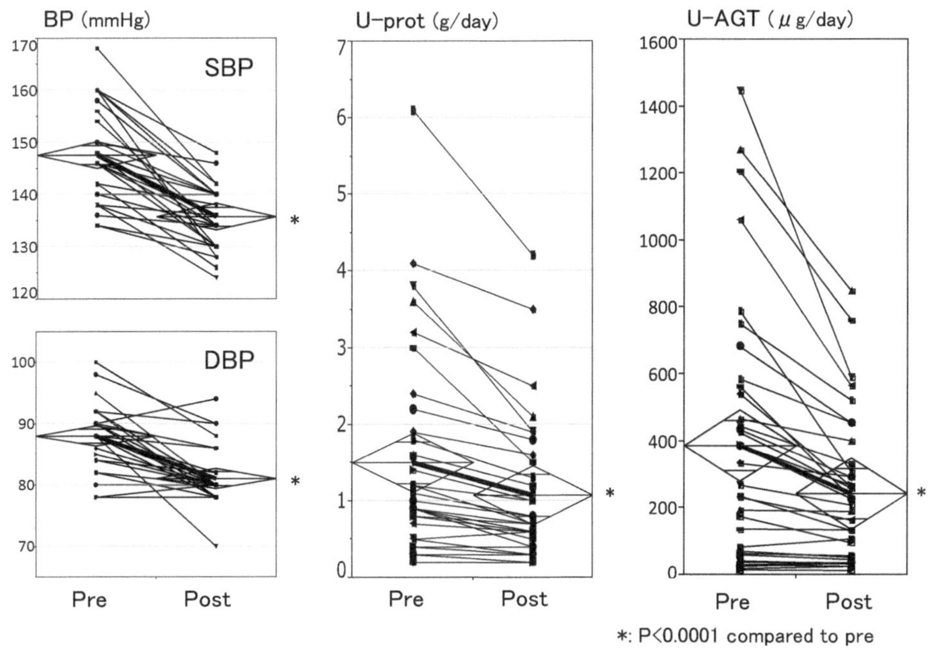

Figure 1. Effect of intensive antihypertensive therapy with ARB/HCTZ.

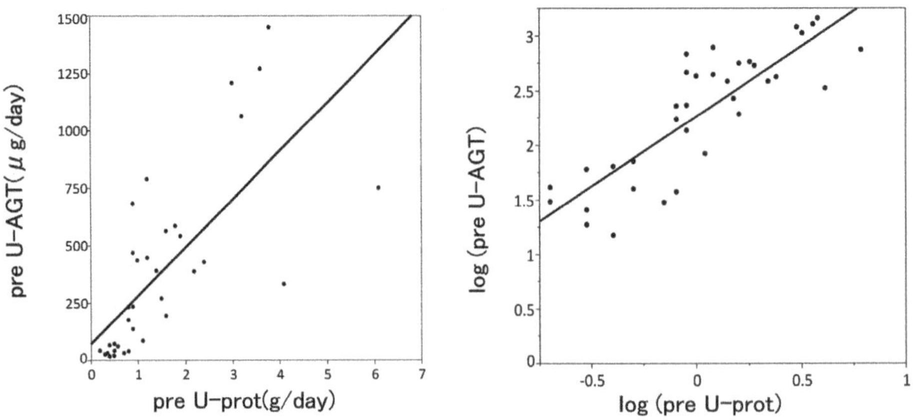

y = 210x +71.5, r=0.72, P<0.0001 y = 1.28x+ 2.27, r=0.84, P<0.0001

Figure 2. Relationship between preU-AGT and preU-prot.

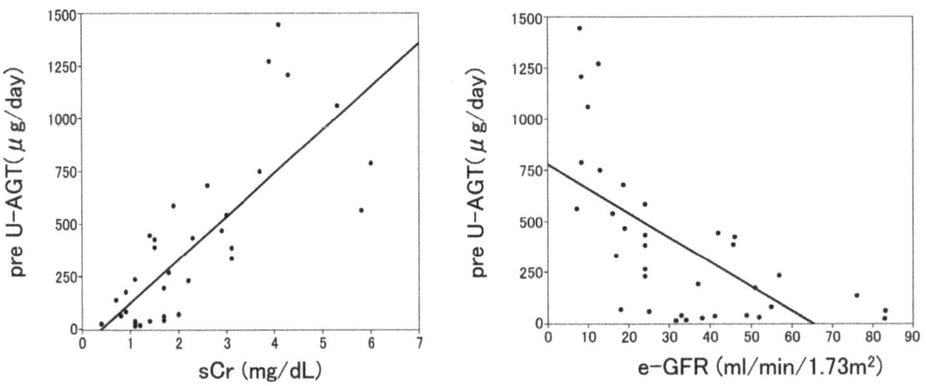

y = 206x −79.3 , r =0.78 , P<0.0001 y = −11.9x+ 779, r = −0.63 , P<0.0001

Figure 3. Relationship between preU-AGT and Cr, and preU-AGT and e-GFR.

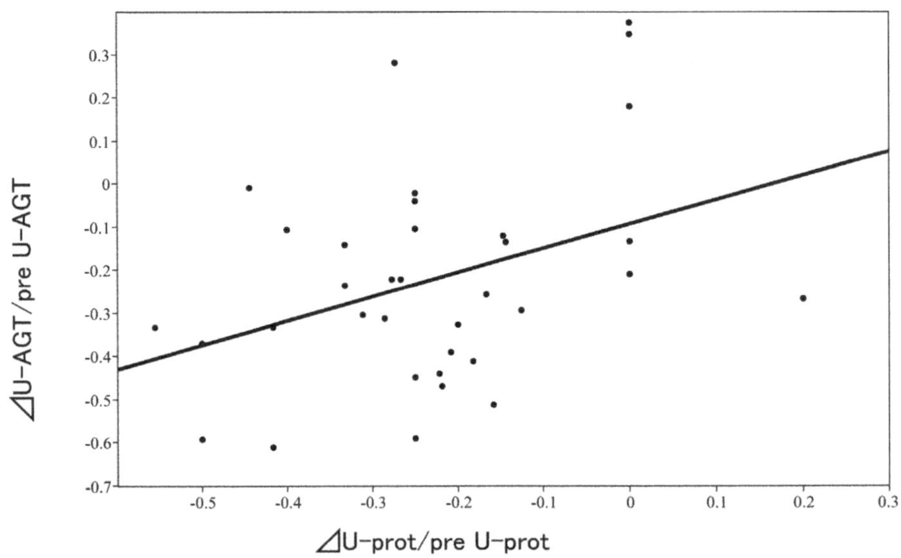

y = 0.561x −0.092 , r = 0.3733, P=0.027

Figure 4. Relationship between ΔU-AGT ratio and ΔU-prot ratio.

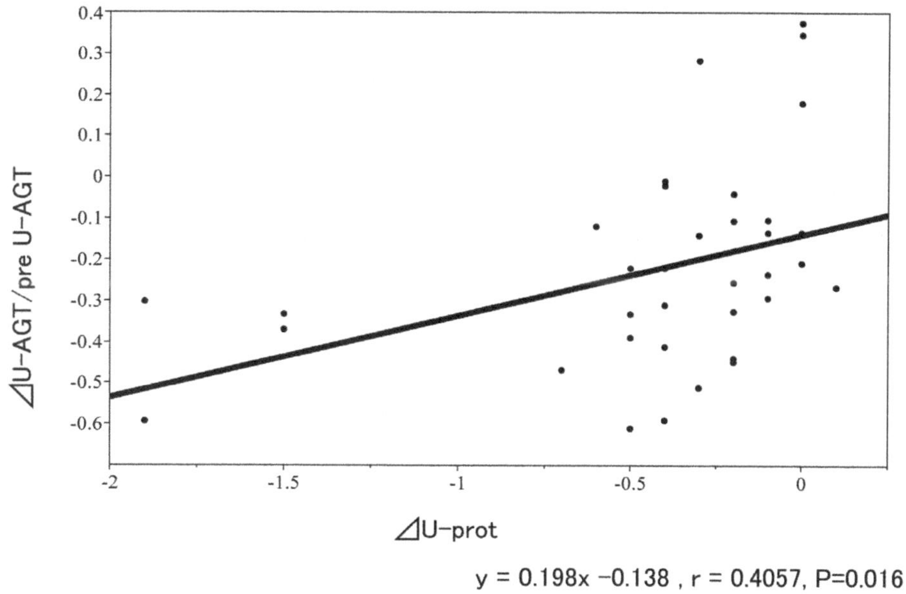

Figure 5. Relationship between ΔU-AGT ratio and ΔU-prot.

Table 2 shows the result of a stepwise regression analysis to explain pre-treatment value of U-AGT. The factors affecting such values were predicted to be pre-treatment U-prot, HbA1c and e-GFR.

Table 3 shows the result of a stepwise regression analysis to explain the reduction in U-AGT. Such predictors include the reduction in U-prot, e-GFR and HbA1c.

4. Discussion

This clinical study presented two major findings. First, U-AGT is substantially increased and positively correlated with U-prot in patients with mild to moderate type 2 diabetic nephropathy, suggesting that this biomarker can be used as a potential surrogate marker for the renal RAS. Second, intensive antihypertensive treatment with ARB plus HCTZ reduces both U-AGT and U-ptot, suggesting that intensive BP lowering may ameliorate an accelerated activity of renal RAS.

Table 2. A stepwise regression analysis to explain pre U-AGT.

Parameters	β value	F	p-value
U-prot (pre)	151.5	24.3	$2.86e^{-5}$
HbA1c	91.55	9.6	0.00419
e-GFR	−5.86	8.7	0.00601
DBP	13.9	3.9	0.0574

Table 3. A stepwise regression analysis to explain ΔU-AGT.

Parameters	β value	F	p-value (p > F)
ΔU-prot	205.6	20.5	$8.15e^{-5}$
e-GFR	2.84	7.2	0.01161
HbA1c	−37.54	5.2	0.03011

4.1. Urinary AGT as a Biomarker for Renal RAS

Notwithstanding that a part of the activity of systemic RAS can be clinically assessed as plasma renin activity (PRA), up until several years ago there was no accurate surrogate biomarker to estimate the activity of the local RAS in the kidney. Assessment of intrarenal RAS status is essential to understand the mechanisms that mediate the pathophysiology of renal function and injury [1,2]. Recent preclinical evidence suggests that intrarenal RAS activity is regulated by changes in local AGT levels [1-4] and that urinary excretion of AGT reflects intrarenal AGT production [3-8]. Following the substantial amount of animal experiments showing that U-AGT can be a new marker of intrarenal RAS status, similar results on the clinical significance of U-AGT have emerged from human studies in patients with CKD including type 1 diabetics with early stage nephropathy and primary glomerulonephritis [9-11,19-21]. Considering that all of those human studies were performed measuring U-AGT levels in a semi-quantitative way, not quantifying the total amount of daily excretion of AGT, the present study carried out quantitative measurement of a 24-hour daily protein excretion and AGT for the purpose of evaluating U-AGT status with more accuracy.

Inasmuch as the present finding does not address "cause & effect" scenario, a close association of U-AGT with U-prot confirms that U-AGT can be used as a biomarker for the increase renal RAS activity. Saito *et al.* demonstrated that urinary AGT levels are increased in type 1diabetic subjects and that the early dissociation between urinary albumin levels and AGT levels may imply increased urinary AGT levels precede increased urinary albumin levels. They proposed that urinary AGT levels may serve as a sensitive early marker for intrarenal RAS activity and can be one of the earliest predictors of diabetic nephropathy in diabetic patients [19]. Similarly, in type 2 diabetic patients, increased urinary levels of AGT have accumulated [20,21]. The mechanisms by which the up-regulated renal AGT has a deleterious effect on renal tissue can be accounted for by the high glucose milieu in diabetic nephropathy, leading to an overproduction of local AII [22].

As to the urinary protein excretion which sometimes reaches the range of nephrotic syndrome in overt diabetic nephropathy, concerns remain about the urinary leakage of AGT from the systemic circulation. However, this is very unlikely because a large molecular weight (MW) substance like AGT, a precursor of AII, (MW: 50 - 60 kDa) in the systemic circulation hardly penetrates basal membrane of glomeruli of the kidney. Indeed, to determine if circulating AGT is a source of urinary AGT, Kobori *et al.* infused human AGT into hypertensive and normotensive rats [6]. However, human AGT was detectable in plasma but not detectable in the urine of rats, indicating quite limited glomerular permeability and/or tubular degradation. In addition, Katsurada *et al.* found that there was a strong correlation between urinary AGT levels and urinary protein levels, but no link was found between plasma AGT and urinary protein levels [23].

In non-diabetic population, Nishiyama *et al.* reported that urinary AGT levels were higher in IgA nephropathy patients than in healthy volunteers and that treatment with an ARB reduced AGT levels, suggesting the significance of urinary AGT as a potential biomarker for local RAS in the kidney [24]. Jang *et al.* also reported that urinary AGT level reflects intrarenal AGT expression and correlates with the extent of proteinuria and renal function, indicating the intrarenal compartment as the main source of urinary AGT in proteinuric IgA nephropathy patients [25]. Recently, Kim *et al.* also support that urinary AGT is a biomarker in patients with IgA nephropathy [26]. These findings strongly endorse the hypothesis that urinary AGT is derived from the AGT produced and secreted by renal tissue, probably the proximal tubules, and is undoubtedly not from plasma. These observations are in good accordance with our present findings and reinforce the notion that urinary AGT is a potential novel biomarker of the intrarenal RAS in CKD patients.

4.2. Effect of Intensive Antihypertensive Treatment on Urinary AGT

Many reports have shown that effective antihypertensive interventions are associated with a decline in U-prot, and contribute to renoprotection [27-31]. However, it is also obvious that treatment with RAS inhibitor, either ACEIs or ARBs, is successful in mitigating CKD in a BP independent manner [10-12]. Although clinical studies to observe the effects of ARB on urinary AGT are scarce and a matter of controversy, it appears that ARB reduces urinary AGT in most of the studies [19-21,24]. There was one controversial report that did not show any association between urinary AGT levels and BP lowering with ARB or ACE-I [32].

The majority of guidelines for the management of hypertension have recommended that combination of multiple antihypertensive agents with different pharmacological mode of action is more efficacious than a single agent alone in terms of renal protection [16,33,34]. Combining ARB with HCTZ exerts a complementary pharmacological effect by suppressing RAS with the former and body fluid system with the latter. A fixed combination formulation of ARB plus HCTZ may be more advantageous because of a better adherence to therapy. Hosoya *et al.* have reported that after switching from the preceding antihypertensive treatment with ARB alone a fixed combination formula tablet of losartan and HCTZ efficiently reduced BP, albumin-creatinine ratio (ACR) and B-type natriuretic peptide (BNP), suggesting that intensive therapy with ARB plus HCTZ has a beneficial effect not only on kidney function but also on cardiac protection [17]. Using the similar clinical interventional method, the present study clarified that the switching therapy from ARB alone to a fixed combination formula of ARB plus HCTZ is effective in reducing in both U-AGT and U-prot.

Whether urinary AGT is a superior biomarker to the recently-reported other urinary RAS components (AII, aldosterone and renin) is still a matter for debate, and future studies will disclose which one would be an appropriate marker to more accurately estimate local RAS activity.

4.3. Limitation of the Study

There are several limitations in this exploratory study. A larger number of patients and a longer observation period with a contol-based prospective design must be carried out in the future evaluation on the role of urinary AGT.

In summary, the present study indicates that increase in urinary AGT is correlated well with urinary protein excretion in patients with type 2 diabetic nephropathy and that intensive antihypertensive treatment ameliorates such abnormalities. These data support the notion that urinary AGT is a potential tool for the determination of intrarenal RAS status and is associated with renal derangement.

5. Acknowledgement

A part of this work was presented at the 55th Annual Meeting of the Japanese Society of Nephrology held in Tokyo, Japan, on June 1st, 2012.

REFERENCES

[1] L. G. Navar, L. M. Harrison-Bernard, A. Nishiyama and H. Kobori, "Regulation of Intrarenal Angiotensin II in Hypertension," *Hypertension*, Vol. 39, 2002, pp. 316-322. doi:10.1161/hy0202.103821

[2] H. Kobori, M. Nangaku, L. G. Navar and A. Nishiyama, "The Intrarenal Renin-Angiotensin System: From Physiology to the Pathobiology of Hypertension and Kidney Disease," *Pharmacological Reviews*, Vol. 59, No. 3, 2007, pp. 251-287. doi:10.1124/pr.59.3.3

[3] H. Kobori, Y. Ozawa, Y. Suzaki, M. C. Prieto-Carrasquero, A. Nishiyama, T. Shoji, E. P. Cohen and L. G. Navar, "Young Scholars Award Lecture: Intratubular Angiotensinogen in Hypertension and Kidney Diseases," *American Journal of Hypertension*, Vol. 19, No. 5, 2006, pp. 541-550. doi:10.1016/j.amjhyper.2005.11.014

[4] H. Kobori, Y. Ozawa, R. Satou, A. Katsurada, K. Miyata, N. Ohashi, N. Hase, Y. Suzaki, C. D. Sigmund and L. G. Navar, "Kidney-Specific Enhancement of ANG II Stimulates Endogenous Intrarenal Angiotensinogen in Genetargeted Mice," *American Journal of Physiology—Renal Physiology*, Vol. 293, No. 3, 2007, pp. F938-F945. doi:10.1152/ajprenal.00146.2007

[5] H. Kobori, L. M. Harrison-Bernard and L. G. Navar, "Urinary Excretion of Angiotensinogen Reflects Intrarenal Angiotensinogen Production," *Kidney International*, Vol. 61, 2002, pp. 579-585. doi:10.1046/j.1523-1755.2002.00155.x

[6] H. Kobori, A. Nishiyama, L. M. Harrison-Bernard and L. G. Navar, "Urinary Angiotensinogen as an Indicator of Intrarenal Angiotensin Status in Hypertension," *Hypertension*, Vol. 41, 2003, pp. 42-49. doi:10.1161/01.HYP.0000050102.90932.CF

[7] H. Kobori, A. B. Alper Jr., R. Shenava, A. Katsurada, T. Saito, N. Ohashi, M. Urushihara, K. Miyata, R. Satou, L. L. Hamm and L. G. Navar, "Urinary Angiotensinogen as a Novel Biomarker of the Intrarenal Renin-Angiotensin System Status in Hypertensive Patients," *Hypertension*, Vol. 53, 2009, pp. 344-350. doi:10.1161/HYPERTENSIONAHA.108.123802

[8] H. Kobori, Y. Ozawa, Y. Suzaki and A. Nishiyama, "Enhanced Intrarenal Angiotensinogen Contributes to Early Renal Injury in Spontaneously Hypertensive Rats," *Journal of the American Society of Nephrology*, Vol. 16, No. 7, 2005, pp. 2073-2080. doi:10.1681/ASN.2004080676

[9] T. Yamamoto, T. Nakagawa, H. Suzuki, N. Ohashi, H. Fukasawa, Y. Fujigaki, A. Kato, Y. Nakamura, F. Suzuki and A. Hishida, "Urinary Angiotensinogen as a Marker of Intrarenal Angiotensin II Activity Associated with Deterioration of Renal Function in Patients with Chronic Kidney Disease," *Journal of the American Society of Nephrology*, Vol. 18, No. 5, 2007, pp. 1558-1565. doi:10.1681/ASN.2006060554

[10] H. Kobori, A. Katsurada, Y. Ozawa, R. Satou, K. Miyata, N. Hase, Y. Suzaki and T. Shoji, "Enhanced Intrarenal Oxidative Stress and Angiotensinogen in IgA Nephropathy Patients," *Biochemical and Biophysical Research Communications*, Vol. 358, No. 1, 2007, pp. 156-163. doi:10.1016/j.bbrc.2007.04.105

[11] M. Takamatsu, M. Urushihara, S. Kondo, M. Shimizu, T. Morioka, T. Oite, H. Kobori and S. Kagami, "Glomerular Angiotensinogen Protein Is Enhanced in Pediatric IgA Nephropathy," *Pediatric Nephrology*, Vol. 23, No. 8, 2008, pp. 1257-1267. doi:10.1007/s00467-008-0801-6

[12] D. Russo, R. Minutolo, A. Pisani, R. Esposito, G. Signoriello, M. Andreucci and M. M. Balletta, "Coadministration of Losartan and Enalapril Exerts Additive Antiproteinuric Effect in IgA Nephropathy," *American Journal of Kidney Diseases*, Vol. 38, No. 1, 2001, pp. 18-25. doi:10.1053/ajkd.2001.25176

[13] K. F. Hilgers and J. F. Mann, "ACE Inhibitors versus AT(1) Receptor Antagonists in Patients with Chronic Renal Disease," *Journal of the American Society of Nephrology*, Vol. 13, No. 4, 2002, pp. 1100-1108.

[14] R. Coppo, L. Peruzzi, A. Amore, A. Piccoli, P. Cochat, R. Stone, M. Kirschstein and T. Linné, "IgACE: A Placebo-Controlled, Randomized Trial of Angiotensin-Converting Enzyme Inhibitors in Children and Young People with IgA Nephropathy and Moderate Proteinuria," *Journal of the American Society of Nephrology*, Vol. 18, No. 6, 2007, pp. 1880-1888. doi:10.1681/ASN.2006040347

[15] G. L. Bakris, M. Williams, L. Dworkin, W. J. Elliott, M. Epstein, R. Toto, K. Tuttle, J. Douglas, W. Hsueh and J. Sower, "Preserving Renal Function on Adults with Hypertension ans Diabetes: A Consensus Approach. National Kidney Foundation Hypertension and Diabetes Executive Committees Working Group," *American Journal of Kidney Diseases*, Vol. 36, No. 3, 2000, pp. 646-661. doi:10.1053/ajkd.2000.16225

[16] B. Waeber, "Achieving Blood Pressure Targets in the Management of Hypertension," *Blood Pressure*, Vol. 10, No. 2, 2001, pp. 6-12. doi:10.1080/080370501750275839-1

[17] T. Hosoya, S. Kuriyama, I. Ohno, T. Kawamura, M. Ogura, M. Ikeda, M. Ishikawa, F. Hayashi, T. Kanai, H. Tomonari, M. Soejima, K. Akaba and G. Tokudome, "Antihypertensive Effect of a Fixed-Dose Combination of Losartan/Hydrochlorothiazide in Patients with Uncontrolled Hypertension: A Multicenter Study," *Clinical and Experimental Nephrology*, Vol. 16, No. 2, 2012, pp. 269-278. doi:10.1007/s10157-011-0564-4

[18] American Diabetes Association, "Diagnosis and Classification of Diabetes Mellitus," *Diabetes Care*, Vol. 35, Suppl. 1, 2012, pp. s64-s71. doi:10.2337/dc12-s064

[19] T. Saito, M. Urushihara, Y. Kotani, S. Kagami and H. Kobori, "Increased Urinary Angiotensinogen Is Precedent

to Increased Urinary Albumin in Patients with Type 1 Diasbetes," *The American Journal of the Medical Sciences*, Vol. 338, 2009, pp. 478-480. doi:10.1097/MAJ.0b013e3181b90c25

[20] S. Ogawa, H. Kobori, N. Ohashi, M. Urushihara, A. Nishiyama, T. Mori, T. Ishizuka, K. Nako and S. Ito, "Angiotensin II Type 1 Receptor Blockers Reduce Urinary Angiotensinogen Excretion and the Levels of Urinary Markers of Oxidative Stress and Inflammation in Patients with Type 2 Diabetic Nephropathy," *Biomark Insights*, Vol. 4, 2009, pp. 97-102.

[21] M. Sawaguchi, S. I. Araki, H. Kobori, M. Urushihara, M. Haneda, D. Koya, A. Kashiwagi, T. Uzu and H. Maegawa, "Association between Urinary Angiotensinogen Levels and Renal and Cardiovascular Prognoses in Patients with Type 2 Diabetes Mellitus," *Journal of Diabetes Investigation*, Vol. 3, No. 3, 2012, pp. 318-324.

[22] D. E. Casarini, "Upregulation of Intrarenal Angiotensinogen in Diabetes," *Hypertension Research*, Vol. 33, 2010, pp. 1174-1181. doi:10.1038/hr.2010.163

[23] A. Katsurada, Y. Hagiwara, K. Miyashita, R. Satou, K. Miyata, N. Ohashi, L. G. Navar and H. Kobori, "Novel Sandwich ELISA for Human Angiotensinogen," *American Journal of Physiology—Renal Physiology*, Vol. 293, No. 3, 2007, pp. F956-F960. doi:10.1152/ajprenal.00090.2007

[24] A. Nishiyama, Y. Konishi, N. Ohasi, T. Morikawa, M. Urushihara, I. Maeda, M. Hamada, M. Kishida, H. Hitomi, N. Shirahashi, H. Kobori and M. Imanishi, "Urinary Angiotensinogen Reflects the Activity of Intrarenal Renin Angiotensin System in Patients with IgA Nephropathy," *Nephrology Dialysis Transplantation*, Vol. 26, No. 1, 2011, pp. 170-177. doi:10.1093/ndt/gfq371

[25] H. R. Jang, S. M. Kim, Y. J. Lee, J. E. Lee, W. Huh, D. J. Kim, H. Y. Oh and Y. G. Kim, "The Origin and the Clinical Significance of Urinary Angiotensinogen in Proteinuric IgA Nephropathy Patients," *Annals of Internal Medicine*, 2011.

[26] Y. G. Kim, S. B. Song, S. H. Lee, J. Y. Moon, K. H. Jeong, T. W. Lee and C. G. Ihm, "Urinary Angiotensinogen as a Predictive Marker in Patients with Immunoglobulin A Nephropathy," *Clinical and Experimental Nephrology*, Vol. 15, No. 5, 2011, pp. 720-726. doi:10.1007/s10157-011-0475-4

[27] B. M. Brenner, M. E. Cooper, D. de Zeeuw, W. F. Keane, W. E. Mitch, H. H. Parving, G. Remuzzi, S. M. Snapinn, Z. Zhang and S. Shahinfar, "Effects of Losartan on Renal and Cardiovascular Outcomes in Patients with Type 2 Diabetes and Nephropathy," *New England Journal of Medicine*, Vol. 345, 2001, pp. 861-869. doi:10.1056/NEJMoa011161

[28] H. H. Parving, H. Lehnert, J. Bröchner-Mortensen, R. Gomis, S. Andersen and P. Arner, "Irbesartan in Patients with Type 2 Diabetes and Microalbuminuria Study Group. The Effect of Irbesartan on the Development of Diabetic Nephropathy in Patients with Type 2 Diabetes," *New England Journal of Medicine*, Vol. 345, 2001, pp. 870-878. doi:10.1056/NEJMoa011489

[29] H. Makino, M. Haneda, T. Babazono, T. Moriya, S. Ito, Y. Iwamoto, R. Kawamori, M. Takeuchi and S. Katayama, "Prevention of Transition from Incipient to Overt Nephropathy with Telmisartan in Patients with Type 2 Diabetes," *Diabetes Care*, Vol. 30, No. 6, 2007, pp. 1577-1578. doi:10.2337/dc06-1998

[30] G. Viberti and N. M. Wheeldon, "MicroAlbuminuria Reduction with VALsartan (MARVAL) Study Investigators. Microalbuminuria Reduction with Valsartan in Patients with Type 2 Diabetes Mellitus: A Blood Pressure-Independent Effect," *Circulation*, Vol. 106, 2002, pp. 672-678. doi:10.1161/01.CIR.0000024416.33113.0A

[31] G. Mancia, G. De Backer, A. Dominiczak, R. Cifkova, R. Fagard, G. Germano, G. Grassi, A. M. Heagerty, S. E. Kjeldsen, S. Laurent, K. Narkiewicz, L. Ruilope, A. Rynkiewicz, R. E. Schmieder, H. A. Boudier, A. Zanchetti, A. Vahanian, J. Camm, R. De Caterina, V. Dean, K. Dickstein, G. Filippatos, C. Funck-Brentano, I. Hellemans, S. D. Kristensen, K. McGregor, U. Sechtem, S. Silber, M. Tendera, P. Widimsky, J. L. Zamorano, S. Erdine, W. Kiowski, E. Agabiti-Rosei, E. Ambrosioni, L. H. Lindholm, M. Viigimaa, S. Adamopoulos, E. Agabiti-Rosei, E. Ambrosioni, V. Bertomeu, D. Clement, S. Erdine, C. Farsang, D. Gaita, G. Lip, J. M. Mallion, A. J. Manolis, P. M. Nilsson, E. O'Brien, P. Ponikowski, J. Redon, F. Ruschitzka, J. Tamargo, P. van Zwieten, B. Waeber and B. Williams, "Management of Arterial Hypertension of the European Society of Hypertension; European Society of Cardiology. 2007 Guidelines for the Management of Arterial Hypertension: The Task Force for the Management of Arterial Hypertension of the European Society of Hypertension (ESH) and of the European Society of Cardiology (ESC)," *Journal of Hypertension*, Vol. 25, 2007, pp. 1105-1187. doi:10.1097/HJH.0b013e3281fc975a

[32] M. van den Heuvel, W. W. Batenburg, S. Jainandunsing, I. M. Garrelds, J. M. G. van Gool, R. A. Feelders, A. H. van den Meiracker and A. H. Jan Danser, "Urinary Renin, but Not Angiotensinogen or Aldosterone, Reflects the Renal Renin-Angiotensin-Aldosterone System Activity and the Efficacy of Renin-Angiotensin-Aldosterone System Blockade in the Kidney," *Journal of Hypertension*, Vol. 29, 2011, pp. 2147-2155. doi:10.1097/HJH.0b013e32834bbcbf

[33] T. Ogihara, K. Kikuchi, H. Matsuoka, T. Fujita, J. Higaki, M. Horiuchi, Y. Imai, T. Imaizumi, S. Ito, H. Iwao, K. Kario, Y. Kawano, S. Kim-Mitsuyama, G. Kimura, H. Matsubara, H. Matsuura, M. Naruse, I. Saito, K. Shimada, K. Shimamoto, H. Suzuki, S. Takishita, N. Tanahashi, T. Tsuchihashi, M. Uchiyama, S. Ueda, H. Ueshima, S. Umemura, T. Ishimitsu and H. Rakugi, "The Japanese Society of Hypertension Guidelines for the Management of Hypertension (JSH 2009)," *Hypertension Research*, Vol. 32, 2009, pp. 11-23. doi:10.1038/hr.2009.34

[34] A. V. Chobanian, G. L. Bakris, H. R. Black, W. C. Cushman, L. A. Green, J. L. Izzo Jr., D. W. Jones, B. J. Materson, S. Oparil, J. T. Wright Jr. and E. J. Roccella, "National Heart, Lung, and Blood Institute Joint National Committee on Prevention, Detection, Evaluation, and Treatment of High Blood Pressure; National High Blood Pressure Education Program Coordinating Committee. The Seventh Report of the Joint National Committee on Prevention, Detection, Evaluation, and Treatment of High Blood Pressure: The JNC 7 Report," *JAMA*, Vol. 289, No. 19, 2003, pp. 2560-2572. doi:10.1001/jama.289.19.2560

12

Variability of Serum Concentration of Calcium, Phosphate and Parathyroid Hormone Depending on Time of Blood Draw for Patients on Nocturnal Home Hemodialysis*

Nasim Shahbazi[1], Pierre A. Brown[2], Ayub Akbari[2,3], Deborah L. Zimmerman[2,3]
[1]Department of Medicine, Division of Nephrology, Thunder Bay Regional Health Sciences Centre, Thunder Bay, Canada
[2]Department of Medicine, Division of Nephrology, Ottawa Hospital, Ottawa, Canada
[3]Kidney Research Centre, Ottawa Hospital Research Institute, Ottawa, Canada
Email: dzimmerman@ottawahospital.on.ca

ABSTRACT

Background: Guidelines for patients treated with conventional hemodialysis patients have been written for target serum levels for calcium (Ca), phosphate (PO_4) and intact parathyroid hormone (iPTH). No guidelines exist for nocturnal home hemodialysis (NHHD) patients for target values or timing of the blood sample draw. We undertook a prospective cohort study to examine the variability in pre, post and clinic (post-post) serum values for Ca, PO_4, and iPTH in NHHD patients to determine if timing of blood draw could affect clinical decisions. **Methods:** Twenty prevalent NHHD patients collected blood pre and post their usual NHHD session with an additional blood sample drawn in clinic (post-post). Median and interquartile range of pre, post and clinic (post-post) values of iPTH, PO_4 and Ca were calculated and compared with Freidman/Wilcoxon test. Serum concentrations were also categorized according to Canadian Society of Nephrology (CSN) guidelines target values for pre and clinic (post-post) samples. The proportion of patients that would be categorized differently by clinic (post-post) samples was determined. **Results:** There was a significant difference between pre-serum values compared to post and clinic (post-post) values. Overall, iPTH, PO_4 and Ca values would be misclassified in 25%, 70% and 50%, respectively if blood was drawn at the clinic visit (post-post) compared to pre-HD as per CSN guidelines. **Conclusions:** Although no specific guideline has been written for NHHD patients, to ensure consistency of management compared to in-centre HD patients, lab values should be drawn pre-HD until clinical evidence suggests that the recommendations should be different for NHHD.

Keywords: Nocturnal Hemodialysis; Calcium; Phosphate; Parathyroid Hormone

1. Introduction

Conventional in-centre hemodialysis (HD) is the most common dialysis modality used to treat patients with end-stage renal disease (ESRD). Despite the widespread acceptance of conventional in-centre HD as the standard of care, patients experience a poor quality of life and have a higher mortality rate compared to general population [1]. In an attempt to reduce morbidity and mortality, a few novel approaches that increase dialysis frequency and/or time have been introduced. Nocturnal home HD is one such modality in which patients typically undergo HD for 3 - 6 nights per week for greater than 5 hours per treatment. This type of HD is associated with an improvement in blood pressure, regression of left ventricular hypertrophy [2] and an improvement in quality of life [3]. Improvements in the control of mineral metabolism parameters such as a decrease in serum phosphate and decrease in the use phosphate binders have also been reported [2,4].

Despite the benefits of nocturnal home hemodialysis, this modality is not without its own challenges for both patients and healthcare providers [5]. One such challenge is the timing of blood draw for laboratory analysis and clinician interpretation of the results. Some HD guidelines have emphasized that target levels for bone mineral markers such as calcium (Ca), phosphate (PO_4) and intact parathyroid hormone (iPTH) be based on samples drawn pre-HD [6]. Since no specific guidelines regarding optimal timing of blood sampling has been published for home nocturnal HD patients, most programs encourage pre-post HD blood collection to be done at home. However, there is variability in this practice pattern in different Canadian centres providing care for nocturnal home

*Conflicts of interest: None of the investigators have any conflicts of interest with respect to this study. The manuscript has not been published previously in whole or in part except in abstract form (WCN 2011).

HD patients based on a Canadian Practice patterns survey. Of the 17 program directors who responded to our survey, a centrifuge was not supplied by 3 programs and a further 3 programs only sometimes provide centrifuges (not published). The reasons cited included cost and patient inconvenience/preference.

To our knowledge, no study has been performed to determine if different clinical decisions would be made in the management of mineral metabolism abnormalities based on the timing of blood sample draw in relationship to the HD treatment in nocturnal home HD patients. Therefore, we conducted a prospective cohort study to examine the variability in pre, post and clinic (post-post) serum values for Ca, PO_4 and iPTH in nocturnal home hemodialysis patients to determine if they were statistically and/or clinically different. The study was approved by The Ottawa Hospital Research Ethics Board.

2. Materials and Methods

Twenty prevalent adult nocturnal home HD patients from our tertiary care centre participated in the study. Patients included were over 18 years old and treated for at least 18 hours/week HD (minimum 6 hours per treatment, 3 days per week). Patients with a successful parathyroid-dectomy (iPTH less that 10 pmol/L) were excluded.

After signing informed consent, patients collected blood pre and post their usual Tuesday nocturnal home HD session. Pre-dialysis samples are collected directly from the arterial needle or catheter lumen prior to initiation of treatment. For post-dialysis samples immediately prior to rinseback, the dialysate flow and the ultrafiltration are turned off. Blood pump speed is reduced to 100 mls/min for 15 seconds; the blood sample is drawn with a vacutainer needle and tube directly from the arterial port. The samples were centrifuged and stored in the patient's fridge overnight. An additional blood sample was collected in clinic on Wednesday (clinic sample or post-post). All samples were analyzed in the Ottawa Hospital laboratory in accordance with the Ottawa Hospital laboratory guidelines. iPTH was analyzed with Beckman Coulter Immunoassay analyzer (coefficient of variation for iPTH; 6.9% at 2.6 pmol/L, 6.9% at 19.9 pmol/L and 5.8% at 59.3 pmol/L). Ca and PO_4 were analyzed with Siemens Vista 1500 analyzer (coefficient of variation for Ca; 2.63% at 1.42 mmol/L, and 2.1% at 2.5 mmol/L, coefficient of variation for PO_4; 3.4% at 0.6 mmol/L and 2.4% at 1.2 mmol/L).

Median and interquartile range of pre, post and clinic (post-post) values of iPTH, PO_4 and Ca were determined. The difference in pre, post and clinic (post-post) samples was examined with Freidman/Wilcoxon test. We also categorized values in each sample of pre and clinic (post-post), as within target and out of target as per Canadian Society of Nephrology guidelines and determined the proportion of patients that were categorized differently by clinic (post-post) samples.

3. Results

The majority of patients were male (60%) with a mean age of 47 years (**Table 1**). The median hemodialysis treatment time was 7.5 hours (IQR 6 - 8 hrs) for the study session and the median interval between pre-HD bloodwork, and clinic (post-post) HD bloodwork was 11.7 hours (IQR 10.7 - 14 hrs). Median time from post-HD bloodwork and post-post HD blood sampling was 5.3 hours (IQR 2.9 - 6.2 hours). Calcium concentration in the dialysate ranged between 1.25 and 1.75 mmol/L (mean 1.45 mmol/L). Six patients (30%) had phosphate added to their dialysate and 6 patients (30%) were taking phosphate binders; either Calcium carbonate or Sevelamer. Nine patients (45%) were taking Calcitriol and 2 patients were also taking Cinacalcet. The majority of patients (9 out of 20, 55%) were using the Fresenius Optiflux 160 or 200 dialyzer, 6 patients (30%) were using the Fresenius F16 dialyzer and 1 patient each (5%) was using the Baxter Exeltra 190 and the Fresenius F6 dialyzer.

Median and interquartile range of pre, post and clinic (post-post) values of iPTH, PO_4 and Ca are shown in **Figures 1-3**. Median pre-HD Ca, PO_4, iPTH values were significantly different compared to median postHD calcium, phosphate and iPTH values respectively. The same was true comparing median pre-HD values with clinic (post-post) values (**Table 2**).

The serum values of iPTH, PO_4 and Ca were also clinically different depending on when the blood sample was drawn (**Tables 3-8**). Overall in our 20 NHHD patients, iPTH, PO4, Ca and values would be misclassified in 25%, 70% and 50% respectively if blood was drawn at the clinic visit (post-post) compared to pre-HD as per target values based on Canadian Society of Nephrology mineral metabolism guidelines. Similarly, if blood was only drawn post-HD, iPTH, PO_4, and Ca values would be misclassified in 40%, 80% and 45% compared to pre-HD values.

Table 1. Baseline characteristics.

Age (years)	47.1 (13.9)
Gender (M:F)	12:8
Cause of ESRD ("N")	GN (9), HTN (2), DM (1), Other (4), Unknown (4)
Number of treatments per week ("N")	3 (4), 4 (3) 5 (6), 6 (7)
Blood pump speed (mls/min)	338 (51)
Dialysate flow (mls/min)	350 (83)
Treatment duration in hours ("N")	6 (6), 7 (1) 8 (12), 9 (1)

Table 2. Median and interquartile range of pre, post and clinic (post-post) values of iPTH, PO_4 and Ca.

	Pre HD median, IQR	**Post HD** median, IQR	**Post post HD** median, IQR	**Pre HD vs post HD**	**Pre HD vs post post HD**
Ca	2.27 (2.12 - 2.32)	2.40 (2.24 - 2.51)	2.41 (2.27 - 2.46)	<0.001	<0.001
PO_4	1.62 (1.18 - 2.06)	0.82 (0.73 - 1.12)	1.00 (0.76 - 1.27)	<0.001	<0.001
iPTH	44.65 (27.60 -70.75)	19.1 (8.85 - 30.5)	25.1 (15.52 - 38.15)	<0.01	<0.001

Table 3. Pre and clinic (post-post) iPTH categorized as within target or out of target as per Canadian society of nephrology guidelines and the proportion of patients in each category.

	Low post post HD iPTH	Normal post post HD iPTH	High post post HD iPTH
Low preHD iPTH (<10.6 pmol/L)	**10%**	0%	0%
Normal preHD iPTH (10.6 - 53 pmol/L)	0%	**55%**	0%
High preHD iPTH (>53 pmol/L)	0%	25%	**10%**

Table 4. Pre and clinic (post-post) PO_4 categroized as within target or out of target as per Canadian society of nephrology guidelines and the proportion of patients in each category.

	Low post post HD PO_4	Normal post post HD PO_4	High post post HD PO_4
Low preHD PO_4 (<0.81 mmol/L)	0%	0%	0%
Normal preHD PO_4 (0.81 - 1.58 mmol/L)	25%	15%	0%
High preHD PO_4 (>1.58 mmol/L)	0%	45%	15%

Table 5. Pre and clinic (post-post) Ca categorized as within target or out of target as per Canadian society of nephrology guidelines and the proportion of patients in each category.

	Low post post HD Ca	Normal post post HD Ca	High post post HD Ca
Low preHD Ca (<2.2 mmol/L)	5%	30%	0%
Normal preHD Ca (2.2 - 2.52 mmol/L)	0%	45%	20%
High preHD Ca (>2.52 mmol/L)	0%	0%	0%

Table 6. Pre and post iPTH categorized as within target and out of target as per Canadian society of nephrology guidelines and the proportion of patients in each category.

	Low post HD iPTH	Normal post HD iPTH	High post HD iPTH
Low preHD iPTH (<10.6 pmol/L)	10%	0%	0%
Normal preHD iPTH (10.6 - 53 pmol/L)	15%	35%	5%
High preHD iPTH (>53 pmol/L)	5%	15%	15%

Table 7. Pre and post PO_4 categorized as within target and out of target as per Canadian society of nephrology guidelines and the proportion of patients in each category.

	Low post HD PO_4	Normal post HD PO_4	High post HD PO_4
Low preHD PO_4 (<0.81 mmol/L)	0%	0%	0%
Normal preHD PO_4 (0.81 - 1.58 mmol/L)	25%	15%	0%
High preHD PO_4 (>1.58 mmol/L)	25%	30%	5%

Table 8. Pre and post Ca categoriezed as within target and out of target as per Canadian society of nephrology guidelines and the proportion of patients in each category.

	Low post HD Ca	Normal post HD Ca	High post HD Ca
Low preHD Ca (<2.2 mmol/L)	**10%**	25%	5%
Normal preHD Ca (2.2 - 2.52 mmol/L)	0%	**45%**	15%
High preHD Ca (>2.52 mmol/L)	0%	0%	**0%**

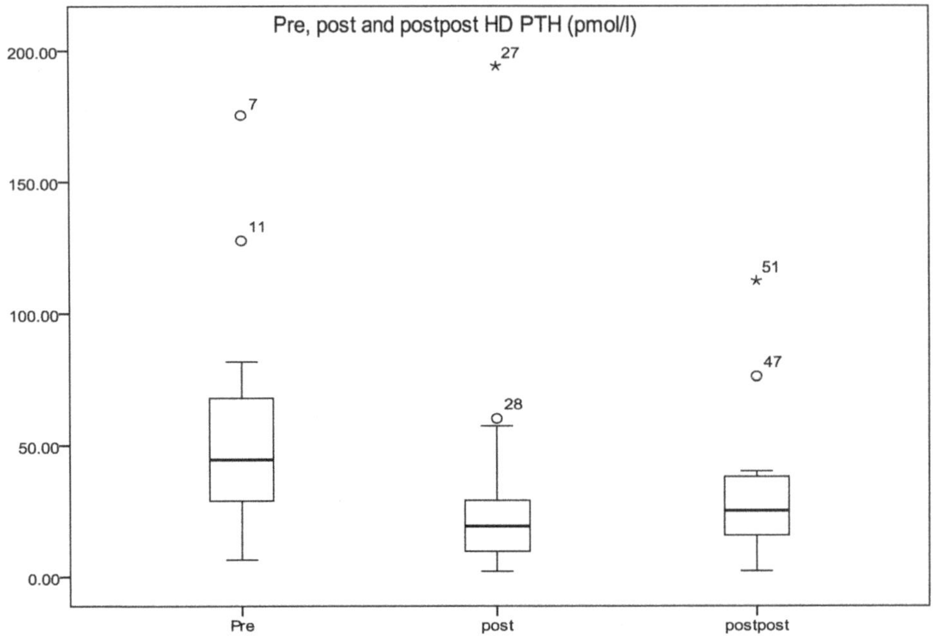

Figure 1. Median and interquartile range of pre, post and clinic (post-post) values of iPTH (outliers are shown as circles).

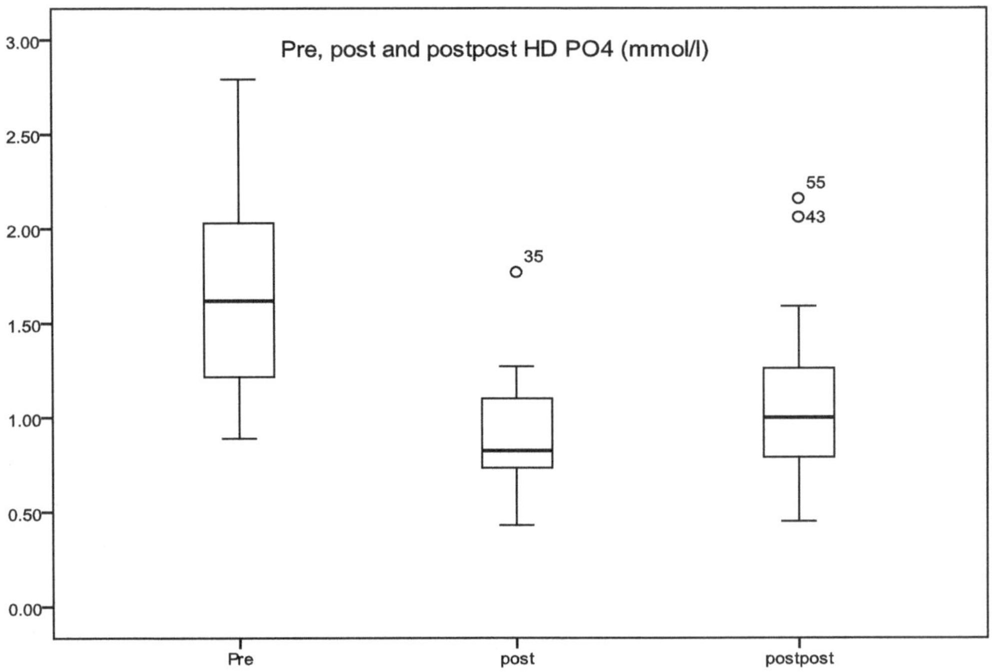

Figure 2. Median and interquartile range of pre, post and clinic (post-post) values of PO_4 (outliers are shown as circles).

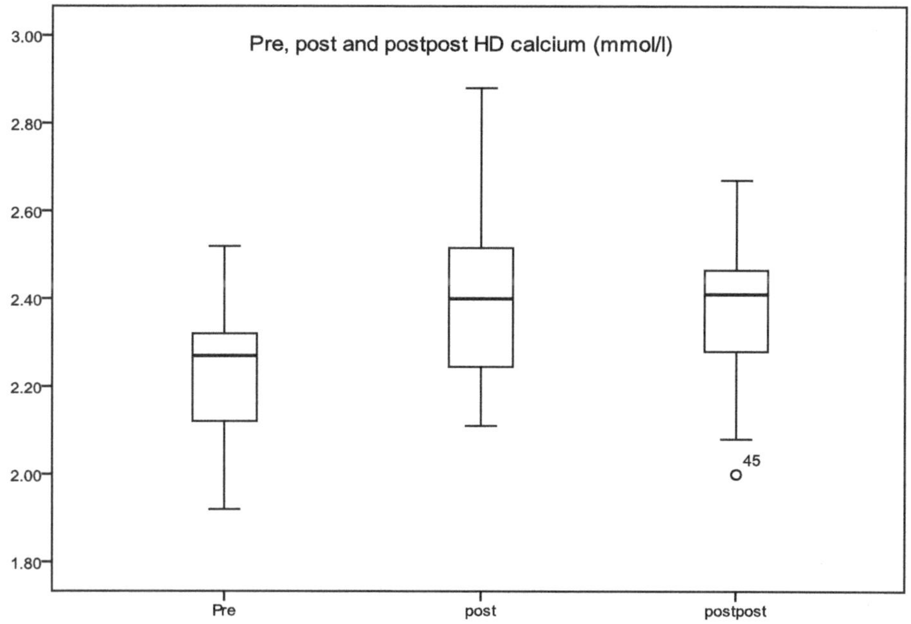

Figure 3. Median and interquartile range of pre, post and clinic (post-post) values of Ca (outliers are shown as circles).

4. Discussion

To our knowledge, this is the first study to compare values of commonly measured mineral metabolism markers pre, post and post-post (clinic visit) dialysis treatment in nocturnal home hemodialysis patients. We have demonstrated that the timing of blood collection has profound effects on the serum concentration of Ca, PO_4 and iPTH in nocturnal home hemodialysis patients that are both clinically and statistically significant. Interventions for the management of mineral metabolism may be applied differently depending on when patients collect their blood samples. This has relevance for patient management but may also affect the interpretation of the results of observational studies in which the timing of blood sample collection may be variable.

Abnormalities in serum calcium, phosphate and parathyroid hormone are common in dialysis dependent patients and constitute part of a systemic syndrome known as chronic kidney disease bone and mineral disorder [7]. An increased risk of fracture, vascular calcification and hospitalization has been associated with altered values of bone metabolism markers [8-10]. Patients with ESRD treated with conventional HD who have abnormal markers of mineral metabolism also appear to be at increased risk for all cause mortality and cardiovascular mortality [10,11].

In an attempt to decrease morbidity and mortality related to mineral metabolism disturbances, clinical practice guidelines (CPG) have been published by the National Kidney Foundation [12], Canadian Society of Nephrology [13], the United Kingdom [14], Caring for Australians with Renal Impairment (CARI) [15], Kidney Disease: Improving Global Outcomes (KDIGO) [16], Renal Association Clinical Practice Guideline [6] and also by the European Best Practice Society [17]. Acceptable values for biochemical markers have been specified; however no discrimination has been made between patients on different dialysis prescriptions. Only some of the guidelines have included a specified timing for blood collection. For example in the CARI guideline, it is recommended that for serum calcium and phosphate measurement, a predialysis blood sample should be sent [15]. The Renal Association Clinical Practice Guideline has also recommended pre-dialysis blood sampling for biochemical and haematological measurements [6]. Similarly not all studies linking different target values for bone metabolism markers to clinical outcomes have clearly specified the timing of blood sampling in their studied population [18,19].

Despite these limitations, to our knowledge blood collection for Ca, PO_4 and iPTH for in-centre hemodialysis patients is typically done predialysis, midweek. However, this may not be true in home nocturnal hemodialysis patients based on a Canadian survey of practice patterns (not published). Although bone mineral metabolism markers have been studied in nocturnal hemodialysis patients, limited data exists in which different target values for Ca, PO_4 and iPTH have been examined with respect to clinically important outcomes such as mortality, vascular calcification or fracture in this patient population. However manipulation of the dialysate in nocturnal HD, compared to conventional HD, is common which may have an affect on serum values depending on the timing of the blood sample collection. The dialysate calcium is often increased above 1.25 mmol/L in order to treat worsening hyperparathyroidism and falling bone mineral density such that hypercalcemia may be present immediately post dialysis [20-21]. This is consistent with our finding that 20% of patients had a high serum calcium post dialysis whether the blood was drawn immediately post dialysis or in the clinic. The transiently high calcium would be expected to suppress serum PTH values [20]. This is consistent with the 35% of patients with a PTH value in a lower category on the post compared to the pre-HD blood work. The longer duration of dialysis associated with nocturnal has been shown to significantly reduce serum phosphate levels and in many reported studies, phosphate has been added to the dialysate. Serum phosphate values would be misclassified as much at 80% of the time if only a post-HD value is used based on our study results.

A CPG has not been specifically written for patients on longer dialysis duration to define optimal mineral metabolism values or suggestions for timing of blood collection that address the uncertainties that exist in target values and the special challenges for patients who undertake their dialysis at home. Our study would suggest that the timing of blood collection has relevance for the interpretation and management of mineral metabolism for nocturnal home hemodialysis patients. The interpretation of studies that are based on this patient population may also be challenging if the timing of blood collection has not been standardized. Although one could argue that the "right numbers"and the "right time" are not known, ultimately the clinician must make treatment decisions on mineral metabolism management that are likely to be altered by timing of blood sample collection such that consistency across renal programs would be desirable.

Our study has a number of limitations. The small patient numbers with different dialysis prescriptions including frequency and duration of the HD treatment, different intervals between pre, post and post-post samples, type of dialyzer and dialysate additives, different medication including phosphate binders and PTH suppressors, all have an impact on the mineral metabolism markers that were examined. However this represents a real patient population with all of the variables that can be manipulated in an attempt to manage mineral metabolism abnormalities in ESRD patients treated with HD. Our study also does not address the potential usefulness of measuring post dialysis serum calcium and phosphate in guiding decisions about dialysis additives. Despite these limitations we believe our sample represents nocturnal home hemodialysis patients of other centres and we have identified the high likelihood of misclassifying patients and making different treatment decisions depending on the timing of the blood sample draw.

In conclusion until outcome data on mineral metabolism management are available in nocturnal hemodialysis patients, for consistency, blood samples should be drawn pre-dialysis similar to in-centre HD patients. This recommendation does not take into account the added convenience to patients of having blood samples drawn in clinic or the potential reduction in costs associated with not providing patients with centrifuges in the home.

5. Acknowledgements

We would like to thank Jessica Wagner (research coordinator), the nurses in the home dialysis unit and the patients for their assistance with this study. Dr. D. Zimmerman receives salary support from the department of medicine at the Ottawa Hospital.

REFERENCES

[1] A. Laupacis, P. Keown, N. Pus, *et al.*, "A Study of the Quality of Life and Cost-Utility of Renal Transplant," *Kidney International*, Vol. 50, No. 1, 1996, pp. 235-242. doi:10.1038/ki.1996.307

[2] B. F. Culleton, M. Walsh, S. W. Klarenbach, *et al.*, "Effect of Frequent Nocturnal Hemodialysis vs Conventional Hemodialysis on Left Ventricular Mass and Quality of Life: A Randomized Controlled Trial," *Journal of the American Medical Association*, Vol. 298, No. 11, 2007, pp. 1291-1299. doi:10.1001/jama.298.11.1291

[3] P. A. McFarlane, A. M. Bayoumi, A. Pierratos and D. A. Redelmeier, "The Quality of Life and Cost Utility of Home Nocturnal and Conventional in-Center Hemodialysis," *Kidney International*, Vol. 64, No. 3, 2003, pp. 1004-1011. doi:10.1046/j.1523-1755.2003.00157.x

[4] M. V. Rocco, R. S. Lockridge Jr, G. J. Beck, *et al.*, "The Effects of Frequent Nocturnal Home Hemodialysis: The Frequent Hemodialysis Network Nocturnal Trial," *Kidney International*, Vol. 80, No. 10, 2011, pp. 1080-1091. doi:10.1038/ki.2011.213

[5] M. John and K. Michael, "Starting a Home Hemodialysis Program," *Seminars in Dialysis*, Vol. 20, No. 1, 2007, pp. 35-39. doi:10.1111/j.1525-139X.2007.00239.x

[6] R. Mactier, N. Hoenich, C. Breen, "Renal Assocition Clinical Practice Guidelines 5th Edition 2009-2012," *Nephron Clinical Practice*, Vol. 118, Suppl. 1, 2011, pp. 241-286.

[7] S. Moe, T. Drueke, J. Cunningham, *et al.*, "Definition, Evaluation, and Classification of Renal Osteodystrophy: A Position Statement from Kidney Disease: Improving Global Outcomes (KDIGO)," *Kidney International*, Vol. 69, No. 11, 2006, pp. 1945-1953. doi:10.1038/sj.ki.5000414

[8] W. G. Goodman, J. Goldin, B. D. Kuizon, *et al.*, "Coronary Artery Calcification in Young Adults with End-Stage Renal Disease Who Are Undergoing Dialysis," *The New England Journal of Medicine*, Vol. 342, No. 20, 2000, pp. 1478-1483. doi:10.1056/NEJM200005183422003

[9] W. Y. Qunibi, C. A. Nolan and J. C. Ayus, "Cardiovas-

cular Calcification in Patients with End-Stage Renal Disease: A Century Old Phenomenon," *Kidney International*, Vol. 62, Suppl. 82, 2002, pp. S73-S80. doi:10.1046/j.1523-1755.62.s82.15.x

[10] G. A. Block, P. S. Klassen, J. M. Lazarus, N. Ofsthun, E. G. Lowrie and G. M. Chertow, "Mineral Metabolism, Mortality, and Morbidity in Maintenance Hemodialysis," *Journal of the American Society of Nephrology*, Vol. 15, No. 8, 2004, pp. 2208-2218. doi:10.1097/01.ASN.0000133041.27682.A2,

[11] M. L. Melamed, J. A. Eustace, L. Plantinga, *et al.*, "Changes in Serum Calcium, Phosphate, and PTH and the Risk of Death in Incident Dialysis Patients: Along Longitudinal Study," *Kidney International*, Vol. 70, 2006, pp. 351-357. doi:10.1038/sj.ki.5001542

[12] National Kidney Foundation, "K/DOQI Clinical Practice Guidelines for Bone Metabolism and Disease in Chronic Kidney Disease," *American Journal of Kidney Diseases*, Vol. 42, Suppl. 3, 2003, pp. S1-S201. doi:10.1016/S0272-6386(03)00553-5

[13] K. Jindal, C. T. Chan, C. Deziel, *et al.*, "Hemodialysis Clinical Practice Guidelines for the Canadian Society of Nephrology," *Journal of the American Society of Nephrology*, Vol. 17, No. 3, 2006, pp. S1-S27.

[14] Joint Specialty Committee on Renal Medicine of the Royal College of Physicians and the Renal Association, and the Royal College of General Practitioners, "Chronic Kidney Disease in Adults: UK Guidelines for Identification, Management and Referral," Royal College of Physicians, London, 2006.

[15] G. Elder, R. Faull, P. Branley and C. Hawley, "Management of Bone Disease, Calcium, Phosphate and Parathyroid Hormone," *Nephrology*, Vol. 11, Suppl. 1, 2006, pp. S230-S261. doi:10.1111/j.1440-1797.2006.00508.x

[16] CKD-MBD Work Group, "KDIGO Clinical Practice Guideline for the Diagnosis, Evaluation, Prevention, and Treatment of Chronic Kidney Disease-Mineral and Bone Disorder (CKD-MBD)," *Kidney International*, Vol. 113, 2009, pp. S1-130.

[17] J. B Cannata-Andía, T. B. Drueke, J. Cunningham, *et al.*, "Clinical Algorithms on Renal Osteodystrophy," *Nephrology Dialysis Transplantation*, Vol. 15, Suppl. 5, 2000, pp. S39-S57.

[18] F. Tentori, M. J. Blayney, J. M. Albert, *et al.*, "Mortality Risk for Dialysis Patients with Different Levels of Serum Calcium, Phosphorus, and PTH: The Dialysis Outcomes and Practice Patterns Study (DOPPS)," *American Journal of Kidney Diseases*, Vol. 52, No. 3, 2008, pp. 519-553. doi:10.1053/j.ajkd.2008.03.020

[19] G. A. Block, P. S. Klassen, J. M. Lazarus, N. Ofsthun, E. G. Lowrie and G. M. Chertow, "Mineral Metabolism, Mortality, and Morbidity in Maintenance Hemodialysis," *Journal of the American Society of Nephrology*, Vol. 15, No. 8, 2004, 2208-2218. doi:10.1097/01.ASN.0000133041.27682.A2

[20] R. M. Lindsay, F. Alhejaili, G. Nesrallah, *et al.*, "Calcium and Phosphate Balance with Quotidian Hemodialysis," *American Journal of Kidney Diseases*, Vol. 42, No. 1, 2003, pp. S24-S29. doi:10.1016/S0272-6386(03)00534-1

[21] N. Toussaint, J. Boddington, R. Simmonds, C. Waldron, C. Soerville and J. Agar, "Calcium Phosphate Metabolism and Bone Mineral Density with Nocturnal Hemodialysis," *Hemodialysis International*, Vol. 10, No. 3, 2006, pp. 280-286. doi:10.1111/j.1542-4758.2006.00109.x

Spouses Who Donate Seem to Be the Winners—A Questionnaire Study of Kidney Donors Long-Term

Annette Lennerling[1,2], Abdul Rashid Qureshi[3], Ingela Fehrman-Ekholm[1,4]
[1]Transplant Institute, Sahlgrenska University Hospital, Gothenburg, Sweden
[2]Institute of Health and Care Sciences, University of Gothenburg, Gothenburg, Sweden
[3]Baxter Novum, CLINTEC, Karolinska Institute, Stockholm, Sweden
[4]Renal Department, Karolinska University Hospital, Stockholm, Sweden
Email: annette.lennerling@vgregion.se

ABSTRACT

Background: Living donor kidney transplantations have been performed at Sahlgrenska University Hospital in Gothenburg, Sweden since 1965. In this study we wanted to explore the living kidney donor's long-term experiences of the donation. **Methods:** Of 1110 consecutive living donors throughout 1965-2005, 823 were available for our questionnaire study. **Results:** Totally 692 replied to the questionnaire, 65% were females. The most common relation to the recipients was siblings (284), parents (262) and spouses (96). Time since donation was median 15 years (2 - 43). The initiative to donate came from the donors themselves in 69%. The dominating motives for donation were a wish to help, worries about the recipient not receiving a transplant and the knowledge that one could live a normal life with one kidney. The majority of the donors, felt well informed about potential risks both short-term and long-term. Depression post donation was reported by few donors, 2.3% and persisting pain by 4.3%. Comparisons between sibling donors and spouse donors show a significant difference ($p < 0.0001$) in the statements; If I donate a kidney "My quality of life will be better" and "The quality of life for the family will be better" more so for spouses. Also spouses seemed to be better informed about risks both for themselves and the recipients ($p < 0.05$). **Conclusions:** Our study shows that the donor population is in good psychosocial health. It is a positive progress that spouses can be living kidney donors—they seem to be the winners.

Keywords: Living Kidney Donors; Long-Term Follow-Up; Motives; Sibling; Spouse; Questionnaire

1. Introduction

Kidney transplantation with an organ from a live donor is the best treatment for the transplant recipient and living donation is increasing in many countries [1,2]. Both short and long term results are better. The recipients are followed closely but the donors check-up vary. Several studies have been published about the better life quality among the living donors compared to background population [3-5]. However, also better psychosocial support has been discussed since some donors have problems post donation [6,7].

In Sweden living kidney donors have been used for kidney transplantation since the start in 1964. Until 31st of December 2011, 3704 living donor kidney transplanttations had been performed and 9238 kidney transplantations from deceased donors. The Transplant Institute at Sahlgrenska University Hospital in Gothenburg is the largest of four kidney transplant centres in Sweden with 1425 (31st of December 2011) living kidney donor transplantations since the start in 1965.

In Sweden, living donors are always the first choice for patients in need of a kidney transplant. The living donor pool has expanded from siblings and parents, to also include spouses, friends, as well as other more distant relatives and anonymous donors. Today live donors constitute about 45% of all kidney transplantations in Sweden. There is no national Swedish donor registry, but a Scandinavian register started in 2004. However, the donors from earlier days are not included. This is a prospective register and limited psychosocial issues are included in the report.

We were interested to know more about the living donors both the physical health status, and the psychosocial well-being. Further we wanted to find out more about their experiences of the donation process, motives for donating, relations with the recipient after donation and present health situation. This living donor study was initiated in 2007. The study was divided in two parts, one medical follow-up-mainly focusing on long-term renal function, and was published in 2011 [8]. In the second part of this study we wanted to explore the donor's experiences of the kidney donation in different aspects in the long term. We here present data and also put focus in comparing the experiences and thoughts from sibling donors and spouse donors. Today the spouse donor is as common as a sibling donor.

2. Subjects and Methods

The study design was cross sectional and the study was performed between the years 2007-2009. We aimed to approach all persons having had a donor nephrectomy performed at Sahlgrenska University Hospital from the start in May 1965 until the end of December in 2005, in total 1112 donors. Of the 1112 donors 13% were deceased, 6% were not possible to identify due to incomplete social security number and 4% were living abroad, thus 823 persons, *i.e.* 77%, were available for the study. Of the 8237/15/2012 donors, 692 participants responded to an author constructed questionnaire. The questionnaire consisted of 50 questions focusing on the living donors experiences of motives, information and health problems. There was no standardized health form added. The questionnaires were sent to the donor by post with one reminder to the non-responders. There was a possibility to reply on-line, which was used by 20% of the donors.

We used a software program for collecting the questionnaire data, the survey tool called Examinare© (www. examinare.com). From this tool descriptive data were obtained. The forms that Examinare© creates are protected by Secure Socket Layer (SSL) and the information between server and browser is encrypted.

The study was approved by the ethical regional board in Gothenburg.

Statistical Methods

Normally-distributed variables were expressed as means ± SD (unless noted otherwise), and non-normally distributed variables were expressed as medians (10th and 90th percentile). Statistical significance was set at the level of $p < 0.05$. Logistic regression analyses were used to study the relative associations of selected markers. All statistical analyses were performed using statistical software Stata version 12.1 (Stata Corp, College station, TX, USA). As p values are not adjusted for multiple testing, they have to be considered as descriptive.

3. Results

3.1. Characteristics of the Donor Population

The response rate for questionnaire was 84%, 692 of the 823 available donors. Of those 65% (n = 447) were females. The median age was 61 years (range 22 - 93). The median age at donation was 47 years (range 21 - 73). The similar trend was found in the non-responders. The relationship to the recipients was sibling (n = 284), parent (n = 262), spouse (n = 96), friend (n = 18), grown-up child (n = 7) and other relation (n = 26).

3.2. Pre-Donation Statements by the Donors

The occupational situation before donation is presented in **Table 1**. A high quantity of the donors 587 (84%) were working at the time of donation, 21 were unemployed, 53 retired, 13 were students and 18 were house wives. None was disability pensioner. The initiative to donate came from the donors themselves in the majority of cases. Thus 474 (69%) offered to donate, the recipients physician asked in 88 (13%) cases, the recipients in 85 (12%) cases. Other family member asked in 20 (3%) cases. The most common motives for donation was the wish to help, worries about the recipient not receiving a transplant and the knowledge that one could live a normal life with one kidney. Generally, the becoming donors felt well informed about risks (76%), short-term complications (69%), and long-term complications (62%). They also felt well informed about recipient risks (73%) and that the given kidney might stop to function or even never function (75%). The donors felt well-informed about the reimbursement system and sick leave regulations (67%). We also asked if the information given was too much but only 3% of the donors stated that.

Table 1. Occupational status and statements by the 692 donors concerning issues before donation.

Response on pre-donation issues	n	%
Working	587	85
Retired	53	8
Students	13	2
Unemployed	21	3
Other activities	18	3
Took the initiative to donate		
Themselves	474	68
The doctor of the recipient	88	13
The recipient	85	12
Other family member	20	3
Other	28	4
Most important motives to donate		
To help	518	75
Worry without a transplantation	497	72
Knowledge: a normal life with one kidney	240	35
Information		
Felt very well-informed about the risks	528	76
Short term complications	478	69
Long term complications	429	62
The recipients risks	502	73
That the given kidney might stop functioning	517	75
Too little information about risks	17	3
Felt well-informed about sick leave and reimbursements	466	67

The experiences following donation are presented in **Table 2**. Time for recovery after donation was 1 - 2 months for 48% of the donors and 5% stated that they had never recovered. Sick leave time was 1 - 3 weeks for 22%, 4 - 7 weeks for 37% and 8 - 12 weeks for 20%. Longer sick leave than 12 weeks were reported by 4%. The reimbursement system functioned completely for 325 donors (47%), partly for 124 (18%) but 98 donors (14%) said they never received anything. However, only 7%, that is 45 donors, considered they still had financial problems due to the donation. No one reported having lost their work due to the donation.

Health problems related to the donation were stated by 12% of the donors. Experienced kidney disease was stated in 2% and 27% had treated hypertension. Depression and diabetes were reported by a few cases, 2% for each and persisting pain problems by 4%.

3.3. Low Pregnancy Frequency among Living Donors

The pregnancy frequency was low, 21 donors (5% of the female donors) had given birth after donation. Most persons were middle-aged at the time of donation and not in childbearing ages. None reported the pregnancy as a problem.

3.4. Spouses versus Siblings as Donors

The three great donor groups are siblings, parents and spouses. From the start only siblings and parents were accepted as live kidney donors but since 1986 spouses were also permitted to donate.

Table 2. Statements by the 692 participants concerning post donation health issues.

Recovery after donation	n	%
1 - 2 months	331	48
3 - 6 months	210	30
6 - 12 months	62	9
More than one year	58	9
Never recovered	31	5
Time for sick leave		
1 - 3 weeks	154	22
4 - 7 weeks	254	37
8 - 12 weeks	140	20
Longer time	37	4
Can't remember	92	13
Experienced health after the donation		
Remaining health problems	79	12
Experienced kidney disease after donation	11	2
Experienced kidney stones	25	4
Developed diabetes	12	2
Had hypertension treatment today	173	27
Had continuous nerve pain	28	5
Muscle weakness in abdomen	58	9
Depression	16	3
Had been pregnant after donation	21	5

A comparison of the responses from the 96 spouses and the 284 siblings were made. In the following questions there were borderline or significant differences. There were no significant differences between the current age of spouses and siblings, **Figure 1**.

The following statements concern the motives for becoming a donor. The parentheses indicate the donor type being closest to the statement.

- Others wanted me to donate (sibling) ($p = 0.05$)
- Waiting-time for a deceased kidney was too long (spouse) ($p = 0.05$)
- A moral duty to donate (sibling) ($p = 0.05$)
- My quality of life would be better (spouse) ($p < 0.0001$)
- The quality of life all the family would be better (spouse) ($p < 0.0001$)

The following statements are about the information prior to donation:

- Well-informed about risks for short term complications (spouse) ($p < 0.05$)
- Well-informed about risks for long-term complications (spouse) ($p < 0.05$)
- Well-informed about complications and risks in the recipients (spouse) ($p < 0.01$)

Statements and experiences after the donation:

- Feeling malaise first week post donation (spouse) ($p < 0.05$)
- Better self-esteem (spouse) ($p < 0.05$)
- Changed to more frequent contact with the recipient (sibling) ($p < 0.01$)
- Would consider to donate again (spouse) ($p < 0.01$)
- Experienced pregnancy, children after the donation (sibling) ($p < 0.001$)

The following statements showed no differences between spouses and siblings regarding motives for donation: a

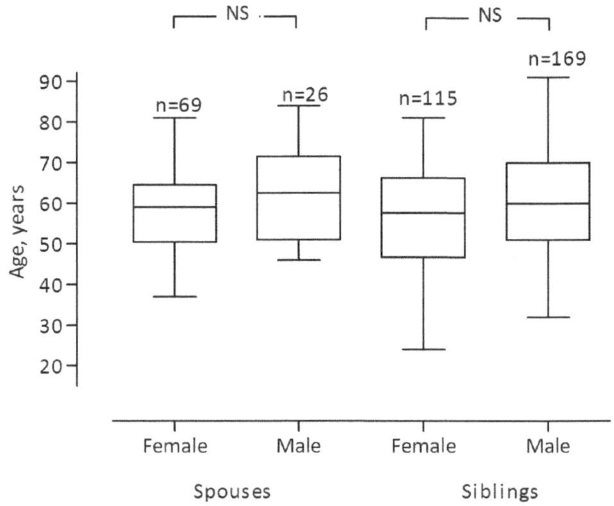

Figure 1. Box plot of the current age of spouses and siblings grouped in males and females.

wish to help, religion, have a normal life with one kidney, the donations would make me a better person, worry for the recipient without a transplant, becoming a better person and seeing no other possibility than donating. Perception about getting information about the following subjects did not differ: re-imbursement system, surgical risks, follow-up routines, and the risk of graft failure for the recipient.

Time for recovery and sick-leave period did not differ between spouses and siblings. Further, there was no difference in percentage regretting the donation or having remaining health problems. Routines for check-ups did not differ either between the two groups.

4. Discussion

The response rate in our study was high with 82%. This has been the case also in earlier Swedish and Norwegian studies on living kidney donors [9,10]. There is a recent French study published on long-term follow-up of 310 living donors and in this study 66% responded [11]. Another published paper from Canada, Australia and Scotland, showed a response rate on 48% [12].

Voluntarism and altruism are prerequisites for living donation. It is encouraging to find that the strongest motive for donation in our study was the wish to help someone in need. This is also in agreement with an interview study performed prior to donation [13].

To donate a kidney is a major surgical event which means risks and a certain recovery time. Time for recovery was 1 - 2 months for half of the donors and sick-leave were 4 - 7 weeks for the majority of the donors. Thus, it is important that the donors are offered the time needed for recovery since 85% of them were working at the time of donation in this study.

Of the responders 12% indicated that they still had some health problem related to the donation, the largest problem being pain which was reported by 4%. Though, we do not know if this pain is due to the donation procedure. However, it is a common problem with chronic pain in the general population, reported to be over 20% in the North American population [14,15]. A recent publication by Owen et al. on pain after nephrectomy show that 12% experienced chronic pain after donation and the donors did not receive adequate treatment [16]. It is noteworthy that pain after surgery is not classified as a major complication according to the Clavien system, where major complication includes an intervention, surgical or radiological [17].

Another finding in our study was that the majority of the donors were satisfied with the given information. Both written and verbal information are given to the donors but we think the information must be more individualised or elaborated to reach every potential donor. Guidelines support the necessity of adequate information [18].

The most interesting part was the comparison between sibling and spouse donors. Today a spouse donor is as common as a sibling donor in Sweden. Who should be preferred? Our study indicates that the spouses donate a kidney to get a better quality of life as well as the quality of life for the family in total. The sibling donors express moral duty as a greater motive. In contrast to a recent published Norwegian study we could not find that the spouse donors had more doubts about the donation [10]. On the contrary, the spouse donors felt well-informed, they knew the expected results, became very satisfied and had an increased self-esteem.

Is psychosocial support necessary? We could find some donors who reported that they did not recover, and some with persisting economical problems. It is important to identify these problems early. On the other hand we do not know if it was the donation process per se or co-existing incidents in their life or pre-donation problems that we were not aware of at the time of donation. A thorough psychosocial investigation before donation is of great importance.

Are check-ups necessary? There was uncertain information about this issue. Some donors stated that they were promised check-ups they never received. About 75% had had some check-ups, which is better than a previous study from Sweden showing that 50% were being controlled [9]. According to our medical study on blood pressure and kidney function made at the same time on these donors we found that two donors had undergone kidney transplantation and that one kidney donor was on dialysis. We also found that two donors had chronic kidney disease stage 4 and may be starting dialysis [8]. Also, the figure of hypertension was in agreement with our clinical finding with 25% having treatment for hypertension. Our aim is that the donors should be offered medical check-ups on a regular basis, with a minimum of every 5th year after the first year post donation [8].

In summary, our study shows that the donor population is in good psychosocial health. It is a positive development that spouses can be living donors. They seem to be the winners.

REFERENCES

[1] J. M. Cecka, "Kidney Transplantation in the United States," Clinical Transplants, Terasaki Foundation Laboratory, Los Angeles, 2008, pp. 1-18.

[2] U. Heemann and L. Renders, "State of Living Kidney Donation in Europe," *Nephrology Dialysis and Transplantation*, Vol. 27, No. 6, 2012, pp. 2166-2170. doi:10.1093/ndt/gfs144

[3] L. Westlie, P. Fauchald, T. Talseth, A. Jacobsen and A. Flatmark, "Quality of Life in Norwegian Kidney Donors," *Nephrology Dialysis Transplantation*, Vol. 8, No.

10, 1993, pp. 1146-1150.

[4] E. M. Johnson, J. K. Anderso, C. Jacobs, *et al.*, "Long-Term Follow-Up of Living Kidney Donors: Quality of Life after Donation," *Transplantation*, Vol. 67, No. 5, 1999, pp. 717-721. doi:10.1097/00007890-199903150-00013

[5] D. Ummel, M. Achille and J. Mekkelholt, "Donors and Recipients of Living Kidney Donation: A Qualitative Metasummary of Their Experiences," *Journal of Transplantation*, Vol. 2011, No. 2011, pp. 1-11. doi:10.1155/2011/626501

[6] S. G. Jowsey and T. D. Schneekloth, "Psychosocial Factors in Living Organ Donation: Clinical and Ethical Challenges," *Transplantation Reviews*, Vol. 22, No. 3, 2008, pp. 192-195. doi:10.1016/j.trre.2008.04.008

[7] A. Lennerling, I. Blohmé, O. Ostraat, H. Lönroth, M. Olausson and G. Nyberg, "Laparoscopic or Open Surgery for Living Donor Nephrectomy," *Nephrology Dialalysis Transplantation*, Vol. 16, No. 2, 2001, pp. 383-386. doi:10.1093/ndt/16.2.383

[8] I. Fehrman-Ekholm, N. Kvarnström, J. Softeland, *et al.*, "Post-Nephrectomy Development of Renal Function in Living Kidney Donors: A Cross-Sectional Retrospective Study," *Nephrology Dialysis Transplantation*, Vol. 26, No. 7, 2011, pp. 2377-2381. doi:10.1093/ndt/gfr161

[9] I. Fehrman-Ekholm, B. Brink, C. Ericsson, C. G. Elinder, F. Dunér and G. Lundgren, "Kidney Donors Don't Regret. Follow-Up of 370 Donors in Stockholm since 1964," *Transplantation*, Vol. 69, No. 10, 2000, pp. 2067-2071. doi:10.1097/00007890-200005270-00016

[10] G. Mjoen, K. Stavern, L. Westlie, *et al.*, "Quality of Life in Kidney Donors," *American Journal of Transplantation*, Vol. 11, No. 6, 2011, pp. 1315-1319. doi:10.1111/j.1600-6143.2011.03517.x

[11] C. Fournier, N. Pallet, Z. Cherqaoui, *et al.*, "Very Long-Term Follow-Up of Living Kidney Donors," *Transplant International*, Vol. 25, No. 4, 2012, pp. 1-6. doi:10.1111/j.1432-2277.2012.01439.x

[12] K. Clemens, N. Boudville, M. A. Dew, *et al.*, "The Long-Term Quality of Life of Living Kidney Donors: A Multicenter Cohort Study," *American Journal of Transplantation*, Vol. 11, No. 3, 2011, pp. 463-469. doi:10.1111/j.1600-6143.2010.03424.x

[13] A. Lennerling, A. Forsberg, K. Meyer and G. Nyberg, "Motives for Becoming a Living Donor," *Nephrology Dialysis and Transplantation*, Vol. 19, No. 6, 2004, pp. 1600-1605. doi:10.1093/ndt/gfh138

[14] J. Hardt, C. Jacobsen, J. Goldberg, R. Nickel and D. Buchwald, "Prevalence of Chronic Pain in a Representative Sample in the United States," *Pain Medicine*, Vol. 9, No. 7, 2008, pp. 803-812. doi:10.1111/j.1526-4637.2008.00425.x

[15] D. Schopflocher, P. Taenzer and R. Jovey, "The Prevalence of Chronic Pain in Canada," *Pain Research and Management*, Vol. 16, No. 6, 2011, pp. 445-450.

[16] M. Owen, P. Lorgelly and M. Serpell, "Chronic Pain Following Donor Nephrectomy—A Study of the Incidence, Nature and Impact of Chronic Post-Nephrectomy Pain," *European Journal of Pain*, Vol. 14, No. 7, 2010, pp. 732-734. doi:10.1016/j.ejpain.2009.11.013

[17] D. Dindo, N. Demartines and P. A. Clavien, "Classification of Surgical Complications: A New Proposal with Evaluation in a Cohort of 6336 Patients and Results of a Survey," *Annals of Surgery*, Vol. 240, No. 2, 2004, pp. 205-209.

[18] The European Parliament and the Council of the European Union, "Directive 2010/45/EU of the European Parliament and of the Council of 7 July 2010 on Standards of Quality and Safety of Human Organs Intended for Transplantation, 2010," 2010. http://eur-lex.europa.eu/LexUriServ/LexUriServ.do?uri=OJ:L:2010:207:0014:0029:EN:PDF

Do We Have a Biocompatible Peritoneal Dialysis Fluid?

Shadi Hassan[1], Batya Kristal[2,3], Khalid Khazim[3], Fadi Hassan[4], Dunia Hassan[5], Kamal Hassan[2,3]
[1]Internal Medicine Department, Carmel Medical Center, Haifa, Israel
[2]Faculty of Medicine in the Galilee, Bar-Ilan University, Safed, Israel
[3]Nephrology and Hypertension Department, Western Galilee Hospital, Nahariya, Israel
[4]Sackler Faculty of Medicine, Tel Aviv University, Tel Aviv, Israel
[5]The Ruth and Bruce Faculty of Medicine, Technion Israel Institute of Technology, Haifa, Israel
Email: drkamalh@hotmail.com, Kamal.Hassan@naharia.health.gov.il

ABSTRACT

Objective: Cardiovascular disease remains the leading cause of morbidity and mortality in patients on maintenance dialysis. Diabetes mellitus, dyslipidemia, hypertension, inflammation and hyperhomocyteinemia are major cardiovascular risk factors. **Aim:** To evaluate the effects of Icodextrin and amino acid peritoneal dialysis fluid (AAPDF) on these major cardiovascular risk factors looking for a more biocompatible PDF formula. **Methods:** 20 adult stable peritoneal dialysis patients were included in the study. 10 patients received 2 L Icodextrin and other 10 patients received 2 L AAPDF in their dialysis prescription for 8 weeks. **Results:** Icodextrin decreased fasting plasma glucose ($p < 0.001$), LDL-C ($p = 0.03$), SBP ($p < 0.01$), DBP ($p < 0.05$) and plasma homocysteine ($p = 0.002$), and increased HDL-C ($p = 0.009$), CRP ($p = 0.035$) and fibrinogen ($p = 0.009$). AAPDF did not affect fasting plasma glucose, LDL-C, HDL-C, CRP and fibrinogen but increased serum albumin ($p = 0.03$), SBP ($p < 0.01$), DBP ($p < 0.05$) and P_{Hcy} ($p = 0.03$). **Conclusions:** A biocompatible PDF should provide not only adequate dialysis and ultrafiltration but should also improve nutritional and metabolic status, blood pressure control and reduce inflammation and plasma homocyteine.

Keywords: Icodextrin; Amino Acids PDF; Homocyteine; Carbohydrates; Lipids; Inflammation

1. Introduction

Cardiovascular disease (CVD) remains the leading cause of morbidity and mortality in end-stage renal disease patients on maintenance dialysis [1]. Diabetes mellitus, dyslipidemia, hypertension, inflammation and hyperhomocyteinemia are major cardiovascular risk factors. Recent studies have suggested that novel risk factors, uremia or dialysis-related, are of great importance, as they act synergistically with the highly prevalent traditional risk factors for CVD in chronic kidney disease (CKD) patients [2]. Glucose based peritoneal dialysis fluids (PDFs) are usually associated with progressive loss of the osmotic gradient, concomitant reduction in ultrafiltration (UF) and to the development of hyperglycemia and dyslipidemia. Dyslipidemia increases the risk of CVD and becomes worse in peritoneal dialysis (PD) patients [3]. Up to 80% of peritoneal dialysis patients are hypertensive [4]. Hypertension plays an important role in the development of CVD in this population [4]. Elevated plasma inflammation markers associated with increased risk for CVD [5]. Almost all (97% - 98%) PD and hemodialysis patients have hyperhomocyteinemia that known to be associated with an increased risk of cardiovascular, cerebrovascular and venous thromboembolic diseases [6-8]. Icodextrin and Amino acid PDF (AAPDF) considered more biocompatible PDFs. Icodextrin PDF is targeted to have more sustained oncotic effect, to reduce plasma glucose and glucose-induced lipid abnormalities, and to avoid the production of glucose degradation products (GDPs) [9,10]. Generally, there is some concern that Icodextrin treatment may induce a subclinical inflammatory response, both intraperitoneally and systemically [10-12]. AAPDF was designed to correct nutriational status by supplying extra nitrogen through the intraperitoneal route [13]. Although the effects of Icodextrin and AAPDF on metabolic status, blood pressure control, inflammation and plasma homocyteine were studied but some issues still controversial. Aim of this study was to evaluate the effects of Icodextrin and AAPDF on these major cardiovascular risk factors.

2. Patients and Methods

Randomly, 20 adult stable PD patients on continuous ambulatory peritoneal dialysis (CAPD) or automated Peritoneal Dialysis (APD) for at least 3 months and with $Kt/V > 1.8$ were included in the study. Demographic and clinical characteristics of the enrolled subjects are listed in **Table 1**. The study protocol was approved by the local

Ethics Committee and all patients gave written informed consent before participating in the study. The patients randomly assigned to receive Icodextrin or AAPDF. Ten patients received 2 L Icodextrin in their dialysis prescription for 8 weeks, the night dwells in CAPD subjects were substituted with 2 L Icodextrin and in APD subjects 2 L from their regular regimen were substituted with 2 L Icodextrin given as last fill. Ten patients received 2 L AAPDF in their dialysis prescription for 8 weeks, the second dwells in CAPD subjects were substituted with 2 L AAPDF and in APD subjects 2 L from their regular regimen were substituted with 2 L AAPDF given at noon. The residual renal function (RRF) was estimated by mean urea and creatinine clearance (C_{UC}) and by the Modification of Diet in Renal Disease (MDRD) equation study [14]. At baseline the standard peritoneal equilibration test (PET) [15], and estimation of Kt/V were performed using PD-Adequest 2.0 for Windows program (Baxter Healthcare Co., Deerfield, IL) [16]. Blood, urine and dialysate analysis were performed in both groups at baseline and 8 weeks. Blood analysis included complete blood count (CBC), glucose, low density lipoprotein cholesterol (LDL-C), high density lipoprotein cholesterol (HDL-C), triglycerides, albumin, CRP, fibrinogen, plasma homocysteine (P_{Hcy}), folic acid, vitamin B12, and PTH. Urine analysis included 24-hour urinary collections for creatinine (mg/dl) (U_{Cr}) and urea (mg/dl) (U_{Urea}). Dialysate analysis included creatinine (mg/dl) (D_{Cr}) and glucose (mg/dl) (D_{Glu}). Daily urinary output (ml/day) (DUO), PET and Kt/V were also evaluated at baseline and 8 weeks. P_{Hcy} was determined using AxSYM Homocysteine assay (Produced by Axis-Shied, Dundee, UK for Abbott laboratories, Abbott park, IL 60064, USA). Statistical methods: Qualitative variables were described as incidences and percentages. Quantitative variables were described as means and standard deviations. Repeated Measures tests were used to evaluate the effects of Icodextrin and AAPDF on RRF, DUO, UF, D/P_{Cr}, D_{Glu}, D_{Cr}, fasting glucose, plasma lipids, plasma inflammation markers, body weight, blood pressure and P_{Hcy}. Repeated Measures tests were also used to evaluate the effects of PD modality, peritoneal membrane characteristics, Kt/V, gender, cause of CKD and hemoglobin on P_{Hcy}. Linear regression was used to evaluate the correlation between P_{Hcy} and RRF, DUO, PD duration, age, body weight, PTH and hemoglobin levels. Linear regression was also used to evaluate the correlation between degree of increment in UF (ΔNet UF) and the degree of reduction in P_{Hcy} (ΔP_{Hcy}) as well as between the degree of increment in D/P_{Cr} ($\Delta D/P_{Cr}$) and ΔP_{Hcy}.

Table 1. Characteristics of the study population.

	Icodextrin group	AAPDF[a] group
Number	10	10
Age (years)	61.3 ± 11.9	59.6 ± 20.0
Male/female	5/5	5/5
CAPD[b]/APD[c]	5/5	5/5
Dialysis duration (months)	29.2 ± 33.6	28.8 ± 17.3
PET[d]: HATs[e]/LATs[f]	5/5	5/5
Kt/V	2.41 ± 0.4	2.39 ± 0.4
Vitamin B12 (pg/ml) (Normal:160 - 680)	598.3 ± 280.3	610.9 ± 330.5
Folic acid (ng/mL) (Normal:150 - 700)	760.0 ± 385.0	771.2 ± 318.1
PTH (pg/ml) (normal:10 - 60)	313 ± 185	301 ± 158
Underlying cause:		
Diabetes mellitus	5	5
Primary hyperoxaluria type 1	2	2
APKD[g]	1	1
Unknown	2	2

a: Amino Acid Peritoneal Dialysis Fluid; b: Continuous ambulatory peritoneal dialysis; c: Automated peritoneal dialysis; d: Peritoneal equilibration test; e: High average transporters; f: Low average transporters; g: Adult Polycystic Kidney Disease.

3. Results

Repeated measures analysis revealed that Icodextrin and AAPDF did not affect the RRF or DUO (**Table 2**). No linear correlation was found between the RRF and P_{Hcy}. Icodextrin increased UF ($p = 0.003$) and D/P_{Cr} ($p < 0.001$) (**Table 2**). Icodextrin, as well AAPDF decreased D_{Glu} ($p = 0.02$) (**Table 2**).

Table 2. Effects of Icodextrin and AAPDF on RRF, DUO, UF, D/P_{Cr} and D_{Glu}.

	Icodextrin group		
	Baseline	8 Weeks	p
P_{Hcy} (μmol/L)	29.1 ± 21.8	14.8 ± 5.3	0.002
C_{UC} (ml/min/1.73m^2)	10.1 ± 2.3	9.5 ± 2.9	n.s.
$eGFR_{MDRD}$ (ml/min/1.73m^2)	8.3 ± 2.4	8.1 ± 2.0	n.s.
DUO (L/day)	0.8 ± 0.4	0.75 ± 0.3	n.s.
UF (L/day)	0.98 ± 0.1	1.22 ± 1.3	0.003
D/P_{Cr}	0.54 ± 0.1	0.79 ± 0.1	<0.001
D_{Glu} (mg/dl)	1035.8 ± 438.1	901.8 ± 354.9	0.016
	AAPDF group		
	Baseline	8 weeks	p
P_{Hcy}[a] (μmol/L)	26.6 ± 17.0	36.4 ± 15.6	0.03
C_{UC}[b] (ml/min/1.73m^2)	10.2 ± 3.7	9.7 ± 3.3	n.s.
$eGFR_{MDRD}$[c] (ml/min/1.73m^2)	8.1 ± 2.3	8.0 ± 2.0	n.s.
DUO[d] (L/day)	0.7 ± 0.3	0.6 ± 0.4	n.s.
UF[e] (L/day)	0.99 ± 0.2	0.97 ± 0.2	n.s.
D/P_{Cr}[f]	0.64 ± 0.1	0.61 ± 0.2	n.s.
D_{Glu}[g] (mg/dl)	981.4 ± 446.8	854.5 ± 435.5	0.02

a: Plasma homocysteine; b: Mean urea and creatinine clearance; c: estimated GFR using the Modification of Diet in Renal Disease equation study; d: Daily Urinary Output; e: Ultrafiltration, f: Dialysate creatinine/plasma creatinine; g: Dialysate glucose level.

The basal levels of HbA_{1C} in the two study groups were similar (4.9% ± 0.7% in Icodextrin group and 5.1% ± 1.5% in AAPDF group). Icodextrin decreased fasting glucose ($p < 0.001$), LDL-C ($p = 0.03$) and triglycerides ($p = 0.04$), and increased HDL-C levels ($p = 0.009$) (**Table 3**). AAPDF did not affect glucose and lipid metabolism (**Table 3**).

Basal levels of inflammation markers were similar in both study groups. Basal serum CRP and fibrinogen levels were elevated in both study groups. Compared to AAPDF, Icodextrin increased serum CRP ($p = 0.035$) and fibrinogen levels ($p = 0.009$) (**Table 3**). AAPDF, in contrast to Icodextrin, increased serum albumin ($p = 0.03$) (**Table 3**). Icodextrin decreased body weight ($p=0.002$), SBP ($p < 0.01$) and DBP ($p < 0.05$) while AAPDF increased body weight ($p = 0.002$), SBP ($p < 0.01$) and DBP ($p < 0.05$) (**Table 3**).

Table 3. Effects of Icodextrin and AAPDF on carbohydrates, lipids, inflammation and blood pressure.

	Icodextrin group		
	Baseline	8 weeks	p
Fasting glucose (mg/dl)	141.1 ± 39.9	119.3 ± 29.1	<0.001
LDL-C (mg/dl)	102.3 ± 33.3	89.6 ± 22.0	0.03
HDL-C (mg/dl)	35.6 ± 10.1	40.7 ± 11.8	0.009
TG (mg/dl)	272.4 ± 67.0	221.4 ± 74.8	0.04
Albumin(gr/dl)	3.6 ± 0.4	3.6 ± 0.3	n.s.
CRP (0 - 5 mg/L)	9.5 ± 6.5	22.4 ± 16.5	0.035
Fibrinogen (200 - 400 mg/dl)	835.1 ± 126.5	1066.1 ± 199.8	0.009
Body weight (kg)	80.4 ± 14.1	78.5 ± 14.7	0.002
SBP (mmHg)	149.5 ± 35.5	131.4 ± 21.9	<0.01
DBP (mmHg)	79.0 ± 14.5	72.8 ± 9.9	<0.05
	AAPDF group		
	Baseline	8 weeks	p
Fasting glucose (mg/dl)	138.4 ± 76.2	142.2 ± 86.6	n.s.
LDL-C[a] (mg/dl)	117.6 ± 25.9	112.97 ± 21.1	n.s.
HDL-C[b] (mg/dl)	42.0 ± 9.4	45.0 ± 11.6	n.s.
TG[c] (mg/dl)	186.4 ± 96.6	176.3 ± 62.7	n.s.
Albumin (gr/dl)	3.5 ± 0.4	4.3 ± 0.5	0.03
CRP (0 - 5 mg/L)	12.6 ± 26.0	10.4 ± 18.3	n.s.
Fibrinogen (200 - 400 mg/dl)	999.6 ± 189.6	973.0 ± 231.4	n.s.
Body weight (kg)	71.6 ± 15.0	72.5 ± 15.0	0.002
SBP[d] (mmHg)	138.7 ± 28.4	146.6 ± 26.4	<0.01
DBP[e] (mmHg)	75.4 ± 12.3	80.1 ± 11.8	<0.05

a: Low density lipoprotein cholesterol; b: High density lipoprotein cholesterol; c: Triglycerides; d: Systolic blood pressure; e: Diastolic blood pressure.

Hyperhomocysteinemia was identified in 84% of the study subjects at baseline. Icodextrin decreased P_{Hcy} ($p = 0.002$) (**Table 2**). AAPDF increased P_{Hcy} ($p = 0.03$) (**Table 2**). Furthermore, in Icodextrin group, a linear correlation was found between the degree of increment in UF (ΔUF) and the degree of reduction in P_{Hcy} (ΔP_{Hcy}) ($p < 0.001$, $R^2 = 0.962$) (**Figure 1**), and between the degree of increment in D/P_{Cr} ($\Delta D/P_{Cr}$) and ΔP_{Hcy} ($p < 0.001$, $R^2 = 0.836$) (**Figure 2**).

Icodextrin decreased P_{Hcy} in both CAPD and APD patients ($p = 0.033$), in low average transporter patients (LATs) ($p = 0.006$), in PD patients with $Kt/V > 2$ ($p = 0.04$) or $Kt/V \leq 2$ ($p = 0.003$) and in non diabetic patients ($p = 0.039$) (**Table 4**). LATs had a higher basal P_{Hcy} compared with high-average transporter patients (HATs) ($p = 0.015$) (**Table 4**). HATs had lower P_{Hcy} which were in the upper normal limits (**Table 4**).

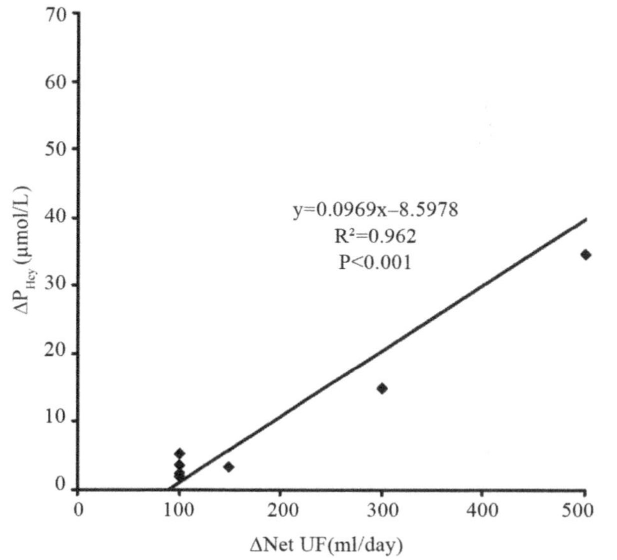

Figure 1. The correlation between ΔP_{Hcy} and ΔNet UF in the extraneal group.

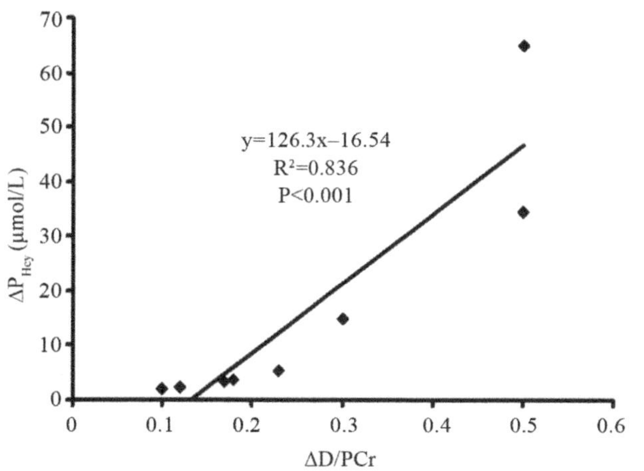

Figure 2. The correlation between ΔP_{Hcy} and $\Delta D/P_{Cr}$ in the extraneal group.

Table 4. Effects of PD[a] modality, peritoneal membrane characteristics, Kt/V, gender and diabetes mellitus on P_{Hcy}.

	P_{Hcy}[b] (μmol/L) in Icodextrin group		
	Baseline	8 weeks	p
CAPD[c]	33.0 ± 26.3	14.7 ± 6.2	0.033
APD[d]	24.3 ± 17.0	14.8 ± 5.0	0.033
p	n.s.		
LATs[e]	46.4 ± 23.2	17.2 ± 5.3	0.006
HATs[f]	15.3 ± 3.0	12.8 ± 5.1	n.s.
P	0.015		
Kt/V ≤ 2	46.9 ± 32.5	19.5 ± 2.7	0.003
Kt/V > 2	20.2 ± 7.3	15.9 ± 6.2	0.04
p	0.05		
DM[g]	24.5 ± 7.9	17.0 ± 7.4	n.s.
Non DM	31.4 ± 6.7	13.7 ± 4.4	0.039
p	n.s.		
	P_{Hcy} (μmol/L) in AAPDF group		
	Baseline	8 weeks	p
CAPD	26.72 ± 7.2	33.6 ± 15.7	n.s.
APD	26.52 ± 24.5	31.12 ± 34.9	n.s.
p	n.s.		
LATs	37.5 ± 18.8	48.5 ± 28.5	n.s.
HATs	15.8 ± 2.1	16.2 ± 3.1	n.s.
p	0.015		
Kt/V ≤ 2	32.3 ± 25.5	38.5 ± 36.6	n.s.
Kt/V > 2	22.8 ± 9.4	28.3 ± 17.9	n.s.
p	0.05		
DM	28.7 ± 5.1	37.0 ± 3.9	n.s.
Non DM	30.0 ± 19.5	38.9 ± 28.4	n.s.
p	n.s.		

a: Peritoneal dialysis; b: Plasma homocysteine; c: Continuous ambulatory peritoneal dialysis; d: Automated peritoneal dialysis, HATs = High average transporters; e: Low average transporters; f: High average transporters; g: Diabetes mellitus.

AAPDF increased P_{Hcy} ($p = 0.03$) (**Table 2**).

Linear regression analysis did not show any correlation between P_{Hcy} and age, gender, body weight, duration of PD, DUO, hemoglobin and PTH levels in both Icodextrin and AAPDF groups.

4. Discussion

Long-term systemic exposure of glucose caused by conventional PD solutions has been well recognized to cause metabolic and cardiovascular abnormalities, which contribute to the morbidities seen in PD patients. Several studies have shown that conventional solutions damage mesothelial cells and peritoneal blood vessels leading to functional impairment [17,18]. Besides its effects on the peritoneal membrane, rapid absorption of glucose during a dwell leads to loss of osmotic gradient and diminished ultrafiltration as well as to the development of hyperglycemia and associated hyperinsulinemia in both diabetic as well as nondiabetic patients [19]. The high levels of dextrose and the lactate acidic buffer make the conventional solutions nonphysiologic and nonbiocompatible. Introducing the newer solutions that designed to be more biocompatible by either, containing physiologic buffer bicarbonate, or having lower GDP concentration, and/or substituting glucose with alternative osmotic agents, like polyglucose or amino acids were targeted to ameliorate the complications of conventional dextrose solutions [20-22]. It is postulated that newer PD solutions containing lower levels of GDPs are less nephrotoxic, and hence may preserve RRF longer. Additionally, the effect of fluid status on preservation of RRF cannot be ignored.

In the present study, Icodextrin and AAPDF did not affect RRF (**Table 2**). Icodextrin improved glucose control and lipid profile including significant decrease in LDL-C and triglyceride levels as well as significant increase in HDL-C (**Table 3**). Similar results were reported by Bredie *et al.* [23].

It is well known that the major reason for the elevation of blood pressure in PD patients is volume overload. Icodextrin improved blood pressure control by improving UF and decreasing body weight (**Tables 2** and **3**).

The effects of Icodextrin on inflammation status in PD patients are controversial [11,12]. Martikainen *et al.* showed that Icodextrin use was resulted in subclinical inflammatory response [11]. In contrast, Lin *et al.* reported that Icodextrin decreased CRP [12]. In this study the basal serum CRP and fibrinogen levels were similar and elevated in both study groups (**Table 3**). Icodextrin use was accompanied by a rise in plasma CRP and fibrinogen levels (**Table 3**). There is a concern that Icodextrin use may induce a subclinical inflammatory response, both intraperitoneally and systemically. Accordingly, Icodextrin that lowered GDPs levels and designed to preserve the peritoneal membrane and to improve glucose and lipid control, seems to intensify systemic inflammation.

Hyperhomocysteinemia was identified in 84% of our study subjects compared to the 97% - 98% reported by Van Guldener [24]. The significant rise in D/P_{Cr} and UF as well as the linear correlations between ΔP_{Hcy} and ΔNetUF, and between ΔP_{Hcy} and $\Delta D/P_{Cr}$ in the Icodextrin group, suggest better peritoneal clearances of Hcy compared to standard glucose-based fluids and AAPDF (**Table 2**, **Figures 1** and **2**). Similar results were reported by Czupryniak *et al.* [25].

It is well known that AAPDF improve nutritional status in malnourished PD patients. Although increased serum albumin levels and did not affect UF, glucose and lipid metabolism, and inflammation status, AAPDF increased body weight, SBP, DBP and P_{Hcy} levels (p =

0.002, $p < 0.01$, $p < 0.05$, $p = 0.03$—respectively) (**Tables 2** and **3**). The increase in P_{Hcy} in the AAPDF group is, most likely, related to methionine, a precursor of Hcy, absorption as well as to the decrease in D/P_{Cr} and UF in the AAPDF group (**Table 2**). Then, AAPDF that introduced to improve nutritional status and survival may contribute to the unfavorable rise of P_{Hcy}. The rise in P_{Hcy} in PD patients treated with AAPDF described also in previous studies [26,27].

End stage renal disease patients are unable to excrete the daily acid load. The standard PDFs, Icodextrin and AAPDF use lactate as a buffer that, by its acidic pH, causes harmful effects on the peritoneal cells [17]. In contrast, bicarbonate-based PDFs include a physiologic buffer with neutral pH, cause less peritoneal damage [28].

The relationships between the PD modality, the peritoneal membrane characteristics and Kt/V, and P_{Hcy} remain a controversial issue [29,30]. Basal P_{Hcy} was elevated and not different in the two study groups and all subgroups apart from HATs (**Table 4**). In the Icodextrin group P_{Hcy} decreased in both PD modalities ($p = 0.033$) (**Table 3**). On the other hand, AAPDF increase P_{Hcy} ($p = 0.033$) (**Table 2**). This may be due to its low osmotic drive and as a result of the absorption of methionine through the peritoneal membrane. These results suggest that the peritoneal membrane characteristics and the composition of the PDF have an important role in the peritoneal elimination of Hcy.

Basal P_{Hcy} in HATs were near normal in both study groups (**Table 4**). It may be related to the higher solute clearances across the peritoneal membrane in HATs.

Basal P_{Hcy} was marginally lower in subjects with $Kt/V > 2$ compared to those with $Kt/V \leq 2$ ($p = 0.05$) (**Table 4**). Icodextrin, but not AAPDF, significantly decreased P_{Hcy} in PD patients with $Kt/V > 2$, in those with $Kt/V \leq 2$ and in non diabetic patients (**Table 4**). Therefore, Icodextrin may influence the atherosclerotic outcomes through Hcy-lowering effects, as it was stated previously by Docloux et al [29].

No associations between age, gender, body weight, duration of PD, hemoglobin, PTH, RRF and DUO and P_{Hcy} were found.

In summary: Higher UF, higher D/P_{Cr}, HATs, $Kt/V > 2$, non diabetic patients and Icodextrin use were associated with decline in P_{Hcy}. Conversely, lower UF, lower D/P_{Cr}, LATs, $Kt/V \leq 2$, diabetic patients and AAPDF use were associated with rise in P_{Hcy}.

Although it exhibited favorable effects on metabolic status, blood pressure control and P_{Hcy} levels, Icodextrin seems to intensify systemic inflammation. On the other hand, although it did not seem to affect adversely the metabolic status and systemic inflammation, AAPDF increased P_{Hcy} and blood pressure.

The results of the present study suggested that the use of Icodextrin and AAPDF was associated with beneficial effects as well as with considerable harmful consequences that may adversely affect the prognosis and survival of PD patients.

5. Conclusion

A new PDF containing a mixture of a biocompatible substance, amino acids without methionine, lower glucose and GDPs content, and neutral pH will provide sustained oncotic effect, adequate dialysis and ultrafiltration as well as will improve nutritional status and metabolic profile, reduce inflammation, plasma homocyteine and blood pressure. A PDF with those properties will preserve the peritoneal membrane and improve the prognosis and survival of peritoneal dialysis patients.

6. Acknowledgements

The authors would like to thank Prof. Ben Ami Sela, Clinical Biochemistry Laboratory-Sheba Medical Center, Tel Hashomer, Israel for his assistance in determination of P_{Hcy}. We also would like to thank Tobie Kuritsky for her assistance in editing our manuscript.

REFERENCES

[1] P. S. Parfrey and J. D. Harnett, "Long Term Cardiac Morbidity and Mortality during Dialysis Therapy," *Advanced Nephrology*, Vol. 23, 1994, pp. 311-330.

[2] S. H. Park, P. Stenvinkel and B. Lindholm, "Cardiovascular Biomarkers in Chronic Kidney Disease," *Journal of Renal Nutrition*, Vol. 22, No. 1, 2012, pp. 120-127. doi:10.1053/j.jrn.2011.10.021

[3] A. H. Mitwalli, A. A. Alam, J. S. Al Wakeel and A. C. Isnani, "Dyslipidemia in Dialysis Patients," *Saudi Journal of Kidney Disease and Transplantation*, Vol. 22, No. 4, 2011, pp. 689-694.

[4] L. M. Ortega and B. J. Materson, "Hypertension in Peritoneal Dialysis Patients: Epidemiology, Pathogenesis, and Treatment," *Journal of the American Society of Hypertension*, Vol. 5, No. 3, 2011, pp. 128-136. doi:10.1016/j.jash.2011.02.004

[5] M. Moriishi and H. Kawanishi, "Icodextrin and Intraperitoneal Inflammation," *Peritoneal Dialysis International*, Vol. 28, Suppl. 3, 2008, pp. S96-S100.

[6] T. Huang, G. Yuan, Z. Zhang, Z. Zou and D. Li, "Cardiovascular Pathogenesis in Hyperhomocysteinemia," *Asia Pacific Journal of Clinical Nutrition*, Vol. 17, No. 1, 2008, pp. 8-16.

[7] C. van Guldener and F. Stam, "Stehouwer CDA. Homocysteine Metabolism in Renal Failure," *Kidney International*, Vol. 59, Suppl. 78, 2001, pp. S234-S237. doi:10.1046/j.1523-1755.2001.07859.x

[8] M. M. Sagheb, M. A. Ostovan, Z. Sohrabi, E. Atabati, G. A. Raisjalai and J. Roozbeh, "Hyperhomocysteinemia and Cardiovascular Risks in Hemodialysis Patients," *Saudi*

Journal of Kidney Diseases and Transplantation, Vol. 21, No. 5, 2010, pp. 863-866.

[9] L. A. Cooker, C. J. Holmes and C. M. Hoff, "Biocompatibility of Icodextrin," *Kidney International*, Vol. 62, Suppl. 81, 2002, pp. S34-S45. doi:10.1046/j.1523-1755.62.s81.6.x

[10] M. Canbakan and G. M. Sahin, "Icodextrine and Insulin Resistance in Continuous Ambulatory Peritoneal Dialysis Patients," *Renal Failure*, Vol. 29, No. 3, 2007, pp. 289-293. doi:10.1080/08860220601166271

[11] T. A. Martikainen, A. M. Teppo, C. Grönhagen-Riska and A. V. Ekstrand, "Glucose-Free Dialysis Solutions: Inductors of Inflammation or Preservers of Peritoneal Membrane?" *Peritoneal Dialysis International*, Vol. 25, No. 5, 2005, pp. 453-460.

[12] W. Lin, Y. C. Chen, M. S. Wu, H. J. Hsu, C. Y. Sun, Y. K.Lin and I. W. Wu, "Icodextrin Dialysate Improves Nutritional and Inflammatory Profiles in Peritoneal Dialysis Patients," *Renal Failure*, Vol. 31, No. 2, 2009, pp. 98-105. doi:10.1080/08860220802595500

[13] F. K. Li, L. Y.Chan , J. C. Woo, *et al.*, "A 3-Year, Prospective, Randomized, Controlled, Study on Amino Acid Dialysate in Patients on CAPD," *American Journal of Kidney Diseases*, Vol. 42, No. 1, 2003, pp. 173-183. doi:10.1016/S0272-6386(03)00421-9

[14] A. S. Levey, J. P. Bosch, J. B. Lewis, T. Greene, N. Rogers and D. Roth, "A More Accurate Method to Estimate Glomerular Filtration Rate from Serum Creatinine: A New Prediction Equation, Modification of Diet in Renal Disease Study Group," *Annals of Internal Medicine*, Vol. 130, No. 6, 1999, pp. 461-470.

[15] Z. J. Twardowski, "Clinical Value of Standardized Equilibration Tests in CAPD Patients," *Blood Purification*, Vol. 7, No. 2-3, 1989, pp. 95-108. doi:10.1159/000169582

[16] G. Amici, S. Mastrosimone, G. Da Rin, C. Bocci and A. Bonadonna, "Clinical Validation of PD Adequest Software: Modeling Error Assessment," *Peritoneal Dialysis International*, Vol. 18, No. 3, 1998, pp. 317-321.

[17] H. Ha, M. R. Yu, H. N. Choi, M. K. Cha, H. S. Kang, M. H. Kim and H. B. Lee, "Effects of Conventional and New Peritoneal Dialysis Solutions on Human Peritoneal Mesothelial Cell Viability and Proliferation," *Peritoneal Dialysis International*, Vol. 20, Suppl. 5, 2000, pp. S10-S18.

[18] R. T. Krediet, M. M. Zweers, A. C. vander Wal and D. J. Struijk, "Neoangiogenesis in the Peritoneal Membrane," *Peritoneal Dialysis International*, Vol. 20, Suppl. 2, 2000, pp. S19-S25.

[19] J. Delarue and C. Maingourd, "Acute Metabolic Effects of Dialysis Fluids during CAPD," *American Journal of Kidney Diseases*, Vol. 37, Suppl. 2, 2001, pp. S103-S107. doi:10.1053/ajkd.2001.20762

[20] N. Posthuma, P. M. ter Wee, A. J. Donker, P. L. Oe, E. M. Peers and H. A. Verbrugh, "Assesement of the Effectiveness, Safety, and Biocompatibility of Icodextrin in Automated Peritoneal Dialysis. The Dextrin in APD in Amsterdam (DIANA) Group," *Peritoneal Dialysis International*, Vol. 20, Suppl. 2, 2000, pp. S106-S113.

[21] T. W. Kao, H. F. Chuang, K. Y. Hung, K. D. Wu and T. J. Tsai, "Rate of Decline of Residual Renal Function is Associated with All-Cause Mortality and Technique Failure in Patients on Long-Term Peritoneal Dialysis," *Nephrology Dialysis Transplantation*, Vol. 24, No. 9, 2009, pp. 2909-2914. doi:10.1093/ndt/gfp056

[22] S. Kim, J. Oh, S. Kim, W. Chung, C. Ahn, S. G. Kim and K. H. Oh, "Benefits of Biocompatible PD Fluid for Preservation of Residual Renal Function in Incident CAPD Patients: A 1-Year Study," *Nephrology Dialysis Transplantation*, Vol. 24, No. 9, 2009, pp. 2899-2908. doi:10.1093/ndt/gfp054

[23] S. J. Bredie, F. H. Bosch, P. N. Demacker, A. F. Stalenhoef and R. Van Leusen, "Effects of Peritoneal Dialysis with an Overnight Icodextrin Dwell on Parameters of Glucose and Lipid Metabolism," *Peritoneal Dialysis International*, Vol. 21, No. 3, 2001, pp. 275-281.

[24] C. Van Guldener, "Why is Homocysteine Elevated in Renal Failure and What Can Be Expected from Homocysteine-Lowering?" *Peritoneal Dialysis International*, Vol. 21, No. 5, 2006, pp. 1161-1166. doi:10.1093/ndt/gfl044

[25] A. Czupryniak, M. Nowicki, G. Chwatko, A. Jander and E. Bald, "Peritoneal Clearance of Homocysteine with Icodextrin or Standard Glucose Solution Exchange," *Nephrology* (*Carlton*), Vol. 10, No. 6, 2005, pp. 571-575.

[26] H. F. Brulez, C. van Guldener, A. J. Donker and P. M. Ter Wee, "The Impact of an Amino Acid-Based Peritoneal Dialysis Fluid on Plasma Total Homocysteine Levels, Lipid Profile and Body Fat Mass," *Nephrology Dialysis Transplantation*, Vol. 14, No. 1, 1999, pp. 154-159. doi:10.1093/ndt/14.1.154

[27] S. Y. Yang, J. W. Huang, K. Y. Shih, *et al.*, "Factors Associated with Increased Plasma Homocysteine in Patients Using an Amino Acid Peritoneal Dialysis Fluid," *Nephrology Dialysis Transplantation*, Vol. 20, No. 1, 2005, pp. 161-166. doi:10.1093/ndt/gfh554

[28] S. Haas, C. P. Schmitt, K. Arbeiter, K. E. Bonzel, M. Fischbach, U. John, A. K. Pieper, T. P. Schaub, J. Passlick-Deetjen and O. Mehls, "Schaefer FImproved Acidosis Correction and Recovery of Mesothelial Cell Mass with Neutral-pH Bicarbonate Dialysis Solution among Children Undergoing Automated Peritoneal Dialysis," *Journal of the American Society of Hypertension*, Vol. 14, No. 10, 2003, pp. 2632-2638. doi:10.1097/01.ASN.0000086475.83211.DF

[29] D. Ducloux, L. Heuze-Lecornu, R. Gibey, C. Bresson-Vautrin, P. Vautrin and J. M. Chalopin, "Dialysis Adequacy and Homocyst(e)ine Concentrations in Peritoneal Dialysis Patients," *Nephrology Dialysis Transplantation*, Vol. 14, No. 3, 1999, pp. 728-731. doi:10.1093/ndt/14.3.728

[30] A. Vychytil, M. Fodinger, M. Papagiannopoulos, *et al.*, "Peritoneal Elimination of Homocysteine Moieties in Continuous Ambulatory Peritoneal Dialysis Patients," *Kidney International*, Vol. 55, No. 5, 1999, pp. 2054-2061. doi:10.1046/j.1523-1755.1999.00437.x

15

Erythropoiesis Stimulating Agents (ESAs) in the Treatment of Cardio-Renal Syndrome Anaemia

Ioannis Koulouridis, Efstathios Koulouridis
Department of Nephrology, General Hospital of Corfu, Corfu, Greece
Email: koulef@otent.gr

ABSTRACT

Coexistence of chronic kidney disease (CKD) and chronic heart failure (CHF) define a recently recognized clinical entity known as cardio-renal syndrome. Sufficient evidence suggests that the two pathological conditions share common pathogenic etiology which is not yet fully defined. Superimposed anaemia is a common finding among patients suffering from cardio-renal syndrome. The combination of CKD, CHF and anaemia increase the probability of death by 6 times compared to normal individuals. Early attempts to restore anaemia either by iron supplementation, erythropoiesis stimulating agents (ESAs) or combination of the two have reported to improve quality of life, morbidity and mortality especially among patients treated by cardiologists. Recent publications of well controlled epidemiological studies failed to prove convincing beneficial effect of the above mentioned therapy moreover skepticism has raised concerning the safety of restoring anaemia among patients with cardio-renal syndrome as well as used medications. There are still unresolved problems concerning the definition of anaemia, by means of hemoglobin level among these patients, the target hemoglobin level and the therapeutic regimen of ESAs administration and iron supplementation. We need much more evidence in order to define an effective and safe treatment strategy correcting anaemia among patients with cardio-renal syndrome.

Keywords: Cardio-Renal Syndrome; Anaemia; Erythropoiesis Stimulating Agents; Adverse Outcomes

1. Introduction

The term cardio-renal syndrome refers to the condition of cardiac and renal failure coexistence when the deterioration of cardiac function implies deterioration of renal function and vice versa. It should not be considered as simple coexistence of two separate pathological conditions but, as a coupled damage of the two organs many of the leading factors are still unknown [1]. According to the consensus conference on cardio-renal syndromes (CRS) held in Venice Italy, 2008 five subtypes of cardio-renal syndromes were recognized [2]. The type 1 or acute cardio-renal syndrome refers to the condition of acute cardiac function worsening which leads to renal injury or dysfunction. The type 2 or chronic cardio-renal syndrome defines the situations of chronic cardiac abnormalities which are coupled with chronic renal dysfunction. The type 3 or acute reno-cardiac syndrome refers to the presence of acute kidney injury which leads to heart injury or dysfunction. The type 4 or chronic reno-cardiac syndrome refers to the presence of chronic kidney disease which leads to chronic cardiac damage or dysfunction and the type 5 or secondary cardio-renal syndrome refers to the presence of systemic pathological conditions affecting simultaneously the two organs such as sepsis, collagen disease, diabetes mellitus, amyloidosis etc. In the present review we shall focus our interest mainly upon the type 2 and type 4 CRS and the effect of anaemia correction upon cardiac and renal function as well as upon patient's final outcome concerning morbidity and mortality.

It is known from the literature that the frequency of kidney disease among patients older than 65 years of age hospitalized for acute decompensated congestive heart failure has been estimated to be 21% where as 41% of them exhibit creatinine levels greater than 1.5 mg/dL [3]. Emergence of acute kidney injury (increment of createnine levels greater than 0.3 mg/dL) during therapeutic manipulation of hospitalized patients suffering from congestive heart failure is estimated to be 27% - 45% even though they exhibited normal creatinine levels at the admission to the hospital [4]. The presence of cardiac failure among patients suffering from chronic kidney disease (CKD) has been estimated in a large epidemiological survey based upon the data of Medicare system and showed that 39.9% of patients exhibited cardiac failure from the first visit and an additional 30.7% developed cardiac failure during the next year [5]. Data from the Acute Decompensated Heart Failure National Registry (ADHERE) study showed that increase of creatinine and blood urea nitrogen levels were the most powerful independent risk factors affecting in-hospital mortality [6]. The detailed effect of kidney injury upon mortality of hospitalized and non-hospitalized patients suffering from congestive heart failure was shown from a meta-analysis of sixteen RCTs including 80,018 patients. This study showed a positive correlation between deterioration of renal function and mortality, moreover each 0.5 mg/dL increment of creatinine exhibited a 15% increment of mortality where as for each 10 ml/min reduction of eGFR observed a 7% increase in mortality [7]. The etiology of increased mortality among patients suffering from cardio-renal syndrome is probably due to increased activity of RAS system, increased sympathetic activity, increased concentration of pro-inflammatory cytokines, deterioration of anaemia, deterioration of left ventricular hypertrophy and myocardial contractility, deranged regulation of extra-cellular volume and final exhaust of the cardiac pump which leads to death [7].

2. Anaemia in Cardio-Renal Syndrome

The frequency of anaemia in cardio-renal syndrome is difficult to be estimated because of lack of universal criteria in defining anaemia among patients with cardiac failure. Most authors accept hemoglobin levels lower than 12 - 12.5 g/dl in order to characterize patients with cardiac failure as anemic [8].

Data from the Organized Program to Initiate Lifesaving Treatment in Hospitalized Patients with Heart Failure ((OPTIMIZE-HF) which included 48,612 patients, showed that 51.2% of them exhibited hemoglobin levels lower than 12.1 g/dL whereas 25% of them exhibited hemoglobin levels between 5 g/dL and 10.7 g/dL. Moreover it was shown that decrease of hemoglobin level by 1 g/dL produced an increase in the likelihood of death by 20% [8].

It is widely accepted that among patients with CKD hemoglobin levels lower than 12 g/dL are compatible with anaemia. According to this definition McClellan *et al.* [9] showed that among 5222 patients with CKD anaemia was present in 47.7% of them. It was shown also that anaemia was inversely correlated with GFR, so patients with GFR levels greater than 60 ml/min/1.73 m^2 exhibited anaemia in a percentage of 26.7% whereas patients with GFR levels lower than 15 ml/min/1.73 m^2 exhibited anaemia in a percentage of 75.5%. The coexistence of cardiac failure, chronic kidney disease and anaemia increases the probability of death by six times compared to healthy individuals [10].

Etiology of anaemia among patients with cardiac failure is attributed to fluid retention and concomitant edema which produce blood dilution as well as to aspirin and antiplatelet drugs which produce chronic occult blood loss. Other causes are reduced absorption of iron, folic acid and vitamin B12 by intestine due to mucosal edema, increased production of inflammatory cytokines such as interleukin 1 or 6 and 18 as well as TNF-α which suppress erythropoiesis and produce cachexia. Another important causative factor of anaemia among these patients is the prescription of angiotensin converting enzyme inhibitors as it is known that Ang-II promotes erythropoiesis in bone marrow. Moreover it is known that converting enzyme is the main catabolic enzyme of the tetra peptide acetyl-N-Ser-Asp-Lys-Pro (AcSDKP) which is a known powerful inhibitor of erythropoiesis so that converting enzyme inhibition leads to increased concentration of AcSDKP with a resultant suppression of effective erythropoiesis [8,10-12].

It has been speculated that patients suffering from cardiorenal syndrome are not deficient of endogenous erythropoietin production. Van der Meer *et al.* [12] showed in a small number of anemic patients, suffering from cardiac failure and CKD, that 29% of them exhibited levels of endogenous erythropoietin greater than expected as well as that these patients exhibited greater mortality rate compared to patients with expected or lower than expected levels of endogenous erythropoietin. This finding suggests that a considerable proportion of patients with cardio-renal anaemia exhibit endogenous erythropoietin resistance.

The most important causative factor of anaemia among patients with CKD is the lack of endogenous erythropoietin, absolute or relative, because it is known that about 40% of patients with CKD exhibit increased levels of bioactive endogenous erythropoietin but reduced response to the hormone action [13]. Other causes of anaemia in CKD patients are the reduced time life of red blood cells, the chronic blood loss from gastrointestinal tract, frequent blood tests, iron deficiency, folate and B12 deficiency, secondary hyperparathyroidism, hypothyroidism, acute or chronic inflammation, aluminum toxicity and hemoglobinopathies [12-14].

3. Restoration of Cardiorenal Anaemia

The exogenous administration of erythropoietin and iron, either solely or in combination, is capable to restore anaemia of cardio-renal syndrome and several earlier publications suggest that improve quality of life, left ventricular ejection fraction and morbidity of these patients but newer randomized controlled trials (RCTs) failed to confirm preliminary enthusiasm, on the contrary it is possible that vigorous attempt to anaemia correction increase all cause mortality, cardiovascular mortality and fatal and nonfatal stroke events [15].

The first disappointing results concerning the correction of anaemia in CKD patients came in 2006 published in the same issue of New England Journal of Medicine and included the Cardiovascular Risk Reduction by early Treatment with Epoetin beta (CREATE) [16] study and the Correction of Hemoglobin and Outcomes in Renal Insufficiency (CHOIR) [17] study.

The CREATE study included 603 patients with CKD stage III-IV (eGFR: 15 - 35 ml/min/1.73 m^2) and mild anaemia (Hb: 11 - 12.5 g/dL), patients randomized in two groups, in group I (n = 301) administered erythropoietin (epoetin beta, NeoRecormone, F. Hoffman-La Roche) with target hemoglobin 13.0 - 15 g/dL, in group II (n = 302) administered erythropoietin only when hemoglobin levels fell below 10.5 g/dL with target hemoglobin lower than 11.5 g/dL. After a three years observation period no difference in cardiovascular events, deterioration of renal function or left ventricular mass index was noted between groups, in contrast more patients from group I than group II reached end stage renal disease (127 vs 111, p = 0.03), general condition and physical activity was improved, as expected, in group I ($p = 0.003$ and $p < 0.001$ respectively).

The CHOIR study included 1432 patients with CKD stage III-IV (eGFR: 27.0 ± 8.7 ml/min/1.73 m^2), patients randomized in two groups, in group I (n = 715) administered epoetin alfa with target hemoglobin 13.5 g/dL and in group II (n = 717) administered epoetin alfa with target hemoglobin 11.3 g/dL. After 16 months Data and Safety Monitoring Board discontinued study because of unfavorable outcomes. The end points of the study were all cause of death, myocardial infarction, hospitalization for decompensated heart failure and stoke. A total of 222 events were recorded, 125 of them in group I (high hemoglobin) and 97 in group II (low hemoglobin) [HR = 1.34 (95% CI 1.03 - 1.74) p = 0.03]. The recorded events were 65 deaths (29.3%), 101 hospitalizations for decompensated heart failure (45.5%), 25 myocardial infarctions (11.3%), and 23 strokes (10.4%) no difference in the improvement of quality of life was justified between groups.

The above mentioned studies prompted the need to contact double blind placebo controlled trials in order to elucidate the effect of anaemia correction in the evolution of kidney disease and cardiac disease among cardio-renal syndrome patients and so emerged the Study of Anemia in Heart Failure Trial (STAMINA-HeFT) and the Trial to Reduce Cardiovascular Events with Aranesp Therapy (TREAT) study.

The STAMINA-HeFT [18] included 319 patients with symptomatic heart failure (EF < 40%) and eGFR < 60 ml/min/1.73 m^2. Patients randomized in two groups in group I (n = 157) administered placebo in order to keep hemoglobin levels about 11.3 g/dL and in group II (n = 162) administered darbepoetin alfa subcutaneously every two weeks for one year with target hemoglobin 14.0 ± 1.0 g/dL. No statistically significant difference in exercise duration and in heart failure severity according to NYHA criteria was noted between the two groups, although a trend toward a reduction of all cause mortality and hospitalization for acute decompensated heart failure was noted in darbepoetin group.

The TREAT [19] study included 4038 patients with CKD stage III-IV (eGFR: 20 - 60 ml/min/1.73 m^2) and diabetes mellitus. Patients randomized in two groups, the darbepoetin alfa group (n = 2012) and the placebo group (n = 2026). Target hemoglobin for the darbepoetin group was 12 g/dL and for the placebo group 9 g/dL, whenever hemoglobin level fell below 9 g/dL in placebo group administered darbepoetin or transfusions but not exceeding hemoglobin level of 11 g/dL. The end points of the study were all cause mortality, non fatal myocardial infarction, congestive heart failure, stroke, hospitalization for myocardial ischemia and end-stage renal disease (ESRD). Death or cardiovascular events occurred in 632 patients of darbepoetin group and in 602 patients in placebo group [HR = 1.06 (95% CI 0.94 - 1.17) p = 0.41], death or ESRD occurred in 652 patients of darbepoetin group and in 618 patients of the placebo group [HR = 1.06 (95% CI 0.95 - 1.19) p = 0.29]. Fatal or nonfatal stroke occurred in 101 patients of the darbepoetin group and in 53 patients of the placebo group [HR = 1.92 (95% CI 1.38 - 2.68) $p < 0.001$]. Blood transfusions needed 297 patients of the darbepoetin group and 496 patients of the placebo group ($p < 0.001$). Only a subtle difference in fatigue was noted among darbepoetin group in relation to the placebo group.

In a later post hoc analysis of the TREAT study Solomon *et al.* [20] compared the outcomes of participants according to their initial response to darbepoetin. The analysis included 1872 patients from the darbepoetin group authors separated 471 patients who after a two weight-based doses of darbepoetin, in a two-week regimen, failed to increase their hemoglobin levels higher than 2% of the initial level. These patients characterized as "poor initial responders" and although they received the higher doses of darbepoetin (median dose 232 μg vs 167 μg, $p < 0.001$) they exhibited the lower levels of hemoglobin throughout the study. Moreover poor initial responders exhibited greater frequency of cardiovascular events [HR = 1.31 (95% CI 1.09 - 1.59)], greater frequency of all-cause mortality [HR = 1.41 (95% CI 1.12 - 1.72)] and greater frequency of stokes [HR = 1.26 (95% CI 0.78 - 2.02)].

More recently published data indicate that erythropoietin dose rather than hemoglobin level is the cause of inverse outcomes among dialysis and non-dialysis patients. Zhang Y *et al.* [21] in an observational study included 35,593 elderly patients of Medicare system, undergoing dialysis (19,034 of them were diabetics) the authors showed that the adjusted 9-month mortality risk for erythropoietin dose between 15,000 U/week and 45,000 U/week was 13% among diabetics (95% CI: 10% - 16%) and 5% among non-diabetics [(95% CI: 2% - 9%) p-value = 0.002]. Koulouridis I *et al.* [22] in a Meta-Regression analysis of 31 RCTs included 12,956 dialysis and non-dialysis patients showed that an increase of ESAs dose (erythropoietina equivalent 10,000 U/week increment) was associated with a higher rate of all cause mortality, Incidence Rate Ratio [IRR = 1.42 (95% CI: 1.10 - 1.83)] but not cardiovascular mortality, [IRR = 1.09 (95% CI: 1.02 - 1.18)].

4. The Holistic Concept of Cardiorenal Patient

In every day clinical practice a controversy exist between cardiologists and nephrologists concerning the correction of anemia among cardiorenal patients. The controversy is primarily relied upon three unresolved items: Firstly what hemoglobin level characterizes a patient with cardiac failure as anemic, secondly what is the target hemoglobin among these patients, thirdly what is the proper therapeutic regimen (dose and frequency of drug administration).

Reports concerning cardiac failure patients suggest that the ideal hemoglobin levels must be at 13 g/dL and preferably between 13.5 g/dL and 14 g/dL but on the other hand, according to KDOQI guidelines [23], ideal hemoglobin levels for CKD patients must be between 11 g/dL and 12 g/dL and under no circumstance should they exceed 13 g/dL because of an increased hazard concerning side effects due to the increased level of hemoglobin or to erythropoiesis stimulating agents by themselves.

Most of the studies concerning cardiac failure patients are observational studies from various centers with a relatively small number of patients and the validation criteria include improvement of exercise duration, heart failure according to NYHA classification, left ventricular ejection fraction and quality of life which confine the efficacy and not the safety of the drags used. On the other hand it has been proved that among CKD patient's hemoglobin levels greater than 12 g/dL are harmful concerning progression of renal disease suggesting that anaemia is a "defense mechanism" which protects glomerulus from further damage and it is possible that these patients are benefited in a narrow limit of hemoglobin level variation [15].

It seems likely that adverse events of anaemia correction are coupled with platelet function and blood viscosity. It has been proven in experimental as well as in clinical studies that hematocrit level greater than 30% leads to increased platelet aggregation and blood viscosity with deleterious effects upon glomerulus blood supply and acceleration of glomerulosclerosis by a concomitant increase of the likelihood of systemic thromboembolic events. Apart from ESAs the correction of anaemia needs to be administered intravenous iron supplementation and it is known that the transferrin-iron complex is filtered through the glomerulus and in the acidic pH of urine dissociates to transferrin and divalent iron ions which via the Fenton reaction produce hydroxyl radicals with resultant oxidative stress and tissue damage [15].

The deleterious effect of full anaemia correction is not restricted only upon the kidney, but also encompasses the rest of the cardio-vascular system because increased blood viscosity is coupled with increased peripheral vascular resistance and increased cardiac after-load whereas the decline of renal function increases extracellular volume and blood pressure with resultant congestive heart failure and left ventricular hypertrophy [15].

The uncertainty of ESAs beneficial effect upon cardiorenal anaemia is much more complicated from the observations of van der Meer *et al.* [12] who investigated 74 anemic patients with congestive heart failure (NYHA class II-IV) and CKD (stage II-III) and found that 29 (39%) of them exhibited endogenous erythropoietin levels lower than expected, 23 (31%) as expected and 22 (29%) higher than expected. Patients with lower levels of endogenous erythropoietin exhibited the lower levels of eGFR which is relevant to reduced erythropoietin production from diseased kidneys on the other hand patients with higher than expected levels of endogenous erythropoietin exhibited increased mortality (log rank: p = 0.024). The multifactorial analysis showed that the ratio O/P (Observed/Predicted) of endogenous erythropoietin emerged as the most powerful independent risk factor of increased mortality even if adjusted to variables such as age, gender, hemoglobin levels, NT-pro-BNP levels and eGFR [HR = 1020 (95% CI 1.004 - 1.036) p = 0.012]. These results suggest that patients with endogenous erythropoietin resistance exhibit higher mortality rate. On the other hand the results of TREAT study showed that patients with exogenous erythropoietin resistance (non-responders) exhibited higher mortality rate than the responders. Taken together these findings suggest the possibility that increasing the dose of erythropoietin in any patient who doesn't respond adequately to the hormone action may aggravate the possibility of inverse outcomes. Although it is only a suggestion because endogenous erythropoietin levels did not estimated in TREAT study it is wise to accept Sandhu A.'s *et al.* [10] opinion that "ESA resistance should not be treated with increase in ESA dose alone".

According to present knowledge there are no convinceing answers to the above mentioned items so it is necessary to conduct prospective controlled trials in order to solve the confliction concerning the beneficial effect of restoring anaemia in patients with cardiorenal syndrome as well as the safety of erythropoietic agents. The

Reduction of Events with Darbepoetin alfa in Heart Failure (RED-HF) [24] trial and EPOCARES study [25] are now in progress and we are waiting with great interest the results to be published. The eligibility criteria in RED-HF trial concerning anaemia in heart failure patients accepted hemoglobin levels between 9.0 g/dL and 12.0 g/dL, the darbepoetin alfa administered subcutaneously every two weeks until hemoglobin levels reached at 13 g/dL and monthly there after, if hemoglobin levels reached 14.5 g/dL darbepoetin stopped and placebo was administered [24]. The eligibility criteria in EPOCARES study accepted hemoglobin levels compatible with mild anemia between 10.3 - 12.6 gr/dL for men and 10.3 - 11.9 gr/dL for women. The study designs encompass three groups of patients with different treatment schedules in order to investigate the hematopoietic and non-hematopoietic effects of erythropoietin [25]. It is obvious that the two studies exhibit considerable discrepancy in anemia definition among CRS patients as well as in target hemoglobin levels.

Meanwhile the Food and Drug Administration (FDA) on June 24, 2011 announced its alert concerning the "Modified dosing recommendations to improve the safe use of Erythropoiesis-Stimulating Agents (ESAs) in chronic kidney disease" according to which stated that: 1) "Using of ESAs to target a hemoglobin level greater than 11 g/dL increases the risk of serious adverse cardiovascular events and has not been shown to provide additional patient benefit"; 2) "No clinical trial to date has identified a hemoglobin target level, ESA dose, or dosing strategy that does not increase these risks". Especially for patients with CKD not on dialysis recommends initiating treatment with ESAs when hemoglobin level is less than 10 g/dL and if the rate of hemoglobin decline indicates the likelihood of red blood cell transfusion in order to avoid alloimmunization and/or other transfusion-related risks. Finally recommends that: "If the hemoglobin level exceeds 10 g/dL, reduce or interrupt the dose of ESA and use the lowest dose of ESA sufficient to reduce the need for red blood cell transfusions".

FDA recommendations refers not only to ESRD patients but also to patients with cardio-renal syndrome anaemia especially type 2 and 4 so it is wise to accept these recommendations in clinical practice when we treat with ESAs patients with cardio-renal syndrome anaemia.

In conclusion we have to pay much more attention in treating cardio-renal anaemia either by erythropoiesis stimulating agents or intravenous iron. It seems likely that, according to FDA, the target hemoglobin must not exceed 11 g/dL. ESAs administration has to begin with the lower recommended doses until target hemoglobin is achieved and then dose titration must be prompted. If patient does not exhibit successful response it is not wise to increase ESAs dose until definite convincing results prove the safety of this strategy.

REFERENCES

[1] C. Longhini, C. Molino and F. Fabbian Cardiorenal, "Syndrome: Still Not a Defined Entity," *Clinical and Experimental Nephrology*, Vol. 14, No. 1, 2010, pp. 12-21. doi:10.1007/s10157-009-0257-4

[2] C. Ronco, P. McCollough, S. D. Anker, I. Anand, N. Aspromonte, S. M.Bagshaw, *et al.*, "For the Acute Dialysis Quality Initiative (ADQI) Consensus Group. Cardio-Renal Syndromes: Report from the Consensus Conference of the Acute Dialysis Quality Initiative," *European Heart Journal*, Vol. 31, No. 6, 2010, pp. 703-711. doi:10.1093/eurheartj/ehp507

[3] H. M. Krumholtz, Y. T. Chen, V. Vaccarino, Y. Wang, M. J. Radford, W. D. Bradford, *et al.*, "Correlates and Impact on Outcomes of Worsening Renal Function in Patients ≥ 65 Years of Age with Heart Failure," *American Journal of Cardiology*, Vol. 85, No. 9, 2000, pp. 1110-1113. doi:10.1016/S0002-9149(00)00705-0

[4] D. E. Forman, J. Butler, Y. Wang, W. T. Abraham, C. M. O'Conor, S. S. Gottlieb, *et al.*, "Incidence, Predictors at Admission, and Impact of Worsening Renal Function among Patients Hospitalized with Heart Failure," *Journal of the American College of Cardiology*, Vol. 43, No. 1, 2004, pp. 61-67. doi:10.1016/j.jacc.2003.07.031

[5] R. N. Foley, A. M. Murray, S. Li, C. A. Herzog, A. M. McBean, P. W. Eggers and A. J. Collins, "Chronic Kidney Disease and the Risk for Cardiovascular Disease, Renal Replacement, and Death in the United States Medicare Population, 1998 to 1999," *Journal of American Society of Nephrology*, Vol. 16, No. 2, 2005, pp. 498-495. doi:10.1681/ASN.2004030203

[6] G. C. Fonarow, K. F. Adams, W. T. Abraham, C. W. Yancy and W. J. Boscardin, "For the ADHERE Scientific Advisory Committee, Study Group, and Investigators. Risk Stratification for In-Hospital Mortality in Acutely Decompensated Heart Failure: Classification and Regression Tree Analysis," *The Journal of the American Medical Association*, Vol. 293, No. 5, 2005, pp. 572-580.

[7] G. L. Smith, J. H. Lichtman, M. B. Bracken, M. G. Shlipak, C. O. Phillips, P. DiCapua, *et al.*, "Renal Impairment and Outcome in Heart Failure. Systematic Review and Meta-Analysis," *Journal of the American College of Cardiology*, Vol. 47, No. 10, 2006, pp. 1987-1996. doi:10.1016/j.jacc.2005.11.084

[8] A. Kazory and E. A. Ross, "Anemia: The Point of Convergence or Divergence for Kidney Disease and Heart Failure," *Journal of the American College of Cardiology*, Vol. 53, No. 8, 2009, pp. 639-647. doi:10.1016/j.jacc.2008.10.046

[9] W. McClellan, S. L. Aronoff, W. K. Bolton, S. Hood, D. L. Lorber, K. L. Tang, *et al.*, "The Prevalence of Anemia in Patients with Chronic Kidney Disease," *Current Medical Research and Opinion*, Vol. 20, No. 9, 2004, pp. 1501-1510. doi:10.1185/030079904X2763

[10] A. Sandhu, S. Soman, M. Hudson and A. Besarab, "Managing Anemia in Patients with Chronic Heart Fail-

ure; What Do We Know?" *Vascular Health and Risk Management*, Vol. 15, No. 6, 2010, pp. 237-252.

[11] D. V. Vlahakos, K. P. Marathias and N. E. Madias, "The Role of the Renin-Angiotensin System in the Regulation of Erythropoiesis," *American Journal of Kidney Diseases*, Vol. 56, No. 3, 2010, pp. 558-565. doi:10.1053/j.ajkd.2009.12.042

[12] P. van der Meer, D. J. Lok, J. L. Januzzi, P. W. de la Porte, E. Lipsic, J. Van Wijngaarden, *et al.*, "Adequacy of Endogenous Erythropoietin Levels and Mortality in Anaemic Heart Failure Patients," *European Heart Journal*, Vol. 29, No. 12, 2008, pp. 1510-1515. doi:10.1093/eurheartj/ehn205

[13] J. W. Eschbach and J. W. Adamson, "Anemia of End-Stage Renal Disease (ESRD)," *Kidney International*, Vol. 28, No. 1, 1985, pp. 1-5. doi:10.1038/ki.1985.109

[14] A. K. Abu-Alfa, "CKD Series: Evaluation and Treatment of Anemia in Chronic Kidney Disease," *Hospital Physician*, Vol. 39, No. 7, 2003, pp. 31-38, 46.

[15] G. Remuzzi and J. R. Ingelfinger, "Correction of Anemia-Payoffs and Problems," *The New England Journal of Medicine*, Vol. 355, No. 20, 2006, pp. 2144-2146. doi:10.1056/NEJMe068233

[16] T. B. Drueke, F. Locatelli, N. Clyne, K. U. Eckardt, I. C. MacDougall, D. Tsakiris, *et al.*, (for the CREATE Investigators), "Normalization of Hemoglobin Level in Patients with Chronic Kidney Disease and Anemia," *The New England Journal of Medicine*, Vol. 355, No. 20, 2006, pp. 2071-2084. doi:10.1056/NEJMoa062276

[17] A. K. Singh, L. Szczech, K. L. Tang, H. Barnhart, S. Sapp, M. Wolfson, *et al.*, (for the CHOIR Investigators), "Correction of Anemia with Epoetin Alfa in Chronic Kidney Disease," *The New England Journal of Medicine*, Vol. 355, No. 20, 2006, pp. 2085-2098. doi:10.1056/NEJMoa065485

[18] J. K. Ghali, I. S. Anand, W. T. Abraham, G. C. Fonarow, B. Greenberg, H. Krum, *et al.*, (for the STAMINA-HeFT Group), "Randomized Double-Blind Trial of Darbepoetin Alfa in Patients with Symptomatic Heart Failure and Anemia," *Circulation*, Vol. 117, No. 4, 2008, pp. 526-535. doi:10.1161/CIRCULATIONAHA.107.698514

[19] M. A. Pfeffer, E. A. Burdmann, C. Y. Chen, M. E. Cooper, D. de Zeeuw, K. U. Eckardt, *et al.*, (for the TREAT Investigators), "A Trial of Darbepoetin Alfa in Type 2 Diabetes and Chronic Kidney Disease," *The New England Journal of Medicine*, Vol. 361, No. 21, 2009, pp. 2019-2032. doi:10.1056/NEJMoa0907845

[20] S. D. Solomon, H. Uno, E. F. Lewis, K. U. Eckardt, J. Lin, E. A. Burdmann, *et al.*, (for the TREAT Investigators), "Erythropoietic Response and Outcomes in Kidney Disease and Type 2 Diabetes," *The New England Journal of Medicine*, Vol. 363, No. 12, 2010, pp. 1146-1155. doi:10.1056/NEJMoa1005109

[21] Y. Zhang, M. Thamer, J. S. Kaufman, D. J. Cotter and M. A. Herman, "High Doses of Epoetin Do Not Lower Mortality and Cardiovascular Risk among Elderly Hemodialysis Patients with Diabetes," *Kidney International*, Vol. 80, No. 6, 2011, pp. 663-669. doi:10.1038/ki.2011.188

[22] I. Koulouridis, M. Alfayez, T. Trikalinos, E. M. Balk and B. L. Jaber, "Dose of Erythropoiesis-Stimulating Agents (ESAs) and Adverse Outcomes in Chronic Kidney Disease (CKD): A Meta-Regression," *Poster Presentation*, *American Society of Nephrology Kidney Week* 2011, 8-13 November 2011, Philadelphia.

[23] National Kidney Foundation KDOQI, "Clinical Practice Guidelines and Clinical Practice Recommendations for Anemia in Chronic Kidney Disease," *American Journal of Kidney Diseases*, Vol. 47, Suppl. 3, 2006, pp. S11-S15. doi:10.1053/j.ajkd.2006.03.010

[24] J. J. V. McMurray, I. S. Anand, R. Diaz, A. P. Maggioni, C. O'Connor, M. A. Pfeffer, *et al.*, (on Behalf of the RED-HF Committees and Investigators), "Design of the Reduction of Events with Darbepoetin Alfa in Heart Failure (RED-HF): A Phase III, Anaemia Correction, Morbidity-Mortality Trial," *European Journal of Heart Failure*, Vol. 11, No. 8, 2009, pp. 795-801. doi:10.1093/eurjhf/hfp098

[25] K. Van der Putten, K. E. Jie, M. E. Emans, J. A. Joles, M. J.Cramer , B. K. Velthuis, *et al.*, "Erythropoietin Treatment in Patients with Combined Heart and Renal Failure: Objectives and Design of the EPOCARES Study," *Journal of Nephrology*, Vol. 23, No. 4, 2010, pp. 363-368.

Acute Renal Failure during Pregnancy

Dong-Su Jeon[1], Tae-Hee Kim[1*], Hae-Hyeog Lee[1], Dong Won Byun[2]
[1]Department of Obstetrics and Gynecology, Soonchunhyang University Bucheon Hospital, Bucheon, South Korea
[2]Division of Endocrinology and Metabolism, Department of Internal Medicine, Soonchunhyang University Hospital, Bucheon, South Korea
Email: *heeobgy@schmc.ac.kr

ABSTRACT

Acute renal failure during pregnancy is a very rare and dangerous medical complication. Here, we report a primigravida at 31 weeks gestation who complained of oliguria, high fever, flank pain, nausea, and vomiting for 3 days. The patient's history was unremarkable. Her laboratory findings and ultrasonography revealed acute renal failure. After delivery, the patient had no complications and normal laboratory findings. Thus, if the gestational age is appropriate to deliver the baby, prompt delivery is important to prevent acute renal failure during pregnancy.

Keywords: Acute Renal Failure; Pregnancy; Delivery; Pyelonephritis

1. Introduction

Acute renal failure during pregnancy presents an important clinical challenge. This disease is uncommon, occurring in only 1 of every 10,000 pregnancies [1]. In recent years, the incidence of acute renal failure has decreased in developed countries, but it continues to be associated with significant mortality and long-term morbidity [2]. Acute renal failure during pregnancy is associated with a high risk for maternal mortality (9% - 55%) [3]. General management of acute renal failure begins with correction of underlying etiological factors and removal of renal toxins [4]. Acute pyelonephritis can lead to acute renal failure in the pregnant women.

Here, we report a patient with acute renal failure during the third trimester of an otherwise uncomplicated pregnancy.

2. Case Report

A 29-year-old woman at 31 weeks gestation of her first pregnancy presented with a history oliguria, high fever, flank pain, nausea, and vomiting for 3 days. The patient's medical history was unremarkable. At the time of admission to our hospital, the patient appeared ill, her body temperature was 38.7˚C, and her pulse rate was 92 beats/min. Her blood pressure was 120/70 mmHg.

Laboratory tests revealed a white blood cell count of 9470/μl, a hemoglobin level of 10.8 g/dl, a platelet count of 156,000/μl, a C-reactive protein level of 16.69 mg/dl, an erythrocyte sedimentation rate of 120 mm/hr, a blood urea nitrogen level of 34.3 mg/dl, and a serum creatinine level of 5.1 mg/ml. Serum protein, calcium, and electrolyte levels were normal, as were the results of liver function studies.

Her abdomen felt soft, but both flanks were tender. The uterus was appropriately enlarged for 31 weeks gestation. The fetal heartbeat was strong at approximately 140 - 160/min. The results of the remaining general physical examinations were normal.

On the second hospital day, labor induction was performed because of renal symptoms. However, labor did not progress well, so the patient underwent an emergency Cesarean delivery of a live male newborn weighing 2090 g. The newborn had no other abnormalities.

We arranged a renal echo study on the first postoperative day, and it showed a bilateral swelling kidney with increased parenchymal echogenicity. The patient received 9 days of ceftriaxone 2.0 g treatment daily and conservative therapy with a good response. On the fourth postoperative day, the serum creatinine level was 0.8 mg/dl, and the patient was discharged. At follow-up, she remained well and renal function values continued to be within normal limits.

3. Discussion

Acute renal failure is an infrequent but life-threatening complication of pregnancy. Since the 1960s, the overall incidence of pregnancy-related acute renal failure has decreased from 1/3000 to 1/15,000 - 1/20,000. Similarly, the proportion of total cases of pregnancy-related acute renal failure has fallen from approximately 20% - 40% in

*Corresponding author.

the 1960s to approximately 2% - 10% in the 1980s [5-7]. Coincident with these declines, little change has been observed in the overall mortality and long-term morbidity rates [4].

Pregnancy has a minimal effect on renal function and is usually not associated with postpartum deterioration or development of end-stage renal disease. In general, no consensus has been established regarding a definition for renal failure during pregnancy, and definitions range from a creatinine level above 0.8 mg/dl to the requirement for dialysis [8].

The pathophysiology of renal failure in pregnancy can be categorized according to anatomical pathology, hemodynamic changes, abnormal substrate handling, and acid-base abnormalities. The most common cause of renal failure in pregnancy is preeclampsia; however, only about 1.5% - 2% of preeclampsia patients develop failure [8]. Renal failure is typically associated with septic abortion, preeclampsia, or uterine hemorrhage from placenta previa or placental abruption.

The initial management of renal failure in pregnancy commences with treatment of the underlying causes. Pyelonephritis can lead to sepsis and acute renal failure in both pregnant and non-pregnant patients; however, an increased risk of acute renal failure exists due to pyelonephritis in pregnancy independent of the presence or absence of sepsis [4]. One historical study showed that 25% of women with pyelonephritis in pregnancy demonstrated a significant decrement in glomerular filtration rate without sepsis [9]. The initial approach to management of our patient was similar to that for acute pyelonephritis management. She was administered antibiotics intravenously.

Our case was considered acute renal failure associated with pyelonephritis. In conclusion, acute renal failure during pregnancy is a rare condition and remains a serious medical complication of pregnancy. The treatment of acute renal failure during pregnancy is correction of underlying disease. Therefore, it is important to quickly find the cause of acute renal failure. We experienced one case of acute renal failure during pregnancy and reported this case with a brief review of relevant literature.

REFERENCES

[1] P. H. Chung, J. S. Abramowicz, D. M. Edgar and D. M. Sherer, "Acute Maternal Obstructive Renal Failure in a Twin Gestation Despite Normal Physiological Pregnancy-Induced Urinary Tract Dilation," *American Journal of Perinatology*, Vol. 11, No. 3, 1994, pp. 242-244. doi:10.1055/s-2008-1040755

[2] N. Pertuiset and J. P. Grunfeld, "Acute Renal Failure in Pregnancy," *Baillière's Clinical Obstetrics and Gynaecology*, Vol. 8, No. 2, 1994, pp. 333-351. doi:10.1016/S0950-3552(05)80324-4

[3] K. R. Goplani, P. R. Shah, D. N. Gera, M. Gumber, M. Dabhi, A. Feroz, *et al.*, "Pregnancy-Related Acute Renal Failure: A Single-Center Experience," *Indian Journal of Nephrology*, Vol. 18, No. 1, 2008, pp. 17-21. doi:10.4103/0971-4065.41283

[4] H. S. Gammill and A. Jeyabalan, "Acute Renal Failure in Pregnancy," *Critical Care Medicine*, Vol. 33, No. 10, 2005, pp. S372-S384. doi:10.1097/01.CCM.0000183155.46886.C6

[5] J. P. Grunfeld and N. Pertuiset, "Acute Renal Failure in Pregnancy: 1987," *American Journal of Kidney Diseases*, Vol. 9, No. 4, 1987, pp. 359-362.

[6] P. Stratta, C. Canavese, M. Dogliani, T. Todros, L. Gagliardi and A. Vercellone, "Pregnancy-Related Acute Renal Failure," *Clinical Nephrology*, Vol. 32, No. 1, 1989, pp. 14-20.

[7] J. H. Turney, C. M. Ellis and F. M. Parsons, "Obstetric Acute Renal Failure 1956-1987," *BJOG: An International Journal of Obstetrics & Gynaecology*, Vol. 96, No. 6, 1989, pp. 679-687. doi:10.1111/j.1471-0528.1989.tb03282.x

[8] C. M. Nzerue, K. Hewan-Lowe and C. Nwawka, "Acute Renal Failure in Pregnancy: A Review of Clinical Outcomes at an Inner-City Hospital from 1986-1996," *Journal of the National Medical Association*, Vol. 90, No. 8, 1998, pp. 486-490.

[9] P. J. Whalley, F. G. Cunningham and F. G. Martin, "Transient Renal Dysfunction Associated with Acute Pyelonephritis of Pregnancy," *Obstetrics & Gynecology*, Vol. 46, No. 2, 1975, pp. 174-177.

Estimation of GFR by MDRD Formula and Its Correlation to Cockcroft-Gault Equation in Five Stages of Chronic Kidney Disease

Absar Ali[1*], Naila Asif[2], Zunaira Rais[2]
[1]Department of Medicine, Aga Khan University, Karachi, Pakistan
[2]Liaquat National Hospital, Karachi, Pakistan
Email: *draliabsar@yahoo.com

ABSTRACT

Background: Purpose of our study was to find out correlation between estimated Glomerular Filtration Rate (GFR) by Modification of Diet in Renal Disease (MDRD) formula and Glomerular Filtration Rate by Cockcroft-Gault equations, in patients with chronic kidney disease (CKD), and to see whether they can be used interchangeably. **Methods:** We conducted a cross section study of 70 patients presented to the nephrology clinic over a period of one year. We compared the Glomerular Filtration Rate by these two formulas in five stages of Chronic Kidney Disease. Abbreviated 4 variable Modification of Diet in Renal Disease formula was used. **Results:** Age range was 15 - 79 years; Male 49%, Female 51%. The correlation (r) between eGFR by MDRD and eGFR by Cockcroft-Gault equation for CKD stages 1 to 5 was 0.64; 0.31; 0.32; 0.67; and 0.45 respectively. The correlation (r) between creatinine clearance by 24 hour urine collection and MDRD formula was 0.84 (P: 0.001). The correlation (r) between creatinine clearance by 24 hour urine collection Cockcroft-Gault equation was 0.79 (P: 0.001). **Conclusion:** We conclude that Cockcroft-Gault equation correlates best with MDRD formula at CKD stages 4 and one. Cockcroft-Gault equation underestimated eGFR in stages 1, 2 and 3 of chronic Kidney Disease.

Keywords: MDRD; Cockcroft-Gault; Chronic Kidney Disease; CKD

1. Introduction

Modification of Diet in Renal Disease (MDRD) formula and Cockcroft-Gault equation are commonly used for estimation of Glomerular Filtration Rate (GFR). Creatinine clearance measurement using 24 hours urine collection is largely abandoned in favor of the MDRD and Cockcroft-Gault formulas, mainly because of the inherited difficulties in accurate collection of 24 hours urine.

Cockcroft-Gault equation remained the most common method for bedside estimation of GFR because it is very easy to use without a calculator or computer. This advantage of Cockcroft-Gault formula is keeping it alive in spite of the rapid popularity of MDRD formula. Numerous studies are done to compare these two equations in various settings. However the data from Asia especially from Pakistan is scanty [1].

Purpose of our study was to find out correlation between the two equations in chronic kidney disease (CKD) in our setting and to see whether they can be used interchangeably. A review of similar studies from other georophical location is also presented.

2. Methods

We conducted a cross section study of 70 patients of age 15 and above who presented to the nephrology clinic of a tertiary care hospital in Karachi Pakistan over a period of 1 year.

Abbreviated four variable MDRD formula was used to estimate GFR using the equation: $186 \times [\text{serum creatinine (mg/dl)}]^{-1.154} \times (\text{age})^{-0.203} \times (0.742 \text{ if female})$. Estimated GFR using the Cockcroft-Gault equation was calculated as follows: $(140 - \text{age}) \times (\text{weight in kg})/\text{serum creatinine (mg/dl)} \times 72 \times (0.85 \text{ if female})$. Measured creatinine clearance was calculated by 24 hour urine collection and using the formula: creatinine excretion (mg/kg/day) divided by serum creatinine (mg/dl) divided by 14.4 (min/d per dl/ml).

Patients with acute renal failure were excluded. All the patients in the study were divided into five groups corresponding to the five stages of chronic kidney disease as follows: Group 1: GFR > 90; Group 2: GFR 90 - 60; Group 3: GFR 30 - 59; Group 4: GFR 15 - 29 and group

*Corresponding author.

5: GFR < 15 ml/min/1.73m^2 [2]. Data was analyzed using SPSS software.

3. Results

Age range was 15 - 79 years. Male were 49%, female were 51%. Mean GFR by MDRD formula for CKD stages 1 to 5 was 111 ± 30, 77 ± 24, 39 ± 9, 21 ± 6 and 13 ± 4 ml/min/1.73m^2 respectively. Mean GFR by Cockcroft-Gault equation for CKD stage 1 to 5 was 119 ± 28, 78 ± 13, 43 ± 7, 23 ± 3 and 12 ± 2 ml/min/1.73m^2 respectively (**Table 1**). The correlation coefficient (r) between eGFR by MDRD and eGFR by Cockcroft-Gault for CKD stages 1 - 5 was 0.64; 0.31; 0.32; 0.67; and 0.45 respectively (**Table 2**).

Mean and median eGFR by MDRD was 48 ± 40 and 32 (58-7) ml/min/1.73m^2 respectively for all patients. Mean and median eGFR by Cockcroft-Gault was 52 ± 42 and 36 (197-7) ml/min/1.73m^2 respectively for all patients (**Table 3**).

The Cockcroft-Gault equation correlated best with MDRD formula at CKD stage four followed by the stage one. The creatinine clearance by 24 urine collection was correlated to the eGFR by MDRD formula. The r value was 0.84 with p value of 0.001. Similarly the creatinine clearance by 24 urine collection was correlated to the eGFR by Cockcroft-Gault equation. The r value was 0.79 with p value of 0.001 (**Table 4**).

Table 1. Mean estimated GFR in each group.

	Groups (CKD Stages)	eGFR by CG ml/min/1.73 m^2	eGFR by MDRD ml/min/1.73m^2
1)	GFR > 90	119 ± 28.1	111 ± 26.2
2)	GFR 60 - 90	78 ± 13.3	77 ± 23.8
3)	GFR 30 - 59	43 ± 7.1	39 ± 9.0
4)	GFR 15 - 29	23 ± 3.1	21 ± 6.0
5)	GFR < 15	13 ± 2.5	13 ± 4.5

CG: Cockcroft-Gault; MDRD: modification of diet in renal disease; CKD: chronic kidney disease.

Table 2. Correlation between eGFR by CG and eGFR by MDRD.

	Groups (CKD Stages)	r	p
1)	GFR > 90	0.64	0.01
2)	GFR 60 - 90	0.31	0.48
3)	GFR 30 - 59	0.32	0.20
4)	GFR 15 - 29	0.67	0.005
5)	GFR < 15	0.45	0.08

CG: Cockcroft-Gault; MDRD: modification of diet in renal disease.

Table 3. Overall average eGFR by CG and MDRD formulas.

	Mean ± SD eGFR ml/min/1.73/m^2	Median eGFR ml/min/1.73m^2
CG	51 ± 42	36 (197-7)
MDRD	48 ± 40	32 (158-7)

CG: Cockcroft-Gault; MDRD: modification of diet in renal disease; eGFR: estimated glomerular filtration rate.

Table 4. Correlation between "24 Hour Urine CrCl" and eGFR by Cockcroft-Gault and MDRD formulas.

Variables	Mean ± SD	r	p
1) 24 hour CrCl 2) eGFR by CG	45 ± 39 51 ± 42	0.84	<0.001
1) 24 hour CrCl 2) eGFR by MDRD	45 ± 39 48 ± 40	0.79	<0.001

CrCl: creatinine clearance; CG: Cockcroft-Gault; MDRD: modification of diet in renal disease; eGFR: estimated glomerular filtration rate.

4. Discussion

Accurate measurement of GFR in chronic kidney disease can not be overemphasized. It is especially important when GFR reaches near stage 3 and 4. The important decision like making AV fistula and initiation of renal replacement therapy are taken at this time.

There are more than eight formulas available to estimate GFR but only two namely Cockcroft-Gault equation and MDRD got the acceptance by the medical community. The Cockcroft-Gault equation was proposed as early as 1976 [2]. Because of its simplicity and bedside use, it was readily accepted by the physicians. The Cockcroft-Gault equation enjoyed this monopoly till the MDRD equation was introduced in 1999 [3].

Twenty four hour urine collection for Creatinine clearance measurement is not the method of choice because of several pitfalls. The most important being the 24 hour urine collection is often not accurate. In addition increased tubular secretion of creatinine in renal failure results in overestimation of GFR.

Using Inulin clearance to measure GFR is very cumbersome and not practical for routine clinical practice. Alternatively, the radioactive and non-radioactive based markers e.g. Iothalamate, Iohexol, DTPA and EDTA are used. The isotope based GFR measurements are thought to be the most accurate but they are costly and not available in many laboratories. Therefore their utility is confined practically to research. Inulin and Isptope methods are used as a gold standard to validate the accuracy of eGFR by MDRD or Cockcroft-Gault equation equations. However we used the traditional 24 hour urine collection to calculate creatinine clearance and compare it with MDRD formula and Cockcroft-Gault equation because of the lack of resources. We were very particular and thorough in giving the instruction to the patients. The strong correlation of 24 hour creatinine clearance to eGFR by Cockcroft-Gault equation as well as MDRD formula goes in favor of our assumption that urine collections were accurate.

MDRD study equation originally required six variables namely Serum Creatinine, Serum Albumin, Serum Urea Nitrogen, Gender, Age and Race. Later a simpler four variable equation was proposed and is considered to be a good as six variable equation [4]. This abbreviated MDRD equation requires Serum Creatinine, Age, Gender and Race only. It does not require Serum Albumin and Serum Urea Nitrogen. The use of standardized serum creatinine in re-expressed 4 variable MDRD formula improves the accuracy [5,6]. Studies have shown that adjustment for body surface area improves the accuracy of Cockcroft-Gault formula [7,8]. The need of this simpler four variable MDRD equation raised due to difficulty of using 6 variable equation on bedside. However still its main drawback remains the need of a computer.

There are a number of studies comparing the MDRD to Cockcroft-Gault formula with variable results. Following is the review of some important studies.

MDRD equation provides unbiased and reasonably accurate estimates across wide range of subgroups when GFR is less than 60 *i.e.* in CKD Stage 3, 4 and 5 [9]. They also proved to be reliable for follow-up in CKD patients in longitudinal studies [10].

MDRD equation performed better than Cockcroft-Gault equation equation in CKD, when GFR was less than 60 $ml/min/1.73m^2$. On the other hand Cockcroft-Gault equation performed better in healthy kidney donors [11]. Cockcroft-Gault equation formula was less precise than MDRD equation in most cases with median GFR of 59.8 $ml/ min/1.73m^2$ [12].

In another study, estimation of GFR in older patients with CKD and mean GFR of 53 $ml/min/1.73m^2$, the Cockcroft-Gault equation was more precise than MDR formula [13]. In diabetic patients MDRD as well as Cockcroft-Gault equation correlated well with isotopic GFR measurements but MDRD equation turned-out to be more accurate [14].

In sick hospitalized patients the performance of MDRD and Cockcroft-Gault equation was compared, using Iodine iothalamate as a control. MDRD equation performed better [15]. MDRD Formula as compare to Cockcroft-Gault formula underestimates GFR in healthy individuals [16].

MDRD formula was more accurate than Cockcroft-Gault equation in ESRD patients. However MDRD formula underestimated GFR when inulin clearance was more than 8 $ml/min/1.73m^2$ and overestimated GFR when inulin clearance was less than 8 $ml/min/1.73m^2$. On the other hand Cockcroft-Gault overestimated GFR when inulin clearance was less than 13 $ml/mim/11.73m^2$ [17].

In patients with CKD but normal serum creatinine, Cockcroft-Gault equation was found to be more accurate than MDRD formula. Measurement of GFR by endogenous and exogenous filtration markers might be the most prudent strategy [18].

5. Conclusion

We conclude that Cockcroft-Gault equation correlates best with MDRD formula at CKD stage 4 and one. Cockcroft-Gault equation overestimated GFR at stages 1, 2, 3. The two formulas may be used interchangeably at stages 4 and 1. Measurement of 24 hour urine creatinine clearance may still be reliable if patients are counseled properly. It is unlikely that MDRD formula will replace Cockcroft-Gault equation in bedside clinical practice soon because the dependency of MDRD formula upon a computer program.

REFERENCES

[1] T. H. Jafar, C. H. Schmid and A. S. Levey, "Serum Creatinine as Marker of Kidney Function in South Asia: A Study of Reduced GFR in Adults in Pakistan," *Clinical Journal of the American Society of Nephrology*, Vol. 16, No. 5, 2005, pp. 1413-1419. doi:10.1681/ASN.2004121100

[2] G. Eknoyan and N. Levin (Co-Chairs Advisory Board of National Kidney Foundation), *et al.*, "K/DOQI Clinical Practice Guidelines for Chronic Kidney Disease: Evaluation, Classification, and Stratification," *American Journal of Kidney Diseases*, Vol. 39, No. 5, 2002, pp. S1-S266. doi:10.1016/S0272-6386(02)70054-1

[3] A. S. Levey, J. P. Bosch, J. B. Levis, T. Greene, N. Rogers and D. Roth, "A More Accurate Method to Estimate Glomerular Filtration Rate from Serum Creatinine: A New Prediction Equation. Modification of Diet in Renal Disease Study Group," *Annals of Internal Medicine*, Vol. 130, No. 6, 1999, pp. 461-470.

[4] D. W. Cockcroft and M. H. Gault, "Prediction of Creatinine Clearance from Serum Creatinine," *Nephron*, Vol. 16, No. 1, 1976, pp. 31-41. doi:10.1159/000180580

[5] G. Rostoker, P. Andrivet, I. Pham, M. Griuncelli and S. Adnot, "A Modified Cockcroft-Gault Formula Taking into Account the Body Surface Area Gives a More Accurate Estimation of the Glomerular Filtration Rate," *Journal of Nephrology*, Vol. 20, No. 5, 2007, pp. 576-585.

[6] A. Schoker, M. A. Hossain, T. Koru-Sengul, D. L. Raju and D. Cockcraft, "Performance of Creatinine Clearance Equation on the Original Cockcraft-Gault Population," *Clinical Nephrology*, Vol. 66, No. 2, 2006, pp. 89-97.

[7] A. S. Levey, J. Coresh, T. Greene, J. Marsh, L. A. Stevens, J. W. Kusek and F. E. Van Lente, "Expressing the Modification of Diet in Renal Disease Study Equation for Estimating GFR with Standardized Serum Creatinine Values," *Clinical Chemistry*, Vol. 53, No. 4, 2007, pp.

7666-7672. doi:10.1373/clinchem.2006.077180

[8] A. S. Levey, J. Coresh, T. Greene, L. A. Stevens, Y. Zhang, S. Hendriksen, *et al.*, "Using Standardized Serum Creatinie Values in the Modification of Diet in Renal Disease Study. Equation for Estimating GFR," *Annals of Internal Medicine*, Vol. 145, No. 4, 2006, pp. 247-254.

[9] L. A. Stevens, J. Coresh, H. I. Feldman, T. Greene, J. P. Lash, R. G. Nelson, *et al.*, "Evaluation of the Modification of Diet in Renal Diease Study Equation in a Large Diverse Population," *Journal of the American Society of Nephrology*, Vol. 18, No. 10, 2007, pp. 2749-2757. doi:10.1681/ASN.2007020199

[10] X. Wang, J. Lewis, L. Appel, D. Cheek, G. Contreras, M. Faulkner, *et al.*, "Validation of Creatinine Based Estimates of GFR When Evaluating Risk Factors in Longitudinal Studies of Kidney Disease," *Journal of the American Society of Nephrology*, Vol. 17, No. 10, 2006, pp. 2900-2909. doi:10.1681/ASN.2005101106

[11] E. D. Poggio, X. Wang, T. Greene, F. Van Lente and P. M. Hall, "Performance of the Modification of Diet in Renal Disease and Cockcroft-Gault Equations in the Estimation of GFR in Health and in Chronic Kidney Disease," *Journal of the American Society of Nephrology*, Vol. 16, No. 2, 2005, pp. 459-466. doi:10.1681/ASN.2004060447

[12] M. Froissart, J. Rossert, E. Jacquot, M. Paillard and P. Houillier, "Predictive Performance of the Modification of Diet in Renal Disease and Cockcroft-Gault Equations for Estimating Renal Function," *Journal of the American Society of Nephrology*, Vol. 16, No. 3, 2005, pp. 763-773. doi:10.1681/ASN.2004070549

[13] E. J. Lamb, M. C. Webb, D. E. Simpson, A. J. Coakley, D. J. Newman and S. E. O'Riordan, "Estimation of GFR in Older Patients with Chronic Renal Insfufficiency: Is the MDRD Formula an Improvement," *Journal of the American Geriatrics Society*, Vol. 51, No. 7, 2003, pp. 1012-1017. doi:10.1046/j.1365-2389.2003.51330.x

[14] V. Rigalleau, C. Lasseur, C. Perlemonine, N. Barthe, C. Raffaitin and E. Liu, "Estimation of GFR in Diabetics: Cockcroft Formula or MDRD Study Equation," *Diabetes Care*, Vol. 28, No. 4, 2005, pp. 838-843. doi:10.2337/diacare.28.4.838

[15] E. D. Poggio, P. C. Nef, X. Wang, T. Greene, F. Van Lente, V. W. Dennis and P. M. Hall, "Performance of Cockcroft-Gault and Modification of Diet in Renal Disease Equations in Estimating GFR in Ill Hospitalized Patients," *American Journal of Kidney Diseases*, Vol. 46, No. 2, 2005, pp. 242-252. doi:10.1053/j.ajkd.2005.04.023

[16] A. D. Rule, T. S. Larson, E. J. Bergs Tralh, J. M. Slezak, S. J. Jacobsen and F. G. Cosio, "Using Serum Creatinine to Estimate GFR: Accuracy in Good Health and in Chronic Kidney Disease," *Annals of Internal Medicine*, Vol. 141, No. 12, 2004, pp. 929-937.

[17] Y. Kuan, M. Hossain, J. Surman, A. M. El Nahas and J. Haylor, "GFR Prediction Using the MDRD and Cockcroft and Gault Equations in Patients with End Stage Renal Disease," *Nephrology Dialysis Transplantation*, Vol. 20, No. 11, 2005, pp. 2394-2401. doi:10.1093/ndt/gfi076

[18] A. G. Boston, F. Kronenberg and E. Ritz, "Predictive Performance of Renal Function for Patients with Chronic Kidney Disease and Normal Serum Creatinine Levels," *Journal of the American Society of Nephrology*, Vol. 13, No. 8, 2002, pp. 2140-2144. doi:10.1097/01.ASN.0000022011.35035.F3

A Case of Severe Hypomagnesaemia*

Gurpreet Anand[1], Martin Konrad[2], Ludwig Theodor Heuss[1], Robert Schorn[1,3#]
[1]Department of Internal Medicine, Spital Zollikerberg, Zollikerberg, Switzerland
[2]Department of General Paediatrics, University Children's Hospital, Münster, Germany
[3]Department of Nephrology and Haemodialysis, Spital Zollikerberg, Zollikerberg, Switzerland
Email: gurpreet.anand@spitalzollikerberg.ch, konradma@uni-muenster.de, ludwigtheodor.heuss@spitalzollikerberg.ch, #robert.schorn@spitalzollikerberg.ch

ABSTRACT

Hypomagnesaemia is a common finding that occurs in hospitalised patients and can be caused by renal or extrarenal wasting. Because it is not routinely tested, even severe hypomagnesaemia can be missed. In cases of extrarenal wasting, the kidney can decrease its magnesium excretion to very low levels. A systematic diagnostic approach allows the proper diagnosis and treatment of hypomagnesaemia. We report on a 72-year-old Caucasian male patient with repeated drops and amyosthenia caused by severe hypomagnesaemia. In this report, we discuss the pathophysiology, clinical signs, diagnostic investigation and treatment of magnesium depletion.

Keywords: Hypocalcaemia; Hypomagnesaemia; Hypokalaemia; Weakness

1. Introduction

Despite the fact that hypomagnesaemia is a frequent finding, ranging from 12% in all hospitalised patients to 60% in an intensive care setting, plasma magnesium is not measured routinely [1,2]. The clinical manifestations of magnesium depletion are rather nonspecific. Early signs include nausea, vomiting, fatigue, weakness, hyperreflexia, carpopedal spasm, tremor and tetany. A prolonged QT interval, ST depression, ventricular arrhythmias and the enhancement of digitalis toxicity are typical cardiac findings [3]. Symptomatic hypomagnesaemia is often associated with hypokalaemia due to urinary potassium wasting and hypocalcaemia due to lower parathyroid hormone secretions, as well as end-organ resistance to its effects. The diagnosis of magnesium depletion is challenging because the clinical manifestation may be absent; additionally, the serum magnesium concentration does not reflect the total body magnesium content.

2. Case Report

A 72-year-old male Caucasian patient presented to the emergency department with a history of progressive amyosthenia developing over eight weeks. Hypocalcaemia and 25-hydroxyvitamin D deficiency had been detected twenty-two days previously, and replacement was started without clinical improvement. The patient had a history of chronic renal failure, coronary artery disease, hypertensive cardiomyopathy and hyperlipidaemia. His medications included aspirin, bisoprolol, losartan, pravastatin, torasemid, pantoprazole, calcium and vitamin D3. There was no evidence of alcohol consumption. His blood pressure was 129/99 mmHg, and his pulse rate was 102 b.p.m. Upon examination, he demonstrated general muscle weakness, absent reflexes in the lower extremities, positive Chvostek's sign and an otherwise normal clinical status. His laboratory analysis showed remarkable results for total serum calcium (1.79 mmol/l), potassium (3.5 mmol/l), 25-hydroxyvitamin D (<30 nmol/l), iPTH (6.3 pmol/l) and creatinine (112 µmol/l). Based on the progressive amyosthenia, positive Chvostek's sign and hypocalcaemia despite the calcium and vitamin D substitution, a magnesium analysis was performed that revealed severe hypomagnesaemia with 0.11 mmol/l (**Figure 1**). Other blood values, including pH and bicarbonate, and the urinary sediment were normal. The loop diuretic and proton pump inhibitor (PPI) were ceased, and a 24-h urine (600 ml) collection yielded the following results: calcium 0.32 mmol/l, magnesium 0.17 mmol/l, phosphate 16.2 mmol/l and creatinine 14.7 mmol/l. Electrocardiography, chest X-ray, head CT-scan and abdominal sonography showed no abnormalities.

The fractional excretion of magnesium (FeMg) was 9.3%, indicating renal magnesium wasting. In the context of hypocalciuria, this raised the suspicion of Gitelman syndrome (GS) or autosomal-dominant renal hypomagnesaemia associated with hypocalciuria (IDH). Because of the reported manifestation of inherited forms of

*Transparency declarations: None to declare.
#Corresponding author.

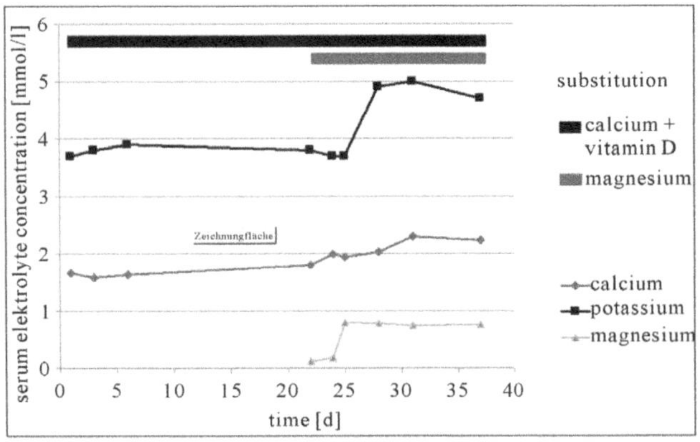

Figure 1. Serum magnesium and calcium levels over time, following calcium and magnesium substitution.

hypomagnesaemia at older ages, despite a negative family history, we performed a genetic analysis that ruled out GS and IDH (no mutations in SLC12A3 or FXYD2). The screened siblings did not demonstrate renal magnesium wasting.

After intravenous magnesium substitution, the clinical picture improved rapidly (**Figure 1**). The follow-up by the family physician showed normal serum magnesium concentrations under oral magnesium substitution despite the restarted loop diuretic and PPI medication.

Concerning the underlying aetiology of the severe magnesium depletion, in this case, we hypothesised a multifactorial aetiology. The degree of hypomagnesaemia induced by loop diuretics is generally mild and associated with hypercalciuria. In theory, increasing calcium reabsorption after stopping the loop diuretic could provoke hypocalciuria. In this case, the concomitant use of a PPI could have induced extrarenal magnesium wasting through decreased intestinal absorption, and the initiation of vitamin D supplementation may have induced a calcium shift into the bones, each of which may have contributed to the development of severe magnesium deficiency.

3. Discussion

Magnesium is the second most common intracellular cation and plays an important role as a cofactor in more than 300 enzymatic reactions. It is also regarded as a natural calcium antagonist. The total magnesium content of an average adult is 24 g. Approximately 60% of the body's magnesium is present in bone, 20% in the muscle and another 20% in the soft tissue and liver. Approximately 99% of total body magnesium is intracellular, with only 1% present in the extracellular space (blood serum or red blood cells (RBC)). Extracellular magnesium exists in three fractions: free/ionised 55% - 70%, protein-bound 20% - 30% and complexed with anions such as phosphate, bicarbonate, citrate or sulphate. Of these fractions, the ionised form has the greatest biological activity and can be measured. Total serum magnesium levels normally range from 0.65 to 1.05 mmol/l [3,4].

Magnesium homeostasis is tightly regulated by the intestine, bone and kidneys. Magnesium is absorbed in the gut and stored in bone minerals, and the excess magnesium is excreted by the kidneys and faeces. The minimal daily intake should be 350 mg for men and 430 mg for women. Magnesium is mainly (80% - 90%) absorbed in the small intestine by a passive transcellular mechanism driven by an electrochemical gradient and solvent drag. A minor fraction is transported via the transcellular transient receptor potential channel melastatin members (TRPM) 6 and 7 [3,4]. The absorption rate of dietary magnesium varies from 24% to 76% and mainly depends on the body magnesium status [5]. The kidney plays a crucial role in magnesium homeostasis, as of the filtered magnesium load (2400 mg daily), 95% is reabsorbed, and only 3% - 5% is excreted. The highest level of reabsorption occurs in the thick ascending limb of the loop of Henle (TAL) and in the proximal tubules in a passive paracellular manner (60% - 70% and 10% - 20%, respectively). In the TAL, the tight junction proteins claudin-16 and claudin-19 are responsible for this transport [4,6]. The final 5% - 10% of the filtered magnesium is reabsorbed in the distal tubule (DCT), where the transient receptor potential melastatin (TRPM) 6 channel plays a pivotal role [6]. The epidermal growth factor (EGF) and oestrogen regulate TRPM 6 activity [4]. The renal excretion of the filtered load can vary from 0.5% to 70%, allowing conservation during states of magnesium deprivation and rapid excretion in cases of excess intake [3].

The measurement of serum magnesium is relatively easy and has become the method of choice to estimate the magnesium content, although it does not reflect the total body stores (only 0.3% of the total body content is present in blood serum). However, magnesium depletion can occur in the setting of a normal serum magnesium concentration, so-called normomagnesaemic magnesium depletion [7]. Haemolysis leads to misinterpretation because the magnesium concentration in RBCs is higher than in serum [3]. The common causes of acquired hypomagnesaemia are listed in **Table 1** [3,8]. A distinction between gastrointestinal and renal losses can be made by measuring the 24-hour FEMg (preferred because of the circadian variation in renal magnesium excretion) or by fractional excretion on a random urine specimen [3,4,9]. FEMg can be calculated from the following formula:

$FEMg = [(UMg \times PCr)/(PMg \times UCr \times 0.7)] \times 100$. In the above equation, U and P refer to the urine and plasma concentrations of magnesium (Mg) and creatinine (Cr). The plasma magnesium concentration is multiplied by 0.7 because only approximately 70% of the circulating magnesium is free (not bound to albumin) and therefore

Table 1. Causes of acquired hypomagnesaemia [3,8].

Gastrointestinal (FEMg < 1% - 2%)

- Decreased dietary intake
  - Malnutrition, alcoholism
- Secretory losses
  - Severe or prolonged chronic diarrhoea
  - Enteric or biliary fistulas
- Reduced absorption
  - Malabsorption, steatorrhoea
  - Small-bowel bypass surgery
  - PPIs
- Saponification in necrotic fat
  - Necrotising acute pancreatitis

Miscellaneous (FEMg < 1% - 2%)

- Magnesium chelation (citrate-rich blood transfusion)
- Redistribution
  - Hungry bone syndrome
  - Refeeding syndrome
- Severe burns
- Excessive lactation, heat, prolonged exercise

Renal (FEMg > 3% - 4%)

- Congenital tubular defects (detailed reviewed in [4])
  - Bartter's syndrome
  - Gitelman syndrome
  - Familial hypomagnesaemia with hypercalciuria and nephrocalcinosis
  - Hypomagnesaemia with secondary hypocalcaemia
  - Isolated autosomal-recessive hypo-magnesaemia
  - Autosomal dominant hypomagnesaemia
  - Isolated dominant hypomagnesaemia
  - EAST syndrome (SeSAME)
- Drug induced
  - Loop diuretics
  - Aminoglycosides
  - Amphotericin B
  - Cyclosporine, tacrolimus
  - Cisplatin
  - EGF antagonists, *i.e.*, cetuximab
  - Foscarnet
  - Pentamidine
  - Alcohol
- Decreased sodium chloride reabsorption
  - Extracellular volume expansion(hyperaldosteronism)
  - Hypercalcaemia
- Osmotic Polyuria (solvent drag)
  - Uncontrolled diabetes
  - Postobstructive diuresis
  - Posttransplant
  - Recovery phase of acute tubular injury

Abbreviations: EGF: Epidermal growth factor; FEMg: fractional excretion of magnesium.

capable of being filtered across the glomerulus. The normal renal response to extrarenal magnesium depletion is to restrict magnesium excretion to very low levels (typically, to <1%) [10]. Thus, the daily excretion of more than 1 mmol or a calculated FEMg above 3% to 4% in a subject with normal renal function indicates renal magnesium wasting [3,10].

A magnesium retention test or loading test can differentiate among patients with hypomagnesaemic and normomagnesaemic deficiencies. After oral loading, the changes in serum magnesium and urinary excretion reflect the intestinal magnesium reabsorption [4]. Parenteral magnesium administration can also identify a functional magnesium deficiency [11]. After a magnesium loading, a urinary excretion of >60% - 70% rules out any relevant magnesium depletion. However, the standardisation and utility of this test are lacking [3,7].

Hypokalaemia, which accompanies 60% of the cases, can be caused by extrarenal (e.g., diarrhoea) and renal loss. Diuretics and a loss of the inhibitory function of magnesium on the ROMK channel promote urinary potassium wasting [7]. Another classical sign of severe hypomagnesaemia is hypocalcaemia, which is induced by the suppression of PTH release, as well as skeletal resistance to PTH [7]. Low calcitriol levels contribute to a fall in calcium concentration as well. Chronic hypomagnesaemia is associated with chondrocalcinosis (magnesium is a co-factor of various pyrophosphatases) and joint swelling.

The method of magnesium repletion varies with the severity of the clinical setting. Severe hypomagnesaemia with tetany or ventricular arrhythmia requires a prompt intravenous substitution followed by oral substitution. Mild or asymptomatic hypomagnesaemia can be substituted orally. The underlying disorder should also be corrected [3,7].

4. Conclusion

The impact of hypomagnesaemia is underestimated because clinicians often fail to measure magnesium [12]. Unexplained muscle weakness, hypocalcaemia and refractory hypokalaemia point to underlying hypomagnesaemia, despite serum magnesium values within the normal limits (normomagnesaemic magnesium depletion). Magnesium depletion can be induced by either renal or extrarenal losses. A 24-hour urinary FEMg can discriminate between these two major mechanisms. Severe hypomagnesaemia requires an intravenous replacement.

REFERENCES

[1] E. T. Wong, R. K. Rude, F. R. Singer, S. T. Shaw Jr., "A High Prevalence of Hypomagnesemia and Hypermagnesemia in Hospitalized Patients," *American Journal of*

Clinical Pathology, Vol. 79, No. 3, 1983, pp. 348-352.

[2] G. M. Tong and R. K. Rude, "Magnesium Deficiency in Critical Illness," *Journal of Intensive Care Medicine*, Vol. 20, No. 1, 2005, 20, pp. 3-17.

[3] W. Jahnen-Dechent and M. Ketteler, "Magnesium Basics," *Clinical Kidney Journal*, Vol. 5, Suppl. 1, 2012, pp. i3-i14. doi:10.1093/ndtplus/sfr163

[4] J. H. F. De Baaij, J. G. J. Hoendderop and R. J. M. Bindels, "Regulation of Magnesium Balance: Lessons Learned from Human Genetic Disease," *Clinical Kidney Journal*, Vol. 5, Suppl. 1, 2012, pp. i15-i24.

[5] L. A. Graham, J. J. Caesar and A. S. Burgen, "Gastrointestinal Absorption and Excretion of Mg^{28} in Man," *Metabolism*, No. 9, 1960, pp. 646-659.

[6] B. Glaudemans, N. V. Knoers, J. G. Hoenderop and R. J. M. Bindels, "New Molecular Players Facilitating Mg^{2+} Reabsorption in the Distal Convoluted Tubule," *Kidney International*, Vol. 77, No. 1, 2010, pp. 17-22. doi:10.1038/ki.2009.358

[7] Z. S. Agus, "Hypomagnesemia," *Journal of the American Society of Nephrology*, Vol. 10, No. 7, 1999, pp. 168-174.

[8] G. Regolisti, A. Cabassi, E. Parenti, U. Maggiore and E. Fiaccadori, "Severe Hypomagnesemia during Long-Term Treatment with a Proton Pump Inhibitor," *American Journal of Kidney Diseases*, Vol. 56, No. 1, 2010, pp. 168-174. doi:10.1053/j.ajkd.2010.03.013

[9] N. V. Knoers, "Inherited Forms of Renal Hypomagnesemia: An Update," *Pediatric Nephrology*, Vol. 24, No. 4, 2009, pp. 695-705. doi:10.1007/s00467-008-0968-x

[10] M. Elisaf, K. Panteli, J. Theodorou and K. C. Siamopoulos, "Fractional Excretion of Magnesium in Normal Subjects and in Patients with Hypomagnesemia," *Magnesium Research*, Vol. 10, No. 4, 1997, pp. 315-320.

[11] P. Hébert, N. Mehta, J. Wang, T. Hindmarsh, G. Jones and P. Cardinal, "Functional Magnesium Deficiency in Critically Ill Patients Identified Using a Magnesium-Loading Test," *Critical Care Medicine*, Vol. 25, No. 5, 1997, pp. 749-755.

[12] R. Whang and K. W. Ryder, "Frequency of Hypomagnesemia and Hypermagnesemia. Requested vs Routine," *Journal of the American Medical Association*, Vol. 263, No. 22, 1990, pp. 3063-3064.

Xanthogranulomatous Pyelonephritis Associated with Crohn's Disease and Primary Hyperparathyroidism

Mekdess Abebe, Wing Mu, Heesuck Suh, Edward P. Nord, Nand K. Wadhwa*
Division of Nephrology, Department of Medicine, School of Medicine, State University of New York at Stony Brook, Stony Brook, USA
Email: *nand.wadhwa@stonybrookmedicine.edu

ABSTRACT

We report on a case of unilateral and diffuse xanthogranulomatous pyelonephritis (XGP) associated with Crohn's disease and primary hyperparathyroidism (HPT). The patient had undiagnosed primary HPT for at least a year prior to presentation. The co-existence of Crohn's disease and primary HPT caused calcium oxalate stone likely by the known mechanism of hypercalcemia and hyperoxaluria respectively. The patient developed XGP, a rare disease, as a result of infected calcium oxalate stone which was treated with antibiotics and unilateral nephrectomy. To the best of our knowledge, this is the first case of XGP associated with Crohn's disease and primary HPT.

Keywords: Xanthogranulomatous Pyelonephritis; Hyperparathyroidism; Crohn's; Hypercalcemia

1. Introduction

XGP is a rare, serious, chronic inflammatory disorder of the kidney and constitutes less than 1% of chronic pyelonephritis. It is characterized by destruction of renal parenchyma and its replacement with granulomatous, abscess and collection of lipid laden macrophage (xanthoma cells) [1]. The disease most frequently presents in middle-aged groups with a predilection for female gender [2]. XGP shares many characteristics with renal neoplasm in terms of its radiologic appearance and its ability to invade adjacent structures. We report a case of unilateral and diffuse XGP due to undiagnosed primary HPT and Crohn's disease leading to unilateral nephrectomy.

2. Case Report

A 46-year-old white woman presented to emergency department with a two week history of right flank pain associated with generalized weakness, dizziness, decreased appetite and weight loss of 50 pounds in the last few months. She also had shortness of breath at minimal exertion. She denied any urinary complaint, fever, nausea or vomiting. Her significant comorbidities included Crohn's disease diagnosed in 2009, small bowel obstruction due to Crohn's disease related stricture resulting in laparoscopic small bowel resection in 2010, chronic pancreatitis and bilateral kidney stones. Patient was not on any medication prior to admission. She was an active smoker but denied alcohol or illegal drug use.

At presentation, the patient was not in any distress. Blood pressure was 97/53 mmHg, pulse 92 beats/minute and temperature was 38.3˚C. She had dry oral mucosa. Abdominal examination showed mildly distended abdomen with right costovertebral angle tenderness. No organomegally was appreciated. The remainder of the physical examination was within normal limits. Laboratory evaluation showed white blood cell count of 11.8×10^3 /mcL, hemoglobin 7.5 g/dL, hematocrit 22.4% and platelet count of 397×10^3 /mcL. Serum chemistry showed a sodium of 134 mEq/L (134 mmol/L), potassium 3.8 mEq/L (3.8 mmol/L), chloride 111 mEq/L (111 mmol/L), bicarbonate 13 mEq/L (13 mmol/L), blood urea nitrogen 60 mg/dL (21.4 mmol/L) , serum creatinine 3.6 mg/dL (275 µmol/L) (her serum creatinine was 0.8 mg/dL (61 µmol/L) 6 months prior to this admission), ionized calcium 5.4 mg/dL (1.35 mmol/L), total calcium 9.8 mg/dL (2.45 mmol/L), corrected calcium for albumin 10.8 mg/dL (2.7 mmol/L), phosphorous 5.2 mg/dL (1.68 mmol/L), albumin 2.8 mg/dL and total protein 6.1 mg/dL. Liver function tests were within normal limits. Anti nuclear antibody was positive at 1:320. Serum protein electrophoresis (SPEP), urine protein electrophoresis (UPEP), C3,

*Corresponding author.

C4, antineutrophil cytoplasmic antibodies, Anti ds DNA antibodies were negative. Urinalysis showed large leukocyte esterase, WBC > 182 and protein 100 mg/dL. Urine culture was negative.

Intravenous ceftriaxone and ciprofloxacin therapy was started for presumed pyelonephritis. Patient also received IV hydration with normal saline and 4 units of packed RBC. Renal ultrasound and non-contrast computed tomography (CT) of the abdomen showed multiple heterogeneous and solid appearing lobular soft tissue masses at the periphery of the mid and lower pole of the right kidney that extends into the peri-renal space which was suspicious for malignancy (**Figure 1**). Bilateral kidney stones were recognized on CT. MRI of the abdomen demonstrated enlarged right kidney with some increased parenchymal signal intensity with poorly defined margin with peri-nephric infection. However, Indium scan revealed no evidence of pyelonephritis or renal abscess. Medical therapy with IV hydration and antibiotics, initially ceftriaxone and ciprofloxacin, later aztreonam for a total of 4 weeks were administered. In view of her hypercalcemia, she was investigated further and was found to have elevated serum PTH of 390 pg/mL. A sestamebi scan and an ultrasound of the neck revealed a right parathyroid adenoma.

Two weeks after admission, because of persistence of the right renal mass, CT guided percutaneous biopsy was performed and revealed 43 cc of turbid fluid which was negative for malignant cells and culture. Further testing of the right kidney function using furosemide renal scan demonstrated residual renal function of <10%. Subsequently, due to suspicion of malignancy in the face of non functioning and possibly infected right kidney, patient underwent right nephrectomy 5 weeks after admission. Gross examination showed a peri-nephric fat adherent to the capsule of the kidney with fat necrosis and diffuse yellow-red hemorrhagic tissue (**Figure 2(A)**). There was also a 2 cm yellow crushable stone at the distal ureter occupying the entire lumen. Histopathology revealed acute and moderate chronic inflammation with focal marked increased interstitial eosinophils and lipid laden macrophage (xanthoma cells) (**Figure 2(B)**), consistent with XGP pyelonephritis. There was also nephrocalcinosis, both polarizable and non-polarizable. Chemical analysis of the stone revealed calcium oxalate stone. Simultaneously right para- thyroidectomy was also performed for parathyroid adenoma. After six weeks of hospital stay, her serum creatinine level was stable at 2.1 mg/dl (160 μmol/L) and was discharged in a stable condition.

3. Discussion

We report on a case of XGP associated with Crohn's disease and primary HPT which was unrecognized for at least a year prior to her present presentation. The coexistence of primary HPT and Crohn's disease caused calcium oxalate stone by the known mechanisms of hypercalcemia and hyperoxaluria respectively. To the best of our knowledge, this is the first case of XGP secondary to Crohn's disease and primary HPT which in turn leads to calcium oxalate stones.

XGP is a rare chronic inflammation of the kidney and constitutes less than 1% of chronic pyelonephritis. It is characterized by destruction of renal parenchyma and its replacement with granulomas, abscesses and collection of lipid laden macrophages (xanthoma cells) [1-3]. Females are more affected than males with a ratio of 1:4, and with a mean age varing from 45 to 55 years [3,4]. Though the exact mechanism of XGP is not clear, a number of predisposing factors have been implicated. The two most common predisposing factors are obstruction and infection of the genitor-urinary system. Calculi frequently stag horn type may be seen from 47% to 100% of cases. It is also more commonly seen in renal transplant recipients and diabetics [4,5]. In our patient, the combination of primary HPT and Crohn's disease leading to kidney stone formation and obstruction, in addition to her gender and age, are the most likely predisposing factors. XGP is commonly associated with *Escherichia coli* and Proteus infection; however bacterial outgrowth from urine culture is not necessary for diagnosis, as in our patient [2,4].

The disease process affects the whole of the kidney in 85% (diffuse form). Focal forms are rare (15%). The lesion is generally unilateral and can affect either kidney with equal frequency. Bilateral lesions are rare and are associated with poor outcome [2,3]. In the present case, a diffuse and unilateral form of XGP is observed. Symptoms are frequently nonspecific and include flank pain, fever, weight loss, anorexia and malaise. Uncommon

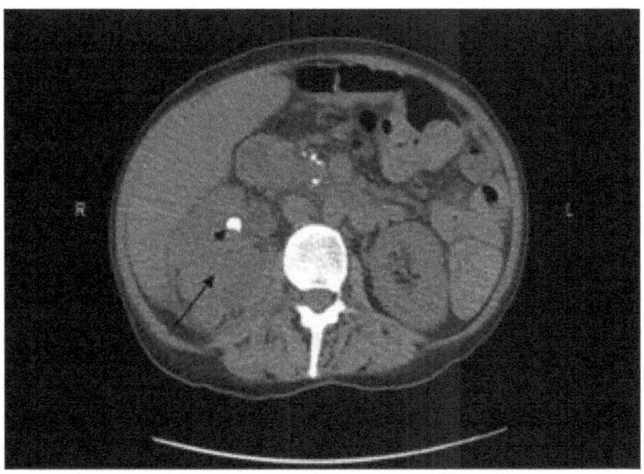

Figure 1. Non-contrast computed tomography of the abdomen and pelvis showing solid appearing soft tissue mass at the periphery of the mid and lower pole of the right kidney extending into the peri-nephric space (arrow) and renal stone (arrow head).

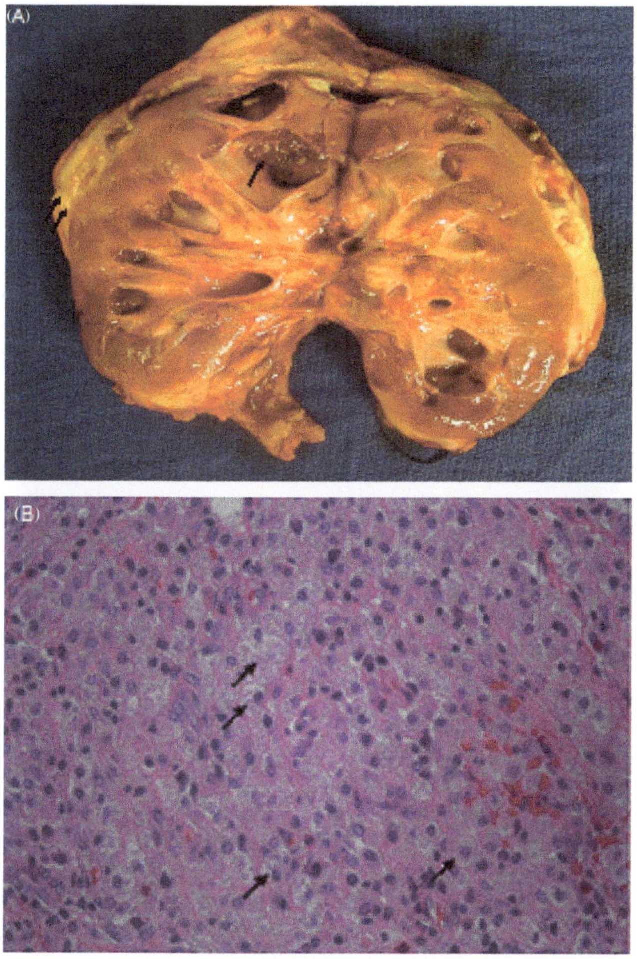

Figure 2. (A) Gross kidney specimen: Fat necrosis and scattered light yellow colored areas (double arrow) with diffuse yellow-red hemorrhagic tissue in the calyces (arrow). (B) Hematoxylin and eosin stain, original magnification ×200, of renal biopsy showing lipid laden macrophage (xanthoma cells) (arrows) and inflammatory cells.

manifestation such as nephro-cutaneous fistula has also been described [6]. Physical exam may reveal palpable and tender flank mass. Clinical findings are easily confused with those of renal tumor in terms of its radiographic appearance and its ability to involve adjacent structures or organs [2,3]. The definitive diagnosis of this entity is achieved only by histopathology examination which shows the presence of lipid laden macrophage (xanthoma cells) [3].

Treatment of XGP consists of nephrectomy after the initial courses of antimicrobial therapy especially in the diffuse form since it is associated with a complete destruction of the kidney [4]. Cases of focal XGP treated with antibiotics alone have also been described [7,8]. Our patient underwent right nephrectomy and was discharged in a stable condition after 6 weeks of hospital stay and her discharge serum creatinine was 2.1 mg/dL (186 μmol/L).

In conclusion, XGP associated with Crohn's disease and primary HPT leading to calcium oxalate stones highlights the importance of early diagnosis of primary HPT and management of kidney stones, thus preventing from potentially incurable renal complications.

REFERENCES

[1] M. Levy, R. Baumal and A. A. Eddy, "Xanthogranulomatous Pyelonephritis in Children. Etiology, Pathogenesis, Clinical and Radiologic Features, and Management," *Clinical Pediatrics*, Vol. 33, No. 6, 1994, pp. 360-366. doi:10.1177/000992289403300609

[2] T. Yoshino and H. Moriyama, "Case of the Diffuse Form of Xanthogranulomatous Pyelonephritis," *Case Reports in Urology*, Vol. 2013, 2013, Article ID: 936035. doi:10.1155/2013/936035

[3] S. Goyal, M. Gupta and R. Goyal, "Xanthogranulomatous Pyelonephritis: A Rare Entity," *North American Journal of Medical Sciences*, Vol. 3, No. 5, 2011, pp. 249-250. http://dx.doi.org/10.4297/najms.2011.3249

[4] L. Li and A. V. Parwani, "Xanthogranulomatous Pyelonephritis," *Archives of Pathology & Laboratory Medicine*, Vol. 135, No. 5, 2011, pp. 671-674.

[5] H. M. Scarpero and J. B. Copley, "Xanthogranulomatous Pyelonephritis in a Renal Recipient," *American Journal of Kidney Diseases*, Vol. 30, No. 6, 1997, pp. 846-848. http://dx.doi.org/10.1016/S0272-6386(97)90092-5

[6] G. Lee and J. H. Hong, "Xanthogranulomatous Pyelonephritis with Nephrocutaneous Fistula Due to *Providencia rettgeri* Infection," *Journal of Medical Microbiology*, Vol. 60, No. 7, 2011, pp. 1050-1052. doi:10.1099/jmm.0.028977-0

[7] C. I. Ho, Y. K. Wen and M. L. Chen, "Xanthogranulomatous Pyelonephritis Successfully Treated with Antibiotics Only," *Journal of the Chinese Medical Association*, Vol. 71, No. 12, 2008, pp. 643-645. doi:10.1016/S1726-4901(09)70008-5

[8] P. S. Brown Jr., M. Dodson, *et al.*, "Xanthogranulomatous Pyelonephritis: Report of Nonsurgical Management of a Case and Review of the Literature," *Clinical Infectious Diseases*, Vol. 22, No. 2, 1996, pp. 308-314. doi:10.1093/clinids/22.2.308

20

Feeding Reduces Serum Concentration of Endogenous Bioactive (1-84), but Not Total Intact Parathyroid Hormone in Female Sprague-Dawley Rats*

Jason R. DeGuire, Hope A. Weiler
School of Dietetics and Human Nutrition, McGill University, Montreal, Canada
Email: hope.weiler@mcgill.ca

ABSTRACT

Background: Interpretation of parathyroid hormone (PTH) measurements requires an understanding of its structural conformation. PTH reflects calcium intake and vitamin D status but is commonly measured in the fasted state using 2nd generation assays, known to cross-react with PTH 7-84 fragments, which is not observed with 3rd generation assays. The objective was to determine if plasma PTH in the fed and non-fed state differ while controlling for diurnal rhythm and the generation of PTH assay. **Methods:** Blood was sampled, 2 d apart, from Sprague-Dawley rats (30 males and 30 females) in both fed and non-fed states at 20 wk of age (weight: 470.2 ± 23.2 g) for measurement of ionized calcium (iCa), total intact (INT) and bioactive 1-84 (BIO) PTH. Differences between groups were tested using a GLIMMIX model with sex and feeding state as fixed effects and individual rats as a random effect. **Results:** Females had a lower iCa than males (F: 1.43 ± 0.01 vs M: 1.46 ± 0.01 mmol/L, P = 0.03). In males and females, there was no difference between fed and non-fed groups when PTH was assessed using the INT PTH assay (M Fed: 21.6 ± 1.3 vs M Non-fed: 22.6 ± 2.3 pmol/L, P = 0.59; F Fed: 19.3 ± 1.5 vs F Non-fed: 22.8 ± 2.9 pmol/L, P = 0.39). However, in females only, PTH measured using the BIO PTH, was significantly lower in the fed group versus the non-fed (Fed: 8.4 ± 0.8 vs Non-fed: 16.7 ± 3.4 pmol/L, P = 0.05). **Conclusions:** These results suggest that fasting elevates BIO PTH in females. Studies related to PTH should consider standardization of fast duration, sex differences, and preferentially use BIO PTH assays.

Keywords: Feeding; Sex; Parathyroid Hormone; Assay; Bioactive; Intact

1. Introduction

Parathyroid hormone (PTH) is the primary determinant of the extent of bone remodeling activity in the skeleton. It regulates bone metabolism and mineralization in addition to maintaining calcium homeostasis in part by binding to the parathyroid hormone 1 receptor in bone and the kidney. Circulating PTH follows a diurnal and circadian rhythm [1-4] and is altered acutely by certain nutrients such as calcium [1,2] and chronically by conjugated linoleic acid (CLA) in healthy and polycystic kidney disease rats [3,4]. Thus when assessing PTH, both timing of sampling and standardized food intake patterns prior to sampling are required in trials designed to assess the physiological response of PTH to diet or supplements. Furthermore, PTH assays have evolved based on their clinical performance in differentiating bone diseases associated with renal failure [5].

First generation assays allowed for the description of circulating PTH immunoreactivity, however, these mainly reacted with PTH fragments without bioactivity. Second generation assays, known as intact PTH (INT), were initially thought to react only with the bioactive form of PTH (1-84) [5]. It was later discovered that these assays cross-reacted with the PTH fragments, notably PTH (7-84), which are suggested to antagonize the calcemic and bone resorptive effects of PTH (1-84). Third generation assays (BIO), with no cross-reactivity with the PTH fragments were thus developed to address the issue of the detection of fragments with biologically opposite effects [5]. Recently, in male and female cynomolgus monkeys, feeding reduced INT PTH suggesting that feeding state should be considered when interpreting PTH values [6]. The objective of this study was to confirm these results in another species and to assess possible differences in feeding state, sex and type of PTH assay used. It was hypothesized that: 1) feeding would reduce both INT and BIO PTH; 2) there would be no sex differences for both

*This research was supported by a collaborative research development grant from the Dairy Farmers of Canada and the Natural Sciences and Engineering Research Council of Canada.

INT and BIO PTH; and 3) INT and BIO PTH assays will yield different values for PTH.

2. Materials and Methods

2.1. Study Protocol and Diets

All procedures and measurements were approved by the University of Manitoba Committee on Animal Care and conformed to Canadian Council on Animal Care guidelines [7]. This study was part of a larger study investigating the effect of CLA on bone and mineral metabolism [4]. Sprague-Dawley rats, (30 males and 30 females), were fed AIN-93G diets [8] from 3 to 20 wk of age with the exception of slightly higher fat content (84 g/kg) in all groups with the control group containing only soybean oil and the other dietary groups receiving 0.5% to 1% CLA. Animals were acclimatized to the housing conditions and housed (12 h light, 12 h dark cycle) in same-sex pairs, fed ad libitum and food disappearance monitored 3 times weekly over the study.

2.2. Assessment of Growth, PTH and Ionized Calcium

Body weight was measured weekly throughout the study using a weigh scale with a dynamic weighing program specifically for animal weighing (SB8001, Mettler-Toledo, Columbus, USA). Length was measured at wk 16 from nose to base of tail in the anesthetized state using isoflurane gas (AErrane®, Baxter, Mississauga, Canada). At the wk 16 time-point, a blood sample of no more than 10% blood volume was taken from the tail vein, between 0800 and 1000h to control for diurnal variation and separated to obtain serum for determination of PTH. Serum samples were stored at −80˚C until analysis. The fed state was a reflection of ad libitum intake during normal nocturnal feeding. Food was removed at 2000 h the night before the non-fed blood sampling 2 days after the fed blood sampling. Blood sampling of fed animals occurred first to ensure clearance of circulating PTH fragments. Moreover, a 2 day period between blood sampling was used to minimize stress to the animals and to allow for a complete feeding cycle in order to prevent any compensatory feeding after the fasting period. Blood was separated at 2000 g to obtain serum for determination of PTH using both second generation INT PTH and third generation BIO PTH using separate ELISA kits specific to rodent PTH (Alpco Diagnostics, Windham, USA). To assess intra- and inter-assay precision of both assays, the coefficient of variation (CV) was calculated from 20 triplicate determinations of two samples each performed in a single assay. For the BIO assay, intra-assay CV ranged from 2.5% - 3.9% and inter-assay CV ranged from 7.8% - 8.9%. For the INT assay, intra-assay CV ranged from 2.1% - 2.4% and inter assay CV ranged from 5.1% - 6.0%. Regarding serum ionized calcium (iCa), samples were measured within 4 h of collection using a Nova analyzer (Model 11, Nova Biomedical, Waltham, USA) with a CV < 1.6%.

2.3. Statistical Analysis

Data was analyzed using SAS statistical package software version 9.2.0 (SAS Institute Inc., Cary, USA). A GLIMMIX model included feeding state, sex, type of assay used and day of sampling combined with the individual animals included as a random factor. Diet was tested as a covariate, but did not significantly affect the results. This relatively new model was used to accommodate the Gaussian and non-Gaussian distribution and unequal variances of the data; all pair wise differences in diet means were tested using Tukey-Kramer approximation and a P-value of ≤0.05 was accepted as significant. Data are presented as mean ± SEM unless otherwise stated.

3. Results

At 20 wk of age, females had 47.5% lower weight than males (F: 323.1 ± 32.6 vs M: 615.2 ± 51.6 g, P < 0.0001), 18.6% lower length (F: 21.5 ± 0.5 vs M: 26.4 ± 0.8 cm, P < 0.0001), and 8.8% less food intake (F: 179.3 ± 22.9 vs M: 196.6 ± 18.0 g, P = 0.003). Fed animals had significantly higher (1.4%) iCa versus non-fed (fed: 1.45 ± 0.01 vs non-fed 1.43 ± 0.01 mmol/L, P = 0.0002). In males, iCa was 2.0% lower in the non-fed group versus fed (M non-fed: 1.43 ± 0.01 vs M fed: 1.46 ± 0.01 mmol/L, P = 0.003). A similar trend was observed in females (1.4% lower), however, it did not reach significance (F fed: 1.44 ± 0.01 vs F non-fed: 1.42 ± 0.01 mmol/L, P = 0.08). There was a significant difference between sexes where females had a 2.1% lower iCa compared to males (F: 1.43 ± 0.01 vs M: 1.46 ± 0.01 mmol/L, P = 0.03).

BIO PTH values were 48.6% lower (P < 0.0001) than INT PTH. In females, there was no difference between fed and non-fed groups when PTH was assessed using the INT assay however, PTH measured using the BIO was lower in the fed group versus the non-fed. In males, there was no difference between fed and non-fed groups when measured with either BIO or INT assays (**Figure 1**).

4. Discussion

The results of the present study indicate that for the biological assessment of PTH, one should take into consideration sex, feeding state, and generation of assay (ELISA) used. The assays used in this study were from

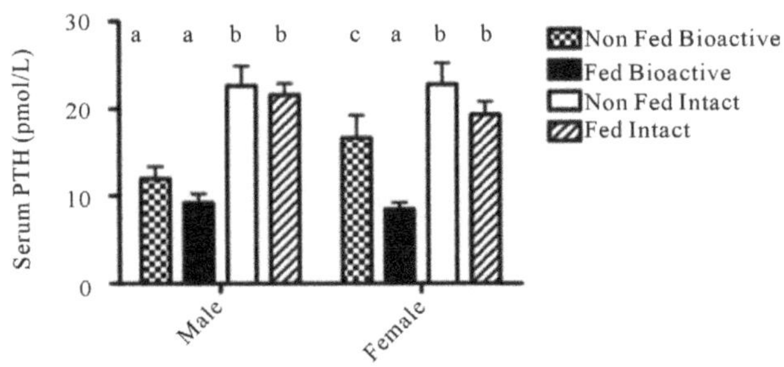

Figure 1. Effect of feeding on endogenous serum PTH concentration assessed using INT and BIO PTH assays in male and female rats. Differences detected using GLIMMIX model with post hoc testing using Tukey-Kramer approximation. Different letters indicate significant differences ($P < 0.05$). Values are mean ± SEM; n = 30 per sex.

the same manufacturer and were similar except for the horseradish peroxidase (HRP) conjugated detection antibody. The detection antibody in the INT assay binds to epitopes within the 13-34 amino acid region of the rat PTH molecule while the detection antibody in the BIO PTH assay binds to an initial amino terminal epitope of amino acids 1-3. Generally, the second-generation INT PTH assay reacts with both the PTH (1-84) and the shorter PTH fragments notably PTH (7-84), which, in a group of renal transplant patients, was reported to account for 44.1% of total plasma PTH [9].

Evidence suggests that PTH (7-84) fragments can lead to skeletal resistance to PTH and inhibit bone resorption and thus display an antagonistic action to PTH (1-84) [9,10]. Moreover, PTH (7-84) fragments have a half-life of ~10 minutes versus ~4 minutes for PTH (1-84) [11]. This could explain in part the higher PTH values measured by the INT PTH assay compared to the BIO PTH assay could reflect the sum of agonist and slow degrading antagonist fragments of PTH. These results are in agreement with Inaba *et al.* where the mean concentrations measured by the BIO PTH and INT PTH assays in healthy Japanese men and women were 62% higher in the INT assay, indicating that the PTH fragments account for ~40% of circulating PTH immunoreactivity [12]. Thus, the results obtained with the second-generation INT assay may not accurately reflect parathyroid function or serum PTH concentration.

Nutritional intake and extended fasting periods (33 to 96 hours) can modulate the circadian rhythm of PTH [13, 14]. Additionally, plasma phosphate (PO_4) and iCa are known to be correlated with PTH [14-19], which emphasizes the importance of meal times, type of food ingested and the resulting flux of PO_4 and iCa on PTH. Serum iCa, PO_4 and $1,25(OH)_2D_3$ are known to regulate serum PTH, and in turn are regulated by changes in PTH [20,21]. An increase in iCa mediates a decrease in PTH secretion within seconds of being detected by calcium receptors in the parathyroid gland and this is accompanied by the breakdown of circulating PTH over the following hours [22]. PO_4 independently increases PTH synthesis and secretion via a post-transcriptional mechanism occurring over a span of hours [23,24], while $1,25(OH)_2D_3$ decreases PTH via inhibition of PTH gene expression [25]. This study has demonstrated that being in a non-fed state for 8 to 10 h is sufficient to decrease iCa, whereas the increase in PTH values were true for the BIO PTH assay only in females. It is possible that the already lower values for BIO PTH in some of the dietary groups of males but not females from the original study [4], precluded detection of differences in INT and BIO PTH between feeding states in males. Nonetheless, BIO PTH values for animals in the control diet were not different between feeding states (Fed 9.1 ± 1.7 vs non-fed 9.8 ± 2.3 pmol/L, $P = 0.81$); the same was true for INT PTH (Fed 22.1 ± 2.3 vs non-fed 21.7 ± 4.6 pmol/L, $P = 0.97$). In addition the iCa values for males were higher than females whereas BIO PTH was lower.

Overall our work contrasts that of Ruh *et al.* who found that in male and female monkeys, withdrawing food increases INT PTH [6]. The animals' food was removed for 7 hours and collected the blood samples in the late afternoon, which would also reflect circadian rhythm near the end of the expected feeding period. One of the reasons for the discrepancy might relate to the use of isoflurane anesthesia in rats, which is known to decrease iCa and increase INT PTH after induction of anesthesia and peaking after 30 minutes of exposure [26]. However, sampling in the rats was rapid within 10 to 15 min total. In summary, the present study suggests that the INT assay could mask the changes in PTH seen with sex and feeding states, at least in rats.

The assessment of PTH is difficult due to its complex metabolic and structural properties. Mallette first proposed that PTH could be considered as a "polyhormone" based on the multiple biological actions of single peptide regions of the PTH molecule [27]. This theory continues to be verified with ongoing discoveries of different forms of circulating PTH [28-30]. This reinforces the importance of careful selection of PTH assays depending on the purpose of the study. As demonstrated in this study, 2nd generation assays yield higher values than 3rd generation assays. Also, they appear to be unable to differentiate differences incurred based on sex although further PTH analyses using assays from different manufacturers is warranted to confirm these results. Future studies related to PTH should consider standardization of fast duration, sex effects, and measure BIO PTH.

5. Acknowledgements

The work was conducted at the University of Manitoba

facilities and the associated Manitoba Institute of Child Health. The authors acknowledge the assistance with feeding and some sample collection and measurement by S. Fitzpatrick, M. Kaur, and R. Mollard and A. Dick. The authors have no conflict of interest.

REFERENCES

[1] T. Fujita, S. Ohgitani and Y. Fujii, "Overnight Suppression of Parathyroid Hormone and Bone Resorption Markers by Active Absorbable Algae Calcium. A Double-Blind Crossover Study," *Calcified Tissue International*, Vol. 60, No. 6, 1997, pp. 506-512. doi:10.1007/s002239900272

[2] W. R. McKane, S. Khosla, K. S. Egan, S. P. Robins, M. F. Burritt and B. L. Riggs, "Role of Calcium Intake in Modulating Age-Related Increases in Parathyroid Function and Bone Resorption," *The Journal of Clinical Endocrinology and Metabolism*, Vol. 81, No. 5, 1996, pp. 1699-1703. doi:10.1210/jc.81.5.1699

[3] H. A. Weiler, S. Austin, S. Fitzpatrick-Wong, E. Nitschmann, N. Bankovic-Calic, R. Mollard, H. Aukema and M. Ogborn, "Conjugated Linoleic Acid Reduces Parathyroid Hormone in Health and in Polycystic Kidney Disease in Rats," *American Journal of Clinical Nutrition*, Vol. 79, No. S6, 2004, pp. S1186-S1189.

[4] H. A. Weiler, S. Fitzpatrick and S. C. Fitzpatrick-Wong, "Dietary Conjugated Linoleic Acid in the cis-9, trans-11 Isoform Reduces Parathyroid Hormone in Male, but Not Female Rats," *Journal Nutritional Biochemistry*, Vol. 19, No. 11, 2008, pp. 762-769. doi:10.1016/j.jnutbio.2007.09.010

[5] P. Gao and P. D'Amour, "Evolution of the Parathyroid Hormone (PTH) Assay—Importance of Circulating PTH Immunoheterogeneity and of Its Regulation," *Clinical Laboratory*, Vol. 51, No. 1-2, 2005, pp. 21-29.

[6] C. Ruh, N. Doyle, P. Oldfield, P. Bednarek and S. Y. Smith, "Effects of Fasting on Endogenous Parathyroid Hormone (PTH) Levels in Cynomolgus Monkeys," *Journal of Bone and Mineral Research*, Vol. 25, No. S1, 2010, pp. S363-S502.

[7] Canadian Council on Animal Care, "Guide to the Care and Use of Experimental Animals," Bradda Printing Services Inc., Ottawa, 1993.

[8] P. G. Reeves, "Components of the AIN-93 Diets as Improvements in the AIN-76A Diet," *Journal of Nutrition*, Vol. 127, No. S5, 1997, pp. S838-S841.

[9] E. Slatopolsky, J. Finch, P. Clay, D. Martin, G. Sicard, G. Singer, P. Gao, T. Cantor and A. Dusso, "A Novel Mechanism for Skeletal Resistance in Uremia," *Kidney International*, Vol. 58, No. 2, 2000, pp. 753-761.

[10] P. Divieti, M. R. John, H. Juppner and F. R. Bringhurst, "Human PTH-(7-84) Inhibits Bone Resorption *in Vitro* via Actions Independent of the Type 1 PTH/PTHrP Receptor," *Endocrinology*, Vol. 143, No. 1, 2002, pp. 171-176. doi:10.1210/en.143.1.171

[11] H. Yamashita, P. Gao, T. Cantor, T. Futata, T. Murakami, S. Uchino, S. Watanabe, H. Kawamoto, M. Fukagawa and S. Noguchi, "Large Carboxy-Terminal Parathyroid Hormone (PTH) Fragment with a Relatively Longer Half-Life than 1-84 PTH is Secreted, Directly From the Parathyroid Gland in Humans," *European Journal of Endocrinology*, Vol. 149, No. 4, 2003, pp. 301-306. doi:10.1530/eje.0.1490301

[12] M. Inaba, K. Nakatsuka, Y. Imanishi, M. Watanabe, Y. Mamiya, E. Ishimura and Y. Nishizawa, "Technical and Clinical Characterization of the Bio-PTH (1-84) Immunochemiluminometric Assay and Comparison with a Second-Generation Assay for Parathyroid Hormone," *Clinical Chemistry*, Vol. 50, No. 2, 2004, pp. 385-390. doi:10.1373/clinchem.2003.026831

[13] A. Schlemmer and C. Hassager, "Acute Fasting Diminishes the Circadian Rhythm of Biochemical Markers of Bone Resorption," *European Journal of Endocrinology*, Vol. 140, No. 4, 1999, pp. 332-337. doi:10.1530/eje.0.1400332

[14] W. D. Fraser, F. C. Logue, J. P. Christie, D. A. Cameron, D. S. Oreilly and G. H. Beastall, "Alteration of the Circadian-Rhythm of Intact Parathyroid-Hormone Following a 96-Hour Fast," *Clinical Endocrinology*, Vol. 40, No. 4, 1994, pp. 523-528.

[15] M. S. Calvo, R. Kumar and H. Heath, "Elevated Secretion and Action of Serum Parathyroid-Hormone in Young-Adults Consuming High Phosphorus, Low Calcium Diets Assembled from Common Foods," *Journal of Clinical Endocrinology & Metabolism*, Vol. 66, No. 4, 1988, pp. 823-829. doi:10.1210/jcem-66-4-823

[16] W. D. Fraser, F. C. Logue, J. P. Christie, S. J. Gallacher, D. Cameron, D. S. J. O'Reilly, G. H. Beastall and I. T. Boyle, "Alteration of the Circadian Rhythm of Intact Parathyroid Hormone and Serum Phosphate in Women with Established Postmenopausal Osteoporosis," *Osteoporosis International*, Vol. 8, No. 2, 1998, pp. 121-126. doi:10.1007/BF02672507

[17] F. C. Logue, W. D. Fraser, D. S. Oreilly and G. H. Beastall, "The Circadian-Rhythm of Intact Parathyroid-Hormone (1-84) and Nephrogenous Cyclic Adenosine-Monophosphate in Normal Men," *Journal of Endocrinology*, Vol. 121, No. 1, 1989, pp. R1-R3. doi:10.1677/joe.0.121R001

[18] M. E. Markowitz, S. Arnaud, J. F. Rosen, M. Thorpy and S. Laximinarayan, "Temporal Interrelationships between the Circadian-Rhythms of Serum Parathyroid-Hormone and Calcium Concentrations," *Journal of Clinical Endocrinology & Metabolism*, Vol. 67, No. 5, 1988, pp. 1068-1073. doi:10.1210/jcem-67-5-1068

[19] M. S. Calvo, R. Kumar and H. Heath, "Persistently Elevated Parathyroid-Hormone Secretion and Action in Young-Women after 4 Weeks of Ingesting High Phosphorus, Low Calcium Diets," *Journal of Clinical Endocrinology & Metabolism*, Vol. 70, No. 5, 1990, pp. 1334-1340. doi:10.1210/jcem-70-5-1334

[20] E. Slatopolsky, A. Brown and A. Dusso, "Pathogenesis of Secondary Hyperparathyroidism," *Kidney International*, Vol. 73, 1999, pp. S14-S19. doi:10.1046/j.1523-1755.1999.07304.x

[21] E. Slatopolsky and J. A. Delmez, "Pathogenesis of Secondary Hyperparathyroidism," *Nephrology Dialysis Trans-*

plantation, Vol. 11, 1996, pp. 130-135. doi:10.1093/ndt/11.supp3.130

[22] E. M. Brown, M. Pollak, C. E. Seidman, J. G. Seidman, D. Riccardi and S. C. Hebert, "Seminars in Medicine of the Beth-Israel-Hospital, Boston—Calcium-Ion-Sensing Cell-Surface Receptors," *New England Journal of Medicine*, Vol. 333, No. 4, 1995, pp. 234-240. doi:10.1056/NEJM199507273330407

[23] E. Reiss, J. M. Canterbury, M. A. Bercovitz and E. L. Kaplan, "Role of Phosphate in Secretion of Parathyroid Hormone in Man," *Journal of Clinical Investigation*, Vol. 49, No. 11, 1970, pp. 2146-2149. doi:10.1172/JCI106432

[24] E. Slatopolsky, A. Dusso and A. J. Brown, "The Role of Phosphorus in the Development of Secondary Hyperparathyroidism and Parathyroid Cell Proliferation in Chronic Renal Failure," *American Journal of the Medical Sciences*, Vol. 317, No. 6, 1999, pp. 370-376. doi:10.1097/00000441-199906000-00004

[25] T. Navehmany, M. M. Friedlaender, H. Mayer and J. Silver, "Calcium Regulates Parathyroid-Hormone Messenger Ribonucleic-Acid (Messenger-Rna), but Not Calcitonin Messenger-Rna *in Vivo* in the Rat—Dominant Role of 1,25-Dihydroxyvitamin-D," *Endocrinology*, Vol. 125, No. 1, 1989, pp. 275-280. doi:10.1210/endo-125-1-275

[26] C. E. Hotchkiss, R. Brommage, M. Du and C. P. Jerome, "The Anesthetic Isoflurane Decreases Ionized Calcium and Increases Parathyroid Hormone and Osteocalcin in Cynomolgus Monkeys," *Bone*, Vol. 23, No. 5, 1998, pp. 479-484. doi:10.1016/S8756-3282(98)00124-0

[27] L. E. Mallette, "The Parathyroid Polyhormones—New Concepts in the Spectrum of Peptide-Hormone Action," *Endocrine Reviews*, Vol. 12, No. 2, 1991, pp. 110-117. doi:10.1210/edrv-12-2-110

[28] P. D'amour, J. H. Brossard, A. Rakel, L. Rousseau, C. Albert and T. Cantor, "Evidence that the Amino-Terminal Composition of Non-(1-84) Parathyroid Hormone Fragments Starts before Position 19," *Clinical Chemistry*, Vol. 51, No. 1, 2005, pp. 169-176. doi:10.1373/clinchem.2004.040485

[29] P. D'amour, J. H. Brossard, L. Rousseau, L. Nguyen-Yamamoto, E. Nassif, C. Lazure, D. Gauthier, J. R. Lavigne and R. J. Zahradnik, "Structure of Non-(1-84) PTH Fragments Secreted by Parathyroid Glands in Primary and Secondary Hyperparathyroidism," *Kidney International*, Vol. 68, No. 3, 2005, pp. 998-1007. doi:10.1111/j.1523-1755.2005.00493.x

[30] A. Rakel, J. H. Brossard, J. V. Patenaude, C. Albert, E. Nassif, T. Cantor, L. Rousseau and P. D'Amour, "Overproduction of an Amino-Terminal Form of PTH Distinct from Human PTH(1-84) in a Case of Severe Primary Hyperparathyroidism: Influence of Medical Treatment and Surgery," *Clinical Endocrinology*, Vol. 62, No. 6, 2005, pp. 721-727.

21

Atypical Presentation of Classical Bartter Syndrome as a Case of Chronic Diarrhea and Failure to Thrive*

Anil Kumar Mohanty, Deepti Damayanty Pradhan, Bijay Kumar Meher, Pradeep Sivraj
Department of Paediatrics, Sardar Vallavbhai Patel Post Graduate Institute of Paediatrics (SCB Medical College), Cuttack, India
Email: bkmeher187@yahoo.co.in

ABSTRACT

The classical Bartter syndrome is an uncommon tubular disorder of autosomal recessive inheritance, characterized by early childhood onset of polyuria, polydipsia, vomiting, dehydration, constipation and salt craving habit. The long-term outlook for patients with Bartter syndrome is not certain. If not properly treated, it may lead to failure to thrive and growth retardation. We herein report a case of 18-month-old girl child who presented chronic diarrhea and failure to thrive and then was diagnosed as a case of classical Bartter syndrome. She was successfully treated with potassium supplementation and ibuprofen therapy.

Keywords: Bartter Syndrome; Chronic Diarrhea; Ibuprofen Therapy

1. Introduction

Bartter Syndrome first described in 1960 but, over the years several phenotypic and genotypic variants of original description of Bartter syndrome have been identified [1,2]. The classical Bartter syndrome (BS) is characterized by early childhood onset with polyuria, polydipsia, vomiting, constipation, salt craving, severe dehydration, failure to thrive and growth retardation [3]. It is an uncommon tubular disorder, characterized by metabolic alkalosis, hyponatremia, hypokalemia, hypochloremia, with hyper-reninemia and hyperaldosteronemia, and normal or low blood pressure associated with increased loss of sodium, potassium, calcium and chloride in the urine [4].

2. Case Report

An 18-month-old female child born out of non-consanguineous marriage presented with history of vomiting, poor feeding, on and off low grade fever, loose motion and weight loss for 3 months. Vomiting was projectile, non-bilious, and 6 - 8 times per day. The loose motion was watery sometimes mucoid 6 - 8 times daily and was continuing for last 3 months and was hospitalized in local hospital twice for dehydration but loose motion did not relieved by treatment. There was no history of decrease in urination. This child was 4th order, term normal vaginal delivery, birth weight being 2800 gm with uneventful perinatal period. Baby was on exclusive breast fed up to 6 months of age and thereafter was on home based cereal diet. Developmental milestones were normal till about 15 months of age then unable to stand and walk and started crawling. In the sibling history, 1st male child died at 4 months and 2nd female child died at 6 months due to unknown reasons, 3rd female child was 5 years old and doing well.

On examination, at admission, the patient was cachectic, afebrile, lethargic, severely dehydrated, having tachycardia, tachypnea, hypotension, weight 5.5 kg, (previous documented weight at 6 months was 6.5 kg and at 1 year was 8 kg.) without stunting, head circumference 45 cm, MAC-10 cm with US/LS ratio of 1.4. (**Figure 1**) She was pale, without having lymphadenopathy, jaundice, cyanosis, clubbing or edema with systemic examinations being normal. Clinical diagnosis at admission was chronic diarrhea with failure to thrive.

On investigation, microcytic hypochromic anemia with normal erythrocyte sedimentation rate (ESR) and normoglycemia, without any features of infection (total leucocyte counts, C-reactive protein, urine microscopy including culture were normal). Stool examination revealed no red blood cells, pus cell, parasites, fat globules and normal level of reducing sugars. Serum albumin was 3 gm/dL. Renal function test revealed normal serum-

*Funding: none; Conflicting interest: none.

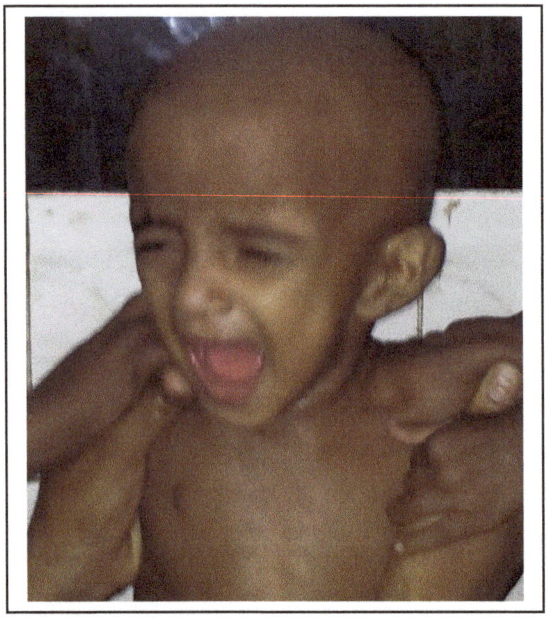

Figure 1. 18-month-old child with failure to thrive and note the irritability of the child.

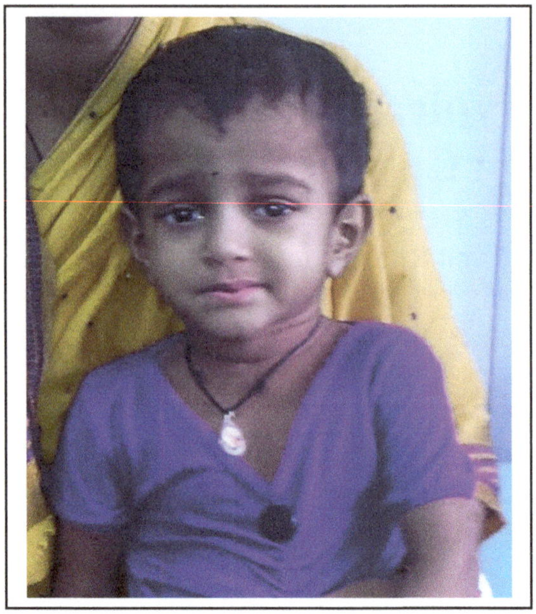

Figure 2. Same child during follow up after 10 months of treatment.

urea, creatinine with hyponatremia (118 mEq/L), hypokalemia (2.9 mEq/L), hypochloremia (85 mEq/L). ABG revealed metabolic alkalosis with pH 7.771; bicarbonate 26 mEq/L. Spot urinary sodium was 184 mEq/L, potassium 14 mEq/L, calcium 12.6 mEq/L, chloride-112 mEq/L. Serum tissue transglutaminase level was normal. Ultrasonogram of abdomen was normal. Bartter syndrome was suspected in the view of metabolic alkalosis with high urinary excretion of chloride, hyponatremia, hypokalemia and hypochloremia and then blood sample was sent for serum renin and aldosterone.

The child was initially managed with intravenous fluids followed by oral rehydration solution (ORS) and F-75 diet. Serum aldosterone and serum renin were found to be raised *i.e.* 551.57 pg/ml (normal 25 - 315 pg/ml) and 87.6 uIU/ml (normal upright-4.4 to-46.1 uIU/ml, supine-2.8- to 39.9 uIU/ml) respectively. Later on child was started on F-100 diet, potassium supplementation and Ibuprofen therapy (30 mg/kg/day). With this treatment, child improved symptomatically (vomiting and stool frequency was reduced, her appetite improved) and she gained 600 gram during the hospital stay. Repeat Serum electrolytes showed normal sodium (137 mEq/L), low normal potassium (3.1 mEq/L), and low normal Calcium (0.9 mEq/L).

During follow up after 4 month there was no diarrhea, weight was increased to 7.7 kg, height 75 cm and serum electrolyte was normal except for low normal potassium level (sodium 139 mEq/L, potassium 3.36 mEq/L, Calcium 1.0 mEq/L). At 10 months follow up, the weight was 9.5 kg, height 82 cm (**Figure 2**) and serum electrolytes were normal.

3. Discussion

Bartter syndrome is rare autosomal recessive renal tubular disorders characterized by hypokalemia, hypochloremia, metabolic alkalosis, and hyperreninemia with normal blood pressure. The underlying renal abnormality results in excessive urinary losses of sodium, chloride, and potassium. The occurrence varies from country to country. Incidence of our country is not known. In Costa Rica, the frequency of neonatal Bartter syndrome is approximately 1.2 cases per 100,000 live births but is higher if all preterm births are considered. Bartter syndrome has traditionally been classified into 3 main clinical variants: neonatal (or antenatal) Bartter syndrome, classical Bartter syndrome, and Gitelman syndrome. Abnormalities of classical Bartter syndrome are all suggestive of a defect related to Cl^- transport in the medullary thick ascending loop of Henle and distal convoluted tubule (DCT). Failure to reabsorb chloride results in a failure to reabsorb sodium and leads to excessive sodium and chloride (salt) delivery to the distal tubules, leading to excessive salt and water loss from the body and activation of renin-angiotensin aldosterone system (RAAS).

Our case presented at 18 months of age with severe dehydration and failure to thrive. We initially treated as a case of diarrhea; child improved symptomatically and again went in for severe dehydration. But the urine output was not impaired even in severe dehydration. Blood and urine investigations revealed increased loss of sodium, potassium, chloride and calcium. After then, serum renin and aldosterone was found high and treated in line of Bartter syndrome, child improved with our treatment. K. Sampatkumar *et al.* [5] in an Indian series of childhood Bartter syndrome had found the mean age of presentation at 6.5 ± 4.9 months with features of vomiting, FTT, polyuria, dehydration, some with fever, irritability, respiratory difficulty, alkalosis, hypokalemia, hypochloremia, hyponatremia. However in their series no diarrhea was reported.

In another case report by P Samayam *et al.* [6] a 5year old child had presented with history of recurrent vomiting, generalized weakness, FTT, dehydration, pallor which was diagnosed to be Bartter syndrome, and treated with Potassium supplements & ibuprofen along with appropriate dietary advice & improved on follow up. However no diarrhea was associated.

P Saravan kumar *et al.* [7] reported a case of neonatal Bartter syndrome which presented at age of 2 months 10 days with diarrhea, vomiting, abdominal distention and FTT since 20 days of life. But diarrhea was controlled with treatment and hypokalemia persisted, so Bartter syndrome was suspected and diagnosed by investigation. However in our case the diarrhea persisted and did not respond to treatment. But diarrhea stopped with treatment of Bartter syndrome in form of potassium supplements and ibuprofen therapy.

4. Conclusions

Bartter syndrome should be suspected in any case of Vomiting and FTT. Also some cases of diarrhea and FTT with normal urination should be strongly suspected.

What is already known?

FTT and persistent vomiting cases should be investigated for Bartter syndrome.

What the study adds?

FTT and chronic diarrhea cases should also be investigated for BS.

Limitation of the study: We could not do genetic analysis of the child. More cases should be studied in future.

5. Contributors

AK overall designed the study. DP & BM case study and follow up, BM & PS preparing manuscript.

REFERENCES

[1] F. C. Bartter, P. Pronove, J. R. Gill and R. C. MacCardle (with tech. assistance of Diller E), "Hyperplasia of the Juxtraglomerular Complex with Hyperaldosteronism and Hypokalemic Alkalosis. A New Syndrome," *The American Journal of Medicine*, Vol. 33, No. 6, 1962, pp. 811-828. http://dx.doi.org/10.1016/0002-9343(62)90214-0

[2] W. Proesmans, "Threading through the Mizmaze of Bartter Syndrom," *Pediatric Nephrology*, Vol. 21, No. 7, 2006, pp. 896-902. http://dx.doi.org/10.1007/s00467-006-0113-7

[3] J. Rodrígu-Soriano, "Bartter and Related Syndromes; the Puzzle Is Almost Solved," *Pediatric Nephrology*, Vol. 12, No. 4, 1998, pp. 315-327. http://dx.doi.org/10.1007/s004670050461

[4] I. Kurtz, "Molecular Pathogenesis of Bartter's and Gitelman's Syndromes," *Kidney International*, Vol. 54, No. 4, 1998, pp. 1396-1410. http://dx.doi.org/10.1046/j.1523-1755.1998.00124.x

[5] K. Sampathkumar, U. Muralidharan, A. Kannan, M. Ramakrishnan and R. Ajeshkumar, "Childhood Bartter's Syndrome: An Indian Case Series," *Indian Journal of Nephrology*, Vol. 20, No. 4, 2010, pp. 207-210. http://dx.doi.org/10.4103/0971-4065.73455

[6] P. Samayam, B. R. Chander and V. R. S. Reddy, "An Unusual Cause of Failure to Thrive in a Child," *The National Medical Journal of India*, Vol. 24, No. 2, 2011, pp. 86-87.

[7] P. S. Kumar, M. Deendayalan, L. Janakiraman and M. Vijakumar, "Neonatal Batter Syndrome," *Indian Pediatrics*, Vol. 43, No. 8, 2006, pp. 735-737.

22

Two-Hour Creatinine Clearance and Glomerular Filtration Rate Estimated from Serum Cystatin C and Creatinine in the Elderly to Preoperative Period

Leopoldo Muniz da Silva, Pedro Thadeu Galvão Vianna, Mariana Takaku, Glênio Bittencourt Mizubuti, Yara Marcondes Machado Castiglia*

Department of Anaesthesiology, Botucatu School of Medicine,
São Paulo State University (UNESP), São Paulo, Brazil
Email: *yarac@fmb.unesp.br

ABSTRACT

Introduction: The utility of estimates of glomerular filtration rate based on creatinine and cystatin C serum levels to assess renal function in older surgical patients remains to be determined. **Objective:** To determine whether 2h-creatinine clearance (CrCl-2h) can be an adequate substitute for glomerular filtration rate estimates obtained by measuring serum cystatin C and creatinine in the elderly at preoperation. **Methods:** A total of 102 consecutive elder patients undergoing pre-anesthesia evaluation for routine surgeries were included. Study subjects were allocated into three groups: Group 1 (G1)—hypertensive diabetic patients, Group 2 (G2)—hypertensive patients, and Group 3 (G3)—non-hypertensive and non-diabetic patients. Two-hour urine collection was performed and CrCl-2h adjusted for ultrasonic residual bladder volume was estimated. GFR was estimated based on creatinine and cystatin C serum levels. Bland-Altman analysis was used to compare methods. **Results:** The mean difference between the evaluated methods and CrCl-2h was <15 $mL \cdot min^{-1} \cdot 1.73\ m^{-2}$ for Cys-GFR, and >20 $mL \cdot min^{-1} \cdot 1.73\ m^{-2}$ for Cr-GFR in all groups. CrCl-2h adjusted for ultrasonic residual bladder volume did not differ from non-adjusted CrCl-2h in none of the groups. **Conclusion:** Two-hour creatinine clearance was not an adequate substitute for GFR estimates based on creatinine and cystatin C serum levels in older patients at preoperation. The ultrasonic assessment of residual bladder volume had no significant influence on the calculation of two-hour creatinine clearance.

Keywords: Renal Function; Creatinine Clearance; Cystatin C; Elderly

1. Introduction

Subclinical renal disease, frequently seen in the diabetic and long-term hypertensive elderly, increases the risk associated with anesthesia and surgery, and enhances the susceptibility of these individuals to intraoperative renal failure, leading to high postoperative mortality rates [1-3].

The collection of urine output over 24 hours is one of the methods that have been used to assess renal function as it eliminates the potential error due to the existence of residual bladder volume, particularly in older people. However, a 24-h urine collection may not be feasible during preoperative evaluation delaying the availability of information for clinical evaluation [4].

In 1988, Cardenas *et al.* [5] described a small portable ultrasound device, specifically designed to determine bladder volumes that can be operated with minimal training. According to these authors, volumes estimated using this noninvasive method correlate with those obtained by urethral catheterization. Thus, the assessment of renal function at 2-h intervals using ultrasound bladder scan to eliminate the bias associated with postmicturition residual volume would be useful for the preoperative evaluation of elderly patients. Among intensive care patients, 2-h creatinine clearance has been demonstrated to be an adequate substitute for 24-h clearance, even in unstable patients [6].

Whether estimates of glomerular filtration rate based on creatinine and cystatin C serum levels are compared with 2-h creatinine clearance to assess renal function in older patients remains to be determined. Despite being an earlier marker of renal failure, cystatin C has not shown

*Corresponding author.

advantages over creatinine in the elderly [7]. Therefore, the purpose of this study was to assess whether creatinine clearance determined by a 2-hour urine collection adjusted for residual bladder volume is an adequate substitute for glomerular filtration rate estimates obtained by measuring serum cystatin C and creatinine in older patients before surgery.

2. Methods

This study was approved by the Committee of Research Ethics of Botucatu Medical School, and written informed consent was obtained from all subjects.

The study population consisted of 102 consecutive elderly patients (≥65 years) who underwent pre-anesthesia evaluation for routine orthopedic, gastrointestinal, vascular, or gynecologic surgery in a tertiary university hospital.

Study subjects were allocated into three groups: Group 1 (G1)—hypertensive diabetic patients, Group 2 (G2)—hypertensive patients, and Group 3 (G3)—non-hypertensive and non-diabetic patients. Patients were considered hypertensive and diabetic when diagnosis and specific treatment for these conditions had been established prior to admission. Patients with heart failure, renal failure requiring dialysis, anuria or kidney transplant were excluded. All patients had surgical diseases and were receiving preoperative in-patient care.

For renal function assessment, post-void residual urine volume was checked using a BVI 5000 ultrasound scanner (Diagnostic Ultrasound Corporation, USA). With the patient lying supine, the scanhead was lubricated with conductive gel (gel pad Sontac 50) and positioned approximately 5 cm above the symphysis pubis. Three scans were performed on each subject and the mean volume from these scans was used as the mean urine volume. Time count was then started. Patients were asked to complete urine collection in a special container for the next two hours. After one hour, a blood sample (15 mL) was obtained for the measurement of creatinine (mg/dL), urea (mg/dL), cystatin C (mg/L), and glycated hemoglobin (%). By the end of the two-hour interval, patients were asked to void in a container. From the total urine volume voided, a sample was collected for creatinine assessment (mg/dL). Ultrasonic residual volume was then measured again. Three readings were taken and the mean volume from these readings was added to the amount collected in the container. Adjusted urine volume was estimated by subtracting the initial residual volume from this sum. Urine output per minute ($mL{\cdot}min^{-1}$) was obtained by dividing the adjusted residual volume by the time elapsed to obtain it. Two-hour creatinine clearance ($mL{\cdot}min^{-1}$), or two-hour glomerular filtration rate (GFR), was estimated from the equation [urine creatinine (mg/dL) × adjusted two-hour urine volume (mL/min^{-1})/blood creatinine (mg/dL)].

Serum cystatin C measurements were performed by latex enhanced reagent (N Latex Cystatin C, Dade Behring, Deerfield, IL, USA) using a Behring BN ProSpec analyser (Dade Behring) and Dade Behring calibrators. The test was performed according to the in- structions of the manufacturer. Serum creatinine was measured by a dry chemistry technique at the Chemistry Laboratory of the hospital.

Creatinine-estimated GFR was calculated by the Cockcroft & Gault formula [8] where (GFR_{CG}) = [140 − age (years) × weight (kg) / 72 × blood creatinine (mg/dL) × 0.85 (if female). GFR from cystatin C was calculated by the Larsson *et al.* formula [9] where ($GFR_{Larsson}$) = [77.24 × cystatin $C^{-1.2623}$ (mg/L)]. GFR and two-hour creatinine clearance were expressed per 1.73 m^{-2} of body surface area by multiplying measured values by 1.73 of body surface area. Anthropometric data, such as age (years), gender, weight (kg), height (m^2) and body mass index (kg/m^2) were collected during preoperative clinical evaluation.

Statistical Analysis

Sample size (n = 102) was calculated to detect a difference of at least 15% between GFR by serum creatinine and two-hour creatinine clearance. Assuming a probability of 5% for a type I error and 20% for a type II error, 34 patients in each group would allow two-tailed comparisons. Median and 25% - 75% percentiles were used as a measure of central tendency and variability due to non-normal distribution of the study data. Categorical variables were reported as absolute values and percentages. Comparisons were performed with the non-parametric Kruskal Wallis test for continuous variables, followed by the a posteriori Dunn test for multiple comparisons if $P > 0.05$. Significance was set at $P < 0.05$. CrCl-2h adjusted for ultrasonic residual bladder volume and not adjusted CrCl-2h was compared by Mann-Whitney test.

Because analysis with correlation and least squares linear regression is fundamentally misleading, Bland and Altman analysis [10] was used to compare the differences between the methods for glomerular filtration rate measurement (Y axis) plotted against their mean (X axis). Bias was defined as the mean value of the differences between methods. If the 95% limits of agreement (mean ± 2SD) between methods were not clinically important, methods were considered interchangeable. The confidence intervals for the 95% limits of agreement were calculated by mean difference ±1.96 standard deviation of the differences. Bland and Altman analysis [10] of the GFR estimates was performed with Medcalc (Medical

Software, Mariakerke, Belgium).

3. Results

Patient median age was 71 years (65 - 88 years). Males accounted for 66.34% of the study population. In diabetic patients, median glycated hemoglobin was 7.2%.

Study groups were homogeneous according to age, gender and body mass index (kg·m^{-2}). There was no statistically significant difference in adjusted urine volume, two-hour creatinine clearance (CrCl-2h), creatinine-estimated glomerular filtration rate (Cr-GFR) and Cystatin-C estimated GFR (Cys-GFR).

The mean differences between the evaluated methods and CrCl-2h were 3.67 mL·min^{-1}·1.73 m^{-2} for Cys-GFR, and 27.44 mL·min^{-1}·1.73 m^{-2} for Cr-GFR in **G1**; 2.29 mL·min^{-1}·1.73 m^{-2} for Cys-GFR and 22.96 mL·min^{-1}·1.73 m^{-2} for Cr-GFR in **G2;** 13.10 mL·min^{-1}·1.73 m^{-2} for Cys-GFR and 40.40 mL·min^{-1}·1.73 m^{-2} for CR-GFR in **G3** (**Figure 1**). Limits of agreement between Cys-GFR - CrCl-2h and Cr-GFR - CrCl-2h were showed in **Table 1**.

CrCl-2h adjusted for ultrasonic residual bladder volume did not differ from non-adjusted CrCl-2h in all patients (**Figure 2**).

4. Discussion

The assessment of renal function using creatinine concentration as a marker has several limitations in the elderly. Two hour-creatinine clearance would then be an important alternative for assessing renal function serially and at short intervals.

In this study, CrCl-2h was compared with glomerular filtration rate and estimates from creatinine and cystatin C. Our data showed that CrCl-2h better agreed with cystatin C-estimated GFR (Larsson equation) than with creatinine-estimated GFR (Cockcroft & Gault equation) in older patients. The mean difference between the evaluated methods and CrCl-2h was < 15 mL·min^{-1}·1.73 m^{-2} for Cys-GFR, and >20 mL·min^{-1}·1.73 m^{-2} for Cr-GFR in all groups. A mean difference between methods of 18 -

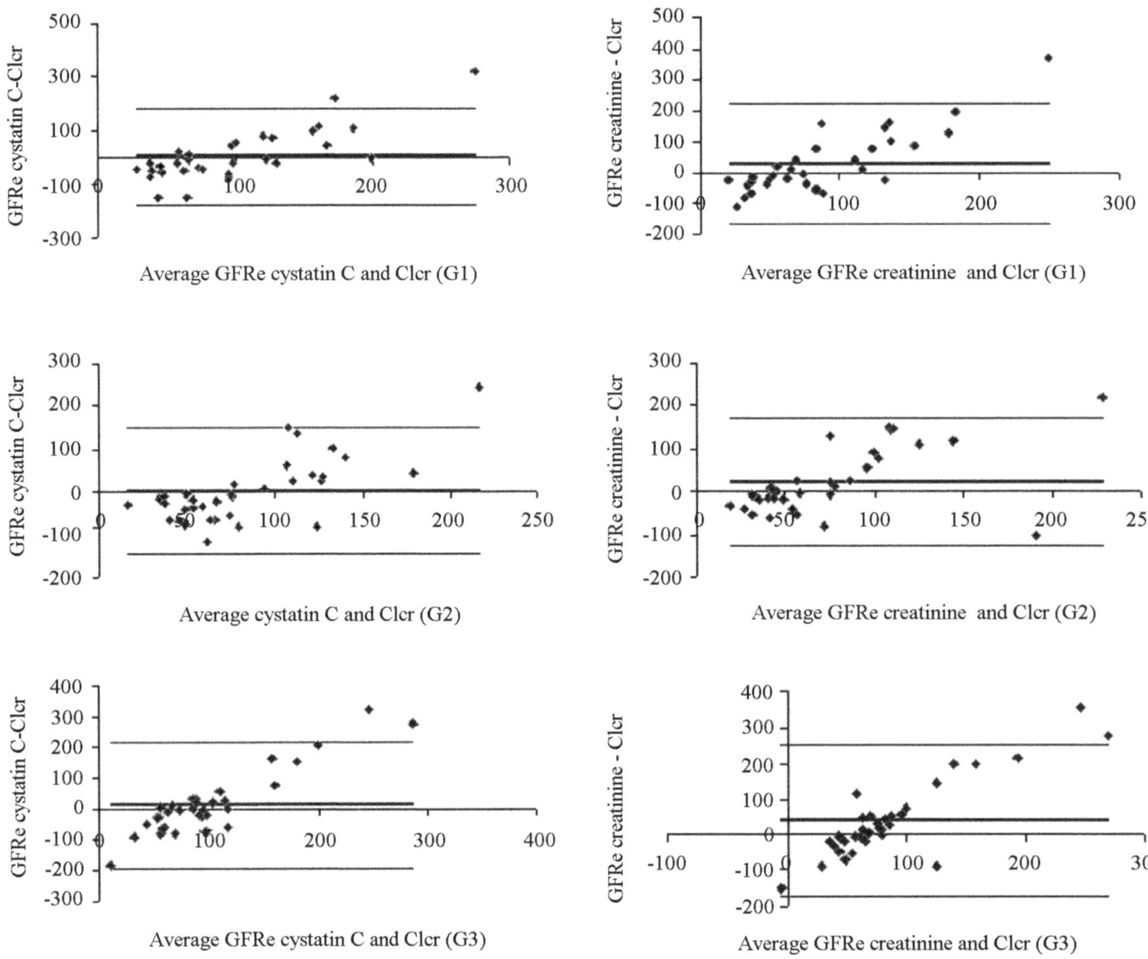

Figure 1. Bland-Altman plot for differences between Cys-GFR, Cr-GFR and two-hour creatinine clearance (CrCl-2h) per group (G1-G3) in the preoperative period. Horizontal lines indicate the mean reflecting the mean difference and the span between +1.96 SD and −1.96 SD of the mean difference between CrCl-2h and the methods evaluated (Cys-GFR and Cr-GFR).

Table 1. Bland-Altman for differences between Cys-GFR, Cr-GFR and two-hour creatinine clearance (CrCl-2h) per group (G1-G3) in the preoperative period. Limits of agreement - Upper limit (+1.96 SD) (CI 95%) and lower limit (−1.96 SD) (CI 95%) (mL·min^{-1}·1.73 m^{-2}).

Limits of agreement	Groups		
Cystatin C-GFR*	G1	G2	G3
Upper limit (CI 95%)	187.50 (131.02; 144.03)	149.58 (99.74; 190.26)	218.60 (155.46; 281.75)
Lower Limit (CI 95%)	−180.26 (−236.77; −126.76)	−145.00 (−194.55; −104.33)	−192.40 (−255.54; −129.26)
Creatinine-GFR*			
Upper limit (CI 95%)	220.73 (161.35; 280.14)	171.62 (125.96; 217.33)	250.51 (183.65; 315.89)
Lower Limit (CI 95%)	−165.85 (−225.25; −106.46)	−125.80 (−171.4; −80.03)	−169.71 (−239.70 ; −107.47)

*mL·min^{-1}·1.73 m^{-2}.

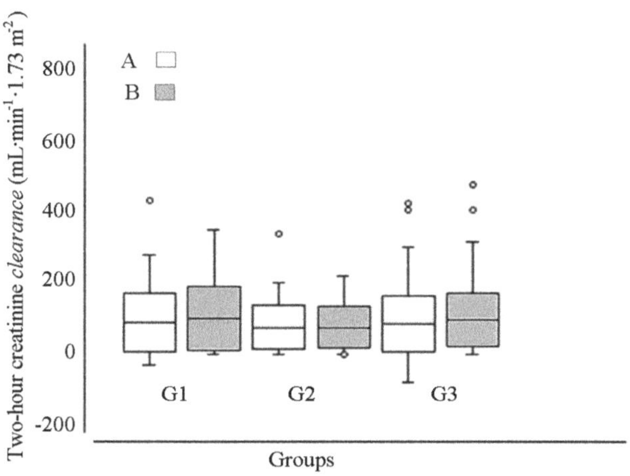

Figure 2. Comparison of CrCl-2h adjusted (B) and not adjusted (A) for ultrasonic residual bladder volume (mL·min^{-1}·1.73 m^{-2}) in elder patients during the preoperative period. Box plots - Bars represent median values, boxes represent interquartile ranges, and whishers show 95% confidence intervals. Mann-Whitney Test: A = B in G1, G3 and G3.

20 mL·min^{-1}·1.73 m^{-2} [6] was considered acceptable. However, although CrCl-2h values showed a better agreement with Cys-GFR, the wide limits of agreement between these methods, which reflect the great variation of the results obtained, did not allow concluding that these methods actually agree and can be used interchangeably.

In intensive care patients, Gutierrez *et al.* [6] found a close correlation between 24-h and 2-h creatinine clearance that remained even with the use of diuretics or in the presence of low or irregular diuresis, suggesting that such methods are interchangeable. These authors further report that 24-h creatinine clearance correlated poorly with GFR estimated by the Cockcroft & Gault equation.

Diabetes and hypertension, which have the kidney as a target organ, tend to worsen renal function in older patients. The diabetic and hypertensive elderly included in this study was receiving preoperative care for routine surgery, and was, therefore, well compensated. Moreover, those who were diabetic had satisfactory previous glycemia control as measured by glycated hemoglobin. This fact may explain why no difference in preoperative renal function was detected among groups.

Studies comparing cystatin C with creatinine measurements have produced conflicting results. While some have demonstrated that cystatin C is more sensitive than creatinine in detecting renal failure [11-13], others have reported no difference between these markers [7,14]. This disparity is likely to be due to differences in study population. In patients with normal or slightly reduced renal function, cystatin C seems to be superior to creatinine. In contrast, in patients with a marked decline in renal function, differences between cystatin C and creatinine are smaller as frequently observed in older patients [11,14].

Because the formula of Cockcroft & Gault may overestimate renal function when GFR >60 mL·min^{-1}·1.73 m^{-2}, cystatin C is clearly more useful in these cases. In this study, in which individuals with markedly reduced renal function were not included and most elderly patients showed GFR >60 mL·min^{-1}·1.73 m^{-2}, cystatin C was a more adequate marker of renal function than CrCl-2h [15]. The Cockcroft & Gault formula might have overestimated GFR, and this would explain the increased difference between mean CrCl-2h and mean Cockcroft & Gault formula values seen in our older patients. However, other studies have demonstrated that cystatin C has no advantages over creatinine in population with GFR < 60 mL·min^{-1}·1.73 m^{-2} [14]. Thus, the severity of pre-existing renal disease should be considered when selecting the method to be used for the assessment of renal function in older patients.

The use of ultrasound to measure residual bladder volume in order to obtain more precise two-hour urine volume estimates is essential in the elderly. In this population, physiological disorders such as prostatic hypoplasia and bladder prolapse can lead to underestimation of the two-hour volume measured. Nonetheless, whether adjusted or not for residual bladder volume, CrCl-2h values did not differ among our patients. An explanation for this finding is that few residual amounts cannot be easily detected by ultrasound examination and this might have influenced the interpretation of the results.

Diurnal variation in diuresis is another factor that has been suggested to interfere with CrCl-2h assessment. However, creatinine clearance estimates obtained at a shorter interval (8 hours) have been demonstrated to be as accurate as 24-h clearances [16].

In conclusion, two-hour creatinine clearance was not an adequate substitute for GFR estimates based on creatinine and cystatin C serum levels in older patients at preoperative period. The ultrasonic assessment of residual bladder volume had no significant influence on the calculation of two-hour creatinine clearance.

REFERENCES

[1] S. Klag, P. K. Whelton, B. L. Randall, *et al.*, "Blood Pressure and End-Stage Renal Disease in Men," *The New England Journal of Medicine*, Vol. 334, No. 1, 1996, pp. 13-18.

[2] M. C. B. S. Benarab, Y. M. M. Castiglia, P. T. G. Vianna, *et al.*, "Two-Hours Evaluation of Renal Function in the Elderly," *Revista Brasileira de Anestesiologia*, Vol. 55, No. 3, 2005, pp. 269-278. http://dx.doi.org/10.1590/S0034-70942005000300003

[3] Y,Yi-sun, C. H. Peng, C. K. Lin, *et al.*, "Use of Serum Cystatin C to Detect Early Decline of Glomerular Filtration Rate in Tape 2 Diabetes," *Intern med.*, Vol. , No. , 2007, pp. 801-806.

[4] J. R. Friedman, D. C. Norman and T. T. Yoshikawa, "Correlation of Estimated Renal Function Parameters Versus 24-Hour Creatinine Clearance in Ambulatory Elderly," *Journal of the American Geriatrics Society*, Vol. 37, No. 2, 1989, pp. 145-149.

[5] D. D. Cardenas, E. Kelly, J. N. Krieger, *et al.*, "Residual Urine Volumes in Patients with Spinal Cord Injury: Measurement with a Portable Ultrasound Instrument," *Archives of Physical Medicine and Rehabilitation*, Vol. 69, No. 7, 1988, pp. 514-516.

[6] M. Gutierrez, G. S. Perez, E. Banderas-Bravo, *et al.*, "Replacement of 24h Creatinine Clearance by 2-h Creatinine in Intensive Care Unit Patients: A Single-Center Study," *Intensive Care Medicine*, Vol. 33, No. 11, 2007, pp. 1900-1906. http://dx.doi.org/10.1007/s00134-007-0745-5

[7] N. J. Van Den Noortgate, W. H. Janssens, J. R. Delanghe, *et al.*, "Serum Cystatin C Concentration Compared with Other Markers of Glomerular Filtration Rate in the Old Old," *Journal of the American Geriatrics Society*, Vol. 50, No. 7, 2002, pp.1278-1282. http://dx.doi.org/10.1046/j.1532-5415.2002.50317.x

[8] D. W. Cockcroft and M. H. Gault, "Prediction of Creatinine Clearance from Serum Creatinine," *Nephron*, Vol. 16, No. 1, 1976, pp. 31-41. http://dx.doi.org/10.1159/000180580

[9] A. Larsson, J. Malm, A. Grubb, *et al.*, "Calculation of Glomerular Filtration Rate Expressed in mL/min from Plasma Cystatin C Values in mg/L," *Scandinavian Journal of Clinical and Laboratory Investigation*, Vol. 64, No. 1, 2004, pp. 25-30.

[10] J. M. Bland and D. G. Altman, "Statistical Methods for Assessing Agreement between Two Methods of Clinical Measurement," *The Lancet*, Vol. 327, No. 8476, 1986, pp. 307-310. http://dx.doi.org/10.1016/S0140-6736(86)90837-8

[11] D. J. Newman, H. Thakkar, R. G. Edwards, *et al.*, "Serum Cystatin C Measured by Automated Immunoassay: A More Sensitive Marker of Changes in GFR than Serum Creatinine," *Kidney International*, Vol. 47, No. , 1995, pp. 312-318. http://dx.doi.org/10.1038/ki.1995.40

[12] B. Stabuc, L. Vrhovec, M. Stabuc-Silih, *et al.*, "Improved Prediction of Decreased Creatinine Clearance by Serum Cystatin C: Use in Cancer Patients before and during Chemotherap," *Clinical Chemistry*, Vol. 1, No. , 2000, pp. 29-34.

[13] D. Fliser and E. Ritz, "Serum Cystatin C Concentration as a Marker of Renal Dysfunction in the Elderly," *American Journal of Kidney Diseases*, Vol. 37, No. 1, 2001, pp. 79-83.

[14] E. Coll, A. Botey, L. Alvarez, *et al.*, "Serum Cystatin C as a New Marker for Noninvasive Estimation of Glmerular Filtration Rate and as a Marker for Early Renal Impairment," *American Journal of Kidney Diseases*, Vol. 36, No. 1, 2000, pp. 29-34. http://dx.doi.org/10.1053/ajkd.2000.8237

[15] T. H. Goldberg and M. S. Fin kelstein, "Difficulties in Estimating Glomerular Filtration Rate in the Elderly," *Archives of Internal Medicine*, Vol. 147, No. 8, 1987, pp. 1430-1433. http://dx.doi.org/10.1001/archinte.1987.00370080066014

[16] S. L. Markantonis and E. Kioupaki-Agathokleusous, "Can Two, Four or Eight-Hour Urine Collections after Voluntary Voiding Be Used Instead of Twenty-Four Collections for the Estimation of Creatinine Clearance in Healthy Subjects?" *Pharmacy World and Science*, Vol. 20, No. 6, 1998, pp. 258-263.

23

Surgical Complications and Evolution of Grafts in Children with Renal Transplantation at Cayetano Heredia National Hospital

Roberto Sanchez[1,2*], **Reyner Loza**[2,3], **Cesar Loza**[2,4], **Luis Zegarra**[1,2]
[1]Surgery and Urology Unit, Department of Surgery, Cayetano Heredia Hospital, Lima, Peru
[2]Renal Transplant Unit, Cayetano Heredia Hospital, Lima, Peru
[3]Paediatric Nephrology Unit, Department of Pediatrics, Cayetano Heredia Hospital, Lima, Peru
[4]Nephrology Service, Department of Medicine, Cayetano Heredia Hospital, Lima, Peru
Email: *robmedic1@hotmail.com

ABSTRACT

Objective: This study aims to determine surgical complications and graft outcome in children undergoing renal transplantation at Cayetano Heredia National Hospital (CHNH). **Materials and Methods:** A case study series focused on the incidence of surgical complications and graft outcome in pediatric patients with end stage renal disease (ESRD) who underwent renal transplant (RT) between December 2007 and March 2011. **Results:** The study described 29 pediatric transplant patients whose average age was 13.69 ± 3.38 (6.2 - 17.9) years. The etiology of end stage renal disease (ESRD) was renal hypoplasia in 12 patients (41.38%), primary glomerulopathy in 10 patients (34.48%), obstructive uropathy in 4 patients (13.79%), vasculitis in 2 patients (6.9%) and hemolytic uremic syndrome (HUS) in 1 (3.45%) patient. There were 11 surgical complications (34.48%): 2 cases of arterial thrombosis, 3 cases of urinary fistula, 3 of lymphocele, 1 of venous thrombosis, urinoma and perineal collection. The follow-up time was 15.84 ± 12.19 months. Graft survival at 12, 24, and 40 months was 89.29%, 77.16% and 77.16%, respectively. **Conclusion:** Surgical complications and graft survival in pediatric renal transplantation in our series did not differ from other published series.

Keywords: Children; Terminal Chronic Renal Disease; Renal Transplantation; Surgical Complications

1. Introduction

ESRD, defined as a permanent loss of the kidneys' ability to filter waste from the circulatory system, is a global public health problem of growing proportions [1]. Its prevalence in the pediatric population fluctuates between 5 to 10 children per million per year. Forty years ago, children with ESRD died. However, current renal replacement (RRT) therapies used in children have changed this bleak picture significantly, enabling almost all children to be treated by dialysis or renal transplantation (RT). RT has been shown to be the therapy of choice for this population, resulting in better long-term survival and quality of life [2]. The costs of transplanted organ maintenance are low compared to other methods of RRT. Dialysis provides only a fraction of normal renal clearance, relieves but does not remove uremic symptoms such as fatigue and anorexia, and does not resolve the anomalies of growth and development. In contrast, RT can provide kidney function equivalent to 40 to 80 per cent of normal renal function [3-8]. Advances in anesthesia, surgical techniques, and the discovery of immunosuppressants have allowed a progressive reduction in the contraindications to this procedure, even though the biological behavior and potential complications in transplanted children differ to those in adults [4,9,10]. Globally, surgical complications affect survival and renal graft loss, so early diagnosis and prompt treatment are important. Surgical complications in renal transplantation are defined as complications that occur during surgery and the postoperative follow-up. They are classified as vascular, urological, and collections and have an incidence ranging from 1% to 38% [9-15]. RT surgery has been performed in Peru since the 1960s. Augusto Hernandez Mendoza, a urologist, performed the first RT, and followed by Raul Romero Torres, who established the transplant unit at the Naval Medical Center

*Corresponding author.

in August 1969. In the same year, the first kidney transplant was carried out under the Peruvian social insurance system [16]. In July 2007, a renal transplant pilot program at Cayetano Heredia National Hospital was funded. In the same year, the CHNH was accredited by the National Organization of Organ and Tissue Transplants (ONDT) as a transplant-donation center, performing its first kidney transplant on December 14, 2007, on a pediatric patient [17]. To date, 51 patients, both adults and children, have received transplants. The aim of the present study was to describe the incidence of surgical complications and evolution of the renal graft in children who received transplants

2. Material and Method

Reviewed twenty-nine medical records of pediatric patients (under 18 years) who received transplants (28 from living donors and 1 from a nonliving donor) between December 2007 and March 2011. Any event that occurred in the intra- and/or postoperative period, classified as vascular, urological, and/or collection, was defined as a surgical complication. In all transplants, lateral anastomosis was performed of the artery and renal vein from the donor to the external iliac vein and artery from the receptor, respectively. For ureteral reimplantation the Politano-Leadbetter technique was performed in 2 patients, and Lich-Gregoir in 27 patients, with posterior ureteral catheterization in a systematic way. The Jackson-Pratt drain was left in the first 22 patients and then laminated to the retro peritoneum. Some patients had a urinary Foley catheter for 5 days. The immunosuppression process used was timoglobulina, daclizumab, and basiliximab induction therapy. The maintenance therapy was tacrolimus (Tac), mycophenolate mofetil (MMF), and prednisone (Pd). The surgical complications found were vascular thrombosis, primary vascular anastomosis failure, lymphocele, urinoma, urinary fistula, perirenal collection, intestinal blockage by adhesions, and secondary adherence to a previous umbilical hernia surgery. Renal graft function was evaluated by measuring creatinine serum and clearance of creatinine. A Doppler ultrasound was performed on the graft 24 hours after transplantation and during follow-up. For the analysis of the graft survival, loss of the graft was considered as a failure. According to Kaplan-Meier survival curves were performed. Data processing and statistical analysis were carried out using Stata version 11.

3. Results

The study population comprised 29 patients, 14 girls and 15 boys. The average age was 13.69 ± 3, 38 (6. 2 - 17. 9) years. Sixteen of the children came from Lima (55.17%) and 13 from other cities in Peru (44.83%)

The etiology of the ESRD in the patients was renal hypoplasia in 12 (41.38%), primary glomerulopathy in 10 (34.48%), obstructive uropathy in 4 (13.8 %), vasculitis in 2 (6.9%), and hemolytic uremic syndrome (HUS) in 1 (3.45%).

At the time of the RT, 19 patients (65.52%) were receiving peritoneal dialysis, 6 patients were receiving hemodialysis (10.69%), and 4 patients (13.79%) both therapies. The average time on dialysis was 3.26 ± 2.20 (0.65 - 7.7) years. The related living donors were mothers in 23 (79.31%) patients, fathers in 3 patients (10.34%), and grandfather in one (3.45%) patient. There was one unrelated living donor (adoptive mother) and a cadaver donor (**Table 1**).

In tests of histocompatibility (HLA), identity between the recipient and donor was as follows: 6/6 in 1 case (3.45%), 5/6 in 4 cases (13.79%), 4/6 in 11 cases (37.94%), 3/6 cases in 10 (34.48%) cases, 1/6 in 2 cases (6.90%), and 0/6 in 1 case (3.45%).

The duration of warm ischemia was 1.85 ± 0.94 (0.83 - 5) minutes, and cold ischemia 173.83 ± 205.11 (49 - 1200) minutes, with a median of 140 minutes. The duration of venous anastomosis was 31.86 ± 10.79 (18 - 60) minutes and for arterial anastomosis 25.66 ± 10.6 (14 - 48) minutes. Nine donors had a double renal artery (31.03%).

Average post-operative hospitalization was 21.52 ± 21.06 (7 - 113) days and the average follow-up period 15.84 ± 12.19 (0 - 39.57) months. The average glomerular filtration rate at the end of the observation period was 76.43 ± 28.86 (23 - 130) ml/min/1.73 m^2. In the follow-up period, the variation of post-transplant weight to basal weight was 7.28 ± 6.57 (−2.4 - 25.9) kg and the average size gain 6.65 ± 5.09 (0 - 20) cm (**Table 2**).

Of the 29 patients, 12 (34.48%) had surgical complications from the procedure and one had intestinal obstruction due to bands and adhesion without repercussion on the renal function of the graft (the patient had a history of surgery for umbilical hernia). Four patients had vascular complications, with arterial thrombosis in 2 patients (6.9%) and venous thrombosis in 1 (3.45%). Both led to loss of the graft. A fourth patient had a double artery with failure in the anastomosis in one; a reanastomosis was performed using the same surgical procedure without complications.

There were 3 urological complications (10.34%), all urinary fistula (in 2 patients they were surgically repaired and in one there was spontaneous closure with the use of a urinary catheter). There were 5 collections, with diagnosis by ultrasound in all cases. Lymphocele occurred in 3 patients (10.34%) (one was resolved by laparoscopic surgery and 2 reabsorbed spontaneously). There was one case of urinoma and another of perirenal collection (**Table 3**). Of the major medical complications, we found

Table 1. Dialysis modality and type of donor in pediatric transplants at the national cayetano heredia hospital.

Dialysis Modality	n	%
Peritoneal dialysis	19	65.52
Hemodialysis	6	20.69
Both	4	13.79
TOTAL	**29**	**100**
Type of donor		
Mother	23	79.31
Father	3	10.34
Grandfather	1	3.45
Non-related donor	1	3.45
Cadaver donor	1	3.45
TOTAL	**29**	**100**

Table 2. Perioperative and evolutionary characteristics of pediatric patients receiving transplants at the national cayetano heredia hospital.

Variable	X ± D.E.
Duration of warm ischemia (minutes)	1.85 ± 0.94
Duration of cold ischemia (minutes)	173.83 ± 205.11
Duration of arterial anastomosis (minutes)	25.66 ± 10.6
Duration of venous anastomosis (minutes)	31.86 ± 10.79
Glomerular filtration rate (ml/min/1.73 m^2) (*)	76.43 ± 28.86
Hospitalization time (days)	21.52 ± 21.06
Variation of weight (kg)	7.28 ± 6.57
Variation of size (cm)	6.65 ± 5.09
Average follow-up (months)	15.84 ± 12.19

*Last control in the follow-up.

Table 3. Surgical complications in pediatric patients undergoing transplant at the National Cayetano Heredia Hospital.

	n	%
Vascular complications	**4**	**13.80**
Arterial thrombosis	2	6.90
Venous thrombosis	1	3.45
Primary anastomosis failure	1	3.45
Urological complications	**3**	**10.34**
Urinary fistula	3	10.34
Collections	**5**	**17.24**
Lymphocele	3	10.34
Urinoma	1	3.45
Perirenal collection	1	3.45
Other	**1**	**3.45**
Intestinal obstruction	1	3.45

that urinary tract infection occurred in 9 patients (34.61%) and a sharp rejection in 7 (26.92%).

The overall graft survival 12, 24, and 40 months after renal transplantation was 89.29% (IC95%: 70.36 - 96.41), 77.16% (IC95%: 51.82 - 90.28), and 77.16% (IC95%: 51, 82 - 90.28) respectively (**Figure 1**). There were 5 graft losses (17.24%) after discharge from hospital with a functioning kidney: 3 due to vascular complications and 2 to medical complications (one due to nephrotoxicity to tacrolimus and the other to lack of adherence to the treatment).

4. Discussion

In our series, the most common etiology of the TCRD was renal hypoplasia, followed by the primary glomerulopathies, similar to that reported by Palacios *et al.* in Chile [4]. In the area covered by the Latin American Pediatric Nephrology Association (ALANEPE), the leading causes are obstructive uropathy and chronic glomerulopathy. In contrast, in the North American Pediatric Registry Transplant Cooperative Study (NAPRTCS), renal hypoplasia and obstructive uropathy are reported as the most frequent [14]. In Argentina, the primary cause in children is hemolytic uremic syndrome [8]. Our incidence of surgical complications was 34.48%, which is similar to figures in the literature, highlighting that we have considered minor surgical complications that are usually not reported by other series such as El Atat *et al.* (30%) and Barba *et al.* in Spain (38%) [11,12]. The incidence of vascular thrombosis was 10.34%, which is comparable with other series such as El Atat *et al.* (18.9%), Palacios *et al.* in Chile (9.2%), and Irtan *et al.* (13.9%) in France. In our series, 2 cases of vascular thrombosis were diagnosed during surgery and 1 on the fifth day post-surgery by a Doppler ultrasound scan [4,11,18]. The urological complication in our series was urinary fistula.

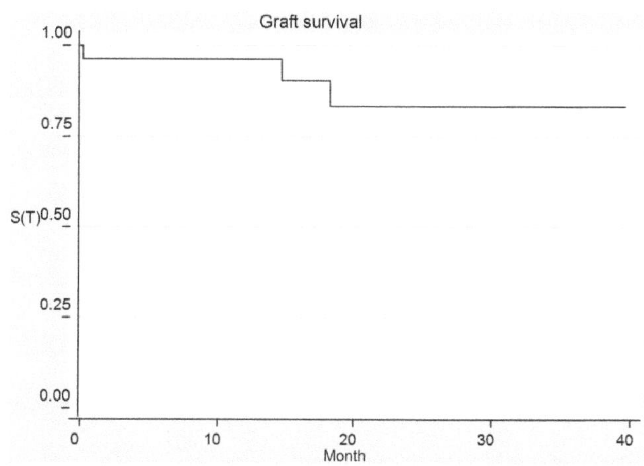

Figure 1. General survival of the graft in pediatric patients undergoing transplant at the National Cayetano Heredia Hospital. Period 2007-2011 (N = 29).

This differs from other reports in the literature, which present problems between 3.1% and 30%, with vesicoureteral reflux being the chief complication [18]. Among the most frequent collections, lymphocele (10.34%) should be highlighted, which differs from that reported in adults (49%) [6]. In all cases, diagnosis and follow-up were by ultrasound. It should be noted that the graft was lost in 17.24% of cases in our study, a similar situation to that reported by other series, for example Palacios (25%). The overall survival rate of the graft was also similar to Palacios' data from Chile and Medeiros' data from Mexico [4,6]. In the NAPRTCS, the survival rate after 1 and 3 years was 96.5% and 91.5%, respectively, and in ALANEPE 96% and 93% [14]. At study the mortality rate of our patients is zero, while Medeiros in Mexico reported a 4.3% mortality rate and the NAPRTCS a rate of 4.8% after 3 years [6].

5. Conclusion

The rates of complications in pediatric renal transplantation surgery in our series and the survival of renal grafts up to 40 months post-surgery do not differ from other international series.

REFERENCES

[1] T. Kalblea, M. Lucanb, G. Nicitac, R. Sellsd, F. J. Burgos, M. Wieselet, *et al.*, "Eau Guidelines on Renal Transplantation," *European Urology*, Vol. 47, No. 2, 2005, pp. 156-166. doi:10.1016/j.eururo.2004.02.009

[2] S. P. McDonald and J. C. Craig, "Long-Term Survival of Children with End-Stage Renal Disease," *The New England Journal of Medicine*, Vol. 350, 2004, pp. 2654-2662. doi:10.1056/NEJMoa031643

[3] B. A. Warady, D. Herbert, E. K. Sullivan, *et al.*, "The 1995 Annual Report of the North American Pediatric Renal Transplant Cooperative Study," *Pediatric Nephrology*, Vol. 11, No. 1, 1997, pp. 49-64. doi:10.1007/s004670050232

[4] J. M. Palacios, P. Rosati, E. Lagos, P. Hevia, S. Rodríguez, O. Jiménez, I. Turu and K. Cuevas, "Pediatric Renal Transplant: The Experience of a Center," *Chilean Review in Surgery*, Vol. 57, 2005, pp. 483-488

[5] A. Guardiola, F. Sánchez, L. Gimeno, *et al.*, "Urological Complications in the Renal Transplant. Study in 250 Cases," *Actas Urológicas Españolas*, Vol. 25, No. 9, 2001, pp. 628-636. doi:10.1016/S0210-4806(01)72688-5

[6] M. Medeiros, B. Romero, S. Valverde, R. Delgadillo, G. Varela and R. Muñoz, "Pediatric Renal Transplant," *Revista de Investigacion Clinica*, Vol. 57, No. 2, 2005, pp. 230-236.

[7] A. E. Da Silveira, M. de Almeida, W. Cosenza, A. C. Amarante, R. de Menezes and E. Schulz, "Renal Transplant in Children: Analytical Study in 25 Cases," *Revista Cirugia Infantil*, Vol. 6, No. 4, 1996, pp. 172-176.

[8] V. Zúñiga and L. Álvarez, "Pediatric Renal Transplantation in the South Central Specialty Services Hospital (HC SAE) from PEMEX (México)," *Mexican Nephrology*, Vol. 22, No. 2, 2001, pp. 75-82.

[9] F. Cano and P. Rosati, "Pediatric Renal Transplant. A Decade of Multicentric Experience," *Revista Chilena de Pediatria*, Vol. 72, No. 6, 2001, pp. 504-515.

[10] O. Salvatierra, "Pediatric Renal Transplantation," *Transplantation Proceedings*, Vol. 31, No. 4, 1999, pp. 1787-1788. doi:10.1016/S0041-1345(99)00168-2

[11] R. El Atat, A. Derouiche, S. Guellouz, T. Gargah, R. Lakhoua and M. Chebil, "Surgical Complications in Pediatric and Adolescent Renal Transplantation," *Saudi Journal of Kidney Diseases and Transplantation*, Vol. 21, 2010, p. 251.

[12] J. Barba, A. Rincón, E. Tolosa, L. Romero, D. Rosell, J. E. Robles, *et al.*, "Surgical Complications in Renal Transplantations and Its Influence in the Survival of the Graft," *Actas Urológicas Españolas*, Vol. 34, No. 3, 2010, pp. 266-273. doi:10.1016/S2173-5786(10)70059-7

[13] S. P. Lapointe, M. Charbit, D. Jan, S. Lortat-Jacob, J. L. Michel, D. Beurton, *et al.*, "Urological Complications after Renal Transplantation Using Ureter Ureteral Anastomosis in Children," *Journal of Urology*, Vol. 166, No. 3, 2001, pp. 1046-1048. doi:10.1016/S0022-5347(05)65916-2

[14] Latin American Pediatric Nephrology Association, *et al.*, "Latin American Registry of Pediatric Renal Transplantation 2004-2008," *Pediatric Transplantation*, Vol. 14, No. 6, 2010, pp. 701-708. doi:10.1111/j.1399-3046.2010.01331.x

[15] P. Fentes, B. Parra, T. Caamaño, *et al.*, "Post Renal Transplant Surgical Complications. Study in 185 Cases," *Actas Urológicas Españolas*, Vol. 29, No. 6, 2005, pp. 578-586. doi:10.1016/S0210-4806(05)73300-3

[16] E. Barboza, "Advances in Surgery in the Last 30 Years," *Revista Diagnostico*, Vol. 47, No. 3, 2008, pp. 13-16.

[17] R.M. No 568-2007/MINSA, "The Pilot Program is Created Renal Transplants from the Ministry of Health," El Peruano, 15 July 2007, 349116.

[18] S. Irtan, A. Maisin, V. Baudouin, Y. Nivoche, R. Azoulay, E. Jacqz-Aigrain, A. El Ghoneimi and Y. Aigrain, "Renal Transplantation in Children: Critical Analysis of Age Related Surgical Complications," *Pediatric Transplantation*, Vol. 14, 2010, pp. 512-519.

24

Late and Reversible Kidney-Lung Failure after Intra-Bladder BCG Therapy

Olivier Mat[1*], Rim Kada[1], Patrick Philippart[2], Quentin Mat[2], Steffy Larroze[2], Myriam Remmelink[3], Selda Aydin[4], Vincent Colombie[5]

[1]Department of Nephrology of EpiCURA, Ath, Belgium
[2]Department of Surgery of EpiCURA, Ath, Belgium
[3]Department of Lung Pathology, Hopital Erasme, Université Libre de Bruxelles, Brussels, Belgium
[4]Department of Renal Pathology, Cliniques Universitaires St-Luc, Université Catholique de Louvain, Brussels, Belgium
[5]Department of Infectious Diseases of EpiCURA, Ath, Belgium
Email: *Olivier.mat@epicura.be

ABSTRACT

We observed a 76-year-old man who presented "acute kidney-lung failure" 9 months after intravesical Bacillus Calmette-Guérin (BCG) adjuvant treatment for a T1 bladder cancer. He had inflammatory infiltration on chest radiography and required dialysis for acute renal failure. A percutaneous renal biopsy was performed and revealed tubulointerstitial nephritis with a moderate eosinophilic infiltrate without granulomatous lesion. After a few days, an open lung biopsy was also done due to respiratory deterioration. The anatomopathologic specimen demonstrated moderate fibrosis with lympho-neutrophilic infiltration and few aspecific granulomatous lesions without caseous necrosis. Sarcoïdosis was suspected and high dose oral methylprednisolone was started. Three weeks later, *Mycobacterium bovis* was identified by Polymerase Chain Reaction on open lung biopsy. He responded well to steroids and tuberculostatic tri-therapy. After one month of immunosuppressive treatment, renal function was resolved and hemodialysis could be discontinued. Despite the frequent use of adjuvant BCG immunotherapy, systemic complications such as hepatitis, pneumonitis, spondylodiscitis or multiorgan failure are rare (<1%). Hematogenous dissemination which occurs a few weeks after traumatic instillations is usually suspected but not demonstrated because of absence of mycobacterium in histological specimen. Our case differs from those previously reported by the simultaneous presence of acid-fast bacilli highlighted on lung samples. We discuss the pathophysiology of BCG complications, the use of prophylactic or therapeutic treatment and recommend guidelines to prevent such complications.

Keywords: Corticosteroids; Hemodialysis; Intravesical BCG; *Mycobacterium bovis*; Pulmonary Granulomatosis; Renal Failure; Tubulointerstitial Nephritis; Urothelial Carcinoma

1. Introduction

Combined intravesical instillations of BCG remain the gold standard for intermediate and high risk non-invasive urothelial carcinoma of the bladder. Although the appearance of hematuria, dysuria or cystitis is possible, regional or systemic complications are exceptional. The hematogenous spread of mycobacterium from the bladder which occurs a few weeks after traumatic instillations is usually suspected but not demonstrated because of absence of pathogen in histological specimen. Our case correlates tubulointerstitial nephritis to mycobacterial infection by the simultaneous presence of acid-fast bacilli highlighted on lung samples.

2. Case Report

In March 2012, a 76-year-old man was admitted to the hospital because of acute renal failure associated with progressive grade II dyspnea and recurrent low grade fever for 3 weeks. He also reported tiredness, an 8 kg weight loss and night sweats. He had a history of arterial hypertension and a non invasive (T1) transitional cell carcinoma (TCC) of the bladder. TCC was first treated during the second half of 2008 by cauterization followed by mitomycin instillations for 6 months. Because of the recurrence of polyps, the patient was treated by cauterization and one month later, he received 10 intravesical

*Corresponding author.

instillations of Baccile Calmette-Guerin (BCG) between November 2010 and July 2011. Current medications were amlodipine 10 mg and acétylsalicylate 100 mg/day. On admission, physical examination was unremarkable excepted fever of 37.9˚C, oliguria and few spread crackles in both lung fields and moderate edema of lower limbs. Regular hemodialysis sessions were initiated based on clinical status and blood sample evaluation.

Laboratory investigation showed hemoglobin 1.2 g/dL, a white blood cell count of 4.6 × 10^3 /µL with moderate inflammatory signs (C-reactive protein 30 mg/L, sedimentation rate 30 mm/h), serum creatinine 699 µmol/L. Electrolytes and Lactatate deshydrogenase were normal, aspartate aminotransferase 51 IU/L , alcaline phosphatase 208 IU/L and gamma glutamyl transferase 269 IU/L. Total protein count 47.7 g/L with protein electrophoresis demonstrates albumin 25.1 g/L and a thin monoclonal peak of gamma-globulin; the myelogram was normal. Serologic screenings for anti-nuclear antibody, antineutrophil cytoplasmic antibody, anti basal membrane antibody, immunoglobin A and hepatitis B or C antibodies were negative. Plasma complement and coagulation tests were also normal. Angiotensine Converting Enzyme was increased at 140 IU/L (range 8.0 - 52.0) and normal Urine analysis showed proteinuria of 0.4 g/L, sterile leucocyturia without hematuria.

The standard chest X-ray demonstrated a bilateral infiltration of the lung fields. Chest computed tomography confirmed an interstitial syndrome with a "ground glass" appearance associated with small mediastinal lymphadenopathies; there was no pleural effusion, nor micro nodular lesion. Bronchoalveolar lavage was performed and demonstrated no specific lesion; the microscopic examination revealed lympho-monocytic cells with rare neutrophils; mycobacterium culture stayed permanently sterile. A purified protein derivate (PPD) skin test was negative despite a 10 IU dose. Transesophageal cardiac echography excluded infectious endocarditis.

An abdominal CT tomography was performed and demonstrated normal kidneys, no hepatic enlargement and moderate splenomegaly. A percutaneous needle biopsy was performed and revealed tubulointerstitial nephritis with a moderate eosinophilic infiltrate without granulomatous lesion (**Figure 1**). Glomeruli and arterioles appeared normal; there was no histological evidence of rapidly progressive glomerulonephritis. Immunofluorescence was negative and electronic microscopy was unremarkable. After a few days, an open lung biopsy was also done due to respiratory deterioration. The anatomopathologic specimen demonstrated moderate fibrosis with lympho-neutrophilic infiltration and few aspecific granulomatous lesions without caseous necrosis or Langhans giant cells (**Figure 2**). Mycotic identification remained negative. Specific mycobacterium culture was started.

Sarcoïdosis was suspected and high dose oral methylprednisolone was started (1 mg/kg/day). The patient's general condition began to improve after two weeks of corticosteroid therapy in conjunction with intermittent extra-renal epuration and a supportive permanent parenteral nutrition. Fever resolved, weight increased, chest infiltrates disappeared. In the same time, the serum creatinine began to decrease as shown in **Figure 3**. After one month of immunosuppressive treatment, renal function resolved and hemodialysis could be discontinued. On day 27, culture of lung biopsy samples in Batec 12B medium grew acid-fast bacilli that were identified as *Mycobacterium bovis* by Polymerase Chain Reaction (Pasteur Institute, Brussels). Cultures of urine, alveolar fluid lavage and blood specimens remained definitely negative. Tuberculostatic agents were promptly initiated as rifadine 600 mg/day, myambutol 1200 mg/2 days, nicotibine 300 mg/day and pyridoxine 250 mg/day. Corticosteroid therapy was gradually reduced and stopped.

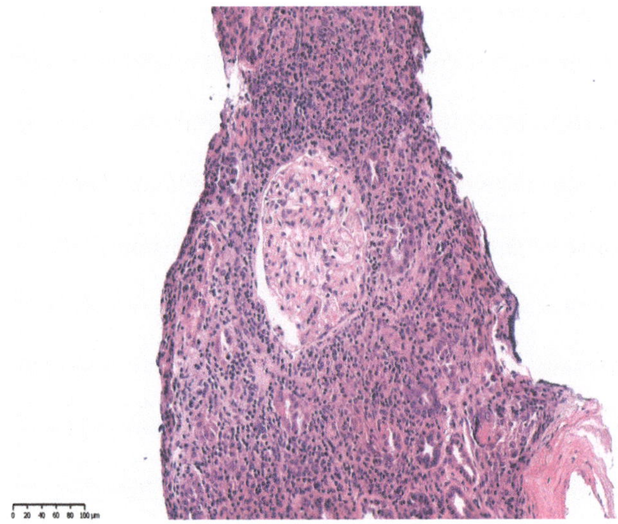

Figure 1. Kidney sample.

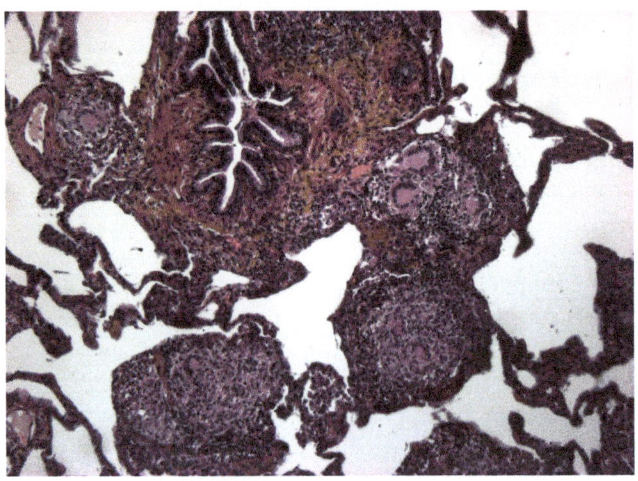

Figure 2. Lung biopsy.

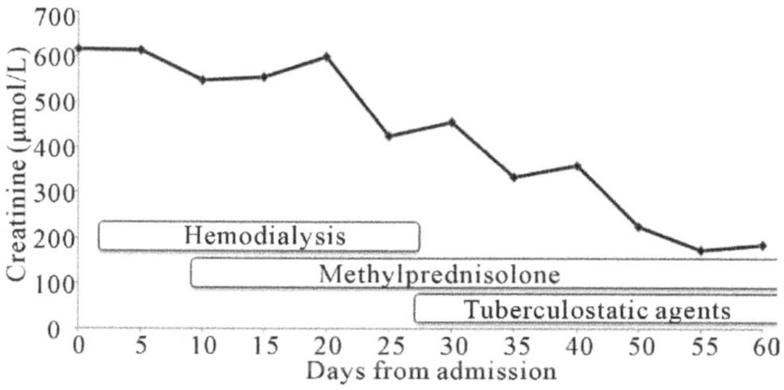

Figure 3. Recovery of renal function under corticosteroid therapy.

The patient is in good condition 6 months after initiation of antituberculosis therapy; chronic renal failure persisted with a serum creatinine of 220 μmol/L.

3. Discussion

Intravesical immunotherapy with BCG has been safely used to treat recurrence of superficial transitional cell carcinoma of the bladder for more than thirty years and remains a cornerstone for the treatment of intermediate and high risk non-invasive urothelial carcinoma of the bladder [1-4]. BCG exerts its antitumor activity through induction of pro-inflammatory cytokines which may explain the flu-like syndrome [4,5] (fever, chills and arthralgia) noted in almost 20% of patients receiving therapy. Regional urological complications can occur as mycobacterium orchi-epidydimitis, prostatis or cystitis. BCG sepsis is a rare (less than 1%, probably due to his high molecular weight) and severe complications with possible multiorgan failure are exceptional [6-9]. Ectopic localizations are also mentioned: hepatitis, pleural abscess or pneumonitis, spondylodiscitis, arthritis, mycotic aneurysms, chorioretinitis and retroperitoneal abscess. The hematogenous dissemination occurs especially after traumatic bladder instillation. Old age, acute bacterial cystitis, cumulative doses are additional risk factors which must be considered before instillations. Prophylactic drug, such as isoniazid, does not seem to reduce side effects of BCG instillations [2,3]. Contraindications include recent bladder surgery or polypectomy, recent radiotherapy treatment, hematuria, active tuberculosis, current immunosuppressive treatment and acute urine tract infection. Renal failure with histological evidence of suspected BCG toxicity is reported in twelve cases found by screening the National Library of Medecine's Medline system. In 9/12 of cases, tubule-interstitial nephritis is presented (5/12 with granuloma) and generally combined with hepatitis; mesangial glomerulonephritis, membranous glomerulonephritis and focal segmental hyalinosis are described as exceptional cases. Mycobacterial infection are usually considered as suspected responsible pathogen but not demonstrated because of absence of mycobacterium in histological specimen. Our case differs from those previously reported by the simultaneous presence of acid-fast bacilli highlighted on lung samples. The evidence of *Mycobacterium bovis* by DNA-rRNA hybridization strengthens the temporal relationship between BCG instillations and kidney-lung impairment despite the unusual delayed onset complications since generally occurring a few weeks after the last instillation [5-7]. Some authors stratified into early- and late-presentation disease [10]. The first one (within 3 months) could be result from systemic infection with proliferation of the organisms causing generalized granulomatous response by repeated instillations. The second one (between 3 months and until more than 1 year) could result from reactivation of infection after successful immunologic control of early dissemination, which is rather the case of our patient. Despite severe presentation of "BCGitis", corticosteroids administration often results in a prompt recovery of both renal and lung functions. The role of corticosteroids in the treatment of the complications of BCG instillations is not clearly defined within randomized studies. Nevertheless, their use seems interesting since the objective of BCG instillation is to induce immune reaction of the host and so we can assume that symptoms may be at least partially related to this mechanism. In the present case, positive culture for *Mycobacterium bovis* questioned the only hypothesis of hypersensitivity reaction, reason why tuberculostatic drugs were added to corticosteroids. We also noted that, despite the absence of tuberculostatic agents during the initial phase of treatment, no proven dissemination of mycobacteria occurred.

4. Conclusion

Unusual complications due to adjuvant BCG immunotherapy mostly occur a few weeks after intravesical treatment. Prevention of these adverse events requires avoiding the risk factors (recent bladder surgery or polypectomy, recent radiotherapy treatment, hematuria, active tuberculosis, current immunosuppressive treatment and acute urinary tract infection) and regular control of renal function during prolonged therapy. Treatment by corticosteroids improves the outcome of patients and the question of tuberculostatic therapy should always be considered. Prophylactic drug, such as isoniazid, does not seem to prevent side effects of BCG instillations.

REFERENCES

[1] A. N. Alexandroff, A. M. Jackson, M. A. O'Donnell and K. James, "BCG Immunotherapy of Bladder Cancer: 20 Years on," *Lancet*, Vol. 353, No. 9165, 1999, pp. 1689-1694. doi:10.1016/S0140-6736(98)07422-4

[2] M. Babjuk, W. Oosterlinck, R. Sylvester, E. Kaasinen, A.

Böhle, J. Palou-Redorta and M. Rouprêt, "EAU Guidelines on Non-Muscle-Invasive Urothelial Carcinoma of the Bladder, the 2011 Update," *European Urology*, Vol. 59, No. 6, 2011, pp. 997-1008. doi:10.1016/j.eururo.2011.03.017

[3] B. B. Houghton, V. Chalasani, D. Hayne, P. Grimison, C. S. Brown, M. I. Patel, I. D. Davis and M. R. Stockler, "Intravesical Chemotherapy Plus Bacilli Calmette-Guérin in Non-Muscle Invasive Bladder Cancer: A Systematic Review with Meta-Analysis," *BJU International*, Vol. 111, No. 6, 2013, pp. 977-983. doi:10.1111/j.1464-410X.2012.11390.x

[4] T. P. Kresowik and T. S. Griffith, "Bacillus Calmette-Guerin Immunotherapy for Urothelial Carcinoma of the Bladder," *Immunotherapy*, Vol. 1, No. 2, 2009, pp. 281-288. doi:10.2217/1750743X.1.2.281

[5] D. L. Lamm, "Complications of Bacillus Calmette-Guérin Immunotherapy," *Urologic Clinics of North America*, Vol. 19, No. 3, 1992, pp. 565-572

[6] M. J. Manzanera Escribano, E. Morales Ruiz, M. Odriozola Grijalba, E. Gutierrez Martínez, A. Rodriguez Antolín and M. Praga Terente, "Acute Renal Failure Due to Interstitial Nephritis after Intravesical Instillation of BCG," *Clinical and Experimental Nephrology*, Vol. 11, No. 3, 2007, pp. 238-240. doi:10.1007/s10157-007-0483-6

[7] S. E. Kennedy, S. Shrikanth and J. A. Charlesworth, "Acute Granulomatous Tubulointerstitial Nephritis Caused by BCG," *Nephrology Dialysis Transplantation*, Vol. 21, No. 5, 2006, pp. 1427-1429. doi:10.1093/ndt/gfk071

[8] C. G. Valentini, V. Bozzoli, A. R. Larici, L. M. Larocca, G. Delogu, G. Leone and L. Pagano, "Systemic Granulomatous Reaction Secondary to Treatment of Bladder Cancer with Bacillus Calmette-Guerin," *Mediterranean Journal of Hematology and Infectious Diseases*, Vol. 4, No. 1, 2012, e2012040. doi:10.4084/mjhid.2012.040

[9] J. D. Colmerano, R. Sanjuan-Jimenez, B. Ramos and P. Morata, "Miliary Pulmonary Tuberculosis Following Intravesical BCG Therapy: Case Report and Literature Review," *Diagnostic Microbiology and Infectious Disease*, Vol. 74, No. 1, 2012, pp. 70-72. doi:10.1016/j.diagmicrobio.2012.05.026

[10] O. Y. Gonzalez, D. M. Musher, I. Brar, S. Furgeson, M. R. Boktour, E. J. Septimus, R. J. Hamill and E. A. Graviss, "Spectrum of Bacille Calmette-Guérin (BCG) Infection after Intravesical BCG Immunotherapy," *Clinical Infectious Diseases*, Vol. 36, No. 2, 2003, pp. 140-148. doi:10.1086/344908

25

A Case of Cytomegalovirus-Induced Arthritis after Lymphocyte-Depleting Therapy for Kidney Allograft Rejection

Richard Fuquay[1*], **James Eric Cooper**[2]
[1]Health Science Center Division of Renal Diseases and Hypertension, University of Colorado Denver, Aurora, USA
[2]Health Science Center Division of Renal Diseases and Hypertension, Transplant Center, University of Colorado Denver, Aurora, USA
Email: {*Richard.Fuquay, James.Cooper}@ucdenver.edu

ABSTRACT

Cytomegalovirus viremia and tissue-invasive disease are common after kidney transplantation. Chemoprophylaxis has made substantial improvement in this clinical problem. Here we report a 29-year-old woman who had kidney allograft rejection and received lymphocyte-depleting therapy. She presented with a new oligo-arthritis that led to 2 successive arthrocenteses. The etiology of the inflammation could not be determined initially. On the second arthrocentesis, a synovial fluid cytomegalovirus polymerase chain reaction test was positive. The patient responded to treatment with valganciclovir, had negative follow-up serum cytomegalovirus polymerase chain reaction tests, and experienced resolution of her joint inflammation. We review briefly the data for cytomegalovirus chemoprophylaxis, preemptive screening, and treatment recommendations.

Keywords: Cytomegalovirus (Mesh); Arthritis (Mesh); Kidney Transplantation (Mesh); Immunosuppression (Mesh); Chemoprevention (Mesh); Valganciclovir (Mesh)

1. Case Report and Methods

A 29-year-old woman with a history of ESRD due to vesico-ureteral reflux underwent living non-related donor kidney transplantation in January 2009. She was seropositive for cytomegalovirus (CMV) IgG antibodies and received a kidney from a CMV seropositive donor. She received 3 days of lymphocyte-depleting induction with thymoglobulin and was placed on maintenance immunosuppression consisting of tacrolimus, myfortic, and prednisone, as well as valganciclovir 450 mg per day for chemoprophylaxis against CMV disease. Serum creatinine (SCr) fell to a nadir of 1.0 mg/dL (normal, 0.4 to 1.2 mg/dL) following transplant. The patient presented with a SCr of 4.15 mg/dL at 4 months and 2 weeks after her transplant surgery. (The patient later admitted to medication nonadherence.) Valganciclovir was stopped due to deteriorating graft function.

On day 1 of her course, the patient was admitted for renal allograft biopsy which revealed Banff IIa rejection with severe interstitial inflammation, focal endothelialitis, and negative staining for C4d. She began a course of lymphocyte-depleting therapy with thymoglobulin 1.5 mg/kg per day, which was changed to muromonab-CD3 (OKT3) 5 mg per day after 3 days due to development of a rash. She received 9 total doses of lymphocyte-depleting therapy for acute rejection, resulting in a new baseline SCr of 2.8 mg/dL.

On day 8 of her course, she experienced abrupt onset of bilateral knee and hip pain, severely limiting her ability to walk. She was afebrile, but had warmth and effusion most pronounced over the right knee. There was no rash. The plasma white blood cell (WBC) count was 25,800 cells/μL (normal, 4.0 to 11.1 cells/μL). Arthrocentesis of the right knee was performed; gram stain revealed no organisms, but heavy neutrophils. The synovial fluid WBC count was 48,400 cells/μL (normal, <200 cells/μL). The fluid was turbid, and there were no crystals.

Cultures of synovial fluid and blood did not grow any organisms. The patient was treated empirically with intravenous ertapenem 500 mg per day and vancomycin 750 mg per day, for a total course of 14 days. Her knee pain slowly improved, and she was able to resume ambulation. She was discharged on day 11 of her course.

On day 17 of her course, the patient was readmitted

*Corresponding author.

with a SCr of 3.9 mg/dL. Repeat allograft biopsy showed Banff Ib rejection with mild interstitial fibrosis and tubular atrophy, resulting in 6 more doses of OKT3. SCr fell to a new baseline of 2.9 - 3.3 mg/dL.

On day 28 of her course, the patient was readmitted for knee pain. A repeat arthrocentesis of the right knee was performed, and the rheumatology consult service saw the patient. The leading diagnoses under consideration were serum sickness reaction, palindromic rheumatoid arthritis, and seronegative spondyloarthropathy. A CMV polymerase chain reaction (PCR) was ordered on the synovial fluid. The synovial fluid CMV PCR was positive at 1660 copies/mL (nl, <100 copies/mL). On day 30, the serum CMV and Epstein-Barr virus (EBV) PCR tests were positive at 113,500 and 71,950 copies/mL, respectively (CMV and EBV PCR normal, <100 copies/mL). HSV PCR was negative. Other negative serologies included HIV, hepatitis B, hepatitis C, and parvovirus IgM.

After the second arthrocentesis, the patient was started on renally-adjusted valganciclovir at 450 mg every other day. She experienced rapid improvement in her joint pain and swelling. The patient completed a three-month course of valganciclovir (adjusted for changes in renal function). She continues to have intermittent pain in the right knee, but there is no warmth or swelling. Subsequent serum PCR screens for CMV showed a nearly 10-fold reduction at 12 days after initiation of valganciclovir, and undetectable levels 48 and 52 days after initiation of treatment. EBV PCR was repeated 6 weeks after start of valganciclovir and found to be negative.

2. Discussion

We present here a case of CMV-induced acute oligoarthritis after lymphocyte-depleting immunosuppression for acute renal allograft rejection. CMV infection is a major cause of morbidity and mortality in the renal transplant population, and CMV pneumonitis was a major cause of death in renal transplant recipients before the availability of chemoprophylaxis [1]. In addition, CMV infection and disease have been found to be associated with acute rejection as well as overall mortality in kidney transplant recipients [2].

Arthritis is a rare manifestation of CMV disease, which to our knowledge has only been described in two renal transplant recipients [3,4] and one bone marrow transplant recipient [5]. Of the two renal transplant patients with CMV arthritis, the earlier patient died without any direct treatment of the CMV disease in 1978. The later patient received first intravenous, and then oral, ganciclovir with resolution of the infection in 1999. Both had synovial fluid aspirations with neutrophilic predominance. The differential diagnosis of acute arthritis in immunocompromised hosts includes, but is not limited to, infectious diseases, metabolic disorders such as gout, connective tissue diseases, and drug reactions including serum sickness. Additionally, idiopathic transudative effusions have been described in a case series of 37 kidney transplant recipients at Indiana University that had 11 cases of arthritis with effusion. Sampling revealed that all effusions were transudative, free of crystals, and had an average WBC count of 28 cells/uL [6]. The differential diagnosis of post-transplant arthralgia is presented in **Table 1**.

To our knowledge, this case is the first to describe successful treatment of CMV-induced arthritis with valganciclovir, the orally available prodrug of ganciclovir. Valganciclovir has an oral bioavailability of 70%, compared to 7% for ganciclovir [10]. A study by Asberg, et al compared the efficacy of oral valganciclovir to intravenous ganciclovir in 321 solid organ transplant recipients with tissue-invasive CMV disease [11]. Patients were randomized to receive 21 days of either 900 mg oral valganciclovir twice daily or 5 mg/kg intravenous ganciclovir twice daily, followed by 49 days of valganci-

Table 1. Differential diagnosis of arthritis in a renal transplant patient.

Etiology of post-transplant arthralgia:	Synovial fluid characteristics [7,8]	Clinical notes
Septic (bacterial, and rarely viral, fungal, or spirochetal)	10,000 to 100,000 wbc/μL; >90% neutrophils; opaque to purulent	Culture sensitivities vary with bacterial organism; other infections require PCR or special culture techniques
Serum sickness	2000 to 75,000 wbc/μL; >50% neutrophils; yellow to opaque	Fever and rash accompany polyarthralgias 1 - 2 weeks after exposure; caused by immune complex deposition and complement activation
Metabolic/crystalline (gout and pseudogout)	>3000 wbc/μL; <50% neutrophils; yellow to opaque	Cyclosporine impairs tubular excretion of uric acid; in one study it caused gout in 24% of renal transplant patients [9]
Autoimmune (RA, lupus)	2,000 to 75,000 wbc/μL; > 50% neutrophils; yellow to opaque	Diagnosis based on American College of Rheumatology
Non-inflammatory	<2000 wbc/μL; <75% neutrophils; yellow +/– bloody	Consider trauma, OA

clovir therapy. At one year of follow up, rates of CMV recurrence were similar between groups (14.8% and 15.5% for valganciclovir and ganciclovir groups, respectively, $p = 0.89$), as was patient survival and renal function.

This case highlights the importance of CMV chemoprophylaxis in heavily immunosuppressed patients. In this case, induction therapy was followed by chemoprophylaxis, but not subsequent courses of lymphocyte-depleting therapy for acute rejection, which led to a complication. Induction therapy or treatment of rejection with lymphocyte-depleting therapy raises the risk of CMV infection and disease. In one study, adding OKT3 treatment as induction therapy raised the incidence of CMV disease from 21% to 59% [23]. USRDS data have shown that recipients of CMV seropositive kidneys who do not receive prophylaxis have increased rates of CMV disease, allograft loss, and healthcare costs [12]. A recent Cochrane review found that prophylaxis for high risk patients reduces CMV infection, disease, and mortality in solid-organ transplant recipients by 39%, 58% and 37%, respectively [13].

In this patient, CMV prophylaxis was withheld in the days following lymphocyte-depleting therapy due to concerns for side effects related to the patient's fluctuating renal function. Valganciclovir is known to cause anemia and leucopenia, but in severe cases involving improper dosing, fatalities have been reported [14]. *In-vitro* studies have shown that ganciclovir inhibits T-lymphocyte activation and proliferation at therapeutic concentrations [15].

The patient may have benefited from a preemptive screening strategy, which has been recommended as an alternative to universal prophylaxis in kidney transplant recipients at risk for CMV infection [16,17]. While prophylaxis has been associated with superior graft and patient survival [18,19], as well as cost and quality of life benefits [20] compared to a preemptive strategy, the latter may be appropriate for patients at risk for CMV disease with contraindications to oral valganciclovir therapy [17,21]. In such an approach, monitoring of the serum C-MV PCR is conducted at regular intervals (often weekly) to detect infections before tissue-invasive disease results [17]. Most CMV infections occur in the first few months after transplantation, or the first few months after CMV prophylaxis is stopped [22].

Treatment of CMV disease usually includes stopping lymphocyte-depleting therapy, reducing the dose of other immunosuppressive medications, and instituting antiviral therapy [14,17]. During treatment, the PCR is followed to verify that the virus is responding to the drug. In rare cases, primarily occurring in donor-positive to recipient-negative transplants, there have been antiviral-resistant CMV strains, with reported adverse outcomes [14, 17].

This case has some notable limitations. No effort was made to establish a histologic diagnosis or conduct immunofluorescence, as the patient improved briskly with valganciclovir. Additionally, it is impossible to definitively exclude culture-negative septic arthritis, a transient EBV mononucleosis, or systemic CMV viremia that "overflowed" into the joints. However, the patient's monoarticular pain, joint effusion, and the positive synovial fluid PCR indicate that the synovium was a focus (if not the only focus) of viral replication. Furthermore, the synovial fluid characteristics such as neutrophilic predominance are consistent with previous biopsy-proven cases of CMV arthritis. Serum sickness was unlikely based on the asymmetry, severity, and rapidity of the arthritis, the lack of rash or fever, and recurrence of symptoms without further drug exposure. Though the CMV PCR was not impressively high, we believe that may have to do with acquisition and handling; CMV is the best explanation for the clinical scenario.

In summary, we have reported a case of CMV-induced oligo-arthritis that followed aggressive immunosuppression for treatment of acute rejection of a kidney allograft. This disease may have been prevented, or diagnosed earlier, through the use of chemoprophylaxis or preemptive screening. Oral valganciclovir is an effective treatment for CMV disease, and other treatment considerations were reviewed.

3. Author Contributions

Richard Fuquay and James Cooper participated in the preparation of the manuscript.

REFERENCES

[1] C. N. Kotton, "Management of Cytomegalovirus Infection in Solid Organ Transplantation," *Nature Reviews Nephrology*, Vol. 6, 2010, pp. 711-721. doi:10.1038/nrneph.2010.141

[2] S. Sagedal, A. Hartmann, K. P. Nordal, K. Osnes, T. Leivestad, A. Foss, M. Degré, P. Fauchald and H. Rollag, "Impact of Early Cytomegalovirus Infection and Disease on Long-Term Recipient and Kidney Graft Survival," *Kidney International*, Vol. 66, 2004, pp. 329-337. doi:10.1111/j.1523-1755.2004.00735.x

[3] C. Contamin, J. P. Brion, F. Bayle, P. Morand, M. Peo'ch and P. Vialtel, "A Case of Arthritis Caused by Cytomegalovirus after Kidney Transplantation," *Transplant Infectious Disease*, Vol. 6, No. 2, 2004, pp. 87-89. doi:10.1111/j.1399-3062.2004.00052.x

[4] H. M. Friedman, T. Pincus, P. Gibilisco, D. Baker, J. P. Glazer, S. A. Plotkin and H. R. Schumacher, "Acute Monoarticular Arthritis Caused by Herpes Simplex Virus and Cytomegalovirus," *The American Journal of Medicine*, Vol. 69, No. 2, 1980, pp. 241-247.

doi:10.1016/0002-9343(80)90384-8

[5] L. J. Burns and R. D. Gingrich, "Cytomegalovirus Infection Presenting as Polyarticular Arthritis Following Autologous BMT," *Bone Marrow Transplant*, Vol. 11, No. 1, 1993, pp. 77-79.

[6] J. D. MacFarlane, R. S. Filo and K. D. Brandt, "Joint Effusions after Kidney Transplantation," *Arthritis & Rheumatism*, Vol. 22, No. 2, 1979, pp. 164-169. doi:10.1002/art.1780220209

[7] J. J. Cush and P. E. Lipsky, "Approach to Articular and Musculoskeletal Disorders," In: D. L. Longo, D. L. Kasper, J. L. Jameson, A. S. Fauci and S. L. Hauser, Eds., *Harrison's Principles of Internal Medicine*, McGraw-Hill, New York, 2012.

[8] S. J. McPhee and M. Papadakis, "Current Medical Diagnosis and Treatment," 51st Edition, McGraw-Hill Medical, New York, 2010.

[9] T. C. Noordzij, K. M. L. Leunissen and J. P. Van Hooff, "Renal Handling of Urate and the Incidence of Gouty Arthritis during Cyclosporine and Diuretic Use," *Transplantation*, Vol. 52, No. 1, 1991, pp. 64-67. doi:10.1097/00007890-199107000-00013

[10] C. E. Chamberlain, S. R. Penzak, R. M. Alfaro, R. Wesley, C. E. Daniels, D. Hale, A. D. Kirk and R. B. Mannon, "Pharmacokinetics of Low and Maintenance Dose Valganciclovir in Kidney Transplant Recipients," *American Journal of Transplantion*, Vol. 8, No. 6, 2008, pp. 1297-1302. doi:10.1111/j.1600-6143.2008.02220.x

[11] A. Asberg, A. Humar, H. Rollag, A. G. Jardine, H. Mouas, M. D. Pescovitz, D. Sgarabotto, M. Tuncer, I. L. Noronha and A. Hartmann, "Oral Valganciclovir Is Noninferior to Intravenous Ganciclovir for the Treatment of Cytomegalovirus Disease in Solid Organ Transplant Recipients," *American Journal of Transplantation*, Vol. 7, No. 9, 2007, pp. 2106-2113. doi:10.1111/j.1600-6143.2007.01910.x

[12] M. A. Schnitzler, J. A. Lowell, K. L. Hardinger, S. B. Boxerman, T. C. Bailey and D. C. Brennan, "The Association of Cytomegalovirus Sero-Pairing with Outcomes and Costs Following Cadaveric Renal Transplantation Prior to the Introduction of Oral Ganciclovir CMV Prophylaxis," *American Journal of Transplantation*, Vol. 3, No. 4, 2003, 445-451. doi:10.1034/j.1600-6143.2003.00069.x

[13] E. M. Hodson, C. A. Jones, A. C. Webster, G. F. Strippoli, P. G. Barclay, K. Kable, D. Vimalachandra and J. C. Craig, "Antiviral Medications to Prevent Cytomegalovirus Disease and Early Death in Recipients of Solid-Organ Transplants: A Systematic Review of Randomised Controlled Trials," *The Lancet*, Vol. 365, No. 9477, 2005, pp. 2105-2115. doi:10.1016/S0140-6736(05)66553-1

[14] A. Asberg, A. Humar, A. G. Jardine, H. Rollag, M. D. Pescovitz, H. Mouas, A. Bignamini, H. Töz, I. Dittmer, M. Montejo and A. Hartmann, "Long-Term Outcomes of CMV Disease Treatment with Valganciclovir versus IV Ganciclovir in Solid Organ Transplant Recipients," *American Journal of Transplantation*, Vol. 9, No. 5, 2009, pp. 1205-1213. doi:10.1111/j.1600-6143.2009.02617.x

[15] M. Battiwalla, Y. Wu, R. P. S. Bajwa, M. Radovic, N. G. Almyroudis, B. H. Segal, P. K. Wallace, R. Nakamura, S. Padmanabhan, T. Hahn and P. L. McCarthy, "Ganciclovir inhibits Lymphocyte Proliferation by Impairing DNA Synthesis," *Biology of Blood and Marrow Transplantion*, Vol. 13, No. 7, 2007, pp. 765-770. doi:10.1016/j.bbmt.2007.03.009

[16] J. A. Khoury, G. A. Storch, D. L. Bohl, R. M. Schuessler, S. M. Torrence, M. Lockwood, M. Gaudreault-Keener, M. J. Koch, B. W. Miller, K. L. Hardinger, M. A. Schnitzler and D. C. Brennan, "Prophylactic versus Preemptive Oral Valganciclovir for the Management of Cytomegalovirus Infection in Adult Renal Transplant Cecipients," *American Journal of Transplantation*, Vol. 6, No. 9, 2006, pp. 2134-2143. doi:10.1111/j.1600-6143.2006.01413.x

[17] C. N. Kotton, D. Kumar, A. M. Caliendo, A. Asberg, S. Chou, D. R. Snydman, U. Allen and A. Humar, "International Consensus Guidelines on the Management of Cytomegalovirus in Solid Organ Transplantation," *Transplantation*, Vol. 89, No. 7, 2010, pp. 779-795. doi:10.1097/TP.0b013e3181cee42f

[18] V. Kliem, L. Fricke, T. Wollbrink, M. Burg, J. Radermacher and F. Rohde, "Improvement in Long-Term Renal Graft Survival due to CMV Prophylaxis with Oral Ganciclovir: Results of a Randomized Clinical Trial," *American Journal of Transplantation*, Vol. 8, No. 5, 2008, pp. 975-983. doi:10.1111/j.1600-6143.2007.02133.x

[19] L. N. Small, J. Lau and D. R. Snydman, "Preventing Post-Organ Transplantation Cytomegalovirus Disease with Ganciclovir: A Meta-Analysis Comparing Prophylactic and Preemptive Therapies," *Clinical Infectious Disease*, Vol. 43, No. 7, 2006, pp. 869-880. doi:10.1086/507337

[20] F. L. Luan, M. Kommareddi and A. O. Ojo, "Universal Prophylaxis Is Cost Effective in Cytomegalovirus Serology-Positive Kidney Transplant Patients," *Transplantation*, Vol. 91, No. 2, 2011, pp. 237-244. doi:10.1097/TP.0b013e318200000c

[21] F. L. Luan, L. J. Stuckey, J. M. Park, D. Kaul, D. Cibrik and A. Ojo, "Six-Month Prophylaxis Is Cost Effective in Transplant Patients at High Risk for Cytomegalovirus Infection," *Journal of American Society of Nephrology*, Vol. 20, No. 11, 2009, pp. 2449-2458. doi:10.1681/ASN.2008111166

[22] D. C. Brennan, "Cytomegalovirus in Renal Transplantation," *Journal of American Society of Nephrology*, Vol. 12, No. 4, 2001, pp. 848-855.

[23] P. L. Hibberd, N. E. Tolkoff-Rubin, A. B. Cosimi, R. T. Schooley, D. Isaacson, M. Doran, A. Delvecchio, F. L. Delmonico, H. Auchincloss Jr. and R. H. Rubin, "Symptomatic Cytomegalovirus Disease in the Cytomegalovirus Antibody Seropositive Renal Transplant Recipient Treated with OKT31,2," *Transplantation*, Vol. 53, No. 1, 1992, pp. 68-72. doi:10.1097/00007890-199201000-00013

Twenty-Two-Year Observation on Urinary Cadmium and β_2-Microglobulin in Inhabitants after Cessation of Cadmium-Exposure in Japan*

Reiko Sato[1#], Teruhiko Kido[1], Hideaki Nakagawa[2], Muneko Nishijo[2], Ryumon Honda[2], Etsuko Kobayashi[3], Yasushi Suwazono[3]
[1]Graduate School of Medical Science, Kanazawa University, Kanazawa, Japan
[2]Kanazawa Medical University, Uchinada, Japan
[3]Graduate School of Medical Science, Chiba University, Chiba, Japan
Email: #totosuki2007@yahoo.co.jp

ABSTRACT

Objective: This is an epidemiological survey that was conducted for 22 years to investigate the physical effects on inhabitants who had been exposed to cadmium (Cd) from processing of remnants discharged at the time of copper refinement. It was possible to obtain findings on physical effects 27 years after Cd exposure. **Materials and Methods:** Of the inhabitants who were 50 years old or younger in 1981 and who were living in the most contaminated area in the Kakehashi River basin, 68 (32 males and 36 females) who underwent all of the 5 screenings during the 22-year period were extracted as subjects. Early morning urine was collected for urinalysis, and Cd and β_2-MG concentrations were determined. **Results:** 27 years after cessation of Cd exposure, it was shown that urinary Cd concentrations were significantly decreased and urinary β_2-MG concentrations were significantly increased. **Conclusion:** Once exposed to Cd, it takes about 30 years for the Cd that remains in the body to decrease by half. Once renal tubular dysfunction occurs after Cd exposure, irreversible aggravation is inevitable.

Keywords: Twenty-Two-Year Observation; Urinary-Cadmium; Urinary-β_2-Microglobulin; Itai-Itai Disease; Biological-Half-Life

1. Introduction

A long-term follow-up survey was conducted to investigate the effects of Cd exposure on the health of inhabitants who had been living in a contaminated region continually in Japan with regard to the following: 1) Cd that remained in the body as determined based on changes in urinary Cd concentration [1], and 2) renal tubular disorder [2], a typical consequence of Cd exposure, based on changes in urinary β_2-microglobulin (β_2-MG) [3,4] concentration.

Once exposed to Cd, about 30 years [5,6] are required to reduce by half the Cd that remains in the body regardless of the amount of exposure. Even after a long period of time, β_2-MG, an index of renal tubular dysfunction caused by exposure, continues to irreversibly increase [7-10] instead of decreasing. It has therefore been suggested that with larger exposure volumes, the risk of development of distressing Itai-itai disease [11-13] may increase infinitely.

The Kakehashi River basin located in Komatsu City, Ishikawa Prefecture, Japan, was contaminated with Cd waste water from the former Ogoya Cupper Mine [14] from 1882 to 1971. The inhabitants of the region were orally exposed to Cd [15] for a long time because they cultivated and consumed rice as a staple food with contaminated water used for irrigation in rice paddies. However, the Ishikawa Prefecture government conducted an health impairment investigation only afterward, in the 1970s.

The physical effects of Cd exposure include renal tubular dysfunction, osteomalacia, osteoporosis, hepatic disorder, hypertension [16], and others. The most severe consequence is Itai-itai disease. The name of this disease

*The authors declare no competing financial interests.
#Corresponding author.

is Japanese, and literally means "ouch-ouch" because even small movements result in fractures due to advanced osteomalacia, making the patient cry (According to autopsy reports, 42 fractures were observed in some cases.).

The Ministry of Health and Welfare of Japan recognized Itai-itai disease as the first mining-related illness in April 1968 [17] and subsequently enacted a law to improve the polluted soil. Based on this law, in 1981 Ishikawa Prefecture improved the soil of the Kakehashi River basin district that was contaminated with Cd. Since the Ogoya Mine had already been closed by this time and its operation suspended, it was declared that Cd exposure had discontinued in this region [18]. At the same time in 1981, the prefectural government investigated health effects [19] only among inhabitants of the Kakehashi River district who were 50 years old or older at that time and also believed to be severely exposed to Cd. In the survey, findings of β_2-MG of 1000 μg/g·Cr [20,21] or higher were judged abnormal. The incidence of abnormal values was 14.3% in males and 18.7% in females who lived in the polluted area, and 6% and 5%, respectively, in those who lived in non-polluted areas, clearly demonstrating a significant difference ($p < 0.01$) [22] between the polluted and non polluted areas. However, the inhabitants who were 50 years of age or younger and assumed to be moderately exposed to Cd were not investigated by Ishikawa Prefecture even though they lived in the same polluted Kakehashi River area. During 22 years from 1986, 5 years after the declaration on the discontinuation of exposure, up to 2008, Kido *et al.* who were concerned about the pollution, conducted a survey 5 times (1986, 1991, 1999, 2003 and 2008) [23,24] to investigate health effects using only excluded inhabitants who were 50 years of age or younger at the time of the former survey. Our study summarizes these investigations.

The objectives of the studies were 1) to investigate the changes in urinary Cd and β_2-MG concentrations in males and females over the 22-year period to determine the excretion of these substances and 2) to determine the relationship between Cd exposure and renal tubular dysfunction on the basis of the correlation of urinary Cd with β_2-MG in males and females over the 22 years. The following methods were used.

2. Materials and Methods

Of all the inhabitants who were 50 years old or younger in 1981 and who were living in the commune, which was one of the most contaminated areas in the Kakehashi River basin, 68 (32 males and 36 females) who under-went all of the 5 screenings during the 22-year period were included as subjects. Inhabitants who neither participated at least once due to their illness or moving were excluded. Early morning urine was collected for urinalysis, and Cd and β_2-MG concentrations were determined. The measured Cd and β_2-MG concentrations were corrected with Cr. As methods of determination, RIA (Radioimmunoassay), flameless atomic absorption spectrophotometry [25] and the Jaffe method were used to determine β_2-MG concentration, Cd concentration, and Cr concentration, respectively. A questionnaire was also used to investigate gender, age, and duration of residence.

β_2-MG is a plasma protein of low molecular weight (11.800 Daltons) and is produced from immunologically competent cells, the liver, and other tissues. Almost 100% of β_2-MG is filtered through the glomeruli of the kidneys and 99.9% of that is reabsorbed in the renal tubules [24-26]. Accordingly, β_2-MG was used as an index of renal tubular dysfunction. Currently, new indexes of renal tubular dysfunction are being described. However, the newest and the most sensitive index as of 1986 was urinary β_2-MG [24,25]. In a long-term follow-up epidemiology survey, it was necessary to employ the same investigation method in the same subjects for 22 years. Therefore, urinary β_2-MG was continuously used as an index of renal tubular dysfunction for the 22-year period.

The results were statically analyzed using analysis of covariance (ANCOVA), Bonferroni and Pearson correlation coefficient. The software used for analysis was SPSS12 OJ for Windows.

The inhabitants participated in the survey of their own free will. The survey in 2008 was granted approval by the Ethics Committee of Kanazawa University (2008, approval No. 166).

3. Results and Discussion

The mean ages of subjects in 2008 were 65 years and 68 years in the case of males and females, respectively. The mean years of residence were 53 years and 46 years, respectively (**Table 1**).

The scales of **Figures 1-3** show concentrations converted to logarithmic values.

Figure 1 shows a graph of average urinary Cd concentrations of 32 males and 36 females during the 22-year period. On t-testing of the difference in average Cd concentrations of male and female urine specimens in 1986 and 2008, the levels of significance were females $p = 0.001$ and males $p = 0.001$, indicating a significant decrease in 2008. The average actual measurements in 1986 were males 6.0 μg/g·Cr and females 8.20 μg/g·Cr, while the 2008 average actual measurements were males 2.30 μg/g·Cr and females 5.70 μg/g·Cr. This graph reflects the biological half-life of Cd, which is about 30 years, though the results also suggest long-term residue of Cd in the body even 27 years after exposure. In addition, the

Table1. Information on tested subjects (Males = 32, Females = 36).

	1986		1991		1999		2003		2008	
	M	F	M	F	M	F	M	F	M	F
Average age	43	46	48	50	56	59	60	62	65	68
Average period of residence	31	24	36	29	44	37	48	41	53	46

M: Males; F: Females.

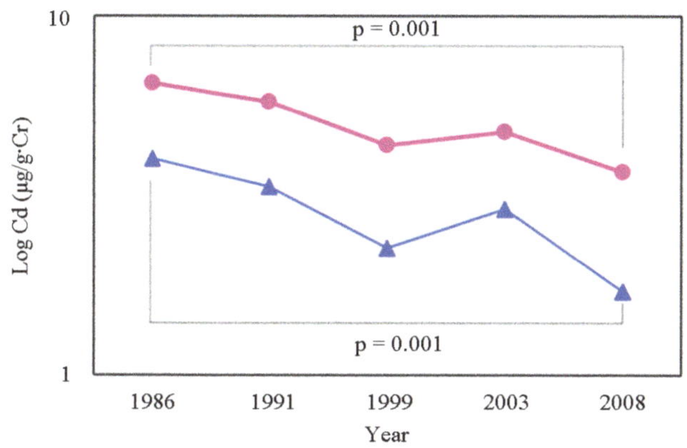

Figure 1. Changes in urinary cadmium concentration (μg/g·Cr) over 22 years in 32 males (Blue) and 36 females (Red).

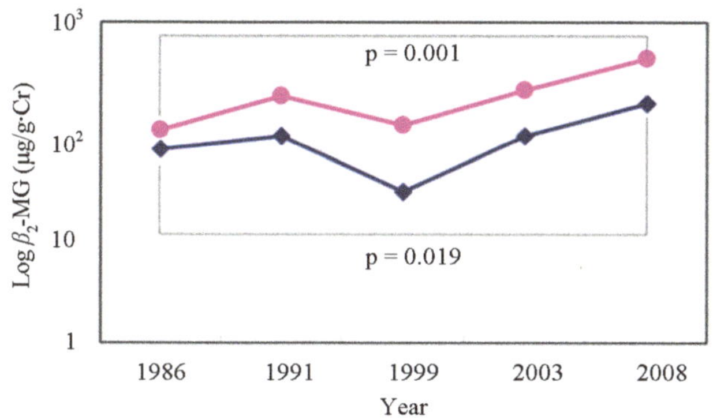

Figure 2. Changes in urinary β_2-MG concentration (μg/g·Cr) over 22 years in males (Blue) and females (Red).

mean concentration in females was clearly higher than that in males, since Cd absorption rate depends on the metallic ion. In conditions of iron deficiency in particular, the absorption rate increases by 20 to 30% compared with normal. The higher incidence of iron deficiency anaemia observed in females [26,27] due to menstruation, giving birth, etc. is cited as a reason why Cd concentration was higher in females than males.

Figure 2 shows a graph of average urinary β_2-MG concentrations of 32 males and 36 females during 22 years. The average actual measurements in 1986 were males 181.0 μg/g·Cr and females 199.0 μg/g·Cr, while the 2008 values were males 224.0 μg/g·Cr and females 268.0 g/g·Cr. On t-testing of the difference in average Cd

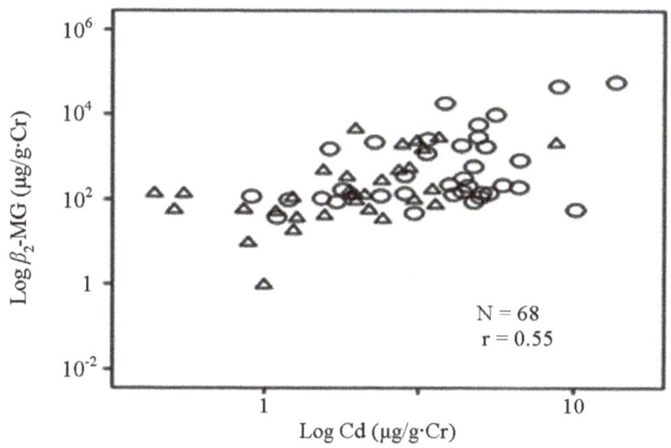

Figure 3. Scatter-plot of correlation between urinary Cd and β2-MG concentrations for 36 females (○) and 32 males (△) in 2008 (r = 0.55: Pearson correlation coefficient, p = 0.000).

concentrations in male and female urine specimens in 1986 and 2008, levels of significance were females p = 0.001 and males p = 0.019. The level significantly increased in both males and females.

These results indicate that, once renal tubular dysfunction occurs after Cd exposure, no cure can be expected and irreversible aggravation is inevitable over time. Fortunately, however, the subject group consisted of those moderately exposed rather than severely exposed to Cd. Since the mean β_2-MG concentration at the time of initial screening in 1986 was 1000 μg/g·Cr or less [18], these individuals had not suffered renal tubular dysfunction, with the exception of several individuals, even though a significant increase in the β_2-MG concentration was noted after 22 years (see **Figure 3**).

In addition, the downward trend in average concentration shown in **Figures 1** and **2** in 1999 is interpreted as the result of physiologically fluctuation, since all values were within normal [24].

To adjust the effects of age or period of residence on the trend in average concentrations of urinary Cd and β_2-MG, analysis of covariance (ANCOVA) analysis was performed and results were shown from **Tables 2-5**. **Table 2** shows the change of urinary Cd concentration during 22 years adjusted by age in males and females. Preliminary parallel tests showed a positive result for females and a negative result for males. Hence, the

Table 2. The change of urinary Cd concentration during 22 years adjusted for age in females.

Year	Urinary Cd (μg/g·Cr) Females (N = 36)		
	GM	SE	p
1986	0.968	0.48	p = 0.002
1991	0.857	0.046	p = 0.027
1999	0.615	0.045	p = 0.001; p = 0.001
2003	0.601	0.045	p = 0.000; p = 0.049
2008	0.419	0.048	

GM: Geometric Mean; SE: Standard Error; p: p-value; A Parallel test for males was negative and positive for females. Hence, a further Bonferroni multiple comparison in ANCOVA analysis was performed for females.

Table 3. The change of urinary Cd concentration during 22 years adjusted for period of residence in males and females.

	Urinary Cd (μg/g·Cr)					
	Males (N = 32)			Females (N = 36)		
Year	GM	SE	p	GM	SE	p
1986	0.670	0.058	p = 0.001	0.925	0.050	p = 0.039
1991	0.563	0.056	p = 0.000	0.824	0.048	
1999	0.343	0.055	p = 0.038	0.626	0.047	p = 0.000; p = 0.038
2003	0.430	0.056	p = 0.000; p = 0.012	0.622	0.048	p = 0.000
2008	0.170	0.057		0.464	0.049	

GM: Geometric Mean; SE: Standard Error; p: p-value; Parallel tests for males and females showed a positive result. Hence, a further Bonferroni multiple comparison in ANCOVA analysis was performed.

Table 4. The change of urinary β_2-MG concentration during 22 years adjusted for age in males and females.

	Urinary β_2-MG (μg/g·Cr)					
	Males (N = 32)			Females (N = 36)		
Year	GM	SE	p	GM	SE	p
1986	1.979	0.131	p = 0.16	2.306	0.121	
1991	2.025	0.126	p = 0.005	2.510	0.116	p = 0.014
1999	1.394	0.124		1.983	0.113	
2003	1.863	0.125	p = 0.001	2.212	0.114	
2008	2.090	0.130		2.377	0.120	

GM: Geometric Mean; SE: Standard Error; p: p-value; Parallel tests for males and females showed a positive result. Hence, a further Bonferroni multiple comparison in ANCOVA analysis was performed.

resulting Bonferroni multiple comparison in ANCOVA analysis for females showed a significant decrease during 22 years (1986 - 2008), without involvement of age. In **Table 3** the change of urinary Cd concentration during 22 years was adjusted by period of residence in males and females. Preliminary parallel tests showed a positive result for both males and females. In the resulting in ANCOVA and Bonferroni multiple comparison analysis, there was a significant decrease in males and females during 22 years (1986 - 2008), without the involvement period of residence. As shown in **Table 4** the change of urinary β_2-MG concentration during 22 years was adjusted by age and preliminary parallel tests showed a positive result in males and females. Hence, the resulting Bonferroni multiple comparison in ANCOVA analysis showed a significant decrease between 1986 to 1999 and

Table 5. The change of urinary β_2-MG concentration during 22 years adjusted for Period of residence in males and females.

	Urinary β_2-MG (μg/g·Cr)						
	Males (N = 32)				Females (N = 36)		
Year	GM	SE	p		GM	SE	p
1986	1.935	0.130	p = 0.038		2.267	0.118	
1991	2.008	0.126		p = 0.009	2.468	0.114	p = 0.038
1999	1.902	0.125			1.999	0.112	
2003	1.877	0.126		p = 0.001	2,230	0.113	
2008	2.129	0.129			2.424	0.117	

GM: Geometric Mean; SE: Standard Erro; p: p-value; A Parallel test for males and females showed a positive result. Hence, a further Bonferroni multiple comparison in ANCOVA analysis was performed.

1991 to 1999, but there was significant increase during 1999 to 2008 in males, with no significant increase in females. However, there was a tendency towards increase during 22 years (1986 - 2008) for both males and females without the involvement of age. **Table 5** shows that urinary β_2-MG concentration during 22 years was adjusted by period of residence. A significant increase was observed between 1999 and 2008 for males, but for females, there was no significant increase without the involvement of period of residence. However, during 22 years (1986 - 2008) there was a tendency to increase in males and females. Therefore, Significant increase were observed for urinary β_2-MG concentration (μg/g·Cr) adjusted by age and period of residence, for males and females. An increasing tendency was observed during 22 years for females. It was revealed that once exposed to Cd, β_2-MG occurs in the body and irreversible

Figure 3 shows a scatter-plot of the correlation between urinary Cd and β_2-MG concentrations for 36 females (○) and 32 males (Δ) in 2008 using the Pearson correlation method. This figure indicates a significant correlation of urinary Cd with β_2-MG in 2008 with a Pearson correlation coefficient of $r = 0.55$ and a significance level of $p = 0.0001$. The relationship of Cd exposure to renal tubular dysfunction indicates that this dysfunction persisted even 27 years after Cd exposure and as long as Cd remained in the body.

4. Conclusion

Our findings clearly indicate the following. Once exposed to Cd, it takes about 30 years for the Cd that remains in the body to decrease by half. Once renal tubular dysfunction occurs after Cd exposure, irreversible aggravation is inevitable. If the Cd exposure volume is larger, the renal tubular dysfunction will be more severe. Therefore, measures to prevent mining pollution are required for mining development in the 21st century so that the tragedy caused by Cd pollution that occurred as a secondary effect of cupper mining development is never repeated. In addition, the first measures to prevent mining pollution is a process of gravel remaining emissions during the refining process. The gravel that contain contaminants is discharged, and appropriate processing of it is the first step in preventing pollution. However, we may be able to find rare metals by carefully sifting this gravel, which has been irresponsibly discharged.

5. Acknowledgements

The authors thank the inhabitants of the Kakehashi area, who had to endure physical examinations over a period of 22 years. Special thanks go to Mr. M. Iga, a historian of Kakehashi town, who is currently 96 years of age. The authors also thank Mr. M. Hino for environmental data on the Kakehashi river stream (Komatsu Environmental Partnership) and Mr. H. Hayashidera.

Finally, we sincerely wish the inhabitants of the Kakehashi area good health and long lives.

6. Author Contributions

Dr. Sato conducted the project. Dr. Nishijo, Dr. Kobayashi, and Dr. Honda analyzed the urinary samples. Dr. Kido and Dr. Nakagawa participated in several health examinations. Dr. Suwazono calculated analytical data.

REFERENCES

[1] T. Kido, "The Relation of Individual Cadmium Concentration in Urine with Total Cadmium Intake in Kakehashi River Basin, Japan," *Toxicology Letters*, Vol. 152, No. 1, 2004, pp. 57-61. http://dx.doi.org/10.1016/j.toxlet.2004.04.001

[2] T. KjellstrÖm, "Renal Effects," In: L. Fridberg, C. G. Elinder, T. KjellstrÖm and G. F Nordberg, Eds., *Cadmium and Health: A Toxicological and Epidemiological*

Appraisal, II. *Effects and Response*, CRC Press, Boca Raton, 1986, pp. 21-110

[3] P. A. Peterson, P. E. Evrin and I. Berggård, "Differentiation of Glomerular, Tubular and Normal Proteinuria: Determinations of Urinary Excretion of β_2-MG, Albumin and Total Protein," *Journal of Clinical Investigation*, Vol. 48, 1969, pp. 1189-1198.

[4] M. Piscator, "Markers of Tubular Dysfunction," *Toxicology Letters*, Vol. 46, 1989, pp. 197-204. http://dx.doi.org/10.1016/0378-4274(89)90128-8

[5] K. Nogawa, "Itai-Itai Disease and Follow-Up Studies," In: J. O. Nriagu Ed., Cadmium in the Environment Part 2 Health Effects," A Wiley-Interscience Publication, New York, 1981, I-37.

[6] K. Aoshima and M. Kasuya, "Itai-Itai Disease a Natural History of Osteomalacia Caused by Urinary Tubular Dysfunction during Exposure to General Environmental Cadmium," *The Journal of Therapy*, Vol. 75, 1993, pp. 1031-1035.

[7] World Health Organization, "Environmental Health Criteria 135 Cadmium—Environmental Aspects," World Health Organization, Geneva, 1992, pp. 174-188.

[8] G. F. Nordberg, *et al.*, "Cadmium and Health. A Toxicological and Epidemiological Appraisal. Vol. I," CRC Press, Boca Raton, 1985, pp. 103-178.

[9] G. F. Nordberg, *et al.*, "Cadmium," In: L. Friberg, C.-G. Elinder, T. KjellstrÖm and G. F. Nordberg, Eds., *Hand Book on the Toxicology of Metals*, 3rd Edition, Elsevier, Amsterdam, 2007.

[10] C.-G. Elinder, "Cadmium and Health. A Toxicological and Epidemiological Appraisal. Chapter 3," CRC Press, Boca Raton, 1985.

[11] K. Iwata, H. Saito, M. Moriyama and A. Nakano, "Renal Tubular Function after Reduction of Environmental Cadmium-Exposure. A Ten-Year Follow up," *Arch Environ Health*, Vol. 43, No. 3, 1993, pp. 157-163. http://dx.doi.org/10.1080/00039896.1993.9940814

[12] G. Nordberg, "Renal Dysfunction Induced by Cadmium-Is It Reversible? Advance in Prevention of Environmental Cadmium Pollution and Countermeasures," *Eiko Laboratory Kanazawa JAPAN*, 1999, pp. 99-102.

[13] Y. Cai, K. Aoshima, T. Katoh, H. Teranishi and M. Kasuya, "Renal Tubular Dysfunction in Male Inhabitants of Cadmium-Polluted Areas in Toyama, Japan-An Eleven-Year Follow-Up Study," *Journal of Epidemiology*, Vol. 11, No. 4, 2001, pp. 180-189. http://dx.doi.org/10.2188/jea.11.180

[14] T. Wada, "Metals and Humans," Asakura Publishers, 1986, pp. 246-258.

[15] K. Nogawa and A. Ishizaki, "Statistical Observations of the Does-Response Relationship of Cadmium Based on Epidemiological Studies in the Kakehashi River Basin," *Environmental Research*, Vol. 15, 1978, pp. 185-198. http://dx.doi.org/10.1016/0013-9351(78)90095-6

[16] M. Kasuya, "Liver Injury by Cadmium," *Kan Tan Sui*, Vol. 10, 1985, pp. 923-928.

[17] J. Matsunami, "Review of Itai-Itai Disease," Katsura Syobou, Japan. 2006, pp. 2-38.

[18] Ishikawa Prefecture Laws and Regulation, "Measurement of Soil in Farmlands of Polluted Areas," Ishikawa Prefecture, 1975. www.pre.ishikawa.jp/reiki/reiki_honbun/enkaku/i101048 8001,html

[19] Ishikawa Prefecture South Kaga Public Health Center, "Research and Induction about Local Health and Environmental during 9 Heisei Year (1997)," Report on Ishikawa Prefecture South Kaga Public Health, 1984, pp. 82-88.

[20] K. Nogawa, Y. Yamada, R. Honda, M. Ishizaki, I. Tsuritani, S. Kawano and T. Kato, "The Relationship between Itai-Itai Disease among Inhabitants of the Jinzu River basin in rice," *Toxicology Letters*, Vol. 17, No. 3, 1983, pp. 263-266. http://dx.doi.org/10.1016/0378-4274(83)90236-9

[21] Y. Kubota, *et al.*, "A Study on Normal Range of Urinary Protein Fraction Concentrations, Albumin, β2-Microgroblin and α1-Microgrobulin among Commounity Inhabitants," *Hokuriku Journal of Public Health*, Vol. 12, 1985, pp. 27-32.

[22] T. Kido, "Studies on Health Effects of Cadmium Exposure in the General Environment," *Japanese Journal of Hygiene*, Vol. 49, No. 6, 1995, pp. 960-972. http://dx.doi.org/10.1265/jjh.49.960

[23] T. Kido, "Progress of Renal Dysfunction in Inhabitants Environmentally Exposed to Cadmium," *Archives of Environmental Health*, Vol. 43, No. 3, 1988, pp. 214-215. http://dx.doi.org/10.1080/00039896.1988.9934935

[24] R. Sato, T. Kido, R. Honda, M. Nishijo, H. Nakagawa, E. Kobayashi and Y. Suwazono, "Seventeen-Year Observation on Urinary Cadmium and β2-Microglobulin in Inhabitants after Cessation of Cadmium-Exposure in Japan," *Bull Environ Contam Toxicol*, Vol. 84, 2010, pp. 363-367. http://dx.doi.org/10.1007/s00128-010-9947-6

[25] R. Honda, *et al.*, "Flameless Atomic Absorption Spectrophotoemetry of Cadmium and Lead in Blood," *Kanazawa Medical University Journal*, Vol. 14, No. 3, 1989, pp. 337-347.

[26] P. A. Peterson, P. E. Evrin and I. Berggård, "Differential of Glomerular, Tubular and Normal Proteinuria: Determinations of Urinary Excretion of β2-MG, Albumin and Total Protein," *Journal of Clinical Investigation*, 1969, pp. 1189-1198.

[27] G. F. Nordberg, L. Friberg, C. Elinder and T. Kjellstrom, "Cadmium and Health. A Toxicological and Epidemiological Appraisal. Vol. 1," CRC Press, Boco Raton, 1985, pp. 103-178.

Acalculous Cholecystitis: An Unusual Manifestation of Cytomegalovirus Disease in Renal Transplant Recipient

Mostapha Habib Allah*, Nour Houda Bassit, Wafaa Fadili, Inass Laouad
Department of Nephrology, Transplantation UHC Mohammed VI, Marrakesh, Morocco
Email: *mostapha82@hotmail.fr, nour-bassit@hotmail.fr, fadili.wafaa@gmail.com, inasslaouad@yahoo.fr

ABSTRACT

Background: Common clinical manifestations of cytomegalovirus (CMV) infection include flu-like symptoms with fever, diarrhea, leukopenia, and elevated liver enzymes. Diagnosis is made by detection of the virus by buffy-coat blood culture or by polymerase chain reaction (PCR) analysis. **Methods:** Here we describe a women renal transplant recipient who presented with acalculous cholecystitis with CMV viremia, anemia and leucopenia tree months after she received a kidney from cadaveric donor. **Results:** Retrospective analysis of peripheral blood by PCR analysis was positive for CMV DNA. Treatement with Intravenous Ganciclovir was started after diagnosis. The role of cholecystectomy in patients diagnosed as having acalculous cholecystitis associated with systemic CMV disease remains unclear. **Conclusions:** Because CMV infection is common in transplant patients, the atypical manifestations of CMV should be considered in the differential diagnosis of posttransplant complications. Detection of CMV DNA in the peripheral blood by PCR analysis may help identify these patients.

Keywords: CMV; Cholecystitis; Kidney; Renal; Transplant

1. Introduction

Cytomegalovirus infection is common in renal transplant recipients in the first 3 - 6 months after transplant [1]. Risk factors in transplant patients include primary exposure to CMV infection at the time of transplantation and the use of antilymphocyte preparations such as OKT3 and antithymocyte globulin [1]. The commonest presenting symptoms of CMV disease include fever, malaise, leukopenia, diarrhea, elevated liver enzymes, and pneumonia in severe cases [1]. With preemptive CMV prophylaxis in transplant recipients, serious manifestations of CMV disease are rarely seen [2]. Here we report a case of renal transplant recipients who experienced unusual manifestations of tissue-invasive CMV disease (cholecystitis). Although CMV is known to cause cholecystitis in patients with acquired immunodeficiency syndrome (AIDS), there is only seven previous cases report in a renal transplant recipient [3-7].

2. Case

A 44-year-old woman, who received a cadaveric renal transplant from a CMV-seropositive donor, presented after 4 months of transplantation with severe right upper quadrant abdominal pain, fever and vomiting. Her immunosuppression consisted of Thymoglobuline, mycofenolate mofetil, prednisolone and cyclosprine. Biochemical results revealed serum creatinine: 132 µmol/l, hemoglobine: 8.3 g/dl, leucopenia: 3040/mm^3 (neutrophile: 2470 and lymphocytes: 400), CRP: 19 mg/l, lipase and liver enzymez are normal.

Cyclosporine residual rate (C0): 222 ng/ml. Abdominal ultrasound revealed sludge and a thinwalled gallbladder. Prior to her transplant, she was CMV seropositive. She didn't receive a prophylaxis against CMV. At that stage her CMV PCR was 1,341,000 copies/mL. She was admitted for treatment with intravenous ganciclovir. After 10 days of antiviral treatment with continued treatment using intravenous ganciclovir. The patient became afebrile, the clinical CMV infection resolved and counts returned to <10,000 copies/mL. At the last follow-up 2 months later, the patient had stable graft function with no recurrence of CMV disease.

3. Discussion

Our case demonstrates that CMV infection of the gallbladder can be a severe disease. Although CMV is

*Corresponding author.

known to cause cholecystitis in patients with AIDS [8], there are only seven previous case reports of CMV cholecystitis in renal transplant recipients [3-7]. Four of those cases required an uncomplicated cholecystectomy [3-6]. There is one previous description of CMV cholecystitis leading to perforation of the gallbladder [6], and two cases described with hemorrhagic CMV cholecystitis postrenal transplantation [7]. The possibility of CMV infection of the gallbladder must be considered in all patients postrenal transplant that present with severe abdominal pain despite a policy of initial antiviral preemptive-prophylaxis. CMV infection is diagnosed by latex agglutination, complement fixation tests, enzyme-linked immunosorbent assay, antigen assay, and polymerase chain reaction. Biopsy is the only way to establish tissue invasion. Treatment is usually indicated for patients having symptoms of viremia or evidence of invasive disease. What remains unclear, though, is the role of cholecystectomy in patients diagnosed as having acalculous cholecystitis associated with systemic CMV disease. Ganciclovir, the most effective antiviral agent against CMV, has no hepatobiliary excretion [9]. Indeed, the gallbladder may serve as a reservoir for CMV, causing recurrent illness in patients treated with ganciclovir. Routine surveillance by PCR analysis of patients at high risk for developing CMV infection, and at the time of atypical clinical presentation, may be helpful in defining atypical cases of CMV-related complications.

4. Conclusion

We suggest that any post-transplant patient with upper abdominal pain should have a CMV-PCR and abdominal imaging.

5. Summary

We report a case of acalculous cholecystitis in renal transplant patients, who appeared with insidious onset, abdominal right upper quadrant pain and fever. CMV acalculous cholecystitis is an uncommon manifestation of CMV disease in renal transplantation, in our knowledge only seven cases were described. It should be considered, especially when abdominal pain and fever are present. Unfortunately, a limited experience in treatment, either medical or surgical, was reported. In our case, the response to medical treatment was successful, disappearing the abdominal pain and the fever.

REFERENCES

[1] P. L. Hibberd and D. R. Snydman, "Cytomegalovirus Infection in Organ Transplant Recipients," *Infectious Disease Clinics of North America*, Vol. 9, No. 4, 1995, pp. 863-877.

[2] P. L. Hibbered, N. E. Tolkoff-Rubin, D. Conti, *et al.*, "Pre-Emptive Ganciclovir Therapy to Prevent Cytomegalovirus Disease in Cytomegalovirus Antibody-Positive Renal Transplant Recipients: A Randomized Controlled Trial," *Annals of Internal Medicine*, Vol. 123, No. 1, 1995, pp. 18-26. doi:10.7326/0003-4819-123-1-199507010-00002

[3] A. Moudgil, S. C. Jordan, *et al.*, "Ureteritis and Cholecystitis: Two Unusual Manifestations of Cytomegalovirus Disease in Renal Transplant Recipients," *Transplantation*, Vol. 64, 1997, pp. 1071-1073. doi:10.1097/00007890-199710150-00021

[4] N. Bagchi, P. Kumar, *et al.*, "Cytomegalovirus Cholecystitis: A Case Report," *Transplantation*, Vol. 75, 2003, pp. 1918-1919. doi:10.1097/01.TP.0000065804.62470.52

[5] D. M. McMullan, O. H. Frazier, *et al.*, "Cytomegalovirus Cholecystitis in a Heart Transplant Recipient," *Transplantation Proceedings*, Vol. 34, No. 4, 2002, pp. 1271-1272. doi:10.1016/S0041-1345(02)02753-7

[6] A. Franco, J. Olivares, *et al.*, "Perforation of the Acalculous Gallbladder in a Renal Transplant Recipient with CMV Infection," *Nefrologia*, Vol. 26, 2006, pp. 619-622

[7] M. Drage, J. Watson, *et al.*, "Acute Cytomegalovirus Cholecystitis Following Renal Transplantation," *American Journal of Transplantation*, Vol. 9, No. 5, 2009, pp. 1249-1252. doi:10.1111/j.1600-6143.2009.02607.x

[8] M. D. Adolf, S. N. Bass, S. K. Lee, *et al.*, "Cytomegaloviral Acalculous Cholecystitis in Acquired Immuno Deficiency Syndrome Patients," *Annals of Surgery*, Vol. 59, 1993, p. 69.

[9] M. A. Jacobson and J. Mills, "Serious Cytomegalovirus Disease in the Acquired Immunodeficiency Syndrome (AIDS)," *Annals of Internal Medicine*, 1988, Vol. 108, No. 4, pp. 585-594. doi:10.7326/0003-4819-108-4-585

Correlation of Surgical Times with Laparoscopic Live Donor Kidney Transplant Outcomes

Sertac Cimen[1], Sanem Guler[2], Ian Alwayn[1], Joseph Lawen[3], Bryce Kiberd[4]
[1]The Division of General Surgery, Dalhousie University, Queen Elizabeth II Health Sciences Centre, Halifax, Canada
[2]Atlantic Centre for Transplantation Research, Dalhousie University, Halifax, Canada
[3]Department of Urology, Dalhousie University, Queen Elizabeth II Health Sciences Centre, Halifax, Canada
[4]Faculty of Medicine, Dalhousie University, Queen Elizabeth II Health Sciences Centre, Halifax, Canada
Email: Bryce.Kiberd@dal.ca

ABSTRACT

Most studies revealed that ischemic time has substantial role in occurrence of delayed graft function (DGF) after deceased donor kidney transplantation. However, less is known about the potential impact of surgical times on early outcomes following live donor kidney transplantation. A retrospective cohort of 189 consecutive laparoscopic live donor kidney transplant (LDKT) recipients from January 2006 to August 2012 was analyzed to reveal the impact of pneumoperitoneum time (PT) and anastomosis time (AT) on donor and recipient length of hospital stay and early graft function (EGF). DGF was observed in 13 (6.8%) patients while slow graft function (SGF) was seen in 27 (14%) of the recipients. The median AT was 28 minutes (interquartile range 23, 35 minutes). AT was associated with DGF (Odds Ratio [OR] 1.044, per minute, 95% CI 1.007, 1.082, p = 0.018). Median recipient length of hospital stay was 8 (interquartile range 7, 11) days. Every 13.5 minutes of longer AT was associated with 1 extra day in hospital. The median PT was 180 minutes (interquartile range 144, 234 minutes). PT was associated with both DGF (OR 1.013 per minute, 95% CI 1.005, 1.021, p = 0.001) and SGF (OR 1.009 per minute, 95% CI 1.002, 1.016, p = 0.016). Every extra hour of PT was associated with 0.42 more days in hospital for the donor. Surgical times may be underestimated variables in dictating use of hospital resources. The effect of surgical times on long term hard outcomes entails further study.

Keywords: Delayed Graft Function; Slow Graft Function; Anastomosis Time; Pneumoperitoneum Time; Kidney Transplantation

1. Introduction

Since its description in 1995 laparoscopic live donor nephrectomy has replaced open donor nephrectomy at many transplant centres [1]. Multiple studies have shown that laparoscopic nephrectomy is considerably gentler for the donor with less postoperative pain, shorter length of hospital stay and improved cosmesis [2,3]. However some studies have shown that the pneumoperitoneum used during laparoscopic donor nephrectomy procedure might impair renal blood flow and prolonged pneumoperitoneum time (PT) can increase the oxidative stress and subsequently cause subtle renal tissue injury [4-6].

In line with this hypothesis, several investigators have reported slower early post-transplant function for laparoscopically retrieved (vs. open) grafts as measured by poor early graft function (EGF) rates [7,8]. This is important because even mild to moderate early graft dysfunction can have a negative impact on long-term graft survival [9].

Studies investigating EGF after kidney transplant from living donors (regardless of the procurement technique) identified prolonged anastomosis time (AT) as another risk factor for the occurrence of poor EGF [10].

In the present study we critically assessed the correlation of PT and AT with the indicators of EGF after laparoscopic live donor kidney transplant (LDKT) surgeries.

2. Materials and Methods

Consecutive laparoscopic LDKT donors and recipients who underwent surgery between January 2006 and August 2012 were identified. Data were extracted retrospectively from the hospital's electronic records. Approval for this study was obtained from our institution's research ethics board.

All donors were admitted the day before surgery. All of the laparoscopic donor nephrectomy procedures were performed by transperitoneal route except for one which was done by retroperitoneoscopic approach. Intravenous fluids, mannitol and furosemide were given as required to help prevent pneumoperitoneum-induced oliguria. The renal vessels were controlled individually by using endoscopic vascular stapler. The graft was extracted through either Pfannensteil incision using an endobag or hand-port. PT was recorded in each case as the time between its initiation and extraction of the graft.

All recipients received induction immunosuppression with either basiliximab or antithymocyte globulin (ATG) and all of them were given methylprednisolone sodium succinate 500 mg intraoperatively. ATG was reserved for those who were repeat transplant recipients or highly sensitized. All received pneumocystis pneumonia and gastric ulcer prophylaxis. For patients already on a proton pump inhibitor pre-transplant, this agent was continued instead of starting ranitidine. Cytomegalovirus (CMV) prophylaxis with valganciclovir was used when the donor was seropositive in a seronegative recipient or when the recipient was induced by ATG. AT was recorded in each case as the time between the end of the cooling period and reperfusion of the kidney. All patients subsequently received were put on oral tacrolimus, mycophenolate and a prednisone tapering dose.

Data extracted for recipients included age, gender, weight, body mass index (BMI), calculated panel reactive antibodies (cPRA), Human Leukocyte Antigen mismatch (HLA MM) status, cause of end stage renal disease (ESRD), diabetes mellitus (DM), AT (minutes), serum creatinine (Cr) pre-transplant and on postoperative day (POD) 5, delayed graft function (DGF), slow graft function (SGF) and duration of hospital stay.

Data extracted for the donors included age, gender, weight, BMI, pre-donation and discharge Cr, duration of hospital stay, PT, side of the retrieved kidney and retrieval technique (laparoscopy/conversion to open donor nephrectomy).

Statistical data are presented as mean and standard deviation (SD) for continuous normally distributed variables, median and interquartile range for continuous variables not normally distributed and percentages for dichotomous variables. Variables associated with DGF (need for dialysis within the first week after kidney transplant) were examined by logistic regression analysis. Since there were a small number of events for DGF, a detailed multivariable linear regression analysis could not be completed. Instead, a univariable logistic regression analysis was done. A binary logistic regression analysis was also performed on whether that patient had SGF which was defined as POD5 creatinine $\geq$265 μmol/L without need of dialysis in the first week post-transplant. A multivariable linear regression analysis was performed for recipient POD5 Cr and duration of hospital stay using both recipient and donor variables. However since >40% of values were missing for cPRA, this variable was not included in the analysis. A multivariable linear regression analysis was performed for the donor duration of hospital stay using donor variables only. Variables that were significant at $p < 0.1$ in a univariable analysis were included into the multivariable models. Overall significance was assumed at $p < 0.05$ level. Statistical analysis was performed by IBM SPSS Statistics software version 20.0 (New York, US).

3. Results

There were 209 consecutive live donor kidney transplant operations. Patients undergoing open nephrectomy were excluded (n = 16) as well as laparoscopic operations without recorded warm ischemic times (n = 4), leaving 189 subjects for evaluation.

Population descriptors are displayed in **Tables 1** and **2** for recipients and donors respectively. Mean ages of the recipients and donors were similar. Donors were more likely female and recipients were more likely men.

Table 1. Recipient descriptors and key results.

Recipient	
Age years mean (SD)	45 (14)
Male	120 (63%)
Body Weight kg Mean (SD)	80 (19)
Body Mass Index kg/m^2 Mean (SD)	28 (6)
HLA Mismatch Mean (SD)	3.1 (1.9)
ESRD	
DM	31 (16%)
Glomerulonephritis	79 (42%)
Interstitial Disease	24 (13%)
PCKD	28 (15%)
Other	27 (14%)
AT minutes	
Mean (SD)	31 (14)
Median (IQR)	28 (23, 35)
Creatinine μmol/L	
Admission	
Mean (SD)	715 (263)
Median (IQR)	666 (521, 885)
POD 5	
Mean (SD)	198 (187)
Median (IQR)	135 (100, 195)
Change day 0 to 5	
Mean (SD)	519 (268)
Median (IQR)	490 (344, 678)
Days in hospital	
Mean (SD)	10.8 (8.2)
Median (IQR)	8 (7, 11)
DGF	13 (6.8%)
SGF	27 (14%)

Table 2. Live donor descriptors and key results.

Donor	
Age years mean (SD)	43 (11)
Male	67 (36%)
Body Weight kg mean (SD)	75 (15)
Body Mass Index kg/m^2	27 (6)
Conversion	6 (3%)
Left	103 (55%)
PT minutes	
Mean (SD)	196 (66)
Median (IQR)	180 (144, 234)
Creatinine μmol/L	
Admission	72 (14)
Discharge	111 (20)
Difference	39 (13)
Days in hospital	
Mean (SD)	5.8 ± 1.7
Median (IQR)	6 (5, 6)

Median and interquartile ranges (IQR) are included for AT (**Figure 1**), PT (**Figure 2**), days in hospital and recipient POD5 Cr since these outcomes were not normally distributed.

DGF was observed in 13 (6.8%) of patients. Significant variables associated with DGF in a binary logistic regression analysis were AT (Odds Ratio [OR] 1.044, per minute, 95% CI 1.007, 1.082, p = 0.018), PT (OR 1.013 per minute, 95% CI 1.005, 1.021, p = 0.001) and pre-transplant Cr (OR 1.003 per μmol/L, 95% CI 1.001, 1.004, p = 0.007). AT and PT were significantly correlated (r = 0.34, p < 0.001) however pre-transplant creatinine was not correlated with AT or PT.

SGF was observed in 27 (14%) of patients. Significant variables associated with SGF in a binary logistic regression analysis were PT (OR 1.009 per minute, 95% CI 1.002, 1.016, p = 0.016), recipient male (OR 9.6, 95% CI 1.2, 76, p = 0.032) and pre-transplant Cr (OR 1.002 per μmol/L, 95% CI 1.000, 1.004, p = 0.014). AT was significant (p = 0.019) in the univariable analysis but not in the multivariable model. No other variables were significant.

In a multivariable linear regression analysis, POD5 Cr was associated with recipient weight (Beta coefficient 1.7 μmol/L per kg, 95% CI 0.3, 3.1, p = 0.018), recipient pre-transplant Cr (0.17 μmol/L per μmol/L, 95% CI 0.07, 0.26, p = 0.001) and AT (3.5 μmol/L per min, 95% CI 1.6, 5.3, p < 0.001). HLA MM, donor gender, donor pre-donation Cr and PT were significant (p < 0.10) in the univariate analysis and were included in the model but were not independent predictors. Therefore every 10 longer minutes of AT was associated with a Cr 35 μmol/L higher on POD5.

For associations with recipient stay in hospital, AT (Beta coefficient 0.073 days per minute, 95% CI 0.017,

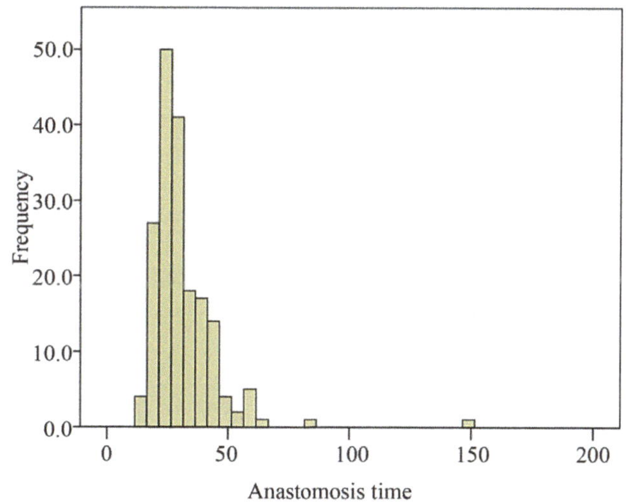

Figure 1. Distribution of anastomosis time among recipient population of the study.

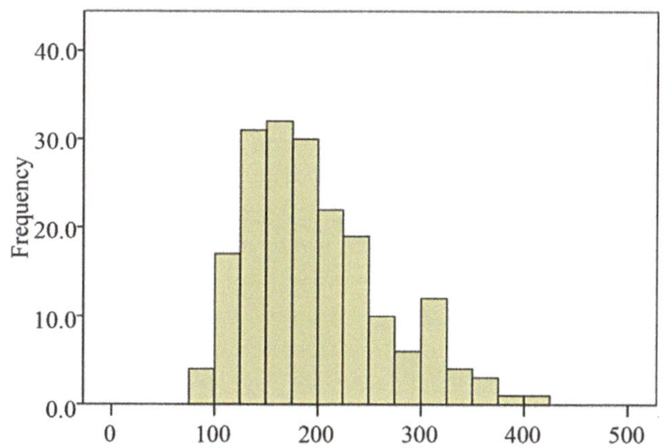

Figure 2. Distribution of pneumoperitoneum time among donor population of the study.

0.13, p = 0.011), HLA MM (0.48 days per MM, 95% CI 0.1, 0.9, p = 0.014), recipient pre-transplant Cr (0.004 days per μmol/L, 95% CI 0.001, 0.007, p = 0.008) and donor age (0.074 days per year, 95% CI 0.005, 0.14, p = 0.035) were significant in a multivariable linear regression analysis. PT was significant in a univariable analysis (p = 0.002) but was not independently significant in the multivariable model. All other variables were not significant. Therefore every 13.5 minutes of longer AT was associated with 1 extra day in hospital.

For associations with donor stay in hospital, only PT (Beta coefficient 0.007 days per min, 95% CI 0.003, 0.011, p < 0.001) and conversion to open surgery (1.4 days, 95% CI 0.05, 2.7, p = 0.42) were significant. Every extra hour of PT was associated with 0.42 more days in hospital for the donor.

4. Discussion

The purpose of this study was to examine the effect of

AT and PT on short term outcomes in laparoscopic LDKT. AT was associated with DGF, higher recipient POD5 serum Cr, and longer recipient stays in hospital. PT was also associated with DGF as well as longer donor hospital stay. Theoretically longer AT and PT could be associated with ischemic injury, longer stays in hospital and possibly poor long term function. We also examined SGF as SGF has been associated with poor long term graft survival in deceased donor kidney transplantation (DDKT) [11,12]. Surprisingly PT but not AT was associated with SGF in our study.

In a recent study regarding impact of AT on the indicators of EGF after DDKT, AT associated with DGF [13]. This report also showed that every 5 minutes of longer AT added 1 extra day to the duration of recipient hospital stay after DDKT. In our current study 13.5 minutes of longer AT leaded to the same result. This significant difference can be explained by the fact that while the former report investigated DDKTs, our current study involved LDKTs.

Sharma *et al.* also evaluated the factors causing DGF after LDKT [14]. In this study, kidneys were predominately procured by standard open approach. Total (retrieval and anastomosis) WIT was found as a major determinant of DGF. Duration of hospital stay was significantly longer in the patient group with DGF when compared with the non-DGF patient group.

In contrast to Sharma *et al.*, our study was exclusively on laparoscopic kidney retrieval. Since almost 30% of the retrieval WIT data were missing, we were unable to calculate the total WIT. On the other hand, WIT associated with retrieval is generally quite short and the median and mean values in our study were both 5 minutes.

Hellegering *et al.* investigated the determinants of poor EGF and showed that prolonged (>45 minutes) total WIT (retrieval and anastomosis) was one of the predictors of poor EGF in either open or laparoscopic LDKT [15]. Brennan *et al.* also examined the risk factors for poor EGF in LDKTs performed after either open or laparoscopic donor nephrectomy [10]. In this study WIT emerged as an independent risk factor for poor EGF, however their WIT included the retrieval WIT.

Conversely Tyson *et al.* studied solely on laparoscopic LDKTs [16]. These authors did not find a correlation between WIT and poor EGF. Nevertheless they only examined the WIT associated with retrieval but not anastomosis.

Abreu *et al.* studied laparoscopically retrieved kidneys [17]. Although their cohort was relatively small (n = 100) and underpowered, they found that total preservation time was more important than AT with regard to graft function. In this study, total preservation time was the sum of total WIT and the cold ischemia time. This study highlights the importance of consistently defining and recording all surgical times.

Some experimental studies indicated that combination of prolonged CO_2 pneumoperitoneum and ischemia during laparoscopic kidney retrieval may increase the risk of early postoperative graft dysfunction [4,18]. In line with these findings, it has been shown that recipients of laparoscopically procured kidneys had higher short-term serum Cr compared to recipients of kidneys procured by open technique [7,19].

Abreu and coworkers examined the impact of PT and CO_2 absorption on early graft function however they did not find any correlation [17]. We did not analyze mean CO_2 absorption or pneumoperitoneum pressures. Nevertheless, as a general principle pneumoperitoneum pressures are rarely higher than 15 mmHg during laparoscopic donor nephrectomy procedures. We investigated the impact of PT on EGF and found that it correlated significantly with both DGF and SGF.

Johnson *et al.* reported that length of hospital stay after laparoscopic donor nephrectomy was significantly longer in cases with prolonged operating time [20]. They ascribed this finding to the impact of prolonged surgery time on other organ systems of the donor. In our analysis, 1 hour of longer PT added 0.42 more days to the hospital stay in the donor.

The limitations of our study are its retrospective nature in addition to missing cPRA, retrieval WIT and pneumoperitoneum pressure data. We did not examine the long-term outcomes such as graft and patient survival as our sample size is quite small. Given the intercorrelation between PT and AT and the relatively small number of events for DGF and SGF, we are not able to predict their independent contributions to early outcomes confidently.

In summary our findings highlight the need for a standardized terminology and accurate documentation of all surgical times. Acknowledging the importance at surgical times is the first step towards finding innovative ways to minimize times and improve the outcomes. Larger studies with longer follow-up periods are needed to examine the impact of AT and PT on long-term patient and graft outcomes.

REFERENCES

[1] L. E. Ratner, L. J. Ciseck, R. G. Moore, F. G. Cigarroa, H. S. Kaufman and L. R. Kavoussi, "Laparoscopic Live Donor Nephrectomy," *Transplantation*, Vol. 60, No. 9, 1995, pp. 1047-1049.

[2] T. L. Merlin, D. F. Scott, M. M. Rao, *et al.*, "The Safety and Efficacy of Laparoscopic Live Donor Nephrectomy: A Systematic Review," *Transplantation*, Vol. 70, No. 12, 2000, pp. 1659-1666. http://dx.doi.org/10.1097/00007890-200012270-00001

[3] N. F. Kok, W. Weimar, I. P. Alwayn and J. N. Ijzermans, "The Current Practice of Live Donor Nephrectomy in

Europe," *Transplantation*, Vol. 82, No. 7, 2006, pp. 892-897.
http://dx.doi.org/10.1097/01.tp.0000235511.19629.0d

[4] G. Akbulut, C. Polat, F. Aktepe, *et al.*, "The Oxidative Effect of Prolonged CO_2 Pneumoperitoneum on Renal Tissue of Rats," *Surgical Endoscopy*, Vol. 18, No. 9, 2004, pp. 1384-1388.
http://dx.doi.org/10.1007/s00464-003-9114-9

[5] E. J. Hazebroek, R. W. de Bruin, N. D. Bouvy, *et al.*, "Long-Term Impact of Pneumoperitoneum Used for Laparoscopic Donor Nephrectomy on Renal Function and Histomorphology in Donor and Recipient Rats," *Annals of Surgery*, Vol. 237, No. 3, 2003, pp. 351-357.
http://dx.doi.org/10.1097/01.SLA.0000055272.96210.A0

[6] E. J. Hazebroek, R. W. de Bruin, N. D. Bouvy, *et al.*, "Short-Term Impact of Carbon Dioxide, Helium and Gasless Laparoscopic Donor Nephrectomy on Renal Function and Histomorphology in Donor and Recipient," *Surgical Endoscopy*, Vol. 16, No. 2, 2002, pp. 245-251.
http://dx.doi.org/10.1007/s00464-001-8169-8

[7] C. Troppmann, D. B. Ormond and R. V. Perez, "Laparoscopic (vs Open) Live Donor Nephrectomy: A UNOS Database Analysis of Early Graft Function and Survival," *American Journal of Transplantation*, Vol. 3, No. 10, 2003, pp. 1295-1301.
http://dx.doi.org/10.1046/j.1600-6143.2003.00216.x

[8] J. M. Nogueira, C. B. Cangro, J. C. Fink, *et al.*, "A Comparison of Recipient Renal Outcomes with Laparoscopic versus Open Live Donor Nephrectomy," *Transplantation*, Vol. 67, No. 5, 1999, pp. 722-728.
http://dx.doi.org/10.1097/00007890-199903150-00014

[9] J. M. Nogueira, A. Haririan, S. C. Jacobs, *et al.*, "The Detrimental Effect of Poor Early Graft Function after Laparoscopic Live Donor Nephrectomy on Graft Outcomes," *American Journal of Transplantation*, Vol. 9, No. 2, 2009, pp. 337-347.
http://dx.doi.org/10.1111/j.1600-6143.2008.02477.x

[10] T. V. Brennan, C. E. Freise, T. F. Fuller, A. Bostrom, S. J. Tomlanovich and S Feng, "Early Graft Function after Living Donor Kidney Transplantation Predicts Rejection But Not Outcomes," *American Journal of Transplantation*, Vol. 4, No. 6, 2004, pp. 971-979.
http://dx.doi.org/10.1111/j.1600-6143.2004.00441.x

[11] N. Smail, J. Tchervenkov, S. Paraskevas, *et al.*, "Impact of Early Graft Function on 10 Year Graft Survival in Recipients of Kidneys from Standard or Expanded Criteria Donors," *Transplantation*, Vol. 96, No. 2, 2013, pp. 176-181. http://dx.doi.org/10.1097/TP.0b013e318297443b

[12] A. Humar, E. M. Johnson, W. D. Payne, *et al.*, "Effect of Initial Slow Graft Function on Renal Allograft Rejection and Survival," *Clinical Transplantation*, Vol. 11, No. 6, 1997, pp. 623-627.

[13] K. Marzouk, J. Lawen, I. Alwayn and B. A. Kiberd, "The Impact of Vascular Anastomosis Time on Early Kidney Transplant Outcomes," *Transplantation Research*, Vol. 2, No. 8, 2013.
http://dx.doi.org/10.1186/2047-1440-2-8

[14] A. K. Sharma, S. L. Tolani, G. L. Rathi, P. Sharma, H. Gupta and R. Gupta, "Evaluation of Factors Causing Delayed Graft Function in Live Related Donor Renal Transplantation," *Saudi Journal of Kidney Diseases and Transplantation*, Vol. 21, No. 2, 2010, pp. 242-245.

[15] J. Hellegering, J. Visser, H. J. Kloke, *et al.*, "Deleterious Influence of Prolonged Warm Ischemia in Living Donor Kidney Transplantation," *Transplantation Proceedings*, Vol. 44, No. 5, 2012, pp. 1222-1226.
http://dx.doi.org/10.1016/j.transproceed.2012.01.118

[16] M. Tyson, E. Castle, P. Andrews, *et al.*, "Early Graft Function after Laparoscopically Procured Living Donor Kidney Transplantation," *Journal of Urology*, Vol. 184, No. 4, 2010, pp. 1434-1439.
http://dx.doi.org/10.1016/j.juro.2010.06.013

[17] S. C. Abreu, D. A. Goldfarb, I. Derweesh, *et al.*, "Factors Related to Delayed Graft Function after Laparoscopic Live Donor Nephrectomy," *Journal of Urology*, Vol. 171 No. 1, 2004, pp. 52-57.
http://dx.doi.org/10.1097/01.ju.0000098819.79442.ce

[18] W. Khoury, K. Jakowlev, A. Fein, H. Orenstein, R. Nakache and A. A. Weinbroum, "Renal Apoptosis Following Carbon Dioxide Pneumoperitoneum in a Rat Model," *Journal of Urology*, Vol. 180, No. 4, 2008, pp. 1554-1558.
http://dx.doi.org/10.1016/j.juro.2008.06.008

[19] L. E. Ratner, L. R. Kavoussi, P. G. Schulam, J. S. Bender, T. H. Magnuson and R. Montgomery, "Comparison of Laparoscopic Live Donor Nephrectomy versus the Standard Open Approach," *Transplantation Proceedings*, Vol. 29, No. 1-2, 1997, pp. 138-139.
http://dx.doi.org/10.1016/S0041-1345(96)00037-1

[20] E. M. Johnson, M. J. Remucal, K. J. Gillingham, R. A. Dahms, J. S. Najarian and A. J. Matas, "Complications and Risks of Living Donor Nephrectomy," *Transplantation*, Vol. 64, No. 8, 1997, pp. 1124-1128.
http://dx.doi.org/10.1097/00007890-199710270-00007

29

Reversal of Severe Volume Deplete Acute Kidney Injury by Rasburicase

Edward P. Nord, Deep Patel, Heesuck Suh, Nand K. Wadhwa
Division of Nephrology, Department of Medicine, School of Medicine,
State University of New York at Stony Brook, Stony Brook, USA
Email: nand.wadhwa@stonybrookmedicine.edu

ABSTRACT

We report on a case of acute kidney injury in a patient with severe volume depletion from high ileostomy output and poor oral intake associated with hyperuricemia and hyperkalemia. The patient presented with similar features on three separate admissions. A conservative management approach was undertaken that included infusion of rasburicase, since the patient refused to undergo hemodialysis on each occasion. Rasburicase is a recombinant urate oxidase enzyme that converts uric acid to allantoin which is five to ten times more soluble than uric acid in urine, thereby enhancing urinary excretion. Rasburicase was administered each time and was followed by a prompt increase in urine output, rapid decrease in serum uric acid level, and recovery of renal function without the need for acute renal replacement therapy. We believe that rasburicase, with a molecular weight of 34 kDa, crossed the glomerular filtration barrier and entered the tubular fluid where it dissolved intra-tubular uric acid, thus relieving obstruction, thereby rapidly enhancing urine excretion and improving renal function. Based on this experience, we propose that rasburicase offers an alternative treatment for acute kidney injury in similar types of settings. To the best of our knowledge this is the first reported case in this situation.

Keywords: Acute Kidney Injury; Rasburicase; Hyperuricemia; Ileostomy

1. Introduction

Patients with ileostomies can acutely develop high volume output states that may be associated with acute kidney injury and life threatening electrolyte and acid base disorders [1]. Traditionally this is treated with intravenous fluid and if indicated, hemodialysis. We report a case where high ileostomy output resulted in severe volume depletion, acute kidney injury, and marked hyperuricemia on three separate occasions. On all three occasions the patient adamantly refused to undergo hemodialysis. Rasburicase, a recombinant urate oxidase enzyme [2] was administered on each of these occasions and was followed by a prompt increase in urine output, rapid decrease in serum uric acid level, and recovery of renal function. We submit that rasburicase administration was responsible for the described course of events and should be considered as an alternate approach to management of acute kidney injury in similar clinical settings.

2. Case Report

A 59-year-old woman presented to the emergency room with nausea, vomiting and fatigue. She reported increased ileostomy output and decreased urine output. Her past medical history was significant for type 2 diabetes mellitus, hyperlipidemia and chronic obstructive airway disease. She had undergone right nephrectomy in 1995 for obstructive nephrolithiasis. Four months prior to this presentation she underwent a total abdominal hysterictomy and bilateral salpingo-ooperectomy for stage 1 A endometrial adenocarcinoma. Her hospital course was complicated by bowel perforation requiring partial ileal resection and ileostomy. Since creation of the ileostomy the patient has had two similar episodes described below, requiring admission to the hospital.

Six weeks prior to the current admission she presented to the emergency room with a 3 day history of nausea, vomiting, high ileostomy output, poor oral intake, and diminished urine output for one day. She denied fever, chills or abdominal pain. Her medications included pioglitazone, pravastatin, fenofibrate, aspirin, tiotropium and astelin nasal spray. Her admission blood pressure was 93/61 mmHg, heart rate 88 beats a minute and regular, temperature 35.9˚C and respiratory rate 16 breaths/min. Her oral mucous membranes were dry. The ileostomy was intact. Initial laboratory data revealed serum sodium (Na^+) 128 mEq/L (128 mmol/L), potassium (K^+) 7.0 mEq/L (7.0

mmol/L), chloride 82 mEq/L (82 mmol/L), and bicarbonate 30 mEq/L (30 mmol/L). Blood urea nitrogen (BUN) was 146 mg/dl (52.1 mmol/L), serum creatinine (SCr) 11.2 mg/dl (990.1 umol/L) (from a baseline value of 0.7 mg/dl, 61.9 umol/L), phosphorus 16.5 mg/dl (5.3 mmol/L), and uric acid 24.4 mg/dl (1.45 mmol/L). No significant abnormalities were noted on EKG. An abdominal computed tomography (CT) scan revealed a kidney on the left with mild perinephric stranding and prominence of the collecting system, without hydronephrosis. She received 2.7 liters of normal saline intravenously and voided 30cc/hr of urine. Hemodialysis was offered but the patient adamantly refused. At this point she received rasburicase 7.5 mg intravenously over 30 minutes (0.08 mg/kg/dose). Her urine output increased to 1300 cc (approximately 130 ml/hr) over the next 10 hours. Fifteen hours following rasburicase infusion, serum K^+ decreased to 3.1 mEq/L (3.1mmol/L), BUN declined to 116 mg/dl (41.4 mmol/L) and SCr 8.67 mg/dl (766.4 umol/L). The serum uric acid level had decreased to 5.4 mg/dl (0.32 mmol/L) within 24 hours. White blood cell count decreased from an admission value of $7.1 \times 10^3/mL^3$ to $2.1 \times 10^3/mL^3$ and spontaneously recovered. The patient was continued on intravenous hydration throughout her ten day hospital stay. Her ileostomy output decreased with diphenoxy/atropine. She was discharged home with a SCr of 1.27 mg/dl (112 umol/L).

Two weeks later, routine laboratory tests revealed a serum of Na^+ 123 mEq/L (123 mmol/L), K^+ 8.5 mEq/L (8.5 mmol/L), chloride 88 mEq/L (88 mmol/L), bicarbonate 21 mEq/L (21 mmol/L), BUN 80 mg/dl (28.6 mmol/L) and SCr 6.37 mg/dl (563.11 umol/L). The patient was again hospitalized with symptoms of nausea, vomiting, decreased oral intake and high ileostomy output. Vital signs revealed blood pressure 104/73mmHg and heart rate 112 beats/min. The physical exam was significant for dry mucous membranes. Repeat laboratory data revealed serum Na^+ 130 mEq/L (130 mmol/L), K^+ 8.0mEq/L (8.0 mmol/L), chloride 88 mEq/L (88 mmol/L), bicarbonate 21 mEq/L (21 mmol/L), SCr 6.30 mg/dl (556.9 umol/L), phosphorus 6.6 mg/dl (2.1 mmol/L), and uric acid 12.1 mg/dl (0.72 mmol/L). Renal sonogram showed the single left kidney with no evidence of hydronephrosis. She was given 2 liters of intravenous normal saline along with three doses of sodium polystyrene sulfonate (30 mg) over4 hours. No increase in urine output was noted. The patient again refused hemodialysis. Rasburicase 11.5 mg (0.13 mg/kg/dose)was infused over 30 minutes. Urine output increased to 920 ml over the next 24 hours. Fifteen hours post rasburicase infusion, serum K^+ was 4.8 mEq/L (4.8 mmol/L), BUN 66 mg/dl (23.6 mmol/L) and SCr 6.23 mg/dl (550 umol/L). Serum uric acid level had decreased to 1.8mg/dl (0.11 mmol/L). Neutropenia evolved which required a single subcutaneous dose of filgastrim (Neupogen) 300 microgram. The patient was discharged after a 7 day hospital stay with a SCr of 1.56 mg/dl (137.9 umol/L) and a normal white blood cell count.

On the current admission, blood pressure was 113/68 mmHg, heart rate 113 beats/min, temperature 35.4°C, and respiratory rate 18 breaths/min with O_2 saturation of 98% on room air. Mucous membranes were dry. Cardiovascular, pulmonary and neurological examinations were unremarkable. Abdominal examination revealed an intact ileostomy, no tenderness, and normal bowel sounds. Laboratory tests showed serum Na^+ 132 mEq/L (132 mmol/L), K^+ 8.1mEq/L (8.1 mmol/L), chloride 95 mEq/L (95.0 mmol/L), bicarbonate 17 mEq/L (17.0 mmol/L), SCr 8.0 mg/dl (707.2 umol/L), phosphorus 7.2 mg/dl (2.3 mmol/L) and uric acid 18.6 mg/dl (1.1 mmol/L). The renal sonogram was unchanged. The patient was given three doses of sodium polystyrene sulfonate (30 gm), and calcium gluconate 1 gm and 50% dextrose (15 gm) and 10 units of regular insulin intravenously. Five liters of normal saline were infused over the initial 24 hours with no urine output. She again refused hemodialysis. A single intravenous dose of rasburicase 6 mg (0.08 mg/kg/dose) was given. Within 24 hours, the urine output increased to 50ml/hr and serum chemistry showed K^+ 3.2 mEq/L (3.2 mmol/L), BUN 76 mg/dl (27.1 mmol/L), SCr 6.67 mg/dl (589.6 umol/L) and uric acid of 4.7 mg/dl (0.28 mmol/L). The white blood cell count decreased from $6.4 \times 10^3/mL^3$ to $2.5 \times 10^3/mL^3$and recovered spontaneously. She continued to receive intravenous hydration until her sixth hospital day at which point she underwent reversal of the ileostomy. The patient was discharged home 1 month later with a SCr of 0.83 mg/dl (73.4 umol/L).

3. Discussion

We report on a case of acute kidney injury in a patient with severe volume depletion from high ileostomy output associated with hyperuricemia and hyperkalemia on three separate admissions. A conservative approach was taken in keeping with the patient's refusal to undergo hemodialysis on each occasion. Administration of rasburicase was followed by a dramatic decrease in serum uric acid level, with a concomitant increase in urine output and significant improvement in renal function on each occasion, alleviating the need for hemodialysis. We submit that rasburicase was responsible for this course of events.

Acute urate nephropathy is most commonly encountered in patients with large tumor burdens who undergo chemotherapy and where there is rapid destruction of tumor cells, the so called "tumor lysis syndrome" [3]. Very elevated serum uric acid levels contributing to acute renal failure has also been described in young infants after cardiovascular surgery [4], and has also been proposed as a risk factor for acute kidney injury in adult patients undergoing high risk cardiac surgery [5,6]. A rise in serum uric acid is also seen in toxic and ischemic acute kidney injury where it is thought to be the result of both increased generation and decreased excretion of uric acid [7]. In all of these settings there is reason to invoke the elevated serum uric acid in the pathogenesis of acute kidney injury.

A number of mechanisms have been proposed by which uric acid may contribute to acute kidney injury. First, the markedly elevated serum uric acid level results in supersaturation of the tubular fluid with precipitation of uric acid and obstruction of the tubular lumina. From micro puncture studies it is known that uric acid precipitates mainly in the distal tubule where uric acid concentration is high and the environment is acidic [8]. Indeed precipitation of uric acid was also noted in the vasa rectae [8]. Second, in an animal model, hyperuricemia has been shown to cause renal vasoconstriction, characterized by a marked increase in resistance primarily of the afferent arteriole [9]. The mechanism by which this occurs appears to be a suppression of nitric oxide production since vasoconstriction can be reversed with L-arginine [10]. Third, uric acid has been shown to stimulate an inflammatory response in vascular smooth muscle cells via proinflammatory cytokines such asMCP-1 [11] Whether any of these mechanisms play a role in acute kidney injury associated with severe volume depletion as described herein, remains to be determined.

Patients with well-functioning ileostomies under steady state conditions can have a 7% to 11% decrease in total body sodium and water [12] reflecting a stable, modest fluid depleted state. With increased ileostomy output and the attendant volume depletion, these individuals can develop sudden acute electrolyte and acid-base disorders [1]. Most commonly, and as observed in our patient, metabolic acidosis ensues due to the high bicarbonate content of the ileostomy fluid. The associated hyperkalemia can be explained by the acute drop in glomerular filtration rate. A paucity of data exists regarding uric acid levels in this setting. In this regard Adler and coworkers [13] reported a series of 133 dehydrated children under the age of 4 years admitted with diarrhea. The majority of children and infants (80%) had transient hyperuricemia that correlated with the serum urea nitrogen level, with a mean serum uric acid level of 12.3 mg/dl (0.73 mmol/L), and range of 2.3 mg/dl (0.14 mmol/L) to 38.0 mg/dl (2.26 mmol/L). Most children had urate crystals in their urine. With volume repletion, uric acid levels returned to normal.

Rasburicase is a recombinant urate oxidase enzyme that converts uric acid to allantoin which is five to ten times more soluble than uric acid in water, thereby enhancing urinary excretion of this product of nucleic acid degradation [2]. Rasburicase, with a molecular weight of 34 kDa, can cross the glomerular filtration barrier and enter the tubular fluid where it can carry out its intended effect [2]. Rasburicase has been reported to be effective in the treatment of renal failure due to obstructive uric acid stones [14]. Both patients in that report did not show any improvement in renal function with intravenous fluid and hemodialysis; rasburicase infusion resulted in brisk diuresis and renal recovery within 24 hours. Repeat abdominal CT scans after rasburicase therapy confirmed complete resolution of uric acid stones with no obstructtion to the urinary tract [14]. A successful outcome following the use of rasburicase has now been reported in an anuric pediatric patient with hyperuricemia in the setting of the hemolytic uremic syndrome [15], and in two teens with acute kidney injury secondary to rhabdomyolysis caused by ecstasy intoxication [16]. In all these settings and now in the patient we report, rasburicase most likely dissolved intra-tubular uric acid, thus relieving obstruction, thereby rapidly enhancing urine excretion and improving renal function.

Acute kidney injury associated with hyperuricemia is traditionally treated with volume expansion and urinary alkalization which favors solubilization of uric acid to urate in the urine. This helps to relieve intra-tubular obstruction. This is based on animal studies where high tubular fluid flow, whether induced by solute or water diuresis, was the primary mechanism of protection in acute urate nephropathy, with alkalization playing a lesser role [17]. Rasburicase rapidly lowers serum uric acid by converting it to a soluble compound allantoin, thereby dramatically decreasing proximal tubular uric acid excretion and preventing its precipitation in the tubular lumen. This mechanism probably holds true both in acute kidney injury related to marked hyperuricemia, and the tumor lysis syndrome (TLS). In addition, rasburicase is freely filtered at the level of the glomerulus and enters the tubular fluid where it can dissolve uric acid crystals and relieve intra tubular obstruction. This ameliorates acute kidney injury associated with acute uric acid nephropathy. Hemodialysis is a treatment of choice in patients with volume overload and hyperkalemia associated with severe hyperuricemia. If there are relative contraindications for access placement such as a severe bleeding disorder and/or refusal by a patient, rasburicase may offer an alternative therapeutic choice as demonstrated in our patient.

In conclusion, we report on a case with acute kidney injury associated with high ileostomy output and secondary hyperuricemia which responded to rasburicase infusion. On three separate occasions, rasburicase infusion led to a dramatic decrease in serum uric acid level over a short period of time, with rapid improvement in renal function. Hemodialysis was obviated in keeping with the patient's request. Based on this limited experience, we propose that rasburicase offers an alternative treatment for acute kidney injury in similar types of settings. Additional clinical studies are needed to confirm this observation.

REFERENCES

[1] W. J. Weise, *et al.*, "Acute Electrolyte and Acid-Base Disorders in Patients with Ileostomies: A Case Series," *American Journal of Kidney Diseases: The Official Journal of the National Kidney Foundation*, Vol. 52, No. 3, 2008, pp. 494-500.

[2] L. Cammalleri and M. Malaguarnera, "Rasburicase Represents a New Tool for Hyperuricemia in Tumor Lysis Syndrome and in Gout," *International Journal of Medical Sciences*, Vol. 4, No. 2, 2007, pp. 83-93. doi:10.7150/ijms.4.83

[3] S. C. Howard, D. P. Jones and C. H. Pui, "The Tumor Lysis Syndrome," *The New England Journal of Medicine*, Vol. 364, No. 19, 2011, pp. 1844-1854. doi:10.1056/NEJMra0904569

[4] R. W. Chesney, *et al.*, "Acute Renal Failure: An Important Complication of Cardiac Surgery in Infants," *The Journal of Pediatrics*, Vol. 87, No. 3, 1975, pp. 381-388. doi:10.1016/S0022-3476(75)80640-8

[5] A. A. Ejaz, *et al.*, "Uric Acid: A Novel Risk Factor for Acute Kidney Injury in High-Risk Cardiac Surgery Patients?" *American Journal of Nephrology*, Vol. 30, No. 5, 2009, pp. 425-429. doi:10.1159/000238824

[6] A. A. Ejaz, *et al.*, "Effect of Uric Acid Lowering Therapy on the Prevention of Acute Kidney Injury in Cardiovascular Surgery," *International Urology and Nephrology*, 2012. doi:10.1007/s11255-012-0192-2

[7] A. A. Ejaz, *et al.*, "Could Uric Acid Have a Role in Acute Renal Failure?" *Clinical Journal of the American Society of Nephrology*, Vol. 2, No. 1, 2007, pp. 16-21. doi:10.2215/CJN.00350106

[8] J. D. Conger, *et al.*, "A Micropuncture Study of the Early Phase of Acute Urate Nephropathy," *The Journal of Clinical Investigation*, Vol. 58, No. 3, 1976, pp. 681-689. doi:10.1172/JCI108514

[9] L. G. Sanchez-Lozada, *et al.*, "Mild Hyperuricemia Induces Glomerular Hypertension in Normal Rats," *American Journal of Physiology. Renal Physiology*, Vol. 283, No. 5, 2002, pp. F1105-F1110.

[10] U. M. Khosla, *et al.*, "Hyperuricemia Induces Endothelial Dysfunction," *Kidney International*, Vol. 67, No. 5, 2005, pp. 1739-1742. doi:10.1111/j.1523-1755.2005.00273.x

[11] J. Kanellis, *et al.*, "Uric Acid Stimulates Monocyte Chemo Attractant Protein-1 Production in Vascular Smooth Muscle Cells via Mitogen-Activated Protein Kinase and Cyclooxygenase-2," *Hypertension*, Vol. 41, No. 6, 2003, pp. 1287-1293. doi:10.1161/01.HYP.0000072820.07472.3B

[12] A. M. Clarke, *et al.*, "Chronic Dehydration and Sodium Depletion in Patients with Established Ileostomies," *Lancet*, Vol. 2, No. 7519, 1967, pp. 740-743. doi:10.1016/S0140-6736(67)91945-9

[13] R. Adler, *et al.*, "Hyperuricemia in Diarrheal Dehydration," *American Journal of Diseases of Children*, Vol. 136, No. 3, 1982, pp. 211-213.

[14] T. P. Segura, *et al.*, "Efficacy of Rasburicase Therapy in Obstructive Renal Failure Secondary to Urolithiasis: A Novel Therapeutic Option," *Nefrologia: Publicacionoficial de la Sociedad Espanola Nefrologia*, Vol. 28, No. 1, 2008, pp. 102-105.

[15] A. A. Acosta and R. J. Hogg, "Rasburicase for Hyperuricemia in Hemolytic Uremic Syndrome," *Pediatric Nephrology*, Vol. 27, No. 2, 2012, pp. 325-329.

[16] P. Y. Lin, *et al.*, "Rasburicase Improves Hyperuricemia in Patients with Acute Kidney Injury Secondary to Rhabdomyolysis Caused by Ecstasy Intoxication and Exertional Heat Stroke," *Pediatric Critical Care Medicine*, Vol. 12, No. 6, 2011, pp. e424-e427.

[17] J. D. Conger and S. A. Falk, "Intrarenal Dynamics in the Pathogenesis and Prevention of Acute Urate Nephropathy," *The Journal of Clinical Investigation*, Vol. 59, No. 5, 1977, pp. 786-793. doi:10.1172/JCI108700

How Safe Is Conversion from Tacrolimus to Its Generic Drug?—A Single Center Experience

Tobias A. Marsen
Nephrology Center and KfH Kidney and Dialysis Center Köln-Lindenthal, Köln, Germany
Email: tobias.marsen@kfh-dialyse.de

ABSTRACT

Background: Generically produced cyclosporine has long been approved in the treatment of organ transplant recipients and several publications have dealt with its use. For tacrolimus, however, very few data exist for safety and efficacy after conversion to its generic in kidney transplant recipients. **Methods:** In this single-center observational study, 14 kidney transplant carriers were converted to generic tacrolimus as part of aftercare, and graft function, fasting tacrolimus levels and the daily tacrolimus dose was pursued for up to 95 weeks. **Results:** Average drug doses changed from 3.64 ± 1.88 mg/day with the original to 3.33 ± 1.72 mg/day after conversion to generic tacrolimus ($p = 0.33$). Tacrolimus fasting levels were 6.23 ± 1.68 ng/ml before and 5.89 ± 1.15 ng/ml after conversion ($p = 0.66$). Average serum creatinine values of 2.26 ± 1.08 mg/dl after conversion did not differ from previous values of 1.99 ± 0.74 mg/dl ($p = 0.15$). **Conclusions:** These data support the assumption, that it is safe to convert stable kidney transplant patients from the original galenic formulation under close scrutiny to the generically produced substance. Conversion is easy to be implemented in the routine follow-up and thus represents an option in the therapy with calcineurin inhibitors, which will contribute to cost reduction in the health system.

Keywords: Kidney; Pharmacoeconomics; Tacrolimus; Transplantation

1. Introduction

Calcineurin inhibitors (CNI) cyclosporine and tacrolimus are milestones in the therapy of organ transplantation. They are the basic immunosuppressants in rejection prophylaxis. Under their use, patient as well as graft survival could be significantly improved.

The lifelong therapy however makes this treatment a most cost-intensive requirement. Upon the expiration of patent protection in 1995 a strong generic market grew for cyclosporine and since 2009 for tacrolimus. Despite all security concerns for generic cyclosporine, its use in the follow-up treatment of organ recipients has been regulated by experts [1] and in many centers now has become the rule. Increasing rates of rejection episodes have not been described [2-4].

Since 2009, tacrolimus, because no longer protected by patents, has been made available as a generic formulation for clinical use, too. Under the increasing pressure on costs in the health system in industrial nations, in Germany by the health insurers and by discounting contracts, there is a growing uncertainty concerning the safety of prescribing generic tacrolimus. To document a practical approach in the use of generically produced tacrolimus, as well as to the diverse needs of all parties to meet and generate no disadvantages for graft survival, 14 stable kidney transplant recipients were followed in a single center cohort study after a shift in favor of a tacrolimus generic. Efficacy and safety parameters for graft function and immunosuppression were obtained.

2. Subjects and Methods

In this single-center observational study we identified 14 patients, 9 male and 5 female with a functioning kidney transplant and a stable graft function under an immunosuppressive therapy with tacrolimus (Prograf®, Astellas Pharma GmbH, Munich, Germany[1]). The mean patient age was 51 ± 16.5 years and the time after transplantation varied from 12 - 138 months, with a mean of 63 months. The patients were switched as part of their routine follow-up care in the nephrologic center in a 1:1 fashion to an equivalent dose of generic tacrolimus (Tacrolimus Hexal®, Hexal AG, Holzkirchen, Germany[2]) as a commercial medication and tracked continuously for 29 - 95

[1]Prograf® composition: Tacrolimus-1-H_2O, Methylhydroxypropylcellulose, Lactose-1-H_2O, Croscarmellose-sodium, Mg-Stearate, Gelatine, Titandioxide, Fe-(III)oxide, Phospholipids.

[2]Tacrolimus Hexal® composition: Tacrolimus-1-H_2O, Methylhydroxypropylcellulose, Lactose-1-H_2O, Croscarmellose-sodium, Mg-Stearate, Gelatine, Titandioxide, Na-dodecylsulfate, Sorbitan laurate, Fe-oxide-hydrate.

weeks (mean 66.4 ± 19.4 weeks). For safety reasons, controls were performed at weekly intervals initially after conversion and were subsequently extended to monthly and to quarterly controls. Longitudinal comparative data were collected for the trough levels of the immunosuppressant prior to and after conversion, as well as for excretory graft function. Routinely clinical data and blood samples were collected after switching and the tacrolimus dose was adapted as necessary. The following routine laboratory parameters were captured: endogenous creatinine clearance, serum creatinine, tacrolimus trough levels (Abbott tacrolimus assay), blood count, differential blood count, absolute lymphocyte number, Na (sodium), K (potassium), Ca (calcium), PO_4 (phosphate), BUN (blood urea nitrogen), uric acid, ALT (alanine aminotransferase), GGT (gamma-glutamyl transpeptidase), AP (alkaline phosphatase), LDH (lactate dehydrogenase), albumin/creatinine ratio, CRP (C-reactive protein), urine sediment (analyzed semi-automatically via urine stix).

Statistical Analysis

To analyze significant changes in tacrolimus trough levels, tacrolimus doses, and serum creatinine values before and after conversion, student paired t-test was used. The level of significance was set to $p < 0.05$. Results are presented as mean ± standard deviation.

3. Results

14 patients (9 male, 5 female) at the age of 25 to 75 years, with a mean of 51 ± 16.5 years, after local ethics votum and informed consent was obtained, were converted to generically manufactured Tacrolimus Hexal® (**Table 1**). This drug is shown to be bioequivalent to the original drug Prograf® in cross-over studies [5]. At the time of conversion, the patients had a functioning-kidney transplant between 12 to 138 months, with a mean of 63 months. The transplant kidney function was stable at the time of conversion in 13 patients, a male patient was confirmed 41 months previously with biopsy proven chronic allograft rejection, which prompted his conversion to Prograf®. Despite conversion he had a continuous decrease in graft function, serum creatinine had increased from 3.7 to 4.2 mg/dl during run-in. Furthermore, a female patient was 36 month prior to conversion also confirmed with biopsy proven chronic-allograft rejection, but during run-in had a much less accelerated course with serum creatinine from 2.55 to 2.6 mg/dl.

Among all patients 10 out of 14 had a concomitant immunosuppression therapy with steroids, 11 out of 14 received mycophenolate mofetil, either MMF (500 - 2000 mg/day) or MMF-sodium (360 - 1440 mg/day), 2 out of 14 were on azathioprine. 5 out of 14 patients were on a dual immunosuppression. During the observation phase the concomitant immunosuppression was not altered in the dose or the choice of preparations. All patients suffered from stable arterial hypertension as concomitant disease, and 4 had NIDDM/IDDM.

After conversion, generic tacrolimus was well tolerated in all patients, there were no symptoms of intolerance, safety laboratory parameters remained unchanged. The average drug doses (**Figure 1**) and tacrolimus levels (**Figure 2**) before and after conversion were not significantly different from each other in the longitudinal course (**Table**

Table 1. Patients individual demographic characteristics (Mean values represent average data for periods "run-in pre conversion" and "follow up after conversion").

Sex	Age (years)	Time since TX (month)	Run-in pre conversion (weeks)	Follow-up after conversion (weeks)	Mean Tac trough level (ng/ml) Post/ pre conversion	Mean Tac dose (mg/day) Post/ pre conversion	Mean creatinine (mg/dl) Post/ pre conversion
Male	45	25	61	79	5.95/5.9	2.0/2.6	1.25/1.21
Male	63	29	65	67	6.92/8.38	3.2/4.0	1.70/1.86
Female	72	88	64	95	5.19/6.66	4.0/4.0	1.24/1.35
Male	31	136	76	75	4.50/6.00	3.0/3.0	1.98/2.07
Female	68	39	76	48	5.75/5.92	4.0/6.0	1.10/1.08
Female	75	56	64	61	6.20/6.62	2.0/2.0	1.45/1.53
Female[a]	63	138	76	51	7.07/5.10	2.67/2.0	3.47/2.30
Female	43	90	29	79	7.66/7.53	5.0/5.3	3.49/2.46
Male	25	76	66	80	3.12/5.68	3.5/2.7	2.21/2.12
Male	66	46	72	86	5.57/5.42	2.0/2.7	2.21/2.32
Male	55	18	68	29	5.40/5.41	7.0/8.4	2.75/2.54
Male[a]	42	92	76	77	5.38/4.56	4.0/3.0	5.48/3.78
Male	33	37	47	35	8.03/6.35	2.3/1.0	1.65/1.70
Male	39	12	46	68	5.78/6.41	3.0/3.7	1.56/1.50

[a]patients have biopsy proven chronic allograft rejection.

2). Also, the mean serum creatinine levels did not differ from the previous values and remained stable over the study period (**Figure 3**).

During the entire observation period dose-adjustments had to be performed with both the originator or generic Tacrolimus Hexal® in 6 out of 14 cases downwards and

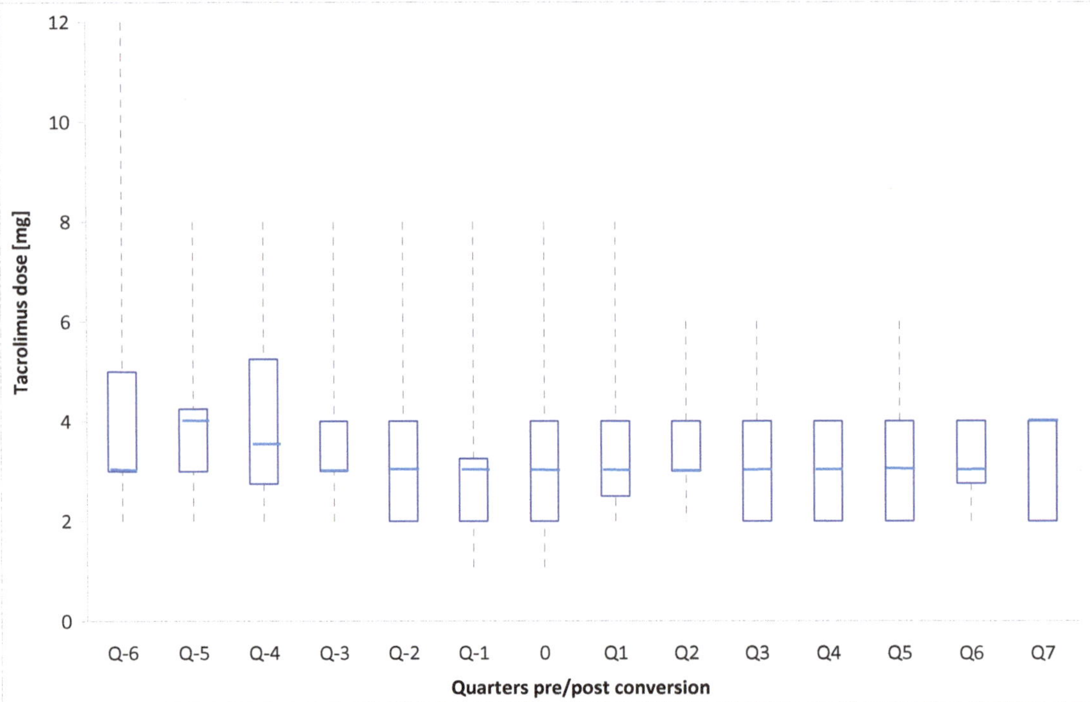

Figure 1. Box-Whisker-plot of tacrolimus daily dose followed 6 quarters before (Q − x) and 7 quarters after (Q x) generic tacrolimus conversion (each quarter represents sampling of 10 patients on average (n_{max} = 13, n_{min} = 6), time of conversion is outlined as 0).

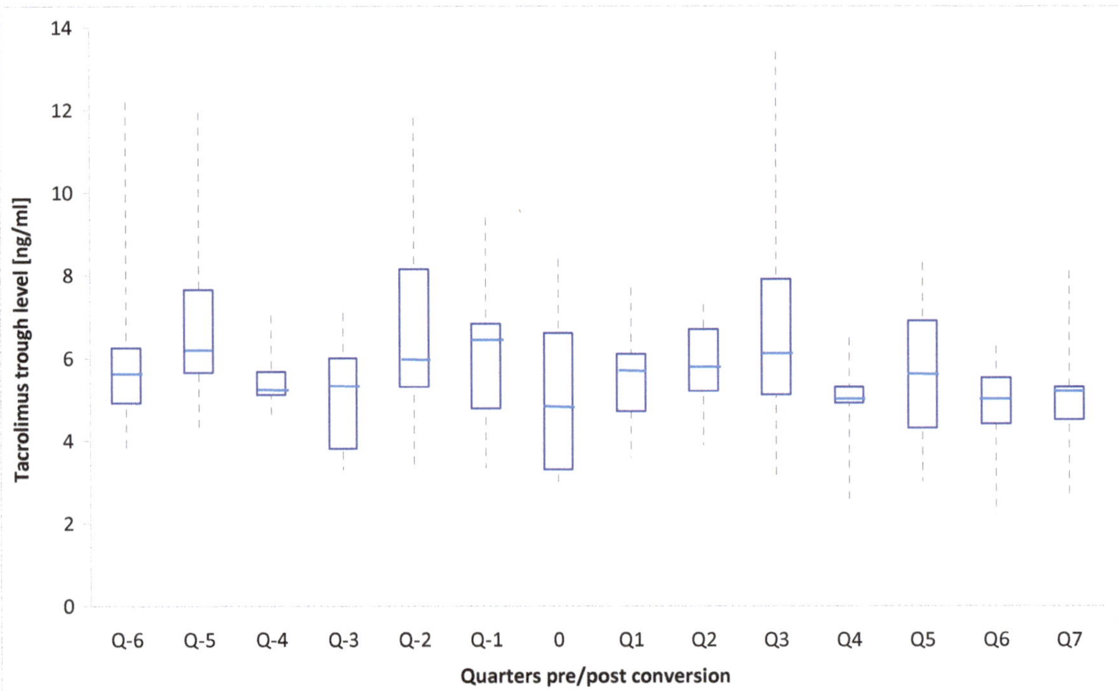

Figure 2. Box-Whisker-plot of mean tacrolimus trough levels of 14 kidney transplant recipients followed 6 quarters before (Q − x) and 7 quarters after (Q x) generic tacrolimus conversion (time of conversion is outlined as 0).

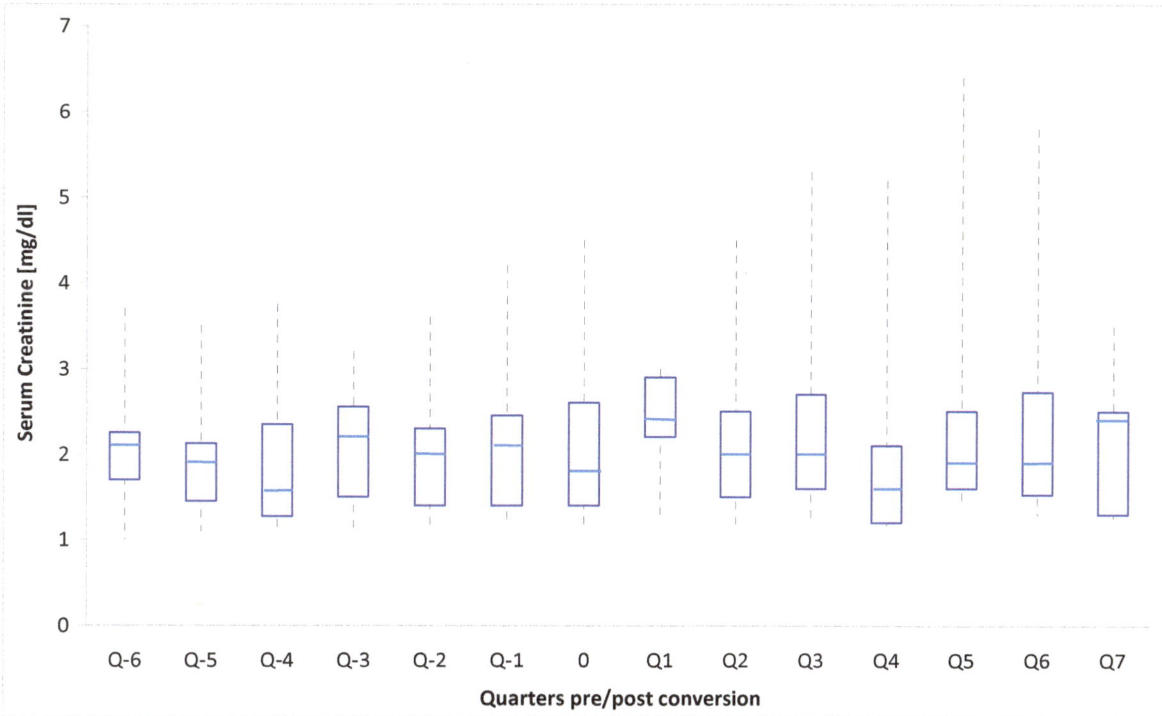

Figure 3. Box-Whisker-plot of mean creatinine levels of 14 maintenance kidney transplant recipients 6 quarters before (Q − x) and 7 quarters after (Q x) generic tacrolimus conversion (each quarter represents sampling of 10 patients on average (n_{max} = 13, n_{min} = 6), time of conversion is outlined as 0).

Table 2. Mean treatment specific patient characteristics (mean ± standard deviation). Mean values represent average data for period length as given in table 1[a].

	Mean Tac trough level [ng/ml]	Mean Tac dose [mg/day]	Mean creatinine [mg/dl] all patients[a]	Mean creatinine [mg/dl] patients with stable function
Pre conversion [weeks] 63.29 ± 13.87	6.23 ± 1.68	3.64 ± 1.88	1.99 ± 0.74	1.80 ± 0.47
Post conversion [weeks] 66.43 ± 19.38	5.90 ± 1.15	3.33 ± 1.72	2.26 ± 1.08	1.89 ± 0.70
p-Value	0.64	0.33	0.15	0.39

[a]patients with biopsy proven chronic allograft rejection included..

in 4 out of 14 upwards, in order to keep blood levels steady. After conversion no immediate dose-adjustments were necessary, however as early as week 9 a single case required a 1 mg daily increase. 4 patients required late dose-adjustments after week 14 - 17, both downwards and upwards, which have to be refered to as the usual titrations under therapy. According to our data, however, post conversion daily doses showed more stable course as pre conversion doses did, with less variation (**Figure 3**).

The excretory kidney function and all safety parameters remained stable without significant deviations compared to previously documented values. Of all patients converted, two individuals showed a continuous increase in serum creatinine levels due to a preceeding biopsy-confirmed chronic allograft rejection.

4. Discussion

The aim of the present study was to demonstrate the safety and efficacy of conversion to generic tacrolimus in stable kidney transplant patients, it was not the aim of the study to generate AUC comparisons, which were generated elsewhere [5]. Moreover, in the context of this cohort study, a practical modality for a change of this critical drug was to be delineated, which could be inserted easily into clinical praoctice, assuring a straight-forward application and a high therapeutic safety.

Critical-dose drugs are known as medications which are controlled via blood levels and in this regard have a narrow therapeutic corridor. Changes in drug preparations should ideally lead only to minor differences in blood levels, so as not to interrupt or decrease drug availability and to flare up the disease to be treated in a critical way. With calcineurin inhibitors (CNI) including tacrolimus, this would ultimately result in an impaired immune suppression and trigger organ rejection episodes. According to KDIGO guidelines for cost reduction, generic treatment of kidney transplant recipients may be admitted, if safety and efficacy could be demonstrated [6, 7]. However, conversions should be implemented by an expert in the handling and control of these therapies.

In only a single report, data for the early controlled conversion in liver and kidney transplant carriers have been documented and demonstrated the bioequivalence in clinical use [8]. The short follow-up period but especially the vigilant therapeutic drug monitoring process in this early post-transplant phase triggered critical discussion, leading to remarks on whether "we are jeopardizing our patients health if we do not perform vigilant therapeutic drug monitoring" during conversion [9]. In contrast the present study on late tacrolimus conversion could easily be integrated into the continuous ambulatory treatment of stable transplant patients and be accomplished. Drug monitoring was performed as usual without jeopardization of transplant survival or the patient's health. There were no reports of compatibility problems. Within 1 - 4 weeks after conversion, security parameters collected for therapeutic safety did not deviate significantly from the previously documented data, as well as the long-term follow-up in 12 of 14 patients revealed no change of graft function. Two patients with biopsy-proven chronic allograft rejection, however, showed a progressive decrease in graft function similar to the run-in phase before the conversion. In these patients, neither the originator nor the generic tacrolimus formulation had made a contribution to achieve a stabilized kidney function.

Despite close supervision, not before week 9 dose adjustment of generically manufactured tacrolimus was required. The probability of occurrence of this behavior is similar to the observation period before conversion, during which only 1 patient had to be reduced in dose. Further 4 patients required late adjustments on weeks 14 - 17, and could be continued without further adjustments thereafter, they may be referred to as usual dose fluctuations. The remaining patients were unchanged and dose-equivalent to the time prior to conversion. All adjustments were made on the basis of fasting blood levels for tacrolimus.

The present findings provide no data on the potential savings of total costs in this population. In a comparison between cyclosporine formulations it has been demonstrated, that, when using the generic, de novo transplant recipients revealed significantly higher total costs for the health system, resulting from the required dose escalation [10]. In contrast, conversion to tacrolimus generic in subjects 70 month after transplantation allows for savings [11]. Rising costs of treatment are primarily generated in the first 2 years after transplantation [12]. They result mainly from rejections, viral infections and delayed graft function with dialysis requirements. After this period, the cost of immunosuppressive therapy come to the fore, and comprise a majority. As shown in the present study, the switch in favor of a generic CNI, assuming a situation with stable graft function and a time point as early as 2 years after transplantation, therefore may provide the possibility of cost reduction by optimizing the cost-intensive continuous immunosuppression.

The study has certain limitations. Designed as an observational study in outpatients, adherence could not be directly validated. Also, the sample size was relatively small. Therefore, the results need to be confirmed in a larger, controlled, prospective trial.

In summary, conversion from original to generic tacrolimus is a straightforward procedure in the follow-up of a stable set of kidney transplant carriers, which in the hands of a skilled and in control of these therapies experienced clinician, can be included easily into clinical practice as part of routine follow-up examinations. It meets the health insurance requirements of cost-efficiant maintenance therapy for graft survival. Furthermore, it puts the after-care nephrologist in a position to implement the relevant budget requirements without disadvantages in the treatment needs and safety. In the future, it may be expected, that the share of generic tacrolimus will grow in size and percentage and catch up with the frequency of the original prescription drug or may overtake it.

5. Conclusion

In renal transplant carriers, stably treated with Prograf®, conversion to a generic tacrolimus can be performed in a straight forward manner. Tacrolimus fasting levels, doses employed and transplant function remain stable, without generating episodes of rejection. Cost savings potential can be fulfilled without causing harm to the patient.

6. Acknowledgements

The author greatly acknowledges the contribution of Michael Maerz, MCSc, for performing the statistical analysis.

REFERENCES

[1] S. Pollard, B. Nashan, A. Johnston, P. Hoyer, P. Belitsky, P. Keown and H. Helderman, "A Pharmacokinetic and Clinical Review of the Potential Clinical Impact of Using

Different Formulations of Cyclosporine A," *Clinical Therapeutics*, Vol. 25, No. 6, 2003, pp. 1654-1669. doi:10.1016/S0149-2918(03)80161-3

[2] W. Carnahan and T. Y. Cooper, "Neoral to Gengraf Conversion in Renal Transplant Recipients," *Transplantation Proceedings*, Vol. 35, No. 4, 2003, pp. 1308-1313. doi:10.1016/S0041-1345(03)00423-8

[3] J. S. Al Wakeel, F. A. Shaheen, M. C. Mathew, H. M. Abouzeinab, A. Al Afi, N. M. Tarif, M. S. Mousawi, T. S. Mahmoud, A. S. Alorrayad, E. A. Fagir, R. S. Dham and D. S. Shaker, "Six-month Clinical Outcome of Cyclosporine Microemulsion Formulation (Sigmasporin Microral) in Stable Renal Transplant Patients Previously Maintained on Sandimmun Neoral," *Transplantation Proceedings*, Vol. 40, No. 7, 2008, pp. 2245-2251. doi:10.1016/j.transproceed.2008.06.044

[4] H. Müller, S. Solari, C. Zuñiga, C. Pedreros, J. Troncoso, C. Morente, R. Ovalle, P. Acosta, T. Chavez and E. Albornoz, "Immunosuppression with Generic Tacrolimus and Mycophenolate Mofetil in Renal Transplant Recipients: Preliminary Report in Chile," *Transplantation Proceedings*, Vol. 40, No. 3, 2008, pp. 705-707. doi:10.1016/j.transproceed.2008.02.056

[5] "Public Assessment Report of the Medicines Evaluation Board in the Netherlands". http://db.cbg-meb.n/mri/par/nih-1340-001-002-003.pdf.

[6] T. R. Türk, O. Witzke and M. Zeier, "KDIGO-Leitlinien Zur Betreuung von Nierentransplantatempfängern," *Nephrologe*, Vol 5, No. 2, 2010, pp. 94-107. doi:10.1007/s11560-009-0369-6

[7] Kidney Disease: Improving Global Outcomes (KDIGO) Transplant Work Group, "KDIGO Clinical Practice Guideline for the Care of Kidney Transplant Recipients," *American Journal of Transplantation*, Vol. 9, Suppl. 3, 2009, pp. S1-S155. doi:10.1111/j.1600-6143.2009.02834.x

[8] J. D. Momper, T. A. Ridenour, K. S. Schonder, R. Shapiro, A. Humar and R. Venkatarmanan, "The Impact of Conversion from Prograf to Generic Tacrolimus in Liver and Kidney Transplant Recipients with Stable Graft Function," *American Journal of Transplantation*, Vol. 11, No. 9, 2011, pp. 1861-1867. doi:10.1111/j.1600-6143.2011.03615.x

[9] G. B. Klintmalm, "Immunosuppression, Generic Drugs and the FDA," *American Journal of Transplantation*, Vol. 11, No. 9, 2011, pp. 1765-1766. doi:10.1111/j.1600-6143.2011.03616.x

[10] J. H. Helderman, N. Kang, A. P. Legoretta and J. Y. Chen, "Healthcare Costs in Renal Transplant Recipients Using Branded versus Generic Cyclosporine," *Applied Health Economics and Health Policy*, Vol. 8, No. 1, 2010, pp. 61-68.

[11] L. M. McDevitt-Potter, B. Sadaka, E. M. Tichy, C. C. Rogers and S. Gabardi, "A Multicenter Experience with Generic Tacrolimus Conversion," *Transplantation*, Vol. 92, No. 6, 2011, pp. 653-657. doi:10.1097/TP.0b013e31822a79ad

[12] E. G. Hagenmeyer, B. Häussler, E. Hempel, G. Grannas, Z. Kaló, A. Kilburg and B. Nashan, "Resource Use and Treatment Costs after Kidney Tranplantation: Impact of Demographic Factors, Comorbidities, and Complications," *Transplantation*, Vol. 77, No. 1, 2004, pp. 1545-1550.

31

Pharmacological Adjuvants to Limit Erythropoietin Stimulating Agents Exposure

Iqbal Masood, Geoffrey Teehan
Department of Nephrology, Lankenau Medical Center and Lankenau Institute for Medical Research, Wynnewood, USA
Email: iqbalmasood@msn.com, gteehan@comcast.net

ABSTRACT

Anemia in chronic kidney disease (CKD) is common, causing morbidity and mortality, and is primarily due to reduced erythropoietin (EPO) release and, to a lesser degree, shortened red cell survival. Erythropoietin Stimulating Agents like epoetin Alfa and darbepoetin alpha are used commonly to treat this form of anemia. Recent evidence suggests increased morbidity and mortality associated with higher hemoglobin in the setting of these agents use. Whether these complications are due to higher dose of erythropoietin or its resistance (*i.e.*, inflammation), or achieving a higher hemoglobin remains unclear. Tightening restrictions on these agents has led to increase interest in the use of non-ESA adjuvants to improve erythropoiesis. This review will highlight the most promising of these agents.

Keywords: Anemia; Chronic Kidney Disease (CKD); End Stage Renal Disease (ESRD); Erythropoiesis Stimulating Agents (ESA); Epoetin Alfa (EPO)

1. Introduction

Anemia in chronic kidney disease (CKD) is common, causing morbidity and mortality, and is primarily due to reduced erythropoietin release and, to a lesser degree, shortened red cell survival [1,2]. The National Health and Nutrition Examination Survey (NHANES) and the Prevalence of Anemia in Early Renal Insufficiency (PAERI) studies suggest the incidence of anemia in CKD stage V is more than 70% [3]. As renal function declines, anemia prevalence increases in CKD, and its associated morbidities generally worsen [4-8].

Since the approval of recombinant human erythropoietin (epoetin Alfa, EPO) by the United States Federal Drug Administration, this and similar therapeutic agents like darbepoetin alpha (DPO) and recently approved once a month agent, methoxy polyethylene glycol-epoetin beta, called Erythropoiesis Stimulating Agents (ESAs) have become the standard of care for the treatment of the erythropoietin-deficient, normocytic anemia that occurs in most patients with CKD. Due to wide spread use of ESA, average hemoglobin in patients with CKD has increased [9]. Recent evidence suggesting increased morbidity and mortality associated with higher hemoglobin levels in the setting of ESA use has spurred interest in pharmacological adjuvants to limit ESA exposure [10-12]. Whether these complications are due to the higher dose of erythropoietin, ESA resistance (*i.e.*, inflammation), or achieving higher hemoglobin, remains unclear.

Nevertheless, all ESAs now come with a "black box warning" recommending physicians to weigh the benefits of ESA use in anemia of CKD to decrease the need for transfusions against the increased risks for serious adverse cardiovascular events. Further, dosing should be individualized to use the lowest dose of ESA sufficient to reduce the need for transfusion. Although a target hemoglobin range is not provided, the insert states that for patients with CKD who are not on dialysis ESA treatment should only begin when the hemoglobin level is less than 10 g/dL and reduce or stop the ESA dose if the hemoglobin level exceeds 10 g/dL. For patients on dialysis, one should initiate ESA treatment when the hemoglobin level is less than 10 g/dL and reduce or interrupt the ESA dose if the hemoglobin level approaches or exceeds 11 g/dl [13].

The 2012 Kidney Disease Improving Global Outcome (KDIGO) [14] recommends the same cut off for ESA initiation in patients with CKD (non-dialysis) and End Stage Renal Disease (ESRD) on dialysis. They also recommend not to use ESA to keep hemoglobin >11.5 mg/dl. Tightening restrictions on these agents has led to the use of non-ESA adjuvants to improve erythropoiesis. This review will highlight the most promising of these agents.

2. Iron

Iron is a vital to hematopoiesis. The extracorporeal process of Hemodialysis (HD) promotes constant blood, and therefore iron loss with such patients, losing an average of 2 g of iron yearly, and subsequent iron deficiency. Reduced iron stores or decreased availability of iron are the most common reasons for resistance to ESA agents [15]. Iron, either IV or oral iron replete lost iron aiding erythropoiesis.

2.1. Diagnosis of Iron Deficiency

Before starting EPO therapy, iron stores must be assessed and non-renal causes of anemia excluded. The evaluation should include testing for fecal occult blood, red blood cell indices, reticulocyte count, serum iron, total iron binding capacity, percent transferrin saturation, serum Ferritin and content of hemoglobin in reticulocyte (where available) [16,17]. Vitamin deficiencies should be corrected in CKD patients [18]. In CKD and ESRD-associated anemia, a different standard is applied to determine adequate iron stores for erythropoiesis [16].

2.2. Absolute Iron Deficiency in CKD

Absolute iron deficiency in CKD occurs when the percent transferrin saturation (TSAT) (plasma iron divided by total iron binding capacityX100) falls below 20%, and the serum Ferritin concentration is under 200 ng/mL (among Hemodialysis patients) or below 100 ng/mL among predialsyis and peritoneal dialysis (PD) patients.

2.3. Functional Iron Deficiency

Functional iron deficiency occurs when adequate iron stores, as defined by conventional criteria, are present, but the iron cannot be mobilized from hepatic and other storage sites to support erythropoiesis even with ESA use. The TSAT is less than 20%, but with elevated ferritin levels (more than 100 - 200 ng/mL). Usually responsive to iron therapy, functional iron deficiency must be differentiated from inflammatory iron block, which may or may not respond to supplemental iron therapy, and can lead to refractory anemia [17]. **Table 1** outlines these iron storage states. The response to ESA and or IV iron may help distinguish between these two.

2.4. A Response to ESA

With increasing dose of ESA, ferritin levels may decrease with increase in hemoglobin levels in patients with functional deficiency but not with inflammatory iron block.

2.5. B Response to Iron

Inflammatory block is suspected if weekly administration of intravenous iron along with increasing dose of ESA fails to increase hematocrit with progressive increase in ferritin concentration. In contrast, patients with functional

Table 1. Different iron states.

Labs	Absolute iron deficiency	Functional iron deficiency	Inflammatory iron block
Ferritin Hemodialysis	<200	>200	>200
Pre-dialysis/PD	<100	>100	>100
Percent saturation	<20	<20	<20
Response to IV iron	++++	++	+/−

iron deficiency, additional intravenous iron with concomitant increases in ESA can be effective in increasing hemoglobin levels, as shown in Dialysis Patients Response to IV Iron with Elevated Ferritin (DRIVE) study [19], in which anemic subjects with elevated ferritin levels (500 - 1200 ng/mL) and low TSAT < 25%, who were on high doses of ESA, were randomly assigned to IV iron or placebo. ESA dose was increased by 25% in all patients at the beginning of study. At six weeks, hemoglobin levels increased more in the active therapy group. Post hoc analysis of DRIVE study showed that none of the iron parameters used in clinical practice is sensitive to predict response to iron supplementation [20].

Hepcidin, a key regulatory protein, controlling intestinal absorption of iron and its distribution throughout the body, may partially explain these observations regarding iron. Produced by the liver, high-circulating hepcidin reduces iron absorption in response to oral or intravenous iron. Conversely, limited iron leads to low hepcidin levels, which allows enhanced intestinal iron absorption and release of storage iron [21,22]. (**Figure 1**). Hepcidin, cleared renally, accumulates in renal failure and may contribute to anemia and ESA hypo response. Administration of oral or intravenous iron leads to increase in hepcidin levels, down regulating intestinal iron absorption. Hepcidin levels fall with ESA therapy improving iron mobilization, as well as with hypoxia and anemia. Levels increase with inflammation. Overall, blood hepcidin levels change in a similar manner to ferritin, decreasing with low iron stores, and increasing as iron storage increases, and in inflammatory states, confounding the evaluation of iron status [23].

Not surprisingly then, Hepcidin levels are elevated significantly in patients on dialysis (and less so in CKD stage II-IV), relative to the general population, correlating directly with ferritin levels and inflammatory markers [24-29]. Hepcidin levels inversely correlate with ESA and fall with initiation of ESA use [24,29].

Elevated hepcidin impairs release of stored iron. Parenteral, but not oral iron, can overcome hepcidin-induced iron blockade [29,30] Studies in CKD and dialysis patients show that intravenous iron improves anemia in most patients, including those with elevated hepcidin levels. Iron use however would over express hepcidin

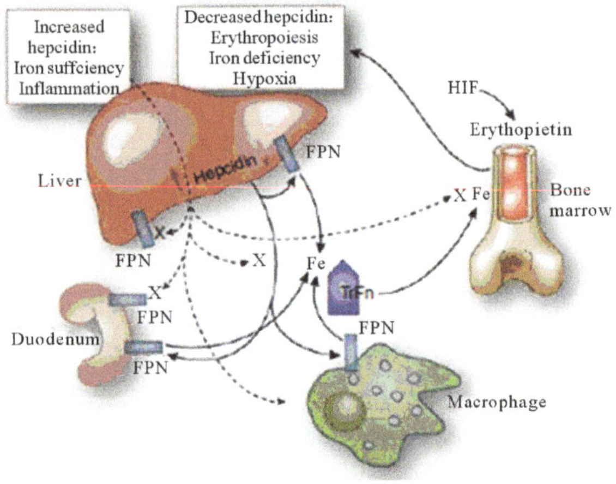

Figure 1. Iron (Fe) sufficiency and inflammation enhance hepcidin production in the liver. Kidney International (2011) 80, 240-244. doi:10. 1038/ki. 2011.141.

further, restricting iron later. Hepcidin and its regulatory pathways are potential therapeutic targets, which could lead to effective treatment of anemia and EPO hypo responsiveness in patients with CKD.

Thus, high hepcidin levels may contribute to the ESA resistance observed in many dialysis patients. Consequently, lowering hepcidin or inhibiting its signaling would release iron from stores, promote erythropoiesis, and prolong red cell survival. This may ultimately be safer than high doses of ESAs with repetitive parenteral iron. Hepcidin and its regulatory pathways are therefore potential therapeutic targets, which could lead to effective treatment of anemia of CKD and ESA hyporesonsiveness.

In animal models, administration of an anti-hepcidin antibody has been shown to treat inflammation-induced anemia when combined with ESA treatment [31].

2.6. IV versus Oral Iron

Iron may be given orally or IV to treat and prevent the development of iron deficiency. A trial of oral iron is often recommended for predialsyis patients, but may be limited by gastrointestinal symptoms and limited efficacy. Intravenous iron is preferred in most patients on PD and hemodialysis patients due to poor GI absorption [32-34].

2.7. Iron in Hemodialysis Patients

Among hemodialysis patients, oral iron usually is ineffective in raising trasferrin saturation or ferritin. In one study, 39 iron-deficient patients starting hemodialysis but not on ESA were randomly assigned to receive oral iron, intravenous iron or none. Those treated with IV iron had a significant increase in hemoglobin levels [32]. MacDougall *et al.* studied 37 HD patients beginning ESA therapy with Epogen (EPO) and found the increase in hemoglobin was greater and the EPO dose requirement were lower among those assigned to IV iron, compared to those receiving either oral or no iron. There was no difference in erythropoietic response to ESA in oral or no iron group [33]. Winard *et al.* prospectively studied 46 patients on EPO, randomized to four different oral iron regimens to give 200 mg of oral iron daily with at least 100 mg of ascorbic acid for 6 months. They found that with compliance, oral iron at the dose used in the study was able to maintain adequate iron status over a short term (less than 6 months) without the need for IV iron Dextran, but eventually IV iron Dextran would be required due to depleted iron stores [34].

Ferumoxytol, an intravenous form of elemental iron, was compared with oral iron by Provenzano *et al.*, and showed a greater increase in mean hemoglobin along with greater increase in TSAT as compared to oral iron, suggesting even in iron-replete patients, those supplemented with IV iron have an enhanced hemoglobin response to EPO with better maintenance of iron stores and lower dosage requirements of EPO [35]. The preferred route of administration of iron in patients with ESRD on HD is intravenous as supported by National Kidney Foundation Disease Outcomes Quality Initiative (NKF KDOQI) of 2006 [36]. Recently published 2012 Kidney Disease Improving Global Outcome (KDIGO) [14] guidelines suggest a trial of IV Iron in patient with ESRD on HD if an increase in hemoglobin is desired without using ESA and if TSAT is <30% and ferritin is <500 ng/ml.

2.8. Iron in Pre-Dialysis Patients

National Kidney Foundation Disease Outcomes Quality Initiative (NKF-KDOQI) guidelines recommend either oral or IV iron for patients with non-ESRD CKD, due to inconsistent data. KDIGO 2012 also recommends a trial of oral iron for 1 - 3 months with the same TSAT of <30% and ferritin of <500 as in ESRD on HD. They also recommended selecting the route of administration based on severity of iron deficiency, response and side effects to prior therapy, patient's compliance and availability of venous access [14].

Contrary to ESRD data, in CKD non-dialysis, multiple trials have failed to show that IV iron is superior to oral iron in hemoglobin response or reduction in EPO dose. In a prospective, controlled trial of 45 anemic patients with non-ESRD CKD, randomized to receive either oral ferrous sulfate (200 mg TID) or intravenous iron Sucrose (300 mg monthly) along with EPO, after an average follow up of 5.2 months, there was no difference in hemoglobin response or EPO dose between the two groups [37]. Another prospective, randomized, controlled trial of 96 non-ESRD CKD patients on EPO, assigned to either IV iron (5 doses of 200 mg Iron Sucrose weekly) or oral iron (ferrous sulfate 325 mg TID), showed that the hemoglobin increased in both groups, but only in the IV iron group did the ferritin increase [38]. In a trial of 75 non-ESRD CKD patients who were ESA naive were randomly assigned to receive either IV Ferric gluconate 250mg weekly for 4 weeks or oral ferrous sulfate 325 mg TID for 42 days. Hemoglobin increased in both groups [39].

In another trial of 182 patients with CKD stage III - V, hemoglobin increase of 1gm or more was more common in the IV treatment group (Sucrose 1 gm in divided doses over 14 days) than in oral iron treatment (ferrous gluconate 325 mg TID for 56 days) [40]. In a phase II trial of Ferumoxytol, 304 patients with CKD were assigned in a 3:1 ratio to two 510-mg doses of intravenous Ferumoxytol or 200mg of elemental iron orally for 21 days. Among patients who were not on ESA, hemoglobin increased significantly with IV ferumoxytol [41]. Thus in non-ESRD CKD, the data are conflicting with regards to the efficacy of IV versus oral iron.

3. Ascorbic Acid

Vitamin C or Ascorbic acid, increases iron release from the reticuloendthelial system, enhancing iron utilization during heme synthesis [42-44]. These findings led to an increased interest in investigating its use in hemodialysis patients with EPO hyporesonsiveness, elevated serum ferritin, and functional iron deficiency. Ascorbic acid levels have been variably reported to be low, normal, or even above normal in dialysis patients. In an observational study Deicher *et al.* failed to show a significant correlation between Vitamin C plasma levels and response to EPO. They concluded that in some hemodialysis patients Vitamin C levels account, at least partially for the response to EPO, particularly those with EPO-hypo responsiveness and functional iron deficiency [45]. Intravenous Vitamin C can overcome ESA resistance and "functional iron deficiency" in HD patients and by limiting iron use, may avoid hemosiderosis [46].

A Meta analysis of randomized controlled trials found that Vitamin C therapy significantly increased hemoglobin levels, decreased EPO dose, and improved trasferrin saturation among hemodialysis patients [47]. These findings were however based on small study sizes with substantial study heterogeneity limiting any solid conclusions about Vitamin C [48-53].

One randomized trial examined patients with EPO-hypo responsiveness and or functional iron deficiency [54]. Among 42 patients the EPO dose exceeded 450 IU/kg per week, the ferritin level was >500 ng/ml, TSAT <50% and the hemoglobin <11.0 g/dl. Subjects were assigned to intravenous Vitamin C (300 mg with dialysis) and standard therapy. After six months, active therapy resulted in significantly higher hemoglobin levels (9.3 - 10.5 g/dl vs 9.3 - 9.6 g/dl in standard group), TSAT level (29% - 37% vs 29%) and lower EPO dose in active group (477 to 429 units/kg per week vs 474 to 447 units/kg per week). No significant adverse effects were reported.

Benz *et al.* showed that once daily ascorbic acid (500 mg) in 21 EPO resistant anemic HD patients significantly decreased ferritin levels and EPO dose requirements while significantly raising hemoglobin and hematocrit. Hemoglobin increased 9% from 11.4% to 12.2% gm/dl ($p = 0.05$), hematocrit increased 10% from 33.3% to 36.7% ($p = 0.05$), and EPO dose requirement decreased 33% from 26,229 to 17,559 U/week ($p = 0.03$). Ferritin levels decreased 21% from 873 to 691 ng/mL ($p = 0.004$). Patients with oxalate levels >27 micromol/L were instructed to stop ascorbic acid treatment, and mean levels decreased from 107 to 19 micromol/L ($p = 0.01$) over a mean time of 71 days [48].

Secondary oxalosis in hemodialysis patients who received IV Vitamin C remains a concern [55,56]. Oxalate levels have been shown to increase modestly after eight weeks of IV Vitamin C [47]. In one study a progressive increase in plasma oxalate levels occurred when 504 mg Vitamin C was given into the arterial line throughout each hemodialysis treatment for 12 weeks [57]. In another study, plasma oxalate levels progressively increased as the dose of Vitamin C was increased from 250 to 500 mg/week. After 6 months, 40 percent of patients attained plasma oxalate levels that exceeded the range that would be associated with calcium oxalate super saturation at usual calcium concentration [58]. Elevated plasma oxalate levels also occur in hemodialysis patients treated with oral Vitamin C [48].

The 2006 KDOQI anemia guidelines in CKD conclude insufficient evidence exists to recommend Vitamin C as an adjuvant to Epoetin therapy [35]. The European Best Practice Guidelines suggested that correction of impaired Vitamin C status can reduce hypo responsiveness to EPO or functional iron deficiency, but do not recommend routine use [59]. The guidelines noted that use of high dose Vitamin C requires monitoring but also commented that the risk of oxalate deposition precludes a recommendation for routine use. Also the 2012 KDIGO guidelines recommend not using VITAMIN C, due to lack of sufficient and long term data to address the safety [14].

Further well controlled trials are needed to determine the role of Vitamin C in anemia of CKD. A short trial of oral or IV Vitamin C may be tried in selected patients with marked EPO hypo responsiveness who are closely monitored for toxicity and efficacy, and should be reserved for the patients who are unable to achieve and maintain target hemoglobin levels despite adequate iron stores and on high epoetin therapy (>450 IU/kg per week). The duration of therapy should not be more than 2 to 6 months.

4. Carnitine

Carnitine is required for the transport of long chain fatty acids into mitochondria. Carnitine also converts acyl CoA which accumulates in renal failure and is toxic, into less toxic acyl Carnitine [60]. Carnitine metabolism is reduced as the glomerular filtration rate falls. Its loss through dialysis has been suggested to result in a Carnitine deficient state. L-Carnitine has been used with or without concomitant ESA [61].

Carnitine increases formation of colony forming unit-serythroid (CFU-E) colonies in cell cultures of mouse bone marrow [62]. It has also been suggested to increase red cell survival by reducing red cell osmotic fragility. However there is no convincing evidence yet about the importance of this in ESRD.

Small case series suggest intravenous or oral L-Carnitine may increase hemoglobin levels or reduce the EPO requirement in patients with renal failure and on dialysis [61-63].

A 2002 metaanalysis of six randomized trials evaluated the efficacy of IV Carnitine supplementation in lowering the required dose of EPO. The EPO dose was found to be significantly lower among those administered Carnitine, with a beneficial response reported in four of the six studies [63].

Only a few randomized, controlled trials of L-Carnitine exist in patients with CKD. One such trial in hemodialysis patients, found that treatment with intravenous L-Carnitine was associated with a 37% reduction in EPO dose without any effect on hematocrit. Neither hematocrit nor EPO dose changed in the control group. A fall in EPO dose was observed in seven of 13 treated patients with maximal benefit by four months [64].

In an open label randomized trial, 55 adult chronic HD patients at a single hemodialysis center were divided into two groups; a group of 20 patients who received 1500 mg/day oral L-Carnitine and a control group of 35 patients. The mean weekly maintenance dose of erythropoietin was not statistically significantly different in L-Carnitine group (80.16 ± 35.61 units/kg) and the control group (91.9 ± 38.21 units/kg, p = 0.20) [65]. In another randomized control trial involving 14 patients, L Carnitine was not associated with a reduction in EPO dose or change in hematocrit over a six month treatment period [66]. In the post-hoc analysis, there was a non-significant trend towards lower EPO dose in patients over the age of 65.

In another study, patients on Hemodialysis received either 5 or 15mg/kg of L Carnitine at each dialysis treatment for 8 months, with IV iron for the first four months with the control group receiving only IV iron. EPO dose did not change over a 4 months period [67]. Mean weekly EPO dose fell by 37% percent among those receiving L-Carnitine.

In two additional randomized trials in which anemia or EPO dose was not the primary endpoint, there was no change in hemoglobin or epogen dose from baseline in patients on L-Carnitine [68,69].

Intravenous L-Carnitine has been well tolerated apart from a small percentage of patients with seizures and has been recommended by some to be used in selected patients with renal failure and EPO resistance, while some have suggested routine use [61]. Treatment with oral Carnitine up to 3 years has been well tolerated [61] with some concern about the accumulation of toxic metabolites of oral L Carnitine in patients with CKD [70,71].

2006 KDOQI guidelines for anemia of CKD concluded that insufficient evidence exists to recommend L-Carnitine [72]. The 2012 KDIGI guideline suggest not using L-Carnitine [14].

5. Pentoxifylline

Pentoxifylline is a methyl xanthine derivative with possible anti inflammatory properties [73,74]. Approved for the treatment of peripheral vascular disease, Pentoxifylline has been shown to suppress IL-2, interferon (INF) gamma, TH1 and TH2-derived cytokines [73].

These findings led to the possible application in EPO-resistant anemia. The benefits of Pentoxifylline were observed in a small study comprised of 16 patients on HD, PD and failing transplants [75]. The mean hemoglobin increased from 9.5 to 11.7 g/dL. Epo dose was reduced in only one patient while remaining the same in the rest. One patient, previously transfusion-dependent, was able to stop transfusion. In another study 7 anemic patients with CKD were treated with Pentoxifylline 400 mg daily for 6 months with the goal of defining the effects of Petoxifylline as an agent with anti-tumor necrosis factor (TNF) alpha properties. Petoxifylline-treated patients at 6 months had significant improvement in hemoglobin with reduction of TNF-alpha concentration [76]. Thus Pentoxifylline by virtue of counteracting anti-erythropoietic cytokines may allow epogen dose reducetions in the anemia of CKD. This should be followed up with a larger prospective study to confirm these findings before consideration for common practice. The 2012 KDIGO guideline suggests not using Pentoxifylline at this time due to lack of high-quality evidence [14].

6. Statins

Statins are a class of drug use to lower cholesterol by inhibiting HMG-CoA redcutase, which plays a central role in the production of cholesterol in the liver. Statins have some anti-inflammatory and antioxidant properties. In a retrospective study, Sirken et al showed mean hemoglobin rose from 10.6 to 12.5 g/dl in 70 hemodialysis patients, with associated 25% reduction in EPO dose, over a mean of 4.7 months after treatment with statin was started [77]. Roughly half of the patients were started on a statin within one month of starting Hemodialysis, limiting generalizabilty. Another study assessed the efficacy of Statins in patients with type 2 diabetes who were on Hemodialysis. The mean EPO dose was significantly lower in statin group [78]. Another prospective study assessed the effects of statin therapy on EPO hypo responsiveness by assessing the anti-inflammatory effects. 30 patients with baseline cholesterol >220 mg/dl were prescribed 10 mg of Atorvastatin for 12 weeks. EPO hypo responsiveness defined by EPO to hematocrit ratio was significantly reduced along with reductions in Interleukin 6 and TNF-alpha level suggesting that statin therapy may benefit patients with EPO hyporesonsiveness [79]. Further investigation of the effects of Statins as an Epo adjuvant is needed. For now Statins cannot be recommended at this time to be used solely for the treatment of anemia, but remain a central weapon in combating cardiovascular disease, the most common cause of death in patients with CKD [80].

7. Androgens

Before the availability of Epogen, androgens were used routinely to treat anemia in patients with dialysis [81-84]. Androgens may increase endogenous erythropoietin production, sensitivity of erythroid progenitors to the effects of erythropoietin and red blood cell survival. Their role as monotherpay for anemia in CKD patients has declined markedly since epoetin alpha was approved. A possible role of androgens in combination with epoetin therapy in dialysis patient has been evaluated in few small studies with EPO with conflicting results.

One study evaluated 15 patients with ESRD, 8 of whom received intramuscular nandrolone decanoate 1000 mg once weekly in combination with EPO with each dialysis session (the remaining 7 received no androgens). The combination was associated with a greater increase in hematocrit values from 24 to 33 percent as well as greater overall response rate defined as having an increase in hematocrit of 1% during a two week period. The authors concluded that androgen therapy significantly augments exogenous Epo, resulting in a lower dose of intravenous EPO [85].

A second trial enrolled 12 hemodialysis patients, randomly assigned to receive EPO 40 units/kg IV three times weekly with or without nandrolone decanoate (2 mg/kg IM weekly) for 16 weeks. The rate of rise of hematocrit did not differ, and only one of six patients receiving nandrolone reached the HCT target of 30 percent as compared to 3 in the Epo-only group [86].

In another longer open label trial, with low dose EPO therapy [87] 19 chronic HD patients were randomly assigned to receive EPO 1500 units with each HD treatment either alone or in combination with nandrolone decanoate 100 mg intramuscularly each week for 26 weeks. With no serious side effects reported, nandrolone group achieved higher final hematocrit values than Epo-alone group (33.2% vs 28.3%) with higher mean increase in hematocrit (8.2% vs 3.5%).

Another study of 32 hemodialysis patients randomly assigned to receive low dose EPO therapy 1000 units subcutaneously at each HD treatment either alone or in combination with nandrolone decanoate 50 mg intramuscularly twice weekly for six months showed no statistically significant rise in HCT in nandrolone group compared with the control group with significant side effects of gynecomastia, hirsutism, menstrual irregularities and increase in liver enzymes and triglycerides [88].

The data on androgens are conflicting; prompting both the NKF-K/DOQI and European Best Practice Guideline to conclude their role is limited and further complicated by unwanted side effects [35,59]. Cost itself also limits the role of androgens. The 2006 KDOQI guidelines for anemia in CKD stated that androgens should not be used as an adjuvant to epoetin alfa [35]. The 2012 KDIGO guidelines recommend not using androgens.

8. N-Acetylecysteine

N-Acetylecysteine (NAC) is used primarily as a mucolytic, for acetaminophen overdoses, and to prevent contrast induced nephropathy [89,90]. Due to lack of benefit in preventing contrast induced nephropathy in a recent trial [91], NAC is falling out of favor, but still recommended by KDIGO 2012 to prevent contrast induced nephropathy in high risk patient [92].

There is growing interest in exploring NAC as an adjuvant to EPO due to its antioxidant properties in patients with CKD. In one study, 49 patients on HD received NAC 200mg three times daily for the first 3 months of dialysis, and were compared to 276 patients who did not receive NAC. During the 4-month study, when the EPO dose was stable, only NAC group had significant increase in hematocrit, accompanied with decrease levels of 8-isoprostane and oxidized low-density lipoprotein, both markers of oxidative stress [93].

To determine the contribution of injectable iron administered to HD patients in causing oxidative stress and the beneficial effects of NAC in reducing it, a prospective double blind, cross over trial was conducted on 14 adult hemodialysis patients [94]. To assess for oxidative stress, lipid peroxidation marker, melondiaaldehyde was measured along with highly sensitive C-reactive protein. Non-invasive assessment of endothelial dysfunction was assessed by digital plethysmography before and after intravenous therapy. NAC was found to reduce oxidative stress along with endothelial dysfunction. Thus by reducing the oxidative stress, NAC may reduce EPO hypo-

Table 2. Summary of different ESA adjuvants.

Agent	Strength of evidence	Recommended by KDOQI or European best practice guideline	Additional comments
Oral iron	Strong for pre-dialysis CKD, not strong for ESRD on HD.	Recommended for initial trial in pre-dialysis CKD/PD.	Limited by GI side effects.
IV iron	Strong: pre-dialysis and ESRD	Recommended for ESRD on dialysis and also for pre-dialysis CKD patients.	IV iron may be able to bypass hepcidin effect.
Ascorbic acid	Mixed. Few small RCTS suggest some benefit.	NKF-KDOQI does not recommend use, European best practice guideline acknowledges benefit but does not recommends it use. KDIGO suggest not using.	Secondary oxalosis may occur. Larger trials needed to confirm benefit. Consider for short course in selected patients with severe EPO resistance.
Carnitine	Mixed, small prospective studies suggest some benefit, while other do not.	NKF-KDOQI: insufficient evidence to suggest its use. KDIGO 2012-Do not suggest.	Expensive, seizure has been reported.
Androgen	Mixed results.	NKF-KDOQI does not suggest use. 2012 KDIGO-does not recommend.	Former agent of choice before ESA as monotherpay. Serious adverse effects including abnormal LFTS, risk of hepatocelullar carcinoma etc.
Statin	Small retrospective and prospective study suggest some benefit.	Not recommended to be used solely for EPO hypo responsiveness.	Many CKD/ESRD patient already on statin to reduce CV morbidity and mortality.
N-Acetyl cysteine	Small prospective studies suggest some benefit.	Not recommended at this time.	Larger trials needed to assess benefit.
Pentoxifylline	Small retrospective studies suggest some benefit.	Not recommended at this time.	Larger trials needed to assess benefit.

responsiveness.

Another small, uncontrolled pilot study enrolled 12 hemodialysis patients treated with 600 mg po BID of NAC showed a 53% reduction in EPO resistance index (weekly EPO dose per Kg/Hematocrit) [95].

These small studies suggest a role for NAC in treating anemia in CKD population, but need larger controlled trial with less confounding factors. Until then, routine use of NAC as an EPO adjuvant cannot be suggested.

9. Summary (Table 2)

The high cost of ESAs and the rising incidence of mor bidity and mortality associated with its use have prompted a search for adjuvants to ESAs to limit cost and potential toxicities in CKD and ESRD-associated anemia. Adequate iron stores are essential for effective erythropoiesis and should be corrected. Use of parenteral, as opposed to oral, iron, particularly in ESRD, can overcome some EPO resistance. Identifying correctable causes of anemia (B12/Folate deficiency, gastrointestinal bleeding) and non-renal causes of anemia (malignancy, hematologic disorders, infections, inflammation) remains vital, as escalating doses of EPO can lead to morbidity and mortality.

Thus far, no one particular adjuvant has proven to be reliably efficacious in improving anemia, reducing ESA dosages, or reducing ESA hyporesonsiveness. IV iron and ESA remain the backbone of all anemia therapy in ESRD. Nevertheless, this review will serve to generate new hypotheses, and may lead to new innovations in anemia management. We believe that Ascorbic Acid, N-Acetyl Cysteine, and targeting hepcidin represent the most promising ways to combat the erythropoietin hypo response, but due to lack of sufficient high quality evidence, should not be routinely use.

REFERENCES

[1] F. Valderrababano, "Erythropoietin in Chronic Renal Failure," *Kidney International*, Vol. 50, No. 4, 1996, pp. 1373-1391. doi:10.1038/ki.1996.452

[2] J. W. Eschbach, "Erythropoietin 1991—An Overview," *American Journal of Kidney Diseases*, Vol. 18, Suppl. 4, 1991, pp. 3-9.

[3] B. C. Astor, P. Muntner, A. Levin, J. A. Eustace and J. Coresh, "Association of Kidney Function with Anemia: The Third National Health and Nutrition Examination Survey (1988-1994)," *Archives of Internal Medicine*, 2002, Vol. 162, No. 12, pp. 1401-1408. doi:10.1001/archinte.162.12.1401

[4] A. Levin, C. R. Thompson, J. Ethier, E. J. Carlisle, S. Tobe, D. Mendelssohn, E. Burgess, K. Jindal, B. Barrett,

J. Singer and O. Djurdjev, "Left Ventricular Mass Index Increase in Early Renal Disease: Impact of Decline in Hemoglobin," *American Journal of Kidney Diseases*, Vol. 34, No. 1, 1999, pp. 125-134. doi:10.1016/S0272-6386(99)70118-6

[5] C. T. Jurkovitz, J. L. Abramson, L. V. Vaccarino, W. S. Weintraub and W. M. McClellan, "Association of High Serum Creatinine and Anemia Increases the Risk of Coronary Events: Results from the Prospective Community-Based Atherosclerosis Risk in Communities (ARIC) Study," *Journal of the American Society of Nephrology*, Vol. 14, No. 11, 2003, pp. 2919-2925. doi:10.1097/01.ASN.0000092138.65211.71

[6] J. L. Abramson, C. T. Jurkovitz, V. Vaccarino, W. S. Weintraub and W. McClellan, "Chronic Kidney Disease, Anemia, and Incident Stroke in a Middle-Aged, Community-Based Population: The ARIC Study," *Kidney International*, Vol. 64, No. 2, 2003, pp. 610-615. doi:10.1046/j.1523-1755.2003.00109.x

[7] M. J. Sarnak, H. Tighiouart, G. Manjunath, B. MacLeod, J. Griffith, D. Salem and A. S. Levey, "Anemia as a Risk Factor for Cardiovascular Disease in the Atherosclerosis Risk in Communities (ARIC) Study," *Journal of the American College of Cardiology*, Vol. 40, No. 1, 2002, pp. 27-33. doi:10.1016/S0735-1097(02)01938-1

[8] W. M. McClellan, W. D. Flanders, R. D. Langston, C. Jurkovitz and R. Presley, "Anemia and Renal Insufficiency Are Independent Risk Factors for Death among Patients with Congestive Heart Failure Admitted to Community Hospitals: A Population-Based Study," *Journal of the American Society of Nephrology*, Vol. 13, No. 7, 2002, pp. 1928-1936. doi:10.1097/01.ASN.0000018409.45834.FA

[9] G. T. Obrador, T. Roberts, W. L. St Peter, E. Frazier, B. J. Pereira and A. Collins, "Trends in Anemia at Initiation of Dialysis in the United States," *Kidney International*, Vol. 60, No. 5, 2001, pp. 1875-1884. doi:10.1046/j.1523-1755.2001.00002.x

[10] M. A. Pfeffer, E. A. Burdmann, C. Y. Chen, M. E. Cooper, D. de Zeeuw, K. U. Eckardt, J. M. Feyzi, P. Ivanovich, R. Kewalramani, A. S. Levey, E. F. Lewis, J. B. McGill, J. J. McMurray, P. Parfrey, H. H. Parving, G. Remuzzi, A. K. Singh, S. D. Solomon and R. Toto, "TREAT Investigators a Trial of Darbepoetin Alfa in Type 2 Diabetes and Chronic Kidney Disease," *New England Journal of Medicine*, Vol. 361, No. 21, 2009, pp. 2019-2032. doi:10.1056/NEJMoa0907845

[11] T. B. Drüeke, F. Locatelli, N. Clyne, K. U. Eckardt, I. C. Macdougall, D. Tsakiris, H. U. Burger and A. Scherhag, "CREATE Investigators Normalization of Hemoglobin Level in Patients with Chronic Kidney Disease and Anemia," *New England Journal of Medicine*, Vol. 355, No. 20, 2006, pp. 2071-2084. doi:10.1056/NEJMoa062276

[12] A. K. Singh, L. Szczech, K. L. Tang, H. Barnhart, S. Sapp, M. Wolfson and D. Reddan, "CHOIR Investigators Correction of Anemia with Epoetin Alfa in Chronic Kidney Disease," *New England Journal of Medicine*, Vol. 355, No. 20, 2006, pp. 2085-2098. doi:10.1056/NEJMoa065485

[13] http://www.fda.gov/Drugs/DrugSafety/ucm259639.htm

[14] "KDIGO Clinical Practice Guideline for Anemia in Chronic Kidney Disease," *Kidney International Supplements*, Vol. 2, Vol. 4, 2012, pp. 279-335.

[15] J. W. Eschbach, J. D. Cook, B. H. Scribner and C. A. Finch, "Iron Balance in Hemodialysis Patients," *Annals of Internal Medicine*, Vol. 87, No. 6, 1977, pp. 710-713.

[16] A. M. Fernández-Rodríguez, M. C. Guindeo-Casasús, T. Molero-Labarta, C. Domínguez-Cabrera, L. Hortal-Casc, P. Pérez-Borges, N. Vega-Díaz, P. Saavedra-Santana and L. Palop-Cubillo, "Diagnosis of Iron Deficiency in Chronic Renal Failure," *American Journal of Kidney Diseases*, Vol. 34, No. 3, 1999, pp. 508-513.

[17] M. Rambod, C. P. Kovesdy, K. Kalantar-Zadeh, "Combined High Serum Ferritin and Low Iron Saturation in Hemodialysis Patients: The Role of Inflammation," *Clinical Journal of the American Society of Nephrology*, Vol. 3, No. 6, 2008, pp. 1691-1701. doi:10.2215/CJN.01070308

[18] F. N. Hutchinson and W. J. Jones, "A Cost-Effectiveness Analysis of Anemia Screening before Erythropoietin in Patients with End Stage Renal Disease," *American Journal of Kidney Diseases*, Vol. 29, No. 5, 1997, pp. 651-657. doi:10.1016/S0272-6386(97)90116-5

[19] D. W. Coyne, T. Kapoian, W. Suki, *et al.*, "Ferric Gluconate Is Highly Efficacious in Anemic Hemodialysis Patients with High Serum Ferritin and Low Transferrin Saturation: Results of the Dialysis Patients' Response to IV Iron with Elevated Ferritin (DRIVE) Study," *Journal of the American Society of Nephrology*, Vol. 18, No. 3, 2007, pp. 975-984. doi:10.1681/ASN.2006091034

[20] A. K. Singh, D. W. Coyne, W. Shapiro, A. R. Rizkala and DRIVE Study Group, "Predictors of the Response to Treatment in Anemic Hemodialysis Patients with High Serum Ferritin and Low Transferrin Saturation," *Kidney International*, Vol. 71, No. 11, 2007, pp. 1163-1171.

[21] G. Nicolas, M. Bennoun, I. Devaux, *et al.*, "Lack of Hepcidin Gene Expression and Severe Tissue Iron Overload in Upstream Stimulatory Factor 2 (USF2) Knockout Mice," *Proceedings of the National Academy of Sciences of the United States of America*, Vol. 98, No. 15, 2001, pp. 8780-8785. doi:10.1073/pnas.151179498

[22] E. Nemeth and T. Ganz, "Regulation of Iron Metabolism by Hepcidin," *Annual Review of Nutrition*, Vol. 26, No. 1, 2006, pp. 323-342. doi:10.1146/annurev.nutr.26.061505.111303

[23] D. Coyne, "Iron Indices: What Do They Really Mean?" *Kidney International*, Vol. 69, 2006, pp. S4-S8. doi:10.1038/sj.ki.5000404

[24] N. Tomosugi, H. Kawabata, R. Wakatabe, *et al.*, "Detection of Serum Hepcidin in Renal Failure and Inflammation by Using ProteinChip System," *Blood*, Vol. 108, No. 4, 2006, pp. 1381-1387. doi:10.1182/blood-2005-10-4043

[25] D. R. Ashby, D. P. Gale, M. Busbridge, *et al.*, "Plasma Hepcidin Levels Are Elevated but Responsive to Erythropoietin Therapy in Renal Disease," *Kidney International*, Vol. 75, No. 9, 2009, pp. 976-981. doi:10.1038/ki.2009.21

[26] J. Zaritsky, B. Young, H. J. Wang, *et al.*, "Hepcidin—A

Potential Novel Biomarker for Iron Status in Chronic Kidney Disease," *Clinical Journal of the American Society of Nephrology*, Vol. 4, No. 6, 2009, pp. 1051-1056 doi:10.2215/CJN.05931108

[27] H. P. Peters, C. M. Laarakkers, D. W. Swinkels, *et al.*, "Serum Hepcidin-25 Levels in Patients with Chronic Kidney Disease Are Independent of Glomerular Filtration Rate," *Nephrology Dialysis Transplantation*, Vol. 25, No. 3, 2010, pp. 848-853. doi:10.1093/ndt/gfp546

[28] G. Weiss, I. Theurl, S. Eder, *et al.*, "Serum Hepcidin Concentration in Chronic Haemodialysis Patients: Associations and Effects of Dialysis, Iron and Erythropoietin Therapy," *European Journal of Clinical Investigation*, Vol. 39, No. 10, 2009, pp. 883-890. doi:10.1111/j.1365-2362.2009.02182.x

[29] B. Ford, C. Eby, M. Scott, *et al.*, "Intra-Individual Variability in Serum Hepcidin Precludes Its Use as a Marker of Iron Status in Hemodialysis Patients," *Kidney International*, Vol. 78, 2010, pp. 769-773. doi:10.1038/ki.2010.254

[30] S. Stancu, L. Barsan, A. Stanciu, *et al.*, "Can the Response to Iron Therapy Be Predicted in Anemic Nondialysis Patients with Chronic Kidney Disease?" *Clinical Journal of the American Society of Nephrology*, Vol. 5, No. 3, 2010, pp. 409-416. doi:10.2215/CJN.04280609

[31] B. J. Sasu, K. S. Cooke, T. L. Arvedson, *et al.*, "Antihepcidin Antibody Treatment Modulates Iron Metabolism and Is Effective in a Mouse Model of Inflammation-Induced Anemia," *Blood*, Vol. 115, No. 17, 2010, pp. 3616-3624. doi:10.1182/blood-2009-09-245977

[32] R. Fudin, J. Jaichenko, A. Shostak, M. Bennett and L. Gotloib, "Nephron Correction of Uremic Iron Deficiency Anemia in Hemodialyzed Patients: A Prospective Study," Vol. 79, No. 3, 1998, pp. 299-305. doi:10.1159/000045053

[33] I. C. MacDougall, B. Tucker, J. Thompson, C. R. Tomson, L. R. Baker and A. E. Raine, "A Randomized Controlled Study of Iron Supplementation in Patients Treated with EPO," *Kidney International*, Vol. 50, No. 5, 1996, pp. 1694-1699. doi:10.1038/ki.1996.487

[34] R. L. Wingard, R. A. Parker, N. Ismail and R. M. Hakim, "Efficacy of Oral Iron Therapy in Patients Receiving Recombinant Human EPO," *American Journal of Kidney Diseases*, Vol. 25, No. 3, 1995, pp. 433-439. doi:10.1016/0272-6386(95)90105-1

[35] R. Provenzano, B. Schiller, M. Rao, D. Coyne, L. Brenner and B. J. Pereira, "Ferumoxytol as an Intravenous Iron Replacement Therapy iN Hemodialysis Patients," *Clinical Journal of the American Society of Nephrology*, Vol. 4, No. 2, 2009, pp. 386-393. doi:10.2215/CJN.02840608

[36] "K/DOQI Clinical Practice Guidelines and Clinical Practice Recommendations for Anemia in Chronic Kidney Disease," *American Journal of Kidney Diseases*, Vol. 47, Suppl. 3, 2006, pp. S1-S3. doi:10.1053/S0272-6386(05)01814-7

[37] J. Stoves, H. Inglis and C. G. Newstead, "A Randomized Study of Oral vs. Intravenous Iron Supplementation in Patients with Progressive Renal Insufficiency Treated with EPO," *Nephrology Dialysis Transplantation*, Vol. 16, No. 5, 2001, pp. 967-974. doi:10.1093/ndt/16.5.967

[38] C. Charytan, W. Ounibi and G. R. Bailie, "Comparison of Intravenous Iron Sucrose to Oral Iron in the Treatment of Anemic Patients with Chronic Kidney Disease Not on Dialysis," *Nephron Clinical Practice*, Vol. 100, No. 3, 2005, pp. c55-c62.

[39] D. B. Van Wyck; M. Roppolo, C. O. Martinez, R. M. Mazey and S. McMurray, "A Randomized, Controlled Trial Comparing IV Iron Sucrose to Oral Iron in Anemic Patients with Non Dialysis-Dependent CKD," *Kidney International*, Vol. 68, No. 6, 2005, pp. 2846-2856 doi:10.1111/j.1523-1755.2005.00758.x

[40] R. Agarwal, A. R. Rizkala, B. Bastani, M. O. Kaskas, D. J. Leehey and A. Besarab, "A Randomized Controlled Trial of Oral versus Intravenous Iron in Chronic Kidney Disease," *American Journal of Nephrology*, Vol. 26, No. 5, 2006, pp. 445-454. doi:10.1159/000096174

[41] B. S. Spinowitz, A. T. Kausz, J. Baptista, S. D. Noble, R. Sothinathan, M. V. Bernardo, L. Brenner and B. J. Pereira, "Ferumoxytol for Treating Iron Deficiency Anemia in CKD," *Journal of the American Society of Nephrology*, Vol. 19, No. 8, 2008, pp. 1599-1605 doi:10.1681/ASN.2007101156

[42] K. R. Bridges and K. E. Hoffman, "The Effects of Ascorbic Acid on the Intracellular Metabolism of Iron and Ferritin," *Journal of Biological Chemistry*, Vol. 261, No. 30, 1986, pp. 14273-14277.

[43] D. A. Lipschitz, T. H. Bothwell, H. C. Seftel, *et al.*, "The Role of Ascorbic Acid in the Metabolism of Storage Iron," *British Journal of Haematology*, Vol. 20, No. 2, 1971, pp. 155-163. doi:10.1111/j.1365-2141.1971.tb07024.x

[44] A. Goldberg, "The Enzymic Formation of Haem by the Incorporation of Iron into Protoporphyrin; Importance of Ascorbic Acid, Ergothioneine and Glutathione," *British Journal of Haematology*, Vol. 5, No. 2, 1959, pp. 150-157. doi:10.1111/j.1365-2141.1959.tb04020.x

[45] R. Deicher, F. Ziai, A. Habicht, *et al.*, "Vitamin C Plasma Level and Response to Erythropoietin in Patients on Maintenance Haemodialysis," *Nephrology Dialysis Transplantation*, 2004, Vol. 19, 2319. doi:10.1093/ndt/gfh260

[46] K. Gastaldello, A. Vereerstraeten, T. Nzame-Nze, J. L. Vanherweghem and C. Tielemans, "Resistance to EPO in Iron-Overloaded Hemodialysis Patients Can Be Overcome by Ascorbic Acid Administration," *Nephrology Dialysis Transplantation*, Vol. 10, Suppl. 6, 1995, pp. 44-47.

[47] D. C. Tarng, Y. H. Wei, T. P. Huang, *et al.*, "Intravenous Ascorbic Acid as an Adjuvant Therapy for Recombinant Erythropoietin in Hemodialysis Patients with Hyperferritinemia," *Kidney International*, Vol. 55, No. 6, 1999, pp. 2477-2486. doi:10.1046/j.1523-1755.1999.00479.x

[48] W. D. Sirover, A. A. Siddiqui and R. L. Benz, "Beneficial Hematologic Effects of Daily Oral Ascorbic Acid Therapy in ESRD Patients with Anemia and Abnormal Iron Homeostasis: A Preliminary Study," *Renal Failure*, Vol. 30, No. 9, 2008, pp. 884-889. doi:10.1080/08860220802353884

[49] K. Keven, S. Kutlay, G. Nergizoglu and S. Ertürk, "Randomized, Crossover Study of the Effect of Vitamin C on EPO Response in Hemodialysis Patients," *American Jour-*

nal of Kidney Diseases, 2003, Vol. 41, No. 6, pp. 1233-1239. doi:10.1016/S0272-6386(03)00356-1

[50] Y. Taji, T. Morimoto, K. Okada, *et al.*, "Effects of Intravenous Ascorbic Acid on Erythropoiesis and Quality of Life in Unselected Hemodialysis Patients," *Journal of Nephrology*, Vol. 17, No. 4, 2004, pp. 537-543.

[51] J. Deira, J. Diego, R. Martínez, *et al.*, "Comparative Study of Intravenous Ascorbic Acid versus Low-Dose Desferroxamine in Patients on Hemodialysis with Hyperferritinemia," *Journal of Nephrology*, Vol. 16, No. 5, 2003, pp. 703-709.

[52] V. Giancaspro, M. Nuzziello, G. Pallotta, *et al.*, "Intravenous Ascorbic Acid in Hemodialysis Patients with Functional Iron Deficiency: A Clinical Trial," *Journal of Nephrology*, Vol. 13, No. 6, 2000, pp. 444-449.

[53] N. Attallah, Y. Osman-Malik, S. Frinak and A. Besarab, "Effect of Intravenous Ascorbic Acid in Hemodialysis Patients with EPO-Hyporesponsive Anemia and Hyperferritinemia," *American Journal of Kidney Diseases*, Vol. 47, No. 4, 2006 pp. 644-654. doi:10.1053/j.ajkd.2005.12.025

[54] V. Deved, P. Poyah, M. T. James, *et al.*, "Ascorbic Acid for Anemia Management in Hemodialysis Patients: A Systematic Review and Meta-Analysis," *American Journal of Kidney Diseases*, Vol. 54, No. 6, 2009, pp. 1089-1097. doi:10.1053/j.ajkd.2009.06.040

[55] P. Balcke, P. Schmidt, J. Zazgornik, *et al.*, "Ascorbic Acid Aggravates Secondary Hyperoxalemia in Patients on Chronic Hemodialysis," *Annals of Internal Medicine*, Vol. 101, No. 3, 1984, pp. 343-344.

[56] C. Pru, J. Eaton and C. Kjellstrand, "Vitamin C Intoxication and Hyperoxalemia in Chronic Hemodialysis Patients," *Nephron*, Vol. 39, No. 2, 1985, pp. 112-116. doi:10.1159/000183353

[57] J. Eiselt, J. Racek, L. Trefil and K. Opatrný Jr., "Effects of a Vitamin E-Modified Dialysis Membrane and Vitamin C Infusion on Oxidative Stress in Hemodialysis Patients," *Artificial Organs*, 2001, Vol. 25, No. 6, pp. 430-436. doi:10.1046/j.1525-1594.2001.025006430.x

[58] C. Canavese, M. Petrarulo, P. Massarenti, *et al.*, "Long-Term, Low-Dose, Intravenous Vitamin C Leads to Plasma Calcium Oxalate Supersaturation in Hemodialysis Patients," *American Journal of Kidney Diseases*, Vol. 45, No. 3, 2005, pp. 540-549. doi:10.1053/j.ajkd.2004.10.025

[59] "SECTION III. Treatment of Renal Anaemia," *Nephrology Dialysis Transplantation*, Vol. 19, Suppl. 2, 2004, pp. ii16-ii31. doi:10.1093/ndt/gfh1026

[60] C. J. Rebouche and H. Seim, "Carnitine Metabolism and Its Regulation in Microorganisms and Mammals," *Annual Review of Nutrition*, Vol. 18, No. 1, 1998, pp. 39-61. doi:10.1146/annurev.nutr.18.1.39

[61] T. A. Golper, S. Goral, B. N. Becker and C. B. Langman, "L-Carnitine Treatment of Anemia," *American Journal of Kidney Diseases*, Vol. 41, Suppl. 42, 2003, pp. S27-S34. doi:10.1016/S0272-6386(03)00114-8

[62] Y. Kitamura, K. Satoh, T. Satoh, *et al.*, "Effect of L-Carnitine on Erythroid Colony Formation in Mouse Bone Marrow Cells," *Nephrology Dialysis Transplantation*, Vol. 20, No. 5, 2005, pp. 981-984. doi:10.1093/ndt/gfh758

[63] J. M. Hurot, M. Cucherat, M. Haugh and D. Fouque, "Effects of L-Carnitine Supplementation in Maintenance Hemodialysis Patients: A Systematic Review," *Journal of the American Society of Nephrology*, Vol. 13, No. 2002, pp. 708-714.

[64] W. D. Labonia, "L-Carnitine Effects on Anemia in Hemodialyzed Patients Treated with Erythropoietin," *American Journal of Kidney Diseases*, 1995, Vol. 26, pp. 757-764. doi:10.1016/0272-6386(95)90439-5

[65] A. A. Sabry, "The Role of Oral L-Carnitine Therapy in Chronic Hemodialysis Patients," *Saudi Journal of Kidney Diseases and Transplantation*, Vol. 21, No. 3, 2010, pp. 454-459.

[66] U. Caruso, L. Leone, E. Cravotto and D. Nava, "Effects of L-Carnitine on Anemia in Aged Hemodialysis Patients Treated with Recombinant Human Erythropoietin: A Pilot Study," *Dialysis & Transplantation*, Vol. 27, 1998, pp. 498-506.

[67] J. Kletzmayr, G. Mayer, E. Legenstein, *et al.*, "Anemia and Carnitine Supplementation in Hemodialyzed Patients," *Kidney International Supplements*, Vol. 55, Suppl. 69, 1999, pp. S93-S96. doi:10.1046/j.1523-1755.1999.055Suppl.69093.x

[68] E. C. Vaux, D. J. Taylor, P. Altmann, *et al.*, "Effects of Carnitine Supplementation on Muscle Metabolism by the Use of Magnetic Resonance Spectroscopy and near-Infrared Spectroscopy in End-Stage Renal Disease," *Nephron Clinical Practice*, Vol. 97, No. 2, 2004, pp. c41-c48. doi:10.1159/000078399

[69] J. Semeniuk, K. F. Shalansky, N. Taylor, *et al.*, "Evaluation of the Effect of Intravenous L-Carnitine on Quality of Life in Chronic Hemodialysis Patients," *Clinical Nephrology*, Vol. 54, No. 6, 2000, pp. 470-477.

[70] A. Evans, "Dialysis-Related Carnitine Disorder and Levocarnitine Pharmacology," *American Journal of Kidney Diseases*, Vol. 41, Suppl. 4, 2003, pp. S13-S26. doi:10.1016/S0272-6386(03)00113-6

[71] M. A. Bain, R. Faull, R. W. Milne and A. M. Evans, "Oral L-Carnitine: Metabolite Formation and Hemodialysis," *Current Drug Metabolism*, Vol. 7, No. 7, 2006, pp. 811-816. doi:10.2174/138920006778520561

[72] G. Eknoyan, D. L. Latos and J. Lindberg, "National Kidney Foundation Carnitine Consensus Conference. Practice Recommendations for the Use of L-Carnitine in Dialysis-Related Carnitine Disorder. National Kidney Foundation Carnitine Consensus Conference," *American Journal of Kidney Diseases*, Vol. 41, No. 4, 2003, pp. 868-876. doi:10.1016/S0272-6386(03)00110-0

[73] J. Bienvenu, C. Doche, M. C. Gutowski, *et al.* "Production of Proinflammatory Cytokines and Cytokines Involved in the TH1/TH2 Balance is Modulated by Pentoxifylline," *Journal of Cardiovascular Pharmacology*, Vol. 25, Suppl. 2, 1995, pp. S80-S84. doi:10.1097/00005344-199500252-00017

[74] N. Benbernou, S. Esnault, G. Potron and M. Guenounou, "Regulatory Effects of Pentoxifylline on T-Helper Cell-Derived Cytokine Production in Human Blood Cells,"

Journal of Cardiovascular Pharmacology, Vol. 25, Suppl. 2, 1995, pp. S75-S79. doi:10.1097/00005344-199500252-00016

[75] J. F. Navarro, C. Mora, J. García, *et al.*, "Effects of Pentoxifylline on the Haematologic Status in Anaemic Patients with Advanced Renal Failure," *Scandinavian Journal of Urology and Nephrology*, Vol. 33, 1999, pp. 121-125. doi:10.1080/003655999750016113

[76] A. Cooper, A. Mikhail, M. W. Lethbridge, *et al.*, "Pentoxifylline Improves Hemoglobin Levels in Patients with Erythropoietin-Resistant Anemia in Renal Failure," *Journal of the American Society of Nephrology*, Vol. 15, No. 7, 2004, pp. 1877-1882. doi:10.1097/01.ASN.0000131523.17045.56

[77] G. Sirken, S. C. Kung and R. Raja, "Decreased Erythropoietin Requirements in Maintenance Hemodialysis Patients with Statin Therapy," *Asaio Journal*, Vol. 49, 2003, pp. 422-425.

[78] K. Tangdhanakanond and R. Raja, "Effect of Statins on EPO Responsiveness in Type 2-Diabetic versus Non-Diabetic Hemodialysis Patients," *Clinical Nephrology*, Vol. 73, No. 1, 2010, pp. 1-6.

[79] C. K. Chiang, S. Y. Yang, Y. S. Peng, S. P. Hsu, M. F. Pai, J. W. Huang, K. Y. Hung and K. D. Wu, "Atorvastatin Increases EPO-Stimulating Agent Hypo Responsiveness in Maintenance Hemodialysis Patients: Role of Anti-Inflammation Effects," *American Journal of Nephrology*, Vol. 29, No. 5, 2009, pp. 392-397. doi:10.1159/000169658

[80] United States Renal Data System, "USRDS 2010 Annual Data Report: Atlas of Chronic Kidney Disease and End-Stage Renal Disease in the United States, National Institutes of Health," National Institute of Diabetes and Digestive and Kidney Diseases, Bethesda, 2010.

[81] J. L. Teruel, R. Marcen, J. Navarro-Antolin, A. Aguilera, G. Fernandez-Juarez and J. Ortuo, "Androgen versus EPO for the Treatment of Anemia in Hemodialyzed Patients: A Prospective Study," *Journal of the American Society of Nephrology*, 1996, Vol. 7, No. 1, pp. 140-144.

[82] A. Gascn, J. J. Belvis, F. Berisa, E. Iglesias, V. Estopin and J. L. Teruel, "Nandrolone Decanoate Is a Good Alternative for the Treatment of Anemia in Elderly Male Patients on Hemodialysis," *Geriatric Nephrology and Urology*, Vol. 9, No. 2, 1999, pp. 67-72. doi:10.1023/A:1008306301255

[83] J. F. Navarro, C. Mora-Fernandez, A. Rivero, M. Macia, E. Gallego, J. Chahin, M. L. Mendez and J. Garcia, "Androgens for the Treatment of Anemia in Peritoneal Dialysis Patients," *Advances in Peritoneal Dialysis*, Vol. 14, 1998, pp. 232-235.

[84] J. F. Navarro, C. Mora, M. Macia and J. Garcia, "Randomized Prospective Comparison between EPO and Androgens in CAPD Patients," *Kidney International*, Vol. 61, No. 4, 2002, pp. 1537-1544. doi:10.1046/j.1523-1755.2002.00271.x

[85] S. H. Ballal, D. T. Domoto, D. C. Polack, P. Marciulonis and K. J. Martin, "Androgens Potentiate the Effects of EPO in the Treatment of Anemia of End-Stage Renal Disease," *American Journal of Kidney Diseases*, Vol. 17, No. 1, 1991, pp. 29-33.

[86] J. S. Bern, M. R. Rudnick and R. M. Cohen, "A Controlled Trial of Recombinant Human Erythropoietin and Nandrolone Decanoate in the Treatment of Anemia in Patients on Hcronic Hemodialysis," *Clinical Nephrology*, Vol. 37, No. 5, 1992, pp. 264-267.

[87] W. J. Gaughan, K. A. Liss, S. R. Dunn, *et al.*, "A 6-Month Study of Low-Dose Recombinant Human Erythropoietin Alone and in Combination with Androgens for the Treatment of Anemia in Chronic Hemodialysis Patients," *American Journal of Kidney Diseases*, Vol. 30, No. 4, 1997, pp. 495-500. doi:10.1016/S0272-6386(97)90307-3

[88] H. Sheashaa, W. Abdel-Razek, A. El-Husseini, *et al.*, "Use of Nandrolone Decanoate as an Adjuvant for Erythropoietin Dose Reduction in Treating Anemia in Patients on Hemodialysis," *Nephron Clinical Practice*, Vol. 99, No. 4, 2005, pp. c102-c106.

[89] A. V. Kshirsagar, C. Poole, A. Mottl, D. Shoham, N. Franceschini, G. Tudor, M. Agrawal, C. Denu-Ciocca, E. Magnus Ohman and W. F. Finn, "N-Acetylcysteine for the Prevention of Radiocontrast Induced Nephropathy: A Meta-Analysis of Prospective Controlled Trials," *Journal of the American Society of Nephrology*, Vol. 15, No. 3, 2004, pp. 761-769. doi:10.1097/01.ASN.0000116241.47678.49

[90] M. J. Smilkstein, G. L. Knapp, K. W. Kulig, B. H. Rumack, "Efficacy of Oral N-Acetylcysteine in the Treatment of Acetaminophen Overdose. Analysis of the National Multicenter Study (1976 to 1985)," *New England Journal of Medicine*, Vol. 319, No. 24, 1988, pp. 1557-1562. doi:10.1056/NEJM198812153192401

[91] ACT Investigators, "Acetylcysteine for Prevention of Renal Outcomes in Patients Undergoing Coronary and Peripheral Vascular Angiography: Main Results from the Randomized Acetylcysteine for Contrast-Induced Nephropathy Trial (ACT)," *Circulation*, Vol. 124, No. 11, 2011, pp. 1250-1259.

[92] "KDIGO Clinical Practice Guideline for Acute Kidney Injury," *Kidney International Supplements*, Vol. 2, No. 1, 2012, pp. 8-12. doi:10.1038/kisup.2012.7

[93] S.-P. Hsu, C.-K. Chiang, S.-Y. Yang and C.-T. Chien, "N-Acetylcysteine for the Management of Anemia and Oxidative Stress in Hemodialysis Patients," *Nephron Clinical Practice*, Vol. 116, No. 3, 2010, pp. c207-c216.

[94] G. Swarnalatha, R. Ram, P. Neela, M. U. Naidu, K. V. Dakshina Murty, "Oxidative Stress in Hemodialysis Patients Receiving Intravenous Iron Therapy and the Role of N-Acetylcysteine in Preventing Oxidative Stress," *Saudi Journal of Kidney Diseases and Transplantation*, 2010, Vol. 21, No. 5, pp. 852-888.

[95] N. A. Finnigan, M. M. Chernick and R. L. Benz, "Nephrology, N-Acetylcysteine (NAC) May Improve Erythropoietin Resistant Anemia (ERA) in Hemodialysis Patients [SA-PO2587] ASN Renal Week 2010 Abstracts."

32

Biomarkers in Acute Kidney Injury

Cai-Mei Zheng[1*], Min-Tser Liao[2,3*], Mei-Yu Lin[4], Lan Lo[4], Chia-Chao Wu[5], Yung-Ho Hsu[1], Yuh-Feng Lin[1], Kuo-Cheng Lu[4#]

[1]Division of Nephrology, Department of Medicine, Taipei Medical University-Shuang Ho Hospital, Taipei Medical University, Chinese Taipei

[2]Department of Pediatrics, Taoyuan Armed Forces General Hospital, Chinese Taipei

[3]Department of Pediatrics, Tri-Service General Hospital, National Defense Medical Center, Chinese Taipei

[4]Department of Medicine, Cardinal Tien Hospital, School of Medicine, Fu Jen Catholic University, New Taipei City, Chinese Taipei

[5]Division of Nephrology, Department of Medicine, Tri-Service General Hospital, National Defense Medical Center, Chinese Taipei

Email: #kuochenglu@gmail.com

ABSTRACT

Acute kidney injury (AKI) is one of the popular topics of discussions due to increasing development of biomarkers recently. The disease progression and prognosis may be determined by these biomarkers detected in blood and urine specimens. Since acute kidney injury is associated with a broad spectrum of disease conditions, prevention and early detection of AKI becomes very important in those clinical settings. Early measurements of AKI biomarkers predict subsequent development of intrinsic AKI, dialysis requirement, duration of intensive care unit stay and finally affect mortality. We, here, discuss the acute kidney injury in different clinical situations and associated natures of biomarkers, which may help us guide to prevent and treat AKI more effectively.

Keywords: Acute Kidney Injury; Critical Care Centers; Biomarkers; Renal Replacement Therapy

1. Introduction

Acute kidney injury (AKI) is one of the major causes of morbidity and mortality encounter in hospitalized patients, especially intensive care centers. Early detection may improve the hospital stay, patients' prognosis and reduce expensive medical costs. Nowadays, different types of bio-markers for acute kidney injury are emerging to play a role in accurate diagnosis, early detection, monitoring therapy and predicting the prognosis. This review discusses the clinical use of biomarkers in acute kidney injury.

2. Definition and Classification of Acute Kidney Injury (AKI)

Acute kidney injury (AKI), a preferred nomenclature to previously termed acute renal failure, refers to a spectrum of disease ranging from a minimal elevation in serum creatinine to anuric renal failure, clinically manifested by changes in blood chemistry and fluid disturbances.

In 2002, the Acute Dialysis Quality Initiative (ADQI) group proposed a definition for AKI stems from criteria for three grades of increasing severity (Risk of acute renal failure, Injury to the kidney, Failure of kidney function) and two outcome classes (Loss of kidney function and End-stage kidney disease) (RIFLE classification) [1,2].

Chertow and colleagues noticed that a rise in serum creatinine of just ≥0.3 mg/dl had a four-fold higher multivariable-adjusted risk of death [3]. The Acute Kidney Injury Network (AKIN) group modified the AKI definition based on RIFLE criteria in 2005 [4]. This new staging system classified the patients with a change in serum creatinine (SCr) concentration ≥ 0.3 mg/dl (≥26.4 μmol/l) within 48 hours as AKIN stage 1, whereas patients receiving renal replacement therapy are included in AKIN Stage 3. RIFLE-Risk classified as Stage 1, RIFLE-Injury and Failure as Stages 2 and 3, respectively; and the two outcome classes RIFLE-Loss and RIFLE-End stage kidney disease has been removed [4] (**Table 1**).

3. Acute Kidney Injury (AKI) in Different Situations

3.1. Community-Acquired AKI

Acute renal injury occurred at the time of hospital admission is regarded as community-acquired AKI and

*These authors equally contributed to this work.

#Corresponding author.

Table 1. Diagnostic criteria for acute kidney injury depend on acute kidney injury (AKIN) network.

Stage	AKIN criteria (2005)	
	Serum creatinine criteria	Urine output criteria
1	↑ SCr ≥ 0.3 mg/dl or ↑ to ≥1.5 - 2-fold from baseline	UO < 0.5 mg/kg/hr ≥ 6 hours
2	↑ SCr ≥ 2 - 3-fold from baseline	UO < 0.5 mg/kg/hr ≥ 12 hours
3	↑ SCr ≥ 3 - 6-fold from baseline, with an acute increase of at least 0.5 mg/dl or individual who received RRT	UO < 0.3 mg/kg/hr ≥ 24 hours

Scr: serum creatinine; UO: urine output [4].

found to be present in about 1% of hospital admissions [5]. The causes of community-acquired AKI also may include pre-renal azotemia, intrinsic renal failure, and post-renal obstruction. The risk factors for developing community-acquired AKI include, old age > 75 yrs, patients with underlying chronic kidney disease (CKD, eGFR < 60 mls/min/1.73m^2), cardiac failure, atherosclerotic peripheral vascular disease, liver disease, diabetes mellitus and patients taking nephrotoxic medications, alternative medical therapies, etc. Other disorders include exercise or heat-stroke related rhabdomyolysis, crush-syndrome from natural disasters such as earthquakes, may also contribute to community-acquired AKI [5].

3.2. Hospital-Acquired AKI

AKI is present in about 7% of all hospitalized patients [6], and more than 30% of critically ill patients experienced AKI [7,8]. The incidence of AKI greatly increased in the hospital settings with improved critical care, increase diagnostic and procedural techniques, and improved management of other organ failures. The risk factors for hospital acquired AKI are sepsis, elder age, pre-existing kidney dysfunction. Since the widespread use of primary percutaneous coronary intervention protocols and intravenous contrast related investigations in intensive care unit, contrast related renal injuries are becomingly known as important risk factor for AKI. Other causes of AKI intensive care units may also include pre-renal azotemia, ischemia, organ failures, toxins, obstruction, etc. The severe AKI in ICU is now considered as a part of a multiple system organ failure (MSOF) complex and its mortality varies over 50-80% in ICU [9, 10]. The natural course of AKI has not been benign as previously thought, and >20% of ICU dialysis survivors progress to CKD and ESRD within 3 - 5 years. In a cohort study, the RIFLE criteria—risk, injury, and failure—found to be associated with inpatient mortality rates of 8.8%, 11.4%, and 26.3%, respectively [11]. Pathophysiology of AKI

The mechanism of acute kidney injury depends on the severity of insults which vary from increased risk, progressive damage to decreased glomerular filtration rate (GFR), kidney failure and death. Abolishment of renal auto-regulation occurs in ischemic renal injury due to imbalance between vasoconstrictors and vasodilators. Diminished renal perfusion may cause elevated of endothelial injury markers, inflammatory mediators like TNF-a, IL-18, etc. with reduced nitric oxide derivatives with resultant endothelial injury. High levels of vasoconstrictors with persistent hypoxia may lead to cellular damage and cell death with reduction in GFR. Necrosis and desquamation of tubular cells result in tubular obstruction, which may further reduce GFR. Local inflammatory mediators may lead to interstitial inflammation, small vessel obstruction and finally, local ischemia [12,13]. Direct nephrotoxic effects may result in decreased GFR in cases of toxic AKI.

A better understanding of the clinical continuum of AKI is needed for better diagnostic and therapeutic measures. The systemic inflammatory response syndrome [14], insulin resistance with hyperglycemia associated injuries [15], and associated oxidative stress may take part in the development of ischemic and toxic AKI in critically ill patients. Since kidney injury itself may also generate oxidative stress, increased oxidative stress biomarkers are found to be elevated [16,17]. Biomarkers of structural injury elevated earlier than those for functional injury during the AKI event. Overall, biomarkers, especially urinary biomarkers of AKI will facilitate earlier diagnosis, provide specific preventative and therapeutic strategies and with the overall improve in outcomes.

4. Types of Biomarkers

An ideal biomarker of AKI would fulfill the following:

- Increase in the urine or blood within minutes or hours

after a renal insult;

- Remains elevated as long as the renal injury persists;
- Correlates quantitatively with the extent of renal injury;
- Decreases proportionally with the renal recovery status.

Urinary biomarkers are regarded more non-invasive, easy to measure, easily obtainable, and clinically earlier detection than blood biomarkers [18,19]. Injury to different segment regions of nephrons may excrete different specific urinary biomarkers. Detection of high-molecular weight protein, like albumin, immunoglobulin, and transferrin in the urine may be associated with glomerular injury. Low-molecular weight proteinuria (e.g. α-1 microglobulin, β-1 microglobulin and retinol binding proteins) [20,21], brush border antigens [20,22,23], urinary enzymes [20,24] and other urinary proteins [25-28] are associated with damage to renal tubules. However, sufficient validation is needed to use these markers for the screening and differentiating the site of injury clinically.

Depend on the time of appearance after AKI, the urinary biomarkers may be classified into biomarkers of structural injury, and those of functional injury. Structural injury biomarkers are those appearing in the urine immediately after tubular cell apoptosis, and include KIM-1, NGAL, NAG, IL-18, and clusterin. Functional injury biomarkers are delayed markers for injury which may indicate global renal dysfunction, and constitutes cystatin C, total protein, albumin and β-2 microglobulin (**Table 2**).

5. Biomarkers under Evaluation in Humans

Recently, more than 20 protein biomarkers have been intensively reviewed in human and animal models of AKI to identify which ones may signal AKI prior to a rise in serum creatinine. Since the gold standard kidney biopsies are not clinically practicable in AKI patients as outcome measures, rise in serum creatinine is still used as clinical outcome. A potential biomarker should increase rapidly in the settings where the timing of renal injury is known (e.g. after cardiopulmonary bypass (CPB) or immediate post-transplant period). The validity of biomarker is assessed most commonly by receiver operating characteristic (ROC) curve, which plots 1 minus specificity of the biomarker on the x-axis against the sensitivity of the biomarker on the y-axis. The area under curve (AUC) is generated from these plots, and an AUC of 1 represents a perfect biomarker and AUC of 0.5 reflects complete lack of accuracy.

5.1. Neutrophil Gelatinase-Associated Lipocalin (NGAL)

Neutrophil gelatinase-associated lipocalin (NGAL) is the one of the most consistant biomarker found during AKI. It is a 25-kDa polypeptide covalently bound to gelatinase from human neutrophils, and predominantly found in proliferating nuclear antigen-positive proximal tubule cells. It is markedly up-regulated in early post-ischemic mouse and rat kidneys [29]. The urinary NGAL protein has been demonstrated to predict the occurrence of ischemic AKI in pediatric and adult patients after cardiac surgery [30,31]. In a prospective study done on pediatric patients undergone cardiopulmonary bypass (CPB) by Mishra *et al.* [30], the urinary NGAL was increased 100 fold and detected within 2 hours of CPB, which precede 50% increase in SCr by 1 - 3 days. In contrast, urinary NGAL did not rise in those patients who did not develop AKI. The area under the receiver operating characteristic curve (AUC-ROC) was 0.99 at 2 hours and 1.00 at 4 hours after CPB [30]. Plasma NGAL was also found to predict morbidity and mortality in pediatric patients who undergo cardiac surgery [32]. Urinary NGAL also was found to be elevated within 1 hour after cardiac surgery in adult patients and revealed the AUC-ROC of 0.74 at 3 hours and 0.8 at 18 hours [31]. In a small prospective study of pediatric and adult kidney transplant patients, urinary NGAL is demonstrated as an excellent predictive marker (AUC-ROC 0.9 at day 0 after transplantation) for the development of delayed graft dysfunction and renal re- placement therapy [33]. Furthermore, a recent study demonstrated that a single urine NGAL measurement in the emergency department could better predict the need for Nephrology consultations, intensive care unit admission, dialysis initiation, or mortality, etc. than could an elevated serum creatinine [34].

5.2. Kidney Injury Molecule-1 (KIM-1)

KIM-1 is an orphan trans-membrane receptor of unknown function. It is undetectable in normal kidney tissue or urine, and is markedly increased in ischemic and nephrotoxic proximal tubule epithelial cell injury, and in renal cell carcinoma [35-37]. In a small cross-sectional study, Han *et al.* [38] demonstrated the elevation of urinary KIM-1 levels within 12 hours after an initial ischemic insult and much earlier than granular casts appearance in established AKI. Higher urinary KIM-1 was also associated with adverse outcomes in these established AKI patients. Urinary KIM-1 was elevated and found to have an AUC-ROC of 0.57 at 2 hours, 0.83 at 12 hours, and 0.78 at 24 hours after pediatric cardiac surgery in a case-control study [39] using the same cohort in the NGAL study previously described [30]. High urinary KIM-1 may also predict the graft loss in renal transplant patients independent of other common risk factors like creatinine clearance, proteinuria, and donor age [40]. Urinary KIM-1 was also proved in some studies to distinguish AKI from CKD and normal [41,42].

Table 2. Biomarkers of acute kidney injury.

Type of biomarkers	Selective sites and associated types of injury
Biomarkers of structural injury	
Kidney injury molecule-1 (KIM-1)	Proximal tubule injury (Ischemic AKI, nephrotoxins, RCC)
n-acetyl glucosaminadase (NAG)	Proximal tubule injury
Neutrophil gelatinase-associated lipocalin (NGAL)*	Tubule and collecting duct injury (Ischemic AKI, nephrotoxins, DRAF)
Interleukin (IL)-18	Tubule injury (AKI, DRAF)
Clusterin	Tubule injury
Biomarkers of functional injury	
Cystatin C*	Glomerular injury; in urine indicates proximal tubule injury
Total protein β2-microglobulin albumin	Glomerular and tubular dysfunction
Brush border antigens	
Adenosine deaminase binding protein	
Carbonic anhydrase	Proximal tubule injury
Other tubular antigens	
Urinary enzymes	
N-acetyl-β-D-glucosaminidase	
Alanine aminopeptidase	
Cathepsin B	Proximal tubule injury
γ-glutamyltransferase	
α-glutathione-S-transferase	
β-glucosidase	Proximal tubule > distal tubule injury
Alkaline phosphatase	
Lactate dehydrogenase	Distal tubule > proximal tubule injury
Others	
Type IV Collagen	Glomerular injury
Gamma-glutamyl transferase (γ-GT)	Tubular epithelium injury
Liver type fatty acid binding protein (L-FABP)	
Retinol binding protein 4 (RBP4)	
Sodium/hydrogen exchanger isoform	Proximal tubule injury
Alpha-glutathione S-transferase (α-GST)	
Exosomal fetuin-A	
Tamm-horsfall glycoprotein	Distal tubule injury
pi-glutathione S-transferase (π-GST)	

*Available in both serum and urine; DRAF: delayed renal allograft function; RCC: renal cell carcinoma; AKI: Acute kidney injury; IL: interleukin; TNF: tumor necrosis factor.

5.3. Interleukin (IL)-18

Interleukin (IL)-18 is a pro-inflammatory cytokine which involve in mediating inflammation process during ischemic, sepsis and nephrotoxic AKI [12]. Since IL-18 serves to recruit the neutrophils during ischemic injury, elevated urine IL-18 have been demonstrated in patients with ischemic acute tubular necrosis (ATN) [43]. In a cross-sectional study, Parikh *et al.* demonstrated that markedly elevated day 0 post-transplantation urinary IL-18 concentration was found in patients with delayed allograft dysfunction (AUC 0.95) [43]. In a prospective study of 138 patients with acute respiratory distress syndrome, elevation of urinary IL-18 could predict AKI one day ahead of serum creatinine with an AUC-ROC 0.73, and also independently predicts mortality in this cohort group [44]. Urinary IL-18 was also found in elevated after CPB, and has an AUC-ROC of 0.61 at 4 hours, 0.75 at 12 hours, and 0.73 at 24 hours following CPB to predict AKI [45]. In the critically ill patients, the urinary IL-18 level was also regarded as an independent predictor of mortality.

5.4. Cystatin C

Cystatin C is a 13kD cysteine protease inhibitor protein that is produced by all nucleated cells into plasma, and freely filtered from glomerulus, completely reabsorbed and not secreted in the tubules. It is less influenced by factors other than glomerular filtration rate (e.g. age, gender, race, or muscle mass) [44]. Several studies have demonstrated that a change in serum and urine Cystatin C is more sensitive than a change in Serum creatinine in predicting a change in glomerular filtration [46-48].

In a prospective study of 85 critically ill patients at high risk to develop AKI, a 50% increase in serum cystatin C was noted one to two days before serum creatinine with an AUC of 0.97 and 0.82 respectively [49]. Furthermore, serum cystatin C also predicts the risk of AKI-associated cardiovascular morbidity and mortality in critically ill patients [50]. In older patients, increased serum cystatin C is also found to be a stronger predictor for the risk of death and cardiovascular events [50,51]. Furthermore, serum cystatin C levels > 1.0 mg/L may also predict cardiovascular events and mortality in participants with serum creatinine-based eGFR > 60 ml/min per 1.73 m^2 [52,53]. Urine cystatin C has also been studied and some studies found that urine Cystatin C performed better for AKI prediction than did serum Cystatin C [54,55]. In addition, increased urinary cystatin C and α1-microglobulin may be early predictors of an unfavorable clinical outcome in ATN, reflected by the requirement for RRT. Severity prediction with these markers could assist in improving the outcome of ATN [55]. Cystatin C also is extensively studied in chronic kidney disease patients. Since serum cystatin C has higher sensitivity and higher negative predictive value in determination of reduced GFR than serum creatinine, many studies examine the serum cystatin C to use clinically in GFR determination [56]. A recent cross-sectional study found that the combined creatinine-cystatin C equation to estimate GFR better than either of these markers alone in chronic kidney disease patients [57]. Although these findings are encouraging, additional studies are further needed for clinical use of serum and urine cystatin-C in acute and chronic renal disease conditions.

6. Biomarker Combinations in Different Clinical Conditions

The ultimate diagnostic goal in AKI is to distinguish pre-renal azotemia, renal AKI (ATN), obstruction, Urinary traction infections, and underlying CKD, etc. Studies are underway to distinguish the various types of AKI by using biomarkers. For example, urinary KIM-1 could distinguish ischemic ATN from pre-renal azotemia and CKD in one study [41], and KIM-1 also found to distinguish AKI from CKD and normal with an AUC of 0.94 [42].

Biomarker combination may be required in improving determination and differentiating the AKI. The sequential appearance of AKI biomarkers has been noted during serial measurements of multiple urinary biomarkers after pediatric cardiac surgery, with urine NGAL peaks at 2 hrs followed by the IL-18 peak at 12 hrs. Urinary IL-18 has a lower AUC (0.74 at 12 hrs) than NGAL (0.99 at 2 hrs) [31,58]. This sequential increase resembles troponin I, CPK and LDH of acute myocardial injury, which may help us to determine the time since injury in AKI. Although NGAL alone can predict AKI in the early hours, the combination of both urinary markers may predict the borderline cases in later periods after surgery. Several biomarker combinations may also predict AKI after adult cardiac surgery (**Figure 1**) [59]. These biomarker combinations have been tested in only small studies and limited clinical situations. Multicenter studies are needed to determine which biomarker combination best predict and determine outcome in AKI.

7. Proposed Biomarker Strategies for Renal Replacement Therapy (RRT) Initiation in AKI

Another hope for biomarkers in AKI is to determine the time to start renal replacement therapy (RRT). Although the results are encouraging for some biomarkers, there still need to create the biomarker-based strategies for RRT initiation. Since wide practice variation in timing of initiating RRT and heterogeneity of AKI in various situations,

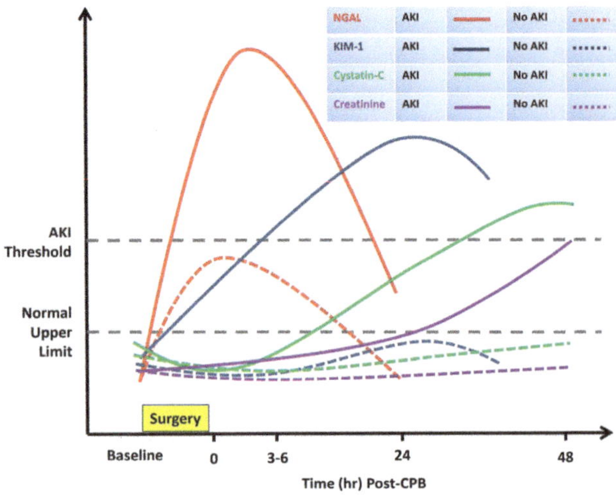

Figure 1. The comparism for the predicted time course of change in urine or serum biomarker levels in AKI and non-AKI patients after cardiac surgery. Patterns of change represent ideal circumstances, which have not been consistently demonstrated in clinical studies. AKI: acute kidney injury; CPB: cardiopulmonary bypass; creatinine: serum creatinine; cystatin-C: serum cystatin-C; KIM-1: urinary kidney injury molecule-1; NGAL: urinary neutrophil gelatinase-associated lipocalin. Modified from [59].

the decision making in initiation of RRT remains subjective in most clinical settings.

An opinion-based clinical algorithm was drawn using RIFLE/AKIN criteria, and several patient-specific factors to decide when to start RRT in critically ill adults [60]. Recently, the well accepted metabolic derangements need for RRT include plasma BUN > 100 mg/dl, hyperkalemia > 6 mEq/L with EKG abnormalities, hypermagnesemia > 8 mEq/L, severe metabolic acidosis pH < 7.15, diuretic resistant fluid overload [61-65]. Some studies demonstrate better renal outcome in patients who start RRT while in RIFLE-Risk or Injury than those who started RRT in RIFLE-Failure status [66,67]. Clinically, it is possible for some RIFLE-Risk and Injury cases to recover spontaneously before complications develop and in these cases RRT may not benefit. And on the other hand, if we could easily categorize these patients in RISK-Risk and Injury cases with severe and sustained renal injury, we can start RRT to provide renal support and to prevent AKI-related complications.

Some studies suggest novel biomarkers like NGAL, Cystatin-C, NAG, KIM-1, and α1-microglobulin can distinguish patients in whom RRT will be needed [55, 68]. A potential use of biomarkers integrated into the clinical decision algorithms to initiate RRT is recently proposed by Cruz *et al.* (**Figure 2**) [69]. In this algorithm, two cut-offs are needed, one represents a high likelihood of needing RRT, and another indicates RRT is very improbable. The first cut-off would identify those AKI patients in whom spontaneous renal recovery is not likely. The second cut-off distinguishes those AKI patients with probable spontaneous renal recovery. These cut-off values may be absolute value or relative change from baseline value, and vary with different clinical settings. Biomarkers are repeatedly measured during conservative therapy to monitor and reassess the disease progress. However, more studies are needed to use these biomarkers effectively in clinical AKI patients.

8. Limitations of Biomarker Use in Clinical Acute Kidney Injury

The heterogeneity of AKI especially in intensive care unit needs more than one biomarker to obtain sufficient sensitivity and specificity for AKI screening. An analysis of multiple biomarkers may need in additional studies before biomarkers may be used in routine clinical practice. Recently, none of the promising biomarkers have been systematically evaluated in the various clinical settings

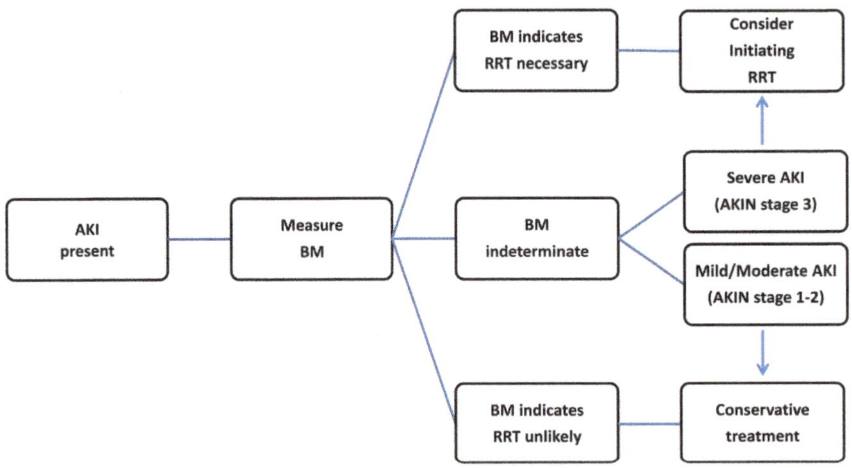

Figure 2. Biomarker-based strategy for renal replacement therapy in AKI patients. AKI: acute kidney injury; BM: biomarker; RRT: renal replacement therapy; AKIN: Acute Kidney Injury Network. Modified from [69].

of AKI. Additionally, no cutoff value that is predictive of AKI has been available nowadays. The role of these biomarkers in association with other comorbidities including sepsis, etc. is not accomplished.

9. Conclusion

Bomarkers of AKI such as NGAL, KIM-1, IL-18 and Cystatin C are now becoming greatest interest among different AKI clinical settings. Early measurements of AKI biomarkers predict subsequent development of intrinsic AKI, dialysis requirement, ICU stay, days of hospital stay and finally affects mortality. Future studies should evaluate biomarker outcomes independent of serum creatinine, and should consider biomarkers as entry criteria for AKI therapeutic protocols. Such an advance would finally find out the gold standard biomarker for AKI, as in case of troponin I for potential myocardial ischemia.

REFERENCES

[1] R. Bellomo, C. Ronco, J. A. Kellum, R. L. Mehta and P. Palevsky, "Acute Renal Failure—Definition, Outcome Measures, Animal Models, Fluid Therapy and Information Technology Needs: The Second International Consensus Conference of the Acute Dialysis Quality Initiative (ADQI) Group," *Critical Care*, Vol. 8, No. 4, 2004, pp. R204-R212. doi:10.1186/cc2872

[2] J. A. Kellum, N. Levin, C. Bouman and N. Lameire, "Developing a Consensus Classification System for Acute Renal Failure," *Current Opinion in Critical Care*, Vol. 8, No. 6, 2002, pp. 509-514. doi:10.1097/00075198-200212000-00005

[3] G. M. Chertow, E. Burdick, M. Honour, J. V. Bonventre and D. W. Bates, "Acute Kidney Injury, Mortality, Length of Stay, and Costs in Hospitalized Patients," *Journal of the American Society of Nephrology*, Vol. 16, No. 11, 2005, pp. 3365-3370. doi:10.1681/ASN.2004090740

[4] R. L. Mehta, J. A. Kellum, S. V. Shah, B. A. Molitoris, C. Ronco, D. G. Warnock and A. Levin, "Acute Kidney Injury Network: Report of an Initiative to Improve Outcomes in Acute Kidney Injury," *Critical Care*, Vol. 11, No. 2, 2007, p. R31. doi:10.1186/cc5713

[5] J. Kaufman, M. Dhakal, B. Patel and R. Hamburger, "Community-Acquired Acute Renal Failure," *American Journal of Kidney Diseases*, Vol. 17, No. 2, 1991, pp. 191-198.

[6] K. Nash, A. Hafeez and S. Hou, "Hospital-Acquired Renal Insufficiency," *American Journal of Kidney Diseases*, Vol. 39, No. 5, 2002, pp. 930-936. doi:10.1053/ajkd.2002.32766

[7] R. L. Mehta, M. T. Pascual, S. Soroko, *et al.*, "Spectrum of Acute Renal Failure in the Intensive Care Unit: The PICARD Experience," *Kidney International*, Vol. 66, No. 4, 2004, pp. 1613-1621. doi:10.1111/j.1523-1755.2004.00927.x

[8] M. Ostermann and R.W. Chang, "Acute Kidney Injury in the Intensive Care Unit According to RIFLE," *Critical Care Medicine*, Vol. 35, No. 8, 2007, pp. 1837-1843. doi:10.1097/01.CCM.0000277041.13090.0A

[9] F. Liano, C. Felipe, M. T. Tenorio, M. Rivera, V. Abraira, J. M. Saez-de-Urturi, J. Ocana, C. Fuentes and S. Severiano, "Long-Term Outcome of Acute Tubular Necrosis: A Contribution to Its Natural History," *Kidney International*, Vol. 71, No. 7, 2007, pp. 679-686. doi:10.1038/sj.ki.5002086

[10] S. M. Bagshaw, K. B. Laupland, C. J. Doig, G. Mortis, G. H. Fick, M. Mucenski, T. Godinez-Luna, L. W. Svenson and T. Rosenal, "Prognosis for Long-Term Survival and Renal Recovery in Critically Ill Patients with Severe Acute Renal Failure: A Population-Based Study," *Critical Care*, Vol. 9, No. 6, 2005, pp. R700-R709. doi:10.1186/cc3879

[11] E. A. Hoste, G. Clermont, A. Kersten, R. Venkataraman, D. C. Angus, D. De Bacquer and J. A. Kellum, "RIFLE Criteria for Acute Kidney Injury Are Associated with Hospital Mortality in Critically Ill Patients: A Cohort Analysis," *Critical Care*, Vol. 10, No. 3, 2006, p. R73. doi:10.1186/cc4915

[12] J. V. Bonventre and J. M. Weinberg, "Recent Advances in the Pathophysiology of Ischemic Acute Renal Failure," *Journal of the American Society of Nephrology*, Vol. 14, No. 8, 2003, pp. 2199-2210. doi:10.1097/01.ASN.0000079785.13922.F6

[13] R. W. Schrier, W. Wang, B. Poole and A. Mitra, "Acute Renal Failure: Definitions, Diagnosis, Pathogenesis, and Therapy," *The Journal of Clinical Investigation*, Vol. 114, No. 1, 2004, pp. 5-14.

[14] M. S. Rangel-Frausto, D. Pittet, M. Costigan, T. Hwang, C. S. Davis and R. P. Wenzel, "The Natural History of the Systemic Inflammatory Response Syndrome (SIRS). A Prospective Study," *Journal of the American Medical Association*, Vol. 273, No. 2, 1995, pp. 117-123. doi:10.1001/jama.1995.03520260039030

[15] G. Van den Berghe, A. Wilmer, G. Hermans, *et al.*, "Intensive Insulin Therapy in the Medical ICU," *The New England Journal of Medicine*, Vol. 354, No. 5, 2006, pp. 449-461. doi:10.1056/NEJMoa052521

[16] J. Himmelfarb, E. McMonagle, S. Freedman, *et al.*, "Oxidative Stress Is Increased in Critically Ill Patients with Acute Renal Failure," *Journal of the American Society of Nephrology*, Vol. 15, No. 9, 2004, pp. 2449-2456. doi:10.1097/01.ASN.0000138232.68452.3B

[17] G. H. Metnitz, M. Fischer, C. Bartens, H. Steltzer, T. Lang and W. Druml, "Impact of Acute Renal Failure on Antioxidant Status in Multiple Organ Failure," *Acta Anaesthesiologica Scandinavica*, Vol. 44, No. 3, 2000, pp. 236-240. doi:10.1034/j.1399-6576.2000.440304.x

[18] P. Devarajan, "Emerging Biomarkers of Acute Kidney Injury," *Contributions to Nephrology*, Vol. 156, 2007, pp. 203-212. doi:10.1159/000102085

[19] P. Devarajan, "Emerging Urinary Biomarkers in the Diagnosis of Acute Kidney Injury," *Expert Opinion on Medical Diagnostics*, Vol. 2, No. 4, 2008, pp. 387-398.

[20] N. E. Tolkoff-Rubin, R. H. Rubin and J. V. Bonventre,

"Noninvasive Renal Diagnostic Studies," *Clinics in Laboratory Medicine*, Vol. 8, No. 3, 1988, pp. 507-526.

[21] C. Bazzi, C. Petrini, V. Rizza, *et al.*, "Urinary Excretion of IgG and Alpha(1)-Microglobulin Predicts Clinical Course Better than Extent of Proteinuria in Membranous Nephropathy," *American Journal of Kidney Diseases*, Vol. 38, No. 2, 2001, pp. 240-248. doi:10.1053/ajkd.2001.26080

[22] N. Taniguchi, M. Tanaka, C. Kishihara, *et al.*, "Determination of Carbonic Anhydrase C and Beta 2-Microglobulin by Radioimmunoassay in Urine of Heavy-Metal-Exposed Subjects and Patients with Renal Tubular Acidosis," *Environmental Research*, Vol. 20, No. 1, 1979, pp. 154-161. doi:10.1016/0013-9351(79)90094-X

[23] A. Mutti, S. Lucertini, P. Valcavi, *et al.*, "Urinary Excretion of Brush-Border Antigen Revealed by Monoclonal Antibody: Early Indicator of Toxic Nephropathy," *Lancet*, Vol. 2, No. 8461, 1985, pp. 914-917. doi:10.1016/S0140-6736(85)90850-5

[24] J. Boldt, T. Brenner, J. Lang, B. Kumle and F. Isgro, "Kidney-Specific Proteins in Elderly Patients Undergoing Cardiac Surgery with Cardiopulmonary Bypass," *Anesthesia and Analgesia*, Vol. 97, No. 6, 2003, pp. 1582-1589. doi:10.1213/01.ANE.0000090146.02929.2E

[25] K. Sugimura, T. Goto, K. Tsuchida, Y. Takemoto, T. Kim and T. Kishimoto, "Production and Activation of Hepatocyte Growth Factor in Acute Renal Failure," *Renal Failure*, Vol. 23, No. 3-4, 2001, pp. 597-603. doi:10.1081/JDI-100104741

[26] F. Mariano, G. Guida, D. Donati, *et al.*, "Production of Platelet-Activating Factor in Patients with Sepsis-Associated Acute Renal Failure," *Nephrology, Dialysis, Transplantation*, Vol. 14, No. 5, 1999, pp. 1150-1157. doi:10.1093/ndt/14.5.1150

[27] H. Zhou, T. Pisitkun, A. Aponte, *et al.*, "Exosomal Fetuin-A Identified by Proteomics: A Novel Urinary Biomarker for Detecting Acute Kidney Injury," *Kidney International*, Vol. 70, No. 10, 2006, pp. 1847-1857. doi:10.1038/sj.ki.5001874

[28] Y. Muramatsu, M. Tsujie, Y. Kohda, *et al.*, "Early Detection of Cysteine Rich Protein 61 (CYR61, CCN1) in Urine Following Renal Ischemic Reperfusion Injury," *Kidney International*, Vol. 62, No. 5, 2002, pp. 1601-1610. doi:10.1046/j.1523-1755.2002.00633.x

[29] J. Mishra, Q. Ma, A. Prada, *et al.*, "Identification of Neutrophil Gelatinase-Associated Lipocalin as a Novel Early Urinary Biomarker for Ischemic Renal Injury," *Journal of the American Society of Nephrology*, Vol. 14, No. 10, 2003, pp. 2534-2543. doi:10.1097/01.ASN.0000088027.54400.C6

[30] J. Mishra, C. Dent, R. Tarabishi, *et al.*, "Neutrophil Gelatinase-Associated Lipocalin (NGAL) as a Biomarker for Acute Renal Injury after Cardiac Surgery," *Lancet*, Vol. 365, No. 9466, 2005, pp. 1231-1238. doi:10.1016/S0140-6736(05)74811-X

[31] G. Wagener, M. Jan, M. Kim, *et al.*, "Association between Increases in Urinary Neutrophil Gelatinase-Associated Lipocalin and Acute Renal Dysfunction after Adult cardiac Surgery," *Anesthesiology*, Vol. 105, No. 3, 2006, pp. 485-491. doi:10.1097/00000542-200609000-00011

[32] C. L. Dent, Q. Ma, S. Dastrala, *et al.*, "Plasma Neutrophil Gelatinase-Associated Lipocalin Predicts Acute Kidney Injury, Morbidity and Mortality after Pediatric Cardiac Surgery: A Prospective Uncontrolled Cohort Study," *Critical Care*, Vol. 11, No. 6, 2007, p. R127. doi:10.1186/cc6192

[33] C. R. Parikh, A. Jani, J. Mishra, *et al.*, "Urine NGAL and IL-18 Are Predictive Biomarkers for Delayed Graft Function Following Kidney Transplantation," *American Journal of Transplantation*, Vol. 6, No. 7, 2006, pp. 1639-1645. doi:10.1111/j.1600-6143.2006.01352.x

[34] T. L. Nickolas, M. J. O'Rourke, J. Yang, *et al.*, "Sensitivity and Specificity of a Single Emergency Department Measurement of Urinary Neutrophil Gelatinase-Associated Lipocalin for Diagnosing Acute Kidney Injury," *Annals of Internal Medicine*, Vol. 148, No. 11, 2008, pp. 810-819.

[35] T. Ichimura, J. V. Bonventre, V. Bailly, *et al.*, "Kidney Injury Molecule-1 (KIM-1), a Putative Epithelial Cell Adhesion Molecule Containing a Novel Immunoglobulin Domain, Is Up-Regulated in Renal Cells after Injury," *The Journal of Biological Chemistry*, Vol. 273, No. 7, 1998, pp. 4135-4142. doi:10.1074/jbc.273.7.4135

[36] T. Ichimura, C. C. Hung, S. A. Yang, J. L. Stevens and J. V. Bonventre, "Kidney Injury Molecule-1: A Tissue and Urinary Biomarker for Nephrotoxicant-Induced Renal Injury," *American Journal of Physiology Renal Physiology*, Vol. 286, No. 3, 2004, pp. F552-F563. doi:10.1152/ajprenal.00285.2002

[37] W. K. Han, A. Alinani, C. L. Wu, *et al.*, "Human Kidney Injury Molecule-1 Is a Tissue and Urinary Tumor Marker of Renal Cell Carcinoma," *Journal of the American Society of Nephrology*, Vol. 16, No. 4, 2005, pp. 1126-1134.

[38] W. K. Han, V. Bailly, R. Abichandani, R. Thadhani and J. V. Bonventre, "Kidney Injury Molecule-1 (KIM-1): A Novel Biomarker for Human Renal Proximal Tubule Injury," *Kidney International*, Vol. 62, No. 1, 2002, pp. 237-244. doi:10.1046/j.1523-1755.2002.00433.x

[39] W. K. Han, S. S. Waikar, A. Johnson, *et al.*, "Urinary Biomarkers in the Early Diagnosis of Acute Kidney Injury," *Kidney International*, Vol. 73, No. 7, 2008, pp. 863-869. doi:10.1038/sj.ki.5002715

[40] M. M. van Timmeren, V. S. Vaidya, R. M. van Ree, *et al.*, "High Urinary Excretion of Kidney Injury Molecule-1 Is an Independent Predictor of Graft Loss in Renal Transplant Recipients," *Transplantation*, Vol. 84, No. 12, 2007, pp. 1625-1630. doi:10.1097/01.tp.0000295982.78039.ef

[41] W. K. Han, V. Bailly, R. Abichandani, R. Thadhani and J. V. Bonventre, "Kidney Injury Molecule-1 (KIM-1): A Novel Biomarker for Human Renal Proximal Tubule Injury," *Kidney International*, Vol. 62, No. 1, 2002, pp. 237-244. doi:10.1046/j.1523-1755.2002.00433.x

[42] M. H. Rosner, "Urinary Biomarkers for the Detection of Renal Injury," *Advances in Clinical Chemistry*, Vol. 49, 2009, pp. 73-97. doi:10.1016/S0065-2423(09)49004-8

[43] C. R. Parikh, A. Jani, V. Y. Melnikov, S. Faubel and C. L. Edelstein, "Urinary Interleukin-18 Is a Marker of Human Acute Tubular Necrosis," *American Journal of Kidney*

Diseases, Vol. 43, No. 3, 2004, pp. 405-414. doi:10.1053/j.ajkd.2003.10.040

[44] C. R. Parikh, E. Abraham, M. Ancukiewicz and C. L. Edelstein, "Urine IL-18 Is an Early Diagnostic Marker for Acute Kidney Injury and Predicts Mortality in the Intensive Care Unit," *Journal of the American Society of Nephrology*, Vol. 16, No. 10, 2005, pp. 3046-3052. doi:10.1681/ASN.2005030236

[45] C. R. Parikh, J. Mishra, H. Thiessen-Philbrook, *et al*., "Urinary IL-18 Is an Early Predictive Biomarker of Acute Kidney Injury after Cardiac Surgery," *Kidney International*, Vol. 70, No. 1, 2006, pp. 199-203. doi:10.1038/sj.ki.5001527

[46] E. Coll, A. Botey, L. Alvarez, *et al*., "Serum Cystatin C as a New Marker for Noninvasive Estimation of Glomerular Filtration Rate and as a Marker for Early Renal Impairment," *American Journal of Kidney Diseases*, Vol. 36, No. 1, 2000, pp. 29-34. doi:10.1053/ajkd.2000.8237

[47] V. R. Dharnidharka, C. Kwon and G. Stevens, "Serum Cystatin C Is Superior to Serum Creatinine as a Marker of Kidney Function: A Meta-Analysis," *American Journal of Kidney Diseases*, Vol. 40, No. 2, 2002, pp. 221-226. doi:10.1053/ajkd.2002.34487

[48] S. Song, M. Meyer, T. R. Turk, *et al*., "Serum Cystatin C in Mouse Models: A Reliable and Precise Marker for Renal Function and Superior to Serum Creatinine," *Nephrology, Dialysis, Transplantation*, Vol. 24, No. 4, 2009, pp. 1157-1161. doi:10.1093/ndt/gfn626

[49] S. Herget-Rosenthal, G. Marggraf, J. Husing, *et al*., "Early Detection of Acute Renal Failure by Serum Cystatin C," *Kidney International*, Vol. 66, No. 3, 2004, pp. 1115-1122. doi:10.1111/j.1523-1755.2004.00861.x

[50] M. G. Shlipak, M. J. Sarnak, R. Katz, *et al*., "Cystatin C and the Risk of Death and Cardiovascular Events among Elderly Persons," *The New England Journal of Medicine*, Vol. 352, No. 20, 2005, pp. 2049-2060. doi:10.1056/NEJMoa043161

[51] M. J. Sarnak, R. Katz, C. O. Stehman-Breen, *et al*., "Cystatin C Concentration as a Risk Factor for Heart Failure in Older Adults," *Annals of Internal Medicine*, Vol. 142, No. 7, 2005, pp. 497-505.

[52] M. G. Shlipak, L. F. Fried, C. Crump, *et al*., "Cardiovascular Disease Risk Status in Elderly Persons with Renal Insufficiency," *Kidney International*, Vol. 62, No. 3, 2002, pp. 997-1004. doi:10.1046/j.1523-1755.2002.00522.x

[53] M. G. Shlipak, R. Katz, M. J. Sarnak, *et al*., "Cystatin C and Prognosis for Cardiovascular and Kidney Outcomes in Elderly Persons without Chronic Kidney Disease," *Annals of Internal Medicine*, Vol. 145, No. 4, 2006, pp. 237-246.

[54] J. L. Koyner, M. R. Bennett, E. M. Worcester, *et al*., "Urinary Cystatin C as an Early Biomarker of Acute Kidney Injury Following Adult Cardiothoracic Surgery," *Kidney International*, Vol. 74, No. 8, 2008, pp. 1059-1069. doi:10.1038/ki.2008.341

[55] S. Herget-Rosenthal, D. Poppen, J. Husing, *et al*., "Prognostic Value of Tubular Proteinuria and Enzymuria in Nonoliguric Acute Tubular Necrosis," *Clinical Chemistry*, Vol. 50, No. 3, 2004, pp. 552-558. doi:10.1373/clinchem.2003.027763

[56] S. Herget-Rosenthal, S. Trabold, F. Pietruck, M. Holtmann, T. Philipp and A. Kribben, "Cystatin C: Efficacy as Screening Test for Reduced Glomerular Filtration Rate," *American Journal of Nephrology*, Vol. 20, No. 2, 2000, pp. 97-102. doi:10.1159/000013564

[57] L. A. Inker, C. H. Schmid, H. Tighiouart, *et al*., "Estimating Glomerular Filtration Rate from Serum Creatinine and Cystatin C," *The New England Journal of Medicine*, Vol. 367, No. 1, 2012, pp. 20-29. doi:10.1056/NEJMoa1114248

[58] C. R. Parikh, J. Mishra, H. Thiessen-Philbrook, *et al*., "Urinary IL-18 Is an Early Predictive Biomarker of Acute Kidney Injury after Cardiac Surgery," *Kidney International*, Vol. 70, No. 1, 2006, pp. 199-203. doi:10.1038/sj.ki.5001527

[59] D. R. McIlroy, G. Wagener and H. T. Lee, "Biomarkers of Acute Kidney Injury: An Evolving Domain," *Anesthesiology*, Vol. 112, No. 4, 2010, pp. 998-1004. doi:10.1097/ALN.0b013e3181cded3f

[60] S. M. Bagshaw, D. N. Cruz, R. T. Gibney and C. Ronco, "A Proposed Algorithm for Initiation of Renal Replacement Therapy in Adult Critically Ill Patients," *Critical Care*, Vol. 13, No. 6, 2009, p. 317. doi:10.1186/cc8037

[61] N. Lameire, "Pathophysiology of Acute Renal Failure in Sepsis," *Acta Clinica Belgica*, Vol. 59, No. 4, 2004, pp. 199-208.

[62] N. Lameire, W. Van Biesen and R. Vanholder, "Acute Renal Failure," *Lancet*, Vol. 380, No. 9857, 2012, p. 1904.

[63] J. A. Foland, J. D. Fortenberry, B. L. Warshaw, *et al*., "Fluid Overload before Continuous Hemofiltration and Survival in Critically Ill Children: A Retrospective Analysis," *Critical Care Medicine*, Vol. 32, No. 8, 2004, pp. 1771-1776. doi:10.1097/01.CCM.0000132897.52737.49

[64] P. Bent, H. K. Tan, R. Bellomo, *et al*., "Early and Intensive Continuous Hemofiltration for Severe Renal Failure after Cardiac Surgery," *The Annals of Thoracic Surgery*, Vol. 71, No. 3, 2001, pp. 832-837. doi:10.1016/S0003-4975(00)02177-9

[65] R. P. Dellinger, J. M. Carlet, H. Masur, *et al*., "Surviving Sepsis Campaign Guidelines for Management of Severe Sepsis and Septic Shock," *Critical Care Medicine*, Vol. 32, No. 3, 2004, pp. 858-873. doi:10.1097/01.CCM.0000117317.18092.E4

[66] M. Bell, E. Liljestam, F. Granath, J. Fryckstedt, A. Ekbom and C. R. Martling, "Optimal Follow-Up Time after Continuous Renal Replacement Therapy in Actual Renal Failure Patients Stratified with the RIFLE Criteria," *Nephrology, Dialysis, Transplantation*, Vol. 20, No. 2, 2005, pp. 354-360. doi:10.1093/ndt/gfh581

[67] C. C. Shiao, V. C. Wu, W. Y. Li, *et al*., "Late Initiation of Renal Replacement Therapy Is Associated with Worse Outcomes in Acute Kidney Injury after Major Abdominal Surgery," *Critical Care*, Vol. 13, No. 5, 2009, p. R171. doi:10.1186/cc8147

[68] V. S. Vaidya, S. S. Waikar, M. A. Ferguson, *et al*., "Urinary Biomarkers for Sensitive and Specific Detection of

Acute Kidney Injury in Humans," *Clinical and Translational Science*, Vol. 1, No. 3, 2008, pp. 200-208. doi:10.1111/j.1752-8062.2008.00053.x

[69] D. N. Cruz, H. R. de Geus and S. M. Bagshaw, "Biomarker Strategies to Predict Need for Renal Replacement Therapy in Acute Kidney Injury," *Seminars in Dialysis*, Vol. 24, No. 2, 2011, pp. 124-131. doi:10.1111/j.1525-139X.2011.00830.x

33

Can Fresh Frozen Plasma Prevent Acute Kidney Injury after Hump-Nosed Viper Bite?

Kolitha H. Sellahewa
Department of Medicine, Melaka Manipal Medical College, Melaka, Malaysia
Email: kolithah@gmail.com

ABSTRACT

Hump-nosed viper bite is the commonest venomous snakebite in Sri Lanka. Acute kidney injury (AKI) in association with coagulopathy is an important cause of mortality. Immunomodulating effects of fresh frozen plasma (FFP) could block the nephrotoxic effects of venom; and by replenishing depleted clotting factors resulting from venom induced consumption coagulopathy could offer an additional benefit in offsetting renal injury triggered by haematological disturbances. In a non-randomised observational study carried out from 2005 to 2008 in adults at the National hospital of Sri Lanka, the mean time for resolution of coagulopathy among 42 patients treated with FFP at the inception of coagulopathy was 4.7 hours compared to 18 patients treated with isotonic Saline among whom the mean time for normalisation of coagulopathy was 6.2 hours. None of these 60 patients developed acute renal failure. A separate cohort of 32 patients with coagulopathy after hump-nosed viper bite who had not received FFP during this study period developed acute renal failure and required haemodialysis. In the absence of safe and effective antivenom for hump-nosed viper in Sri Lanka, FFP may be a therapeutic option. FFP if given early to selected patients at inception of coagulopathy may prevent AKI and serve to save lives after hump-nosed viper bites.

Keywords: Hump-Nosed Viper Bite; Acute Kidney Injury; Fresh Frozen Plasma

1. Introduction

Hump-nosed viper bite is the most common venomous snakebite in Sri Lanka responsible for 22% - 77% of all snakebites [1-3]. Until recently it was considered to be a moderately venomous snake, however many deaths have been reported from time to time particularly in the recent past, so that it is now considered a highly venomous snake [4]. Even though systemic effects are rare these do occur, the commonest of which is coagulopathy [5-8]. All the reported deaths from hump-nosed viper bite had coagulopathy and acute kidney injury (AKI). The only antidote for snakebite is antivenom. In Sri Lanka polyspecific antivenom is used which is imported from India and is raised against the venoms of *Naja naja*, *Bungarus caeruleus*, *Daboia russelii*, and *Echis carinatus*, but not against hump-nosed viper (*Hypnale* spp.). The currently available antivenom is ineffective for hump nosed viper bite and is associated with a high incidence of adverse reactions including anaphylaxis and death [9-12]. In the absence of safe and effective antivenom for hump nosed viper bite a search for optional pharmacotherapeutic interventions addressing the critical clinical effects of systemic envenomation responsible for mortality was performed.

2. Hypothesis

Fresh frozen plasma (FFP) by immunomodulation could prevent venom mediated renal injury by acting at a site lower down the cascade of events that eventually lead to tissue injury. FFP by replenishing depleted clotting factors may also be useful in correcting the coagulopathy.

3. Method

An observational study was carried out at the National Hospital of Sri Lanka from March 2005 to June 2008.

3.1. Patients

All patients admitted to one adult medical unit with a diagnosis of having been bitten by hump-nosed vipers that developed coagulopathy were studied. Only those patients who brought the dead or live snakes that were identified as hump-nosed vipers by the attending physician were included in the study. However species identification as *H. hypnale*, *H. nepa*, or *H. zara* was not done. Coagulopathy was inferred by the detection of a positive 20 minute whole blood clotting test (20WBCT) which was performed in all patients on admission and then every 4 hours up to 24 hours. 20WBCT was performed by adding 3 ml of blood to a clean dry glass test tube and leaving it undisturbed for 20 minutes. At The end of 20 minutes the tube was tilted, if the blood flowed the test was considered positive and if a clot was formed and blood did not flow the test was deemed negative.

3.2. Investigations

Detailed haematological and biochemical investigations were done in the patients with a positive 20WBCT. These constituted full blood count, prothrombin time (PT), activated partial thromboplastin time (APTT), blood urea nitrogen, serum creatinine, and serum electrolytes. Blood samples were collected for PT and international normalized ratio (PT/INR) and APTT by adding 1.8 ml of whole blood into a bottle which contained 0.2 ml of prothrombin citrate. These tests were repeated daily. All laboratory analyses were done in the hospital laboratory.

3.3. Interventions

The patients who developed coagulopathy received either an infusion of FFP at a dose of 15 ml/kg body weight or isotonic Saline. Saline infusion was adjusted to maintain an hourly urine output of 0.5 ml/kg body weight. The patients were not randomised, and the decision to use FFP or Saline was ad hoc at the discretion of the physician on an individualised clinical judgement of the overall clinical condition of the patient. Written informed consent was taken from all the patients prior to intervention. 20WBCTs were then repeated 4 hourly up to 24 hours after the intervention. FFP was repeated every 4 hours until the coagulopathy was normalised.

3.4. Monitoring and Documentation

In all the patients the clinical status, vital signs, fluid intake, and hourly urine output were monitored. The clinical features and its progression or resolution after intervention were observed and documented. Decision to discharge patients included in the study was made by the same admitting physician.

4. Results

4.1. Patients and Treatment

All patients were adolescents and adults with an age range of 14 - 69 years. The mean age was 37.3 years. 74.2% were males and 25.8% were females. During the study period 60 patients developed coagulopathy. 42 were treated with FFP and 18 with isotonic Saline.

4.2. Outcome

The mean times for normalization of coagulopathy in the two groups were 4.7 hours and 6.2 hours respectively. In both these groups none developed acute renal failure (ARF) as evidenced by oliguria, elevated blood urea and a rise in the serum creatinine. Mean duration of hospital stay was also similar at 89.3 and 89.3 hours. All the 60 patients except one developed coagulopathy within 24 hours of the bite and was intervened soon after the detection of the first positive 20WBCT. One patient developed hematuria after 48 hours despite the 20WBCTs have been normal within the first 24 hours after the bite. None of the 42 patients treated with FFP developed any adverse sensitivity reactions. During this study period 32 patients who had developed ARF were transferred from the regional base hospital to this same unit for haemodialysis. All 32 patients were bitten by hump nosed vipers (*Hypnale* spp.) and were identified as such by the physician in the base hospital. Perusal of case records from the transferring base hospital revealed that all the 32 transferred patients had developed coagulopathy within the first 24 hours after the bite but none had received FFP.

Out of the 32 patients with ARF 31 recovered after haemodialysis. One patient a 38-year-old woman took a longer time to recover from ARF and required haemodialysis for 2 weeks. Her blood urea and serum creatinine normalised and had an adequate urine output but had low grade pyrexia. She died 10 days after recovering from the ARF and a post mortem examination revealed cerebral aspergillosis. She was dialysed for longer than usual and the source of infection was likely the catheter used for vascular access in the neck.

5. Discussion

The most consistent effects of envenomation by the hump nosed viper are local pain and swelling of the bitten limb [13]. Systemic effects are rare and unpredictable. Coagulopathy is the most common systemic effect occurring after hump-nosed viper bite. Overt bleeding of clinical significance such as haematuria, bleeding per rectum, and hematemesis are unusual and coagulopathy is usually detected by laboratory tests of the clotting status.

AKI has been reported in as many as 10% among 302 patients after bites of *H. hypnale* [10]. Association of coagulopathy with AKI has been independently reported by several workers [14-19]. It is likely that common pathophysiological mechanisms are responsible for both these important systemic complications of hump-nosed viper bite. Hump-nosed viper venom contains procoagulant, nephrotoxic, myotoxic and cytotoxic properties. AKI is caused primarily by nephrotoxicity rather than myoglobinuria or haemoglobinuria [15,19]. The procoagulant effects and venom induced consumption coagulopathy can also contribute to renal injury by the deposition of fibrin in the renal microcirculation and microvascular coagulation [19]. Fibrinogen degradation products can perpetuate the bleeding tendency by its antihaemostatic effects. These pathogenic mechanisms associated with the haemostatic disturbances seen could be important contributors to AKI apart for the primary venom induced nephrotoxicity. It may even be more important than the direct nephrotoxicity unlike AKI after *Daboia russelli* bites [20]. Interestingly coagulopathy was the earliest systemic manifestation among all the patients who developed ARF in this series. Arguably early correction of coagulopathy may prevent AKI in view of the observation that none of the 42 patients with coagulopathy who received FFP developed ARF; while all the 32 patients with coagulopathy who had not received FFP developed ARF. Whether this observation was a chance occurrence or was causally related to the intervention needs to be ascertained. However all the 18 patients with coagulopathy who were treated with only isotonic saline also recovered completely none of whom developed ARF even though it took a longer time for correction of coagulopathy (mean 6.2 hours) when compared with the group treated with FFP (mean 4.7).

The immunoglobulins in FFP could potentially by immunomodulation prevent nephrotoxin-induced primary renal injury. FFP is an accepted modality of intervention for consumption coagulopathy in a variety of clinical situations. In a similar way FFP by replenishing clotting factors could reverse venom induced consumption coagulopathy and arrest the cascading adverse consequences. Any added benefit in the prevention of AKI could be related to the impact of FFP on the haematopathogenic mechanisms implicated in AKI. In this study coagulopathy normalised earlier in those treated with FFP when compared with the patients who received only isotonic Saline.

6. Conclusions

Death due to hump-nosed viper bite though rare does occur. The primary cause for mortality is from complications associated with AKI. All patients who developed ARF developed coagulopathy within 48 hours of the bite. All who developed ARF had coagulopathy before the advent of clinical and biochemical features of ARF. It is possible that early correction of coagulopathy with FFP could prevent AKI and related adverse clinical outcomes.

The 20WBCT detects coagulopathy and can be used as a reliable and early predictor of systemic envenomation. It can easily be done at the bedside without depending on laboratories in resource poor settings where snake bite is common. Owing to the rarity and unpredictability of systemic manifestations and the recognized potential for a fatal outcome in patients with coagulopathy it is prudent that 20WBCT is monitored in all envenomed patients irrespective of the clinical status on presentation. Observation for at least 48 hours is advocated owing to the possibility of delayed or recurrent manifestation of coagulopathy. Patients who develop coagulopathy as evidenced by a positive 20WBCT should be selected for intensive monitoring and aggressive therapy aimed in the early detection, and treatment of venom induced consumption coagulopathy and thereby retards the advent of acute renal failure.

Thai Red Cross Malayan Pit Viper antivenom because of the close phylogenetic relationship between *H. hypnale* and *C. rhodostoma* may be useful in the treatment of hump nosed viper bite [10,21]. This however is not available in Sri Lanka. The only currently available antivenom in Sri Lanka is indicated for bites from *N. naja*, *B. caeruleus*, *D. russelii*, and *E. carinatus*, but not hump-nosed viper (*Hypnale* spp.). In the absence of safe and effective antivenom or any other specific therapy for hump-nosed viper bite in Sri Lanka I would advocate the use of FFP for selected patients as a safe and probably effective option to reduce morbidity and mortality from hump nosed viper bite in the Sri Lankan setting. This assertion is based on a consideration of the recognized pathogenic mechanisms implicated in hump-nosed viper venom-induced AKI and coagulopathy and application of the known pharmacological benefits of FFP for immunomodulation and consumption coagulopathy to offset these adverse consequences. Personal experience and the observation that none of the patients in this series developed ARF when FFP was used early at the inception of coagulopathy tend to support this contention. A well designed large double blind randomized controlled trial is recommended to test this hypothesis further.

Until the availability of safe and efficacious antivenom for hump-nosed viper envenomed patients, practicing clinicians have two options to reduce mortality due to hump-nosed viper envenoming in Sri Lanka.

1) Not offer any specific therapy and adopt a passive approach to management resigned to detect ARF early by monitoring renal function and offering dialysis once ARF is established. This intervention is expensive, not available for all, and attended with potential complications including fatalities.

2) Monitor 20WBCT and detect coagulopathy early. Select patients with coagulopathy for intensive monitoring of hemostatic attributes, renal function, and aggressive Intervention with FFP very early at the inception of coagulopathy. Thrombocytopenia in association with a positive 20WBCT in this clinical setting implies venom induced consumption coagulopathy and should be treated as such. Determination of APTT, PT, D-Dimmers, fibrinogen degradation products and fibrinogen assays will only serve to increase the precision of the diagnosis. However in resource poor settings none of these tests are

necessary to manage the patients. On the contrary these tests can add to the cost of management and delay interventions, albeit with disastrous and often fatal consequences. The aims of intervention with FFP are to prevent nephrotoxicity and promote the early correction of coagulopathy with the intended hypothetical benefit of averting the advent of ARF and thereby reduce mortality.

7. Limitations

A major drawback is that this is not a randomized controlled trial and devoid of statistical evaluation of the data. Decision to treat some patients with FFP was on the investigators experience in providing individualized care in the routine case management decision making process rather than on defined criteria. The patients who developed ARF were initially managed in a regional hospital and admitted under the care of the investigating physician only after the advent of ARF which required the mixing of results from two cohorts of patients.

8. Acknowledgements

I am thankful to all the patients who participated in this study and acknowledge with gratitude the support and co-operation extended by all the junior physicians, nurses, the laboratory and support staff at the National hospital of Sri Lanka where the study was done. I appreciate the assistance of Shazana Binti Mohd Selva for the literature search.

REFERENCES

[1] A. De Silva, "Snakebites in Anuradhapura District," *The Snake*, Vol. 13, 1981, pp. 117-130.

[2] S. L. Seneviratne, C. J. Opanayaka, N. S. Ratnayake, K. E. Kumara, A. M. Sugathadasa, N. Weerasuriya, W. A. Wickrama, S. B. Gunatilake and H. J. de Silva, "Use of Antivenom Serum in Snake Bite: A Prospective Study of Hospital Practice in the Gampaha District," *Ceylon Medical Journal*, Vol. 45, No. 2, 2000, pp. 65-68.

[3] A. Kasturiratne, A. R. Wickremasinghe, N. de Silv, N. K. Gunawardena, A. Pathmeswaran, R. Premaratna, L. Savioli, D. G. Lalloo and H. J. de Silva, "Estimating the Global Burden of Snakebite: A Literature Analysis and Modelling Based on Regional Estimates of Envenoming and Deaths," *PLoS Medicine*, Vol. 5, No. 11, 2008, p. e218. doi:10.1371/journal.pmed.0050218

[4] D. I. Simpson and R. L. Norris, "Snakes of Medical Importance in India: Is the Concept of 'Big 4' Still Relevant and Useful?" *Wilderness and Environmental Medicine*, Vol. 18, No. 1, 2007, pp. 2-9. doi:10.1580/06-WEME-CO-023R1.1

[5] A. P. Premawardena, S. L. Seneviratne, S. B. Gunatilake and H. J. De Silva, "Excessive Fibrinolysis: The Coagulopathy Following Merrem's Hump-Nosed Viper (*Hypnale hypnale*) Bites," *American Journal of Tropical Medicine and Hygiene*, Vol. 58, No. 6, 1998, pp. 821-823.

[6] A. De Silva, A. S. B.Wijekoon and L. Jayasena, "Haemostatic Dysfunction and Acute Renal Failure Following Envenoming by Merrem's Hump-Nosed Viper (*Hypnale hypnale*) in Sri Lanka: The First Authenticated Case," *Transactions of the Royal Society of Tropical Medicine and Hygiene*, Vol. 88, No. 2, 1994, pp. 209-212. doi:10.1016/0035-9203(94)90301-8

[7] A. Premawardena, S. L. Seneviratne, S. Jayanthi, S. B. Gunathilake and H. J. de Silva, "Coagulopathy and Fibrinolysis Following the Bite of a Hump-Nosed Viper (*Hypnale hypnale*)," *Transactions of the Royal Society of Tropical Medicine and Hygiene*, Vol. 90, 1996, pp. 290-293.

[8] J. K. Joseph, I. D. Simpson, N. C. S. Menon, M. P. Jose, K. J. Kulkarni, G. B. Raghavendra and D. A. Warrell, "First Authenticated Cases of Life-Threatening Envenoming by the Hump-Nosed Pitviper (*Hypnale hypnale*) in India," *Transactions of the Royal Society of Tropical Medicine and Hygiene*, Vol. 101, No. 1, 2007, pp. 85-90. doi:10.1016/j.trstmh.2006.03.008

[9] H. J. de Silva, M. M. D. Fonseka, S. B. Gunatilake, S. A. M. Kularatne and K. H. Sellahewa, "Anti-Venom for Snakebite in Sri Lanka: We Need an Effective, Low Reactogenic, Affordable and Polyvalent AVS," *Ceylon Medical Journal*, Vol. 40, 2002, pp. 43-45.

[10] C. A. Ariaratnam, V. Thuraisingam, S. A. M. Kularatne, M. H. R. Sheriff, R. D. G. Theakston, A. de Silva and D. A. Warrell, "Frequent and Potentially Fatal Envenoming by Hump-Nosed Pit Vipers (*Hypnale hypnale* and *H. nepa*) in Sri Lanka: Lack of Effective Antivenom," *Transactions of the Royal Society of Tropical Medicine and Hygiene*, Vol. 102, No. 11, 2008, pp. 1120-1126.

[11] I. B. Gawarammana and D. E. Keyler, "Dealing with Adverse Reactions to Snake Antivenom," *The Ceylon Medical Journal*, Vol. 56, No. 3, 2011, pp. 87-90.

[12] K. H. Sellahewa, G. Gunawarden and M. P. Kumararathne, "Efficacy of Antivenom in the Treatment of Severe Local Envenomation by the Hump-Nosed Viper (*Hypnale hypnale*)," *American Journal of Tropical Medicine and Hygiene*, Vol. 53, No. 3, 1995, pp. 260-262.

[13] K. H. Sellahewa and M. P. Kumararatne, "Envenomation by the Hump-Nosed Viper (*Hypnalehypnale*)," *American Journal of Tropical Medicine and Hygiene*, Vol. 51, No. 6, 1994, pp. 823-825.

[14] A. De Silva, A. S. B. Wijekoon and L. Jayasena, "Haemostatic Dysfunction and Acute Renal Failure Following Envenoming by Merrem's Hump-Nosed Viper (*Hypnale hypnale*) in Sri Lanka: The First Authenticated Case," *Transactions of the Royal Society of Tropical Medicine and Hygiene*, Vol. 88, No. 2, 1994, pp. 209-212. doi:10.1016/0035-9203(94)90301-8

[15] K. Maduwage, K. Kularatne, A. Wazil and I. Gawarammana, "Coagulopthy, Acute Kidney Injury and Death Following Hypnale Zaraenvenoming—The First Case Report from Sri Lanka," *Toxicon*, Vol. 58, No. 8, 2011, pp. 641-643. doi:10.1016/j.toxicon.2011.09.014

[16] T. Varagunam and R. G. Panabokke, "Bilateral Necrosis of the Kidneys Following Snakebite," *Postgraduate Me-*

dical Journal, Vol. 46, 1970, pp. 449-451. doi:10.1136/pgmj.46.537.449

[17] L. Dharmaratne and U. Gunawardena, "Generalised Bleeding Tendency and Acute Renal Failure Following Merrem's Hump-Nosed Viper Bite," *Journal of Ceylon College Physicians*, 1989, pp. 21-22.

[18] H. Karunatilake, T. Nayakarathna, S. atapattu, T. Saparamadu and S. Dharmasena, "Thrombotic Microangiopathy and Fibrinolysis after Hump Nosed Viper Envenomation," *Ceylon Medical Journal*, Vol. 57, No. 1, 2012, pp. 45-46. doi:10.4038/cmj.v57i1.4204

[19] N. Herath, A. Wazil, S. Kularatne, N. Ratnatunga, K. Weerakoon, S. Badurdeen, P. Rajakrishna, N. Nanayakkara and D. Dharmagunawardane, "Thrombotic Microangiopathy and Acute Kidney Injury in Hump-Nosedviper (Hypnale species) Envenoming: A Descriptive Study in Sri Lanka," *Toxicon*, Vol. 60, No. 1, 2012, pp. 61-65. doi:10.1016/j.toxicon.2012.03.015

[20] M. Gunatilake, R. L. Jayakody, P. Angunawela and A. de Tissera, "Direct Nephrotoxic Effects Produced by Venoms of Sri Lankan Cobra, Russell's Viperand Hump Nosed Viper," *The Ceylon Journal of Medical Science*, 46, 2003, pp. 61-66.

[21] C. H. Tan, P. K. Leong, S. Y. Fung, S. M. Sim, G. Ponnudurai, C. Ariaratnam, S. Khomvilai, V. Sitprija and N. H. Tan, "Cross Neutralization of *Hypnale hypnale* (Hump-Nosed Pit Viper) Venom by Polyvalent and Monovalent Malayan Pit Viper Antivenoms *in Vitro* and in Arodent Model," *Acta Tropica*, Vol. 117, No. 2, 2011, pp. 119-124. doi:10.1016/j.actatropica.2010.11.001

The Efficacy and Safety of Saxagliptin in Haemodialysis Patients*

Abdul Halim Abdul Gafor[1], Azrina Abdul Kadir[1], Rizna Abdul Cader[1], Rozita Mohd[1], Kong Wei Yen[1], Rohana Abdul Ghani[2], Shamsul Azhar Shah[3], Norella C. T. Kong[1]
[1]Department Nephrology Unit, Department of Medicine, University Kebangsaan Malaysia Medical Centre, Kuala Lumpur, Malaysia
[2]Endocrine Unit, Department of Medicine, University Kebangsaan Malaysia Medical Centre, Kuala Lumpur, Malaysia
[3]Department of Epidemiology and Biostatistics, University Kebangsaan Malaysia Medical Centre, Kuala Lumpur, Malaysia
Email: halimgafor@gmail.com

ABSTRACT

Introduction: Good glycaemic control without causing excessive hypoglycaemia reduced the risk of macrovascular and microvascular complications in type 2 DM patients on regular haemodialysis (HD). The objectives of this study were to assess the efficacy and safety of add-on saxagliptin to insulin therapy in blood sugar control compared to insulin therapy alone in diabetic patients undergoing HD. **Design and Methods:** In this prospective open-labelled randomized controlled trial, HD patients with type 2 DM and on stable insulin therapy with HbA1c 7% - 13% were randomized to receive add-on saxagliptin 2.5 mg once daily to insulin therapy or insulin therapy only for 12 weeks. **Results:** 24 patients were randomized into each arm equally. Baseline and week-12 serum HbA1c, fructosamine, fasting blood glucose (FBS) and mean self monitoring blood glucose (SMBG) were comparable in the groups. Reduction of HbA1c and mean SMBG were significant in both groups. There was a significant drop in fructosamine levels ($p = 0.004$) and trend of lower FBS ($p = 0.097$) in add-on saxagliptin group but not in insulin alone group. The incidence of hypoglycaemia was the same in both groups. **Conclusion:** Add-on saxagliptin to insulin is comparable to insulin therapy alone in blood sugar control in regular HD patients and is safe and generally well tolerated. Add-on saxagliptin group may have more persistent and less fluctuation of glucose control compared to insulin only group.

Keywords: Fructosamine; Fasting Blood Sugar; HbA1c; Haemodialysis; Saxagliptin; Type 2 Diabetes Mellitus

1. Introduction

Type 2 diabetes mellitus (DM) is a chronic disease characterized by reduced insulin sensitivity and deficient insulin secretion by pancreatic β-cells [1,2]. These defects lead to elevated fasting plasma glucose and postprandial plasma glucose levels, which increase the risk of diabetes-related microvascular and macrovascular complications [3,4].

End stage renal disease (ESRD) is a major problem in both developed and developing countries. In the year 2010, DM was the cause of ESRD in 56% of all patients accepted for dialysis in Malaysia [5]. The various and opposing effects of ESRD and dialysis can make blood glucose levels fluctuate widely, placing patients at risk of hyperglycaemia and hypoglycaemia [6]. Uraemia complicates glycaemic control by affecting the secretion, clearance, and peripheral tissue sensitivity of insulin [6]. Haemodialysis (HD) further alters insulin secretion, clearance and resistance as the result of periodic improvement in uraemia, acidosis, and phosphate handling [6].

To our knowledge data are scarce on how diabetes should best be treated in ESRD. The importance of glycaemic control in survival benefits among dialysis patients is still in grey area. A seven years observational study by Oomichi, T. *et al.* revealed that high HbA1C levels were associated higher mortality rates in diabetic HD patients [7]. Contrary, Williams, M.E. *et al.* failed to show any correlation between HbA1c with 12-month mortality rate [8]. Therefore it is important to individual-

*Conflict of interest statement: The authors have declared that no conflict of interest exists.

ize the HbA1c target in ESRD patients, perhaps becoming less stringent based on age, co morbidity, life expectancy and the presence of risk factors for the occurrence of hypoglycaemia.

In patients with type 2 DM and chronic kidney disease (CKD), antihyperglycaemic treatment options are limited and often associated with undesirable side effects [9-11]. Metformin is contraindicated in patients with CKD because of the increased risk of lactic acidosis. Thiazolidinediones must be used with caution as they tend to increase fluid retention and can be associated with congestive heart failure. Insulin and sulphonylureas increase the risk for hypoglycaemia and often result in weight gain. Furthermore, patients with CKD may be at inherent risk for hypoglycaemia because of effects of renal disease on glucose metabolism including decreased insulin clearance and impaired gluconeogenesis in the kidney [12,13].

Dipeptidyl peptidase-4 (DPP-4) inhibitors and incretin mimetics are newer antihyperglycaemic agents, which may become more frequently used in patients with type 2 DM and CKD [14]. DPP-4 inhibitors slow the degradation and the inactivation of the incretins [15-17]. The incretins account for approximately 50% to 70% of the postprandial insulin secretion in healthy individuals [18]. DPP-4 inhibitors increase insulin secretion and decrease glucagon concentration in a glucose-dependent manner, which improves fasting plasma glucose and postprandial glucose [15]. DPP4-inhibitors have a favourable tolerability profile compared with other antidiabetic agents. DPP-4 inhibitors are neutral for the following risks: hypoglycaemia, weight gain, gastrointestinal symptoms, heart failure or oedema, fractures, and drug-drug interactions [19].

The primary objective of this study was to assess the efficacy of add-on saxagliptin to insulin therapy in blood sugar control compared to insulin therapy alone in regular HD patients with type 2 DM. Efficacy were defined by HbA1C, fructosamine, fasting blood sugar (FBS) profiles and mean self monitoring blood glucose (SMBG).

The secondary objective of this study was to assess the safety of add-on saxagliptin to insulin therapy compared to insulin therapy alone in regular haemodialysis patients with type 2 diabetes mellitus. Safety in this study was defined as number of episode of hypoglycaemia. Hypoglycaemia was defined as 1) asymptomatic hypoglycaemia (measured plasma glucose measurement <3.9 mmol/l [20]), 2) documented symptomatic hypoglycaemia (sweating, giddiness, palpitations, confusion, measured plasma glucose measurement <3.9 mmol/l, without concomitant hypotensive episodes), and 3) severe hypoglycaemia (an event requiring assistance of another person to actively administer carbohydrate, glucagons or resuscitative actions).

2. Patients and Methods

This was a prospective open labelled randomized control trial involving patients with type 2 DM undergoing HD. This study was approved by the Research and Ethical Committee of this hospital. Informed and written consents were obtained from all the patients. The inclusion and exclusion criteria were listed in **Table 1**. The patients were randomized using block of three equally into either insulin only group or add-on saxagliptin to insulin group (saxagliptin 2.5 mg daily + insulin) and treated for 12 weeks.

Patients were provided with a glucometer and diary, and instructed to monitor their fingerstick capillary glucose (DXT) at least three times a week (one fasting and two pre-meals of either pre-lunch or pre-dinner DXT) and record any hypoglycaemic event. Patient's adherence, diaries, glycaemic control and self-monitored blood glucose levels were reviewed at every visit. Insulin titration was done at every visit based on titration schedule to adhere (**Table 2**). Patients will be reviewed at week 2, 4, 8 and 12. In between the visits, phone calls were made to the HD centres and patients enquiring regarding hypoglycaemic symptoms and DXT readings.

The dosage and duration of treatment were supplied in exact quantities for the 12 weeks study period. Study medication was taken orally, immediately before or with a meal during non-dialysis day. During dialysis day, saxagliptin 2.5 mg was taken after completion of the HD. Compliance and adherence to treatment were assessed by interview and pill counting. Any hypoglycaemic symptom and adverse effects were enquired and recorded.

Statistical Analysis

Data (non-parametric) was expressed as median and interquartile range. The efficacy profile of saxagliptin versus insulin was analysed using Mann-Whitney U test. The changes of parameters in each group were analysed using Friedman test. The safety profile was analysed using Fischer Exact test. A p value of <0.05 was considered as significant. All statistical analyses were performed using the Statistical Package for the Social Sciences version 20.0 (SPSS, Chicago, IL, USA).

3. Results

After screening of a total of 540 patients from our HD clinic, 172 diabetic patients were identified and out of this, 24 patients who met the inclusion criteria were recruited and randomized into two groups, insulin only group and add-on saxagliptin to insulin group (12 patients in each arm).

Table 1. Inclusion and exclusion criteria.

Inclusion	Exclusion
1) Age ≥ 18 years old 2) Type 2 DM 3) ESRD undergoing HD 4) HbA1c: 7% - 13% 5) Stable dose of short acting basal bolus insulin (10 - 80 units/day) for at least for 4 weeks 6) Willingness to give written consent and comply with the study protocol	1) Type 1 DM 2) History of diabetic ketoacidosis or hyperosmolar hyperglycaemic state within the past 6 months 3) Secondary cause of diabetes (e.g. steroid-induced) 4) New York Heart Association stage III/IV congestive heart failure and or known left ventricular ejection fraction ≤40% 5) Cardiovascular events including myocardial infarction and unstable angina within the past 6 months 6) Acute kidney injury 7) History of renal transplant 8) Anaemia with haemoglobin <10 g/dl 9) Any other severe coexisting disease such as, but not limited to, chronic liver disease, psychiatric disorders, malignancy 10) Repeated fasting blood sugar (FBS > 15 mmol/l) 11) Pregnant or lactating women 12) History of alcohol or drug abuse within the previous year

Table 2. Insulin adjustment during study period.

Pre-meal blood glucose (mmol/l)	Action
<4	Reduce insulin dose by 2 units
4 - 7	Maintain current dose
>7 AND no hypoglycaemic episode	Increase insulin dose by 2 units

The demographic data and baseline clinical characteristics were tabulated in **Table 3**. Baseline and end of study parameters between the two groups were tabulated in **Table 4**. **Table 5** revealed the intra-group changes of parameters within each group.

There were 2 patients each group developed hypoglycaemia (p = 1.00). There was no patient developed uncontrolled hyperglycaemia, diabetic ketoacidosis or hyperosmolar hyperglycaemic state in both groups.

4. Discussion

Saxagliptin, a new DPP-4 inhibitor has been evaluated in initial therapy of type 2 DM both as a single agent and in combination with other oral antidiabetic agents [18, 21-24]. It is currently available as a once daily oral medication, usually dosed at 5 mg daily [18]. Saxagliptin is rapidly and extensively absorbed after oral dosing and can be taken with or without food. It is excreted by both renal and hepatic pathways. In patients with renal dysfunction evidenced by a creatinine clearance of ≤50 mL/min, dose reduction to 2.5 mg daily is also recommended [21]. A 4-hour HD session removed 23% of the saxagliptin dose and therefore it should be taken following HD [22].

Serial HbA1c measurements are the standard of care in diabetic patients without renal failure. However, factors such as the shorter red life span of red blood cells, iron deficiency, recent transfusion, and use of erythropoietin-stimulating agents can cause underestimation of glucose control in renal failure patients [23]. Despite these limitations, the HbA1c level is considered a reasonable measure of glycaemic control in ESRD [6].

Both groups had comparable baseline and end of study HbA1c levels. The reductions of HbA1c were significant in both groups. Barnett *et al.* reported greater reductions in mean HbA1c from baseline to week 24 in the add-on saxagliptin group compared to placebo group in a population with normal kidney function [24]. Nowicki *et al.* in a subgroup of 36 ESRD patients treated with saxagliptin + insulin/OHA versus placebo + insulin/ OHA reported similar reduction mean HbA1c between both groups [25]. Unlike our study, not all of the 36 patients were on insulin.

Glycated fructosamine and albumin are other measures of glycaemic control with some advantages over HbA1c in dialysis patients. However, they are not readily available and can be affected by conditions that alter protein metabolism, including ESRD [26-29]. Fructosamine was chosen in this study as it reflects very recent (1 - 3 weeks) glycaemic control, therefore potentially lessening the confounding effect of shortened red cell survival or of high red cell turnover seen with HbA1c levels. Fructosamiane levels were the same in between both groups at baseline and at end of study period. Anyhow, we noted that, the reduction of fructosamine levels were only significant in add-on saxagliptin group and not in insulin alone group. As fructosamine can detect shorter duration control of glucose, we suggested that add-on saxagliptin group had more persistent and less fluctuation of glucose control compared to insulin only group.

There was no significant difference in FBS in between the groups. Anyhow, we noted that there was a trend of lower FBS in add-on saxagliptin group. Barnett *et al.* showed not statistically significant reduction of serum FBS in the add-on saxagliptin group compared to pla-

Table 3. Comparison of baseline demographic and clinical characteristics between both study groups.

	Insulin only	Add-on saxagliptin to insulin	p value
Age (in years)	61 (53.75 - 66)	68 (54.5 - 72)	0.287
Gender(male:female)	8:4	6:6	0.68
Race (Malay:Chinese:Indian)	8:4:0	9:1:2	0.173
BMI (kg/m^2)	25.5 (23.4 - 28.6)	25 (20.7 - 30.8)	0.619
Baseline Co-Morbidities (%)			
Hypertension	11 (92.3%)	12 (100%)	1.00
Dyslipidaemia	12 (100%)	11 (92.3%)	1.00
Cerebrovascular disease	3 (25%)	4 (33.3%)	1.00
Ischaemic heart disease	1 (8.3%)	2 (16.7%)	1.00
SBP (mmHg)	141.5 (129 - 154.3)	141 (129.5 - 149.5)	1.00
DBP (mmHg)	75.5 (68.3 - 82.5)	65 (60 - 82.8)	0.16

Data are expressed as median (IQR). IQR = interquartile range; BMI: Body Mass Index; SBP: Systolic blood pressure; DBP: Diastolic blood pressure.

Table 4. Baseline and end of study parameters.

Characteristic	Baseline			End of study		
	Insulin only	Add-on saxagliptin	p value	Insulin only	Add-on saxagliptin	p value
HbA1c (%)	8.85 (7.1 - 10.3)	8.45 (7.5 - 10.5)	1.00	7.20 (5.90 - 8.70)	7.00 (5.80 - 8.50)	0.56
Fructosamine (umol/l)	420 (366 - 487)	482 (416 - 592.3)	0.104	366 (324 - 410)	395 (351 - 431)	0.33
Fasting blood sugar (mmol/l)	12.6 (10 - 15.7)	12.6 (7.9 - 19.4)	0.976	8.60 (6.93 - 13.58)	7.40 (5.50 - 10.40)	0.43
Mean SMBG, (mmol/l)	11.3 (8.2 - 12.7)	11.4 (8.5 - 14)	0.799	8.10 (6.83 - 10.40)	8.50 (7.30 - 9.70)	0.97
Haemoglobin (g/dL)	11.95 (11.2 - 13.4)	11.9 (10.9 - 12.3)	0.41	11.1 (10.4 - 12.3)	12.1 (10.0 - 13.3)	0.39
Albumin (g/L)	41 (38.3 - 43.8)	40.5 (38.3 - 44.3)	1.00	40.0 (38.3 - 42.5)	42.0 (40.0 - 46.0)	0.12
Insulin requirement (unit)/day	42 (28.5 - 44)	30 (21 - 37.5)	0.128	44.0 (30.0 - 58.0)	32.0 (24.0 - 36.0)	0.40

Data are expressed as median (IQR). IQR = interquartile range.

Table 5. Parameters within each group.

		Baseline	Week 2	Week 4	Week 8	Week 12	p value
HbA1c (%)	Insulin only	8.85 (7.1 - 10.3)	—	8.15 (6.63 - 10.53)	8.05 (7.13 - 9.13)	7.20 (5.90 - 8.70)	0.046
	Add-on Saxagliptin to insulin	8.45 (7.5 - 10.5)	—	7.6 (6.38 - 8.83)	8 (7.33 - 9.1)	7.00 (5.80 - 8.50)	0.001
Fructosamine (umol/l)	Insulin only	420 (366 - 487)	416.0 (378.8 - 464.8)	394.5 (350.3 - 441.3)	410 (360 - 473)	366 (324 - 410)	0.092
	Add-on Saxagliptin to insulin	482 (416 - 592.3)	425.5 (383.3 - 504.8)	454.5 (376.5 - 475.5)	444 (374 - 465)	395 (351 - 431)	0.004
FBS (mmol/l)	Insulin only	12.6 (10 - 15.7)	8.85 (7.1 - 12.9)	9.8 (5.6 - 13.2)	9.05 (7.9 - 12.1)	8.60 (6.93 - 13.58)	0.856
	Add-on Saxagliptin to insulin	12.6 (7.9 - 19.4)	10.5 (6.9 - 11.8)	8.8 (6.9 - 12.4)	9.4 (6.8 - 12.9)	7.40 (5.50 - 10.40)	0.097
Mean SMBG (mmol/l)	Insulin only	11.3 (8.2 - 12.7)	—	8.4 (7.9 - 11.4)	8.05 (8 - 12.6)	8.10 (6.83 - 10.40)	0.045
	Add-on Saxagliptin to insulin	11.4 (8.5 - 14)	—	9.4 (8.4 - 11.8)	10.2 (8.5 - 10.8)	8.50 (7.30 - 9.70)	0.025
Insulin requirement (unit/day)	Insulin only	42 (28.5 - 44)	46 (30 - 49.5)	44 (30 - 56)	42 (30 - 55.5)	44.0 (30.0 - 58.0)	<0.001
	Add-on Saxagliptin to insulin	30 (21 - 37.5)	32 (28.5 - 46)	32 (26 - 45)	33 (26 - 45)	32.0 (24.0 - 36.0)	0.039

Data are expressed as median (IQR). IQR = interquartile range.

cebo in a population of patients with normal kidney function [23]. Nowicki *et al.* reported an increment of adjusted mean FBS from baseline to week 12 for the saxagliptin group, though the difference was not statistically significant [24]. Although, there was no statistical reduction, we believed there was a possible clinical benefit in add-on saxagliptin group with reduction of median FBS from 12.6 to 7.4 mmol/l.

Both groups had comparable baseline and end of study SMBG. Both groups also showed significantly lower SMBG at the end of study period.

There were statistically significant increments of insulin requirement in both groups. This was necessary to prevent hyperglycaemia as majority of the patients had suboptimal glycaemic control on randomization. There was also possible bias as the investigators were not blinded. However, bias was minimized as the insulin dose titration was to follow strict insulin schedule to adhere. Nevertheless, there were no significant differences in insulin increment in between groups and therefore it did not interfere with the efficacy results.

The incidence of hypoglycaemia was the same in both groups. There was no patient had severe hypoglycaemia which required other persons or medical assistance for administration of glucose. The most common adverse reactions reported in of saxagliptin- treated patients were upper respiratory tract infection, headache, nasopharyngitis and urinary tract infection [18,30,31]. Analysis of pooled data also showed no significant weight gain or effect on lipid profile compared to placebo [18,30-33].

The strength of this study relies on its prospective and randomized controlled trial producing homogenous population of type 2 DM on regular HD. However, this study involved a small size and relatively short duration of study period and therefore we may underestimate the safety and tolerability profile. A larger and longer duration of study may provide answers to its safety and tolerability among our HD patients in the future.

5. Conclusion

As a conclusion, add-on saxagliptin to insulin is comparable to insulin therapy alone in blood sugar control in regular haemodialysis patients and is safe and generally well tolerated. Add-on saxagliptin group may have more persistent and less fluctuation of glucose control compared to insulin only group. Thus, saxagliptin may have an important role in the treatment of type 2 DM patients on HD.

6. Acknowledgement

We would like to thank the Dean of the Faculty of Medicine, Universiti Kebangsaan Malaysia, for allowing us to publish these data.

REFERENCES

[1] American Diabetes Association, "Standards of Medical Care in Diabetes—2010," *Diabetes Care*, Vol. 33, Suppl. 1, 2010, pp. S11-S61. doi:10.2337/dc10-S011

[2] Z. H. Israili, "Advances in the Treatment of Type 2 Diabetes Mellitus," *American Journal of Therapeutics*, Vol. 18, No. 2, 2011, pp. 117-152. doi:10.1097/MJT.0b013e3181afbf51

[3] M. J. Fowler, "Microvascular and Macrovascular Complications of Diabetes," *Clinical Diabetes*, Vol. 26, No. 2, 2008, pp. 77-82.

[4] D. M. Nathan, J. B. Buse, M. B. Davidson, *et al.*, "American Diabetes Association; European Association for the Study of Diabetes. Medical Management of Hyperglycemia in Type 2 Diabetes: A Consensus Algorithm for the Initiation and Adjustment of Therapy: A Consensus Statement of the American Diabetes Association and the European Association for the Study of Diabetes," *Diabetes Care*, Vol. 32, No. 1, 2009, pp. 193-203. doi:10.2337/dc08-9025

[5] L. Y. Ngo, *et al.*, "18th Report of the Malaysian Dialysis and Transplant Registry All Renal Replacement Therapy in Malaysia," The National Renal Registry, Kuala Lumpur, 2010, pp. 1-3.

[6] K. Shrishrimal, P. Hart and F. Michota, "Managing Diabetes in Hemodialysis Patients: Observations and Recommendations," *Cleveland Clinic Journal of Medicine*, Vol. 76, No. 11, 2009, pp. 649-655. doi:10.3949/ccjm.76a.09054

[7] T. Oomichi, M. Emoto, T. Tabata, T. Morioka, Y. Tsujimoto, H. Tahara, T. Shoji and Y. Nishizawa, "Impact of Glycemic Control on Survival of Diabetic Patients on Chronic Regular Hemodialysis: A 7-Year Observational Study," *Diabetes Care*, Vol. 29, No. 29, 2006, pp. 1496-1500. doi:10.2337/dc05-1887

[8] M. E. Williams, E. Lacson Jr., M. Teng, N. Ofsthun and J. M. Lazarus, "Hemodialyzed Type I and Type II Diabetic Patients in the US: Characteristics, Glycemic Control, and Survival," *Kidney International*, Vol. 70, No. 8, 2006, pp. 1503-1509. doi:10.1038/sj.ki.5001789

[9] KDOQI, "KDOQI Clinical Practice Guidelines and Clinical Practice Recommendations for Diabetes and Chronic Kidney Disease," *American Journal of Kidney Diseases*, Vol. 49, No. 2, 2007, pp. S12-S154. doi:10.1053/j.ajkd.2006.12.005

[10] J. F. Yale, "Oral Antihyperglycemic Agents and Renal Disease: New Agents, New Concepts," *Journal of the American Society of Nephrology*, Vol. 16, Suppl. 1, 2005, pp. S7-S10. doi:10.1681/ASN.2004110974

[11] N. D. Lubowsky, R. Siegel and A. G. Pittas, "Management of Glycemia in Patients with Diabetes Mellitus and CKD," *American Journal of Kidney Diseases*, Vol. 50, No. 5, 2007, pp. 865-879. doi:10.1053/j.ajkd.2007.08.012

[12] K. Rave, T. Heise, A. Pfutzner, L. Heinemann and P. T. Sawicki, "Impact of Diabetic Nephropathy on Pharmacodynamic and Pharmacokinetic Properties of Insulin in Type 1 Diabetic Patients," *Diabetes Care*, Vol. 24, No. 5,

2001, pp. 886-890. doi:10.2337/diacarc.24.5.886

[13] M. Stumvoll, "Glucose Production by the Human Kidney—Its Importance Has Been Underestimated," *Nephrology Dialysis Transplantation*, Vol. 13, No. 12, 1998, pp. 2996-2999. doi:10.1093/ndt/13.12.2996

[14] D. J. Drucker and M. A. Nauck, "GLP-1R Agonists (Incretin Mimetics) and DPP-4 Inhibitors (Incretin Enhancers) for the Treatment of Type 2 Diabetes," *Lancet*, Vol. 368, No. 9548, 2006, pp. 1696-1705. doi:10.1016/S0140-6736(06)69705-5

[15] A. A. Tahrani, M. K. Piya and A. H. Barnett, "Saxagliptin: A New DPP-4 Inhibitor for the Treatment of Type 2 Diabetes Mellitus," *Advances in Therapy*, Vol. 26, No. 3, 2009, pp. 249-262. doi:10.1007/s12325-009-0014-9

[16] D. J. Drucker, "The Role of Gut Hormones in Glucose Homeostasis," *Journal of Clinical Investigation*, Vol. 117, No. 1, 2007, pp. 24-32. doi:10.1172/JCI30076

[17] A. Barnett, "DPP-4 Inhibitors and Their Potential Role in the Management of Type 2 Diabetes," *International Journal of Clinical Practice*, Vol. 60, No. 11, 2006, pp. 1454-1470. doi:10.1111/j.1742-1241.2006.01178.x

[18] J. Rosenstock, C. Aguilar-Salinas and E. Klein, "CV181-011 Study Investigators. Effect of Saxagliptin Monotherapy in Treatment-Naive Patients with Type 2 Diabetes," *Current Medical Research and Opinion*, Vol. 25, No. 10, 2009, pp. 2401-2411. doi:10.1185/03007990903178735

[19] B. J. Goldstein, M. N. Feinglos, J. K. Lunceford, J. Johnson and D. E. Williams-Herman, "Effect of Initial Combination Therapy with Sitagliptin, a Dipeptidyl Peptidase-4 Inhibitor, and Metformin on Glycemic Control in Patients with Type 2 Diabetes," *Diabetes Care*, Vol. 30, No. 8, 2007, pp. 1979-1987. doi:10.2337/dc07-0627

[20] American Diabetes Association Workgroup on Hypoglycemia, "Defining and Reporting Hypoglycemia in Diabetes," *Diabetes Care*, Vol. 28, No. 5, 2005, pp. 1245-1249. doi:10.2337/diacare.28.5.1245

[21] Onglyza (Saxagliptin) Full Prescribing Information. http://packageinserts.bms.com/pi/pi_onglyza.pdf

[22] D. Boulton, A. Tang, C. Patel, L. Li, X. H. Xu, E. Frevert and D. Kornhauser, "Pharmacokinetics of the Dipeptidyl Peptidase-4 Inhibitor Saxagliptin in Subjects with Renal Impairment," *Endocrine Abstracts*, Vol. 20, 2009, p. 357.

[23] M. S. Joy, W. T. Cefali, S. L. Hogan and P. H. Nachman, "Long-Term Glycemic Control Measurements in Diabetic Patients Receiving Hemodialysis," *American Journal of Kidney Diseases*, Vol. 39, No. 2, 2002, pp. 297-307. doi:10.1053/ajkd.2002.30549

[24] A. H. Barnett, B. Charbonnel, M. Donovan and D. Fleming, "Effect of Saxagliptin as Add-On Therapy in Patients with Poorly Controlled Type 2 Diabetes on Insulin Alone or Insulin Combined with Metformin," *Current Medical Research & Opinion*, Vol. 28, No. 4, 2012, pp. 1-12. doi:10.1185/03007995.2012.665046

[25] M. Nowicki, I. Rychlik, H. Haller, M. L. Warren, L. Suchower and I. G. Nilsson, "Saxagliptin Improves Glycemic Control and Is Well Tolerated in Patients with Type 2 Diabetes Mellitus (T2DM) and Renal Impairment Compared with Placebo," *Diabetes, Obesity and Metabolism*, Vol. 13, No. 6, 2011, pp. 523-532. doi:10.1111/j.1463-1326.2011.01382.x

[26] E. Lamb, T. R. Venton, W. R. Cattell and A. Dawnay, "Serum Glycated Albumin and Fructosamine in Renal Dialysis Patients," *Nephron*, Vol. 64, No. 1, 1993, pp. 82-88. doi:10.1159/000187283

[27] M. Inaba, S. Okuno, Y. Kumeda, *et al.*, "Osaka CKD Expert Research Group. Glycated Albumin Is a Better Glycemic Indicator than Glycated Hemoglobin Values in Hemodialysis Patients with Diabetes: Effect of Anemia and Erythropoietin Injection," *Journal of the American Society of Nephrology*, Vol. 18, No. 3, 2007, pp. 896-903. doi:10.1681/ASN.2006070772

[28] C. Constanti, J. M. Simo, J. Joven and J. Camps, "Serum Fructosamine Concentration in Patients with Nephrotic Syndrome and with Cirrhosis of the Liver: The Influence of Hypoalbuminaemia and Hypergammaglobulinaemia," *Annals of Clinical Biochemistry*, Vol. 29, No. 4, 1992, pp. 437-442.

[29] H. C. Ford, W. C. Lim and M. J. Crooke, "Hemoglobin A1 and Serum Fructosamine Levels in Hyperthyroidism," *Clinica Chimica Acta*, Vol. 166, No. 2-3, 1987, pp. 317-321. doi:10.1016/0009-8981(87)90435-9

[30] M. Jadzinsky, A. Pfützner and E. Paz-Pacheco, "CV181-039 Investigators. Saxagliptin Given in Combination with Metformin as Initial Therapy Improves Glycemic Control in Patients with Type 2 Diabetes Compared with Either Monotherapy: A Randomized Controlled Trial," *Journal of Diabetes, Obesity and Metabolism*, Vol. 11, No. 6, 2009, pp. 611-622. doi:10.1111/j.1463-1326.2009.01056.x

[31] R. A. De Fronzo, M. Hissa, A. J. Garber, *et al.*, "Saxagliptin 014 Study Group. The Efficacy and Safety of Saxagliptin When Added to Metformin Therapy in Patients with Inadequately Controlled Type 2 Diabetes on Metformin Alone," *Diabetes Care*, Vol. 32, No. 9, 2009, pp. 1649-1655. doi:10.2337/dc08-1984

[32] A. R. Chacra, G. H. Tan, A. Apanovitch, S. Ravichandran, J. List and R. Chen, "Saxagliptin Added to a Submaximal Dose of Sulphonylurea Improves Glycaemic Control Compared with Uptitration of Sulphonylurea in Patients with Type 2 Diabetes: A Randomised Controlled Trial," *International Journal of Clinical Practice*, Vol. 63, No. 9, 2009, pp. 1395-1406. doi:10.1111/j.1742-1241.2009.02143.x

[33] P. Hollander, J. Li, E. Allen and R. Chen, "CV181-013 Investigators. Saxagliptin Added to a Thiazolidinedione Improves Glycemic Control in Patients with Type 2 Diabetes and Inadequate Control on Thiazolidinedione Alone," *The Journal of Clinical Endocrinology & Metabolism*, Vol. 94, No. 12, 2009, pp. 4810-4819. doi:10.1210/jc.2009-0550

A Case of Type I Hepatorenal Syndrome Treated with Vasopressin

Laura Connor[1], Geoffrey Teehan[2,3]
[1]Department of Internal Medicine, Lankenau Medical Center, Wynnewood, USA
[2]Department of Nephrology, Lankenau Medical Center, Wynnewood, USA
[3]Lankenau Institute of Medical Research, Wynnewood, USA
Email: connorl@mlhs.org

ABSTRACT

Hepatorenal syndrome (HRS) is a grave complication of end-stage liver disease and is associated with a very high mortality. This case report described a 42-year-old female with advanced alcohol-induced cirrhosis who developed HRS that was initially treated with Midodrine and Octreotide but renal function continued to deteriorate. Vasopressin therapy was added and HRS was successfully reversed. There are few data available on the use of vasopressin for HRS and this case supports its use in treatment of HRS, particularly in countries where the more widely studied Terlipressin is unavailable. This case also demonstrates that a patient failing one medical therapy for HRS may respond to an alternative or adjunctive therapy. Therefore, this should be attempted to increase the patient's chance of survival.

Keywords: Hepatorenal Syndrome; Vasopressin

1. Introduction

Hepatorenal syndrome (HRS) is a grave complication of end-stage liver disease and is associated with a very high mortality. It is characterized by arterial vasodilation of the splanchnic vessels leading to pronounced renal vasoconstriction, marked reduction in renal blood flow and glomerular filtration rate [1]. HRS is classified into two types based on the rate of progression of the renal dysfunction. Type 1 is characterized by an abrupt onset and a rapid progression of renal failure over a period of two weeks or less with a median survival of one to two weeks. Type 2 causes a more slowly progressive renal failure, typically over months with a median survival of about six months [2]. Management of HRS is challenging since the ideal treatment is liver transplantation, which is usually difficult to accomplish in a short timeframe. Therefore, patients with HRS are typically managed medically with the goal to improve renal function and survival as a bridge to transplantation. In Europe, the Vasopressin analogue Terlipressin, has been used successfully. Unfortunately, this medication is costly and not available in many countries, including North America [1]. Here, we present a case of Type 1 Hepatorenal Syndrome that is successfully reversed with vasopressin.

2. Case Report

A 43-year-old female with no significant past medical history presented to the emergency department complaining of bilateral lower extremity edema, abdominal pain, nausea, and vomiting that had progressively worsened over the past month. Review of systems was positive for jaundice, increased abdominal girth, fevers, and occasional hematochezia and hematemesis. She had been taking three to four grams of Acetaminophen daily for the past three months for rib pain, and been consuming two to three alcoholic drinks per day, three to four times a week. She was admitted to the hospital February 2011 for investigation of her symptoms.

The workup disclosed probable alcohol-induced cirrhosis compounded by concomitant use of acetaminophen. On hospital day 9, the patient's urine output declined to 14 cc/hr and urine sodium was low (<10 meq/l) suggesting Hepatorenal Syndrome despite a stable creatinine. She was treated with Octreotide and Midodrine for 5 days while the serum creatinine remained stable. On hospital day 18, the patient developed acute kidney injury with creatinine increasing from 1.0 mg/dl to 1.3 mg/dl. The etiology was either pre-renal from increasing diuretics versus hepatorenal syndrome. Urine sodium was low (<10 meq/l), however serum creatinine improved with holding diuretics and giving an intravenous fluid challenge. Creatinine returned to baseline and diuretics were resumed on hospital day 21. On hospital day 23, urine output decreased to 23 cc/hr despite diuretics so Octreotide and Midodrine were again initiated for treatment of possible HRS. By hospital day 25, creatinine rose to 1.2 mg/dl and the patient continued to be diuretic resistant. Urine sodium was found to be 87 meq/l in the setting of diuretic use. The following day creatinine was 1.3 mg/dl, diuretics were discontinued and urine sodium was <10 meq/l consistent with hepatorenal syndrome. Octreotide, midodrine and albumin were continued. Despite being on this therapy for eleven days, creatinine continued to rise from 1.0 mg/dl to 3.6 mg/dl during this time period. There were no obvious nephrotoxic exposures, episodes of low blood pressure, nor any evidence of urinary retention.

Failing Octreotide and Midodrine therapy and being an unsuitable candidate for liver transplantation due to alcohol use, on hospital day 33, she was transferred to the intensive care unit to begin Vasopressin infusion. Octreotide, Midodrine and albumin were continued as ongoing adjunctive therapy. Vasopressin was initially administered at 0.02 units/min. The following morning creatinine rose from 3.6 mg/dl to 3.8 mg/dl and vasopressin was increased to 0.04 units/min. After approximately 48 to 72 hours of vasopressin infusion, serum creatinine began to trend down. Vasopressin therapy was continued for 12 days until creatinine was 1.2 mg/dl, near baseline of 0.8 mg/dl. Vasopression dose was decreased by 50% for one day, then removed completely. Creatinine remained stable after being off vasopressin for 48 hours at which point Octreotide and Midodrine were discontinued. Creatinine continued to remain stable and was 1.1 mg/dl at the time of discharge. At two and ten weeks post-hospital discharge, creatinine had returned and remained stable at baseline of 0.8 mg/dl.

During treatment with Vasopressin, no improvement in liver function tests or coagulation factors occurred. Child-Pugh score was 10 before and after treatment with vasopressin. MELD score decreased from 33 to 21 from beginning to end of treatment owing to the decrease in serum creatinine achieved.

In summary, a 43-year-old female who presented with bilateral lower extremity edema, abdominal pain and increased girth, nausea and vomiting was found to have end-stage liver disease secondary to alcohol. During her hospitalization she developed type 1 hepatorenal syndrome. Initially she was treated with Midodrine, Octreotide and albumin but renal function continued to decline. Vasopressin was added and her renal function recovered to baseline.

3. Discussion

The only definitive therapy to reverse renal failure in hepatorenal syndrome is successful liver transplantation. HRS carries a very poor prognosis with high mortality rate, which makes liver transplantation often not possible before the disease is fatal [3]. There are several pharmacologic therapies that have been shown to improve renal function in patients with HRS. These treatments can be used to improve survival until a transplant is possible.

Data suggests that the combination of Midodrine, a selective α-1 adrenergic agonist and systemic vasoconstrictor, and Octreotide, a somatostatin analog and inhibitor of endogenous vasodialators, to be effective in prolonging survival in HRS [4,5]. One study using Octreotide alone did prove to be effective in the treatment of HRS [6]. Results of these studies are summarized in **Table 1** [4-6]. A benefit to using the combination of oral Midodrine and subcutaneous Octerotide is the ability to use this therapy in the outpatient setting [3]. In this presented case, however, treatment with Midodrine,

Table 1. Summary of studies involving midodrine and octreotide for treatment of HRS.

Author	Study Design	Participants	Treatment	Outcomes
Angeli [4]	Prospective, single center	13 patients with type 1 HRS	Midodrine + octreotide + albumin vs dopamine + albumin	Midodrine and octreotide in *combination* with intravenous albumin lowered serum creatinine, increased GFR, and increased urine volume in 5 of 5 patients compared to 1 of 8 patients treated with dopamine and albumin.
Esrailian [5]	Retrospective, single center	81 patients with type 1 HRS	Midodrine + octreotid vs untreated controls	40% of patients treated with midodrine and octreotide had sustained reduction in serum creatinine compared to 10% in untreated controls. 30-day survival was 57% in treated patients compared to 29% in untreated controls.
Pomier-Layragues [6]	Prospective, randomized, double-blind, cross-over, single center	19 patient with type 1 or type 2 HRS	Octreotide + albumin vs placebo + albumin	Octreotide did not prove to be effective in the treatment of HRS

Octreotide, and albumin did not reverse HRS and renal function continued to deteriorate on therapy. Our patient was not a candidate for a liver transplant causing us to search for another treatment alternative.

Many studies have shown promising results using vasopressin analogs (Terlipressin and Ornipressin) particularly for prolonging survival in the rapidly fatal type 1 HRS. Vasoconstriction of the splanchnic vascular bed is believed to be responsible for the reversal of HRS by ultimately decreasing compensatory renal vasoconstriction and increasing renal perfusion [3]. Terlipressin and Ornipressin are unavailable in many countries, including the United States. Although Terlipressin has been more widely studied, the wide availability of Vasopression in countries where Terlipressin is unavailable has led to its use in treatment of HRS. A summary of studies using Vasopressin and its analogs can be found in **Table 2** [7-18].

Little data exists on Vasopressin for HRS and this case further supports its use in treatment of HRS. Specifically in this case, Vasopressin, in conjunction with Midodrine,

Table 2. Summary of studies involving vasopressin and vasopressin analogs in treatment of HRS.

Author	Study Design	Participants	Treatment	Outcomes
Moreau [7]	Retrospective, multicenter	99 patients with type I HRS	Terlipressin	64% of patients had improved renal function. Survival rate was 40% at 1 month.
Halimi [8]	Retrospective, multicenter	19 patients with type 1 HRS; 2 patients with Type 2 HRS	Terlipressin	72% of patients had improved renal function. Long term survival was achieved in two patients.
Sanyal [9]	Prospective, randomized, double-blind, placebo-controlled, multicenter	56 patients with type 1 HRS	Terlipressin vs placebo + albumin	HRS reversal was achieved in 34% treated with Terlipressin versus 13% treated with placebo plus albumin. Reversal of HRS significantly improved survival at 180 days
Solanki [10]	Prospective, randomized. single-blind, single center	24 patients with type 1 HRS	Terlipressin vs placebo	5 of 12 patients treated with Terlipressin survived to day 15 versus 0 of 12 patients in the placebo group
Narahara [11]	Prospective, multicenter, open-label	8 patients with type 1 HRS	Terlipressin + albumin	75% of patients had a complete response (Cr $\leq$ 1.5 mg/dl) to treatment. Median survival was 35 days.
Testro [12]	Retrospective, single center	49 patients with type 1 HRS; 20 patients with type 2 HRS	Terlipressin + albumin	37 of 49 (77.5%) patients with Type 1 HRS and 4 of 20 (20%) patients with Type 2 HRS responded to treatment. 17 of 49 (35%) patients with Type 1 HRS and 4 of 20 (20%) patients with Type 2 HRS achieved long-term survival.
Neri [13]	Prospective, randomized, multicenter	52 patients with type 1 HRS	Terlipressin + albumin vs albumin	80% of patients treated with Terlipressin plus albumin demonstrated a complete response (Cr $\leq$ 1.5 mg/dl) compared to 19% of patients treated with albumin alone. Reversal of HRS was strongly associated with improved survival.
Martin-Llahi [14]	Prospective, randomized, multicenter	35 patients with type 1 HRS; 11 patients with type 2 HRS	Terlipressin + albumin vs albumin	Terlipressin plus albumin improved renal function compared to albumin alone (45% vs 8.7%). No significant different in 3-month survival between terlipressin plus albumin vs albumin montherapy (27% vs 19%).
Ortega [15]	Prospective, observational, single center	16 patients with type 1 HRS; 5 patients with type 2 HRS	Terlipressin + albumin vs terlipressin	A complete response was seen in 77% of patients receiving terlipressin plus albumin compared to 25% of patients treated with terlipressin alone. Occurrence of complete response was associated with an improved survival.
Guevera [16]	Prospective, nonrandomized, single center	16 patient with HRS (Type not specified)	Ornipressin + albumin	Ornipression plus albumin was successful at reversing HRS with 15 days of treatment. Three patients developed ischemic complications.
Gulberg [17]	Prospective, nonrandomized, single center	7 patients with type 1 HRS	Ornipressin + dopamine	HRS reverted in 4 of 7 patients treated with ornipressin plus dopamine. 3 of 7 survived to transplantation.
Kiser [18]	Retrospective observations, single center	32 patients with type 1 HRS; 11 patients with type 2 HRS	Vasopressin + octreotide vs vasopressin vs octreotide	Complete response occurred in 42% of patients treated with vasopressin plus octreotide, 38% of patients treated with vasopressin alone and 0% of patients treated with octreotide alone. Survival was improved in patients treated with vasopressin and they were more likely to receive a liver transplant

Octreotide and albumin successfully reversed HRS. This case also demonstrates that a patient failing one medical therapy for HRS may respond to an alternative or adjunctive therapy; therefore these methods should be attempted to increase the patient's chance of survival.

4. Conclusion

In conclusion, we have reported a case of type 1 HRS that is successfully treated with vasopressin. There are studies in Europe using terlipressin that have shown some success, however, terlipressin is not available in many countries. Since terlipressin is not available in the United States, vasopressin is used as an alternative and is successful in this reported case. We would advocate the use of vasopressin where terlipressin is unavailable, particularly when other available treatments are failing to reverse renal failure.

REFERENCES

[1] C. Alessandria, A. Ottobrelli, W. Debernardi-Venon, L. Todros, M. T. Cerenzia, S. Martini, *et al.*, "Noradrenalin vs Terlipressin in Patients with Hepatorenal Syndrome: A Prospective, Randomized, Unblinded, Pilot Study," *Journal of Hepatology*, Vol. 47, No. 4, 2007, pp. 499-505. doi:10.1016/j.jhep.2007.04.010

[2] S. J. Munozo, "The Hepatorenal Syndrome," *Medical Clinics of North America*, Vol. 92, No. 4, 2008, pp. 813-837. doi:10.1016/j.mcna.2008.03.007

[3] T. H. Kiser, R. Maclaren and D. N. Fish, "Treatment of Hepatorenal Syndrome," *Pharmacotherapy*, Vol. 29, No. 10, 2009, pp. 1196-1211. doi:10.1592/phco.29.10.1196

[4] P. Angeli, R. Volpin, G. Gerunda, R. Craighero, P. Roner, R. Merenda, *et al.*, "Reversal of Type 1 Hepatorenal Syndrome with the Administration of Midodrine and Octreotide," *Hepatology*, Vol. 29, No. 6, 1999, pp. 1690-1697. doi:10.1002/hep.510290629

[5] E. Esrailian, E. R. Pantangco, N. L Kyulo, K. Q. Hu and B. A. Runyon, "Octreotide/Midodrine Therapy Significantly Improves Renal Function and 30-Day Survival in Patients with Type 1 Hepatorenal Syndrome," *Digestive Diseases and Sciences*, Vol. 52, No. 3, 2007, pp. 742-748. doi:10.1007/s10620-006-9312-0

[6] G. Pomier-Layragues, S. C. Paquin, Z. Hassoun, M. Lafortune and A. Tran, "Octreotide in Hepatorenal Syndrome: A Ransomized Double-Blind, Placebo-Controlled, Corssover Study," *Hepatology*, Vol. 38, No. 1, 2003, pp. 238-243. doi:10.1053/jhep.2003.50276

[7] R. Moreau, F. Durand, T. Poynard, C. Duhamel, J. P. Cervoni, P. Ichai, *et al.*, "Terlipressin in Patients with Cirrhosis and Type 1 Hepatorenal Syndrome: A Retroepsctive Mulitcenter Study," *Gastroenterology*, Vol. 122, No. 4, 2002, pp. 923-930. doi:10.1053/gast.2002.32364

[8] C. Halimi, P. Bonnard, D. Bernard, P. Mathurin, A. Mofredj, V. Martino, *et al.*, "Effect of Terlipressin (Glypressin) on Hepatorenal Syndrome in Cirrhotic Patients: Results of a Multicentre Pilot Study," *European Journal of Gastroenterology & Hepatology*, Vol. 14, No. 2, 2002, pp. 153-158. doi:10.1097/00042737-200202000-00009

[9] A. J. Sanyal, T. Boyer, G. Garcia-Tsao, F. Regenstein, L. Rossaro, B. Appenrodt, *et al.*, "A Randomized, Prospective, Double-Blind, Placebo-Controlled, Trial of Terlipressin for Type 1 Hepatorenal Syndrome," *Gastroenterology*, Vol. 143, No. 5, 2008, pp. 1360-1368. doi:10.1053/j.gastro.2008.02.014

[10] P. Solanki, A. Chawla, R. Garg, R. Gupta, M. Jain and S. K. Sarin, "Beneficial Effects of Terlipressin in Hepatorenal Syndrome: A Prospective, Randomized Placebo-Controlled Clinical Trial," *Journal of Gastroenterology Hepatology*, Vol. 18, No. 2, 2003, pp. 152-156. doi:10.1046/j.1440-1746.2003.02934.x

[11] Y. Narahara, H. Kanazawa, C. Sakamoto, H. Maruyama, O. Yokosuka, S. Mochida, *et al.*, "The Efficacy and Safety of Terlipressin and Albumin in Patients with Type 1 Hepatorenal Syndrome: A Multicenter, Open-Label, Explorative Study," *Journal of Gastroenterology*, Vol. 47, No. 3, 2011, pp. 313-320. doi:10.1007/s00535-011-0485-8

[12] A. G. Testro, S. Wongseelashote, P. W. Angus and P. J. Gow, "Long-Term Outcome of Patients Treated with Terlipressin for Types 1 and 2 Hepatorenal Syndrome," *Journal of Gastroenterology and Hepatology*, Vol. 23, No. 10, 2008, pp. 1535-1540. doi:10.1111/j.1440-1746.2007.05176.x

[13] S. Neri, D. Pulvirenti, M. Malaguarnera, B. M. Cosimo, G. Bertino, L. Ignaccolo, *et al.*, "Terlipressin and Albumin in Patients with Cirrhosis and Type I Hepatorenal Syndrome," *Digestive Diseases and Sciences*, Vol. 53, No. 3, 2008, pp. 830-835. doi:10.1007/s10620-007-9919-9

[14] M. Martin-Llahi, M. N. Pepin, M. Guevara, F. Diaz, A. Torre, A. Monescillo, *et al.*, "Terlipressin and Albumine vs. Albumin in Patients with Cirrhosis and Hepatorenal Syndrome: A Randomized Study," *Gastroenterology*, Vol. 134, No. 5, 2008, pp. 1353-1359. doi:10.1053/j.gastro.2008.02.024

[15] R. Ortega, P. Gines, J. Uriz, A. Cardenas, B. Calahorra, D. De Las Heras, *et al.*, "Terlipressin Therapy with and without Albumin for Patients with Hepatorenal Syndrome: Results of a Prospective, Nonrandomized Study," *Hepatology*, Vol. 36, No. 4, 2002, pp. 941-941. doi:10.1053/jhep.2002.35819

[16] M. Guevera, P. Gines, G. Fernandez-Esparrach, P. Sort, J. M. Salmero, W. Jimenez, *et al.*, "Reversibility of Hepatorenal Syndrome by Prolonged Administration of Ornipressin and Plasma Volume Expansion," *Hepatology*, Vol. 27, No. 1, 1998, pp. 35-41. doi:10.1002/hep.510270107

[17] V. Gulberg, M. Blizer and A. L. Gerbes, "Long-Term Therapy and Retreatment of Hepatorenal Syndrome Type 1 with Ornipressin and Dopamine," *Hepatology*, Vol. 30, No. 4, 1999, pp. 870-875. doi:10.1002/hep.510300430

[18] T. H. Kiser, D. N. Fish, M. D. Obritsch, R. Jung, R. MacLaren and C. R. Rarikh, "Vasopressin, Not Octreotide, May Be Beneficial in the Treatment of Hepatorenal Syndrome: A Retrospective Study," *Nephrology Dialysis Transplantation*, Vol. 20, No. 9, 2005, pp.1813-1820. doi:10.1093/ndt/gfh930

Dimethylarginine Dimethylaminohydrolase 2 Gene Polymorphism and Its Association with Asymmetrical Dimethyl Arginine in Hemodialyzed Patients*

Mochamad Yusuf[1,2,3], Mochammad Thaha[3,4], Raden Mohammad Yogiarto[1], Muhammad Aminuddin[1], Raden Mohammad Yogiantoro[4], Retno Handajani[2], Yasuhiko Tomino[3]

[1]Cardiology and Vascular Medicine Department, Faculty of Medicine, Airlangga University, Surabaya, Indonesia
[2]Tropical Disease Center, Airlangga University, Surabaya, Indonesia
[3]Division of Nephrology, Departement of Internal Medicine, Juntendo University Faculty of Medicine, Tokyo, Japan
[4]Nephrology-Hypertension Division, Internal Medicine Departement, Faculty of Medicine, Airlangga University, Surabaya, Indonesia
Email: yusuf_505@yahoo.com, yusuf_505@unair.ac.id

ABSTRACT

Introduction: Patients with CKD have elevated plasma levels of Asymmetrical Dimethyl Arginine (ADMA), impaired EDRF/NO responses in isolated resistance vessels, and a marked increase in the frequency of cardiovascular events that are predicated by plasma levels of ADMA. ADMA is considered as a risk factor for endothelial dysfunction, progression of chronic kidney disease and a marked increase in the frequency of cardiovascular events that are predicated by plasma levels of ADMA. Elevated ADMA in CKD have been related to a combination of a reduced renal ADMA excretion and a reduced catabolism of ADMA by dimethylarginine dimethylaminohydrolase (DDAH). The current study was undertaken to determine whether there is a correlation between ADMA and SNPs at −449 DDAH 2. **Subjects and Methods:** It was a cross sectional analytic study, 56 hemodialysis patients and 30 healthy individuals were enrolled. Based on its etiology, HD patients group was further divided in to hypertension (HT) subgroup and non-HT subgroup. Genotyping of the polymorphisms was performed using PCR-based SNP detection methods based on 5'-exonuclease activity assays for rs805305. **Results:** Heterozygotes were observed as the most abundant genotypes in both groups, followed by GG genotype in the HD patients (30%) and CC (27%) healthy individuals. Among the HT subgroup, the mean plasma levels of ADMA were sequentially higher from genotypes CC, G/C and GG (p = 0.037). Further multiple comparisons between groups using post hoc test showed results that genotype GG and CC were different at 0.05 level of significance. These findings were not found among non HT subgroup. **Conclusion:** Genetic variation in the DDAH 2 genes is significantly associated with serum ADMA levels in hypertensive HD patients. We observed that carriage of a G at position −449 in the promoter region of the DDAH 2 gene is associated with higher ADMA levels.

Keywords: ADMA; DDAH; Gene Polymorphism

1. Introduction

Atherosclerotic cardiovascular diseases (CVD) are major causes of morbidity and mortality in patients receiving ongoing hemodialysis (HD) [1,2]. Despite its increasing incidence and the accelerated worsening of atherosclerosis in patients on chronic hemodialysis, the proportion of individuals with chronic kidney disease (CKD) receiving appropriate cardiovascular (CV) risk modification treatment is lower than that in the general population [3]. In metabolic disorders associated with atherosclerosis (dyslipidemia, hypertension (HT) and diabetes mellitus), a reduced endothelium-mediated nitric oxide (NO)-dependent vasodilation has been observed, which may contribute to the initiation and progression of atherosclerosis associated with these disorders [4].

The mechanisms of endothelial vasodilator dysfunction (EVD) are likely multi-factorial [5]. Evidences from both animal models and clinical studies suggests that accumulation of the endogenous nitric-oxide synthase (NOS) inhibitors, ADMA and *N*Gmethyl-L-arginine (L-NMMA) contributes to reducing nitric oxide (NO) [6,7].

*Potential conflict of interest: No potential conflict of interest relevant to this article was reported.

Plasma levels of ADMA are inversely related to the vascular NO bioavailability and ADMA is an independent determinant of the vascular redox-state [8,9]. ADMA is also a risk factor for EVD, CV mortality and progression of CKD [8,10].

The co-localization of DDAH 2 and NOS at several sites supports the hypothesis that DDAH may regulate NOS activity by controlling the metabolism of ADMA [11]. As DDAH 2 regulates ADMA levels, it is believable that functional DDAH 2 gene polymorphisms may account for the variation in ADMA levels [12]. ADMA levels may be genetically determined by a promoter polymorphism in a regulatory gene encoding DDAH 2 [13]. However, the functional significance has not been determined previously in chronic HD patients. Therefore, the current study was undertaken to determine whether or not there is a correlation between single nucleotide polymorphisms (SNPs) at −449 (promoter region) DDAH 2 with ADMA plama levels in HD patients.

2. Patients and Methods

2.1. Study Population and Dialysis Protocol

Fifty-six patients with a creatinine clearance of less than 15 ml/min per 1.73 m^2 who had been on chronic HD treatment for more than 3 months were recruited for the present study. Thirty-four HD patients (60.7%) were male. Clinical practice was not changed or modified for the purpose of the study. As the control group, 30 healthy individuals paramedics who had no cardiovascular clinical risk factors (HT, diabetes, dyslipidemia, smoking, family history of premature coronary artery disease or CKD), were enrolled. Five healthy individuals (16.7%) as controls were male.

All participants (patients and controls) signed the Free and Informed Consent Form and the study was approved by the Ethics Committee of Al Irsyad Hospital, Surabaya, Indonesia. It was an analytic cross-sectional study. Clinical and demographic details were also collected.

All patients underwent dialysis twice a week for 4 weeks using a commercially available dialyser (type F6-8 HPS polysulfone semi-synthetic, fresenius GMBH, Germany). Each HD session lasted 4 hours.

Blood pressure (BP) was measured using standard mercury sphygmomanometers after participants had been sitting for at least 10 min. Hypertension was defined as blood pressure ≥ 140/90 mmHg at the time of recruitment, history of hypertension before HD, or the use of anti-hypertensive medication to have BP ≤ 130/80 mmHg. Hypertension was considered as an etiology of CKD if a patient had chronic hypertension before HD, and still had hypertension after HD.

The clinical features of HD patients are shown in **Table 1**. The predominant causes of CKD were hypertension (35 patients, 62,5%) and diabetes (10 patients, 17.9%). Other etiologies such as infection, glomerulonephritis and kidney stone were less than 10% (**Figure 1**).

Table 1. Clinical features of HD patients.

Clinical features of HD patients (Mean ± SD)	
Age	43.52 ± 10.93
BMI	21.88 ± 3.73
Hb	10.07 ± 0.85
Serum creatinine	9.03 ± 1.11
Systolic blood pressure	146.61 ± 15.29
Diastolic blood pressure	90.71 ± 7.83
ADMA	0.84 ± 0.21

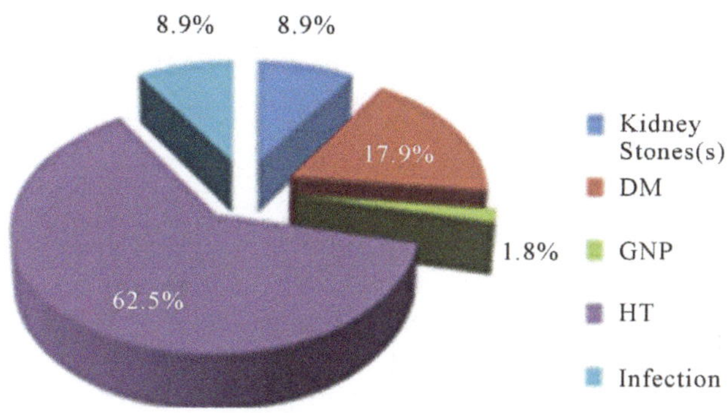

Figure 1. Etiologies of CKD in HD patients.

2.2. Blood Sampling

Venous blood samples were drawn from the arterial-venous fistula 10 minutes before the first HD session in a week. Peripheral whole blood was obtained from 30 healthy individuals. Blood samples were 3 ml for each participant without additives. Plasma was immediately separated by centrifugation at 800 g for 15 minutes, and then was stored at −20˚C prior to use.

2.3. Determination of ADMA

ADMA was measured using an enzyme-linked immunosorbent assay (DLD Diagnostika, Hamburg, Germany) as previously reported [14]. The plasma HCY concentration was measured using The AxSYM HCY assay (Abbott USA), that is a fluorescence polarization immunoassay in the accordance with the procedure previously published [15,16].

2.4. Genomic DNA

Genomic DNA was extracted from whole blood with a commercially available DNA isolation kit (QIAmp DNA blood Mini kit, Qiagen GmBH, Crawley, West Sussex,

UK). Genotyping of the polymorphisms was performed using PCR-based SNP detection methods (Applied Biosystems, Carlsbad, USA) based on 5'-exonuclease activity assays for rs805305 (−449 G/C) [17,18]. Allelic variation was assessed in each participant.

3. Statistics

All variables were examined for normal distribution using the Kolmogorov-Smirnov test. Normally distributed variables were presented as mean ± SD. Pearson correlation was undertaken for associations of clinical covariates with ADMA levels. Distribution differences of gene polymorphism between the groups were analyzed using Mann-Whitney Test. One way Anova and post hoc test were also used to analyze signicant difference between the genotypes within subgroups.

4. Results

4.1. Correlation of ADMA and eGFR in HD Patients

Before performing a parametric correlation test (Pearson), a Kolmogorov-Smirnov test was performed, and the results were normal distribution (ADMA: 0.95; eGFR: 1.05). The Pearson correlation test showed a weak ($p = 0.134$) non-significant correlation between estimated glomerular filtration rate (eGFR) and ADMA in HD patients.

4.2. Gene Polymorphism Distribution HD Patients and Healthy Individuals

Gene polymorphisms were assesed among healthy individuals and HD patients. Heterozygotes were observed as the most abundant genotypes in both groups (70% in healthy individuals and 55% in HD patients), followed by GG genotype in the HD patients (30%), while CC (27%) were the second most common genotype polymorphism in the healthy individuals (**Tables 2** and **3**). Using the Mann-Whitney U test, a significant polymorphism distribution between both groups was sought, and the result was 0.006. There was a significant difference in polymorphism distribution among both groups.

4.3. Subgroups within HD Patients

The HD patients were divided into two subgroups. The subgroups were categorized based on the etiology of the CKD in HD patients. One subgroup was a hypertension subgroup (35 of 56 HD patients samples). The other was a non-HT subgroup, a subgroup of HD patients in which the etiologies of CKD were DM, infection, glomerulonephritis and kidney stone (21 of 56 HD patients samples). There was no significant difference in the distribution of DDAH gene polymorphism among subgroups, as the results of Mann-Whitney test was 0.364.

Table 2. Polymorphism in healthy individuals.

	Frequency	%	Valid %	Cumulative %
Valid GG	1	3.3	3.3	3.3
Heterozygote	21	70.0	70.0	73.3
CC	8	26.7	26.7	100.0
Total	30	100.0	100.0	

Table 3. Polymorphism in HD patients.

	Frequency	%	Valid %	Cumulative %
Valid GG	17	30.4	30.4	30.4
Heterozygote	31	55.4	55.4	85.7
CC	8	14.3	14.3	100.0
Total	56	100.0	100.0	

4.3.1. Subgroup Hypertension Analysis

As the most frequent cause of CKD in this study, DDAH gene polymorphisms and the levels of plasma ADMA were analyzed, including as to whether or not there were differences between genotypes. The distribution of polymorphism is shown in **Table 4**.

The table also reveals that the mean plasma levels of ADMA were sequentially higher from genotypes CC, G/C and GG. These different findings between genotypes were confirmed statistically using a one-way anova test with the results of 0.037. Further multiple comparisons between groups using post hoc test showed results that genotype GG and CC were different at 0.05 level of significance (**Table 5**).

4.3.2. Subgroup Non-Hypertension Analysis

The gene polymorphism distributions and their correlation with plasma levels of ADMA were also analyzed in non-hypertension HD patients. Compared to the HT subgroup, there was a similar composition of gene polymorphism frequency among Non-HT (**Table 6**). But, when statistical tests were used to define association between mean plasma levels of ADMA and DDAH gene polymorphism, there were no significant differences found between groups of genotypes; either by using the Anova test ($p = 0.322$), or using the multiple comparison post hoc test ($p > 0.05$).

5. Discussion

There are considerable data on the role of ADMA in hemodialysis patients and likewise on the association of DDAH gene polymorphism and ADMA in certain popu-

Table 4. ADMA levels among HT subgroups.

	N	Mean	Std deviation	Std Error	95% confidence interval for mean		Min	Max
					Lower bound	Upper bound		
GG	11	0.9491	0.18157	0.05475	0.8271	1.0711	0.80	1.45
Heterozygote	21	0.8248	0.16540	0.03609	0.7495	0.9000	0.60	1.30
CC	3	0.6800	0.12124	0.07000	0.3788	0.9812	0.61	0.82
Total	35	0.8514	0.18103	0.03060	0.7892	0.9136	0.60	1.45

ADMA.

Table 5. Multiple comparison of ADMA levels among DDAH gene polymorphisms.

(I) DDAH	(J) DDAH	Mean difference (I-J)	Standard error	Sig.	95% confidence interval	
					Lower bound	Upper bound
GG	G/C	0.12433	0.06263	0.056	−0.0033	0.2519
	CC	0.26909*	0.10961	0.020	0.0458	0.4924
G/C	GG	−0.12433	0.06263	0.056	−0.2519	0.0033
	CC	0.14476	0.10387	0.173	−0.0668	0.3563
CC	GG	−0.26909*	0.10961	0.020	−0.4924	−0.0458
	G/C	−0.14476	0.10387	0.173	−0.3563	0.0668

Dependent Variable: ADMA; LSD. *The mean difference is significant at the 0.05 level.

Table 6. ADMA levels among Non-HT & HD patients.

	N	Mean	Std deviation	Std error	95% confidence interval for mean		Min	Max
					Lower bound	Upper bound		
GG	6	0.6950	0.38935	0.15895	0.2864	1.1036	0.00	1.05
Heterozygote	10	0.9010	0.21153	0.06689	0.7497	1.0523	0.56	1.17
CC	5	0.7840	0.13278	0.05938	0.6191	0.9489	0.57	0.92
Total	21	0.8143	0.26423	0.05766	0.6940	0.9346	0.00	1.17

ADMA.

lations. Nonetheless, later studies have not only drawn different conclusions (DDAH isoforms, *invitro*/*invivo*, human/animal), but also have found opposite results. In this study, we described the correlation between a novel genetic polymorphism DDAH 2 and ADMA in hypertensive HD patients. The study also revealed a significant distribution difference in DDAH polymorphism between healthy individuals and hemodialysis patients. We believe that this is the first study that has reported such correlations among HD patients.

In the first evaluation, we examined the correlation of estimated glomerular filtration rate (eGFR) and ADMA. There was no significant correlation between eGFR and ADMA. An inverse relationship between plasma ADMA and glomerular filtration rate (GFR) was apparent in patients with coronary artery disease, which has been implicated in their increased cardiovascular risk [19]. However, it has been questioned whether elevated circulating levels of ADMA are merely a marker of kidney disease, coinciding with serum creatinine, or part of the pathophysiological process [20]. Indeed, plasma levels of SDMA correlated more closely with parameters of renal function than did plasma levels of ADMA [21].

ADMA is a naturally-occurring non-selective inhibitor of NOS, and Free ADMA ≥ 80% is actively metabolized by the intracellular enzyme DDAH [11,22]. DDAH is most likely a key determinant of plasma ADMA concentration [14]. Thus, DDAH plays a crucial role in the regulation of NO synthesis via modulating endogenous ADMA levels [23]. Alterations in DDAH activity may effect vascular structure, as well as vascular reactivity [24]. As research has progressed, DDAH has emerged as an important regulator of NO bioavailability and the integrity of renal and vascular function [10].

In higher organisms, including humans, two isoforms of DDAH exist which have distinct tissue distributions but similar enzymatic activity [25]. Based on tissue messenger ribonucleic acid (mRNA) levels, it has been suggested that the expression pattern of DDAH 1 overlaps more closely with the expression pattern of neuronal NOS, whereas DDAH 2 expression has greater similarities with endothelial NOS expression [26,27]. However, it is still unclear which DDAH isoform represents the principal methylarginine-metabolizing enzyme.

Both groups, the HD patients and the healthy individuals, showed a significant difference in the distribution DDAH 2 gene polymorphism. They shared the same most abundant genotype, which was G/C, followed by GG in the HD group and CC in the healthy indivduals group. The polymorphisms were in the non-coding part of the gene, putatively affecting promoter activity, designated DDAH 2 −449. Although our study may not have been adequately powered to detect outcome variations, these findings implied possible functionality polymerphism in the DDAH 2 promoter. As DDAH 2 regulates ADMA levels, it is plausible to think that functional DDAH 2 gene polymorphisms may account for variation in ADMA levels [12]. Data suggest that expression of DDAH 2 may be affected by polymorphisms of the promoter region [17].

For the primary analysis, the HD patients group was divided into a HT subgroup and a Non-HT subgroup. In the subgroup HT, we demonstrated correlations of ADMA with the carriage of the DDAH 2 −449 G allele, where plasma level of ADMA in GG > G/C > CC. Average blood pressure of containing −449 G allele (GG and G/C) was also higher than that of CC allele. O'Dwyer *et al.* recently reported that the −449G allele of the DDAH 2 gene was associated with increased ADMA concentrations [13]. Higher prevalence of hypertension with an odds ratio of 1.80 (95%CI: 1.29 - 2.49, $p < 0.001$) for individuals homozygous for the −449G allele was also reported [18]. In the secondary analysis, we could not find any correlation of ADMA and DDAH 2 gene polymorphism among non-hypertensive HD patients.

Oxidative stress is defined as tissue damage caused by the disequilibrium between pro-oxidants and anti-oxidants [28]. Vascular oxidative stress is a major factor in the pathogenesis of atherosclerosis [29]. One of the main effects of oxidative stress is the decrease in the biological activity of NO [28]. Among the mechanisms for impaired NO synthesis is the accumulation of the endogenous NOS inhibitor asymmetric ADMA [7]. ADMA inhibits all three isoforms of nitric oxide synthase and therefore has the potential to produce diverse biological effects, particularly in the cardiovascular system [26,30]. Some studies of human subjects with essential HT report elevated plasma levels of ADMA [31,32]. Investigations of ADMA concentration by independent methods in patients with renal failure, have identified plasma ADMA concentration as a strong independent predictor of disease progression. Of particular interest was the finding that a 0.1 μmol/L increase in plasma ADMA was associated with a 20% increase in cardiovascular event rate [7,33].

The enzyme DDAH specifically hydrolyzes these asymmetrically methylated arginine residues to citrulline and methylamines [34,35]. Several groups have demonstrated that modulating DDAH activity can have a profound effect on endothelial NO production [7,36,37]. Two isoforms of DDAH have been identified. Since DDAH 2 is the predominant isoform expressed in the cardiovascular system and since hypercholesterolemia impaired endothelial DDAH activity while DDAH 1 protein expression remained unchanged [23,38,39], DDAH 2 gene polymorphism was studied in the present study. The finding that the gene for DDAH is evolutionarily well conserved suggests that the enzyme confers an important survival advantage [10]. And it can be postulated that genetic variations in DDAH that affect the ability of the enzyme to metabolize ADMA might increase cardiovascular risk in patients with renal failure and might also determine, in part, the rate of disease progression [26].

Growing and irresistable epidemiological evidence links ED with cardiorenal syndrome. Recently, a human study, using artery and vein graft suggests that ADMA may be directly implicated in the regulation of the vascular redox state of atherosclerosis by affecting superoxide generation and NO bioavailability [8]. Therefore, any therapeutic modulation of ADMA levels, via genetic modification of DDAH expression or activity, may represent a new strategy for the treatment of cardiovascular disorders, including in HD patients.

6. Conclusions

Genetic variation in the DDAH 2 genes is significantly associated with serum ADMA levels in hypertensive HD patients. We observed that carriage of a G at position −449 in the promoter region of the DDAH 2 gene is associated with higher ADMA levels.

Further studies are required to determine the pathophysiological significance of elevated serum ADMA in HD patients and to better understand how DDAH gene variation influences ADMA levels. And we propose that a polymorphism at position −449 in the DDAH 2 may be functional and that it has the potential to be used as a marker for susceptibility to cardiovascular events among hypertensive hemodialyzed patients.

7. Limitations

This study has some limitations. The number of patients was relatively small, we used only one marker of oxidative stress and we did not evaluate other factors potentially involved in endothelial dysfunction. Furthermore, our study was limited by its cross-sectional design, allowing no causal interferences.

REFERENCES

[1] M. Fujisawa, R. Haramaki, H. Miyazaki, T. Imaizumi and S. Okuda, "Role of Lipoprotein (a) and TGF-β1 in Atherosclerosis of Hemodialysis Patients," *Journal of the American Society of Nephrology*, Vol. 11, No. 10, 2000, pp. 1889-1895.

[2] A. Lindner, B. Charra, D. Sherrard and B. Scribner, "Accelerated Atherosclerosis in Prolonged Maintenance Hemodialysis," *New England Journal of Medicine*, Vol. 290, No. 13, 1974, pp. 697-701.

[3] K. Ma, E. Greene and L. Raij, "Cardiovascular Risk Factors in Chronic Renal Failure and Hemodialysis Populations," *American Journal of Kidney Diseases*, Vol. 19, No. 6, 1992, pp. 505-513.

[4] J. Cooke and V. Dzau, "Derangements of the Nitric Oxide Synthase Pathway, L-Arginine, and Cardiovascular Diseases," *Circulation*, Vol. 96, No. 2, 1997, pp. 379-382.

[5] A. Ito, P. S. Tsao, S. Adimoolam, M. Kimoto, T. Ogawa and J. P. Cooke, "Novel Mechanism for Endothelial Dysfunction: Dysregulation of Dimethylarginine Dimethylaminohydrolase," *Circulation*, Vol. 99, No. 24, 1999, pp. 3092-3095.

[6] R. M. J. Palmer, A. G. Ferrige and S. Moncada, "Nitric Oxide Release Accounts for the Biological Activity of Endothelium-Derived Relaxing Factor," *Nature*, Vol. 327, 1987, pp. 524-526. doi:10.1038/327524a0

[7] A. J. Pope, K. Karrupiah, P. N. Kearns, Y. Xia and A. J. Cardounel, "Role of Dimethylarginine Dimethylaminohydrolases in the Regulation of Endothelial Nitric Oxide Production," *Journal of Biological Chemistry*, Vol. 284, No. 51, 2009, pp. 35338-35347.

[8] C. Antoniades, C. Shirodaria, P. Leeson, A. Antonopoulos, N. Warrick, T. Van-Assche, *et al.*, "Association of Plasma Asymmetrical Dimethylarginine (ADMA) with Elevated Vascular Superoxide Production and Endothelial Nitric Oxide Synthase Uncoupling: Implications for Endothelial Function in Human Atherosclerosis," *European Heart Journal*, Vol. 30, No. 9, 2009, pp. 1142-1150.

[9] R. Maas, K. Quitzau, E. Schwedhelm, L. Spieker, W. Rafflenbeul, A. Steenpass, *et al.*, "Asymmetrical Dimethylarginine (ADMA) and Coronary Endothelial Function in Patients with Coronary Artery Disease and Mild Hypercholesterolemia," *Atherosclerosis*, Vol. 191, No. 1, 2007, pp. 211-219.

[10] F. Palm, M. L. Onozato, Z. Luo and C. S. Wilcox, "Dimethylarginine Dimethylaminohydrolase (DDAH): Expression, Regulation, and Function in the Cardiovascular and Renal Systems," *Heart and Circulatory Physiology: American Journal of Physiology*, Vol. 293, No. 6, 2007, pp. H3227-H3245.

[11] C. Tran, J. Leiper and P. Vallance, "The DDAH/ADMA/NOS Pathway," *Atherosclerosis Supplements*, Vol. 4, No. 4, 2003, pp. 33-40.

[12] R. Ryan, J. Thornton, E. Duggan, E. McGovern, M. J. O'Dwyer, A. W. Ryan, *et al.*, "Gene Polymorphism and Requirement for Vasopressor Infusion after Cardiac Surgery," *Annals of Thoracic Surgery*, Vol. 82, No. 3, 2006, pp. 895-901.

[13] M. O'Dwyer, F. Dempsey, V. Crowley, D. Kelleher, R. McManus and T. Ryan, "Septic Shock Is Correlated with Asymmetrical Dimethyl Arginine Levels, Which May Be Influenced by a Polymorphism in the Dimethylarginine Dimethylaminohydrolase II Gene: A Prospective Observational Study," *Critical Care*, Vol. 10, No. 5, 2006, p. R139.

[14] R. Maas, "Pharmacotherapies and Their Influence on Asymmetric Dimethylargine (ADMA)," *Vascular Medicine*, Vol. 1, Suppl. 1, 2005, pp. S49-S57.

[15] M. Thaha, Widodo, M. Yogiantoro and Y. Tomino, "Intravenous N-Acetylcysteine during Hemodialysis Reduces Asymmetric Dimethylarginine Levels in End-Stage Renal Disease Patients," *Clinical Nephrology*, Vol. 69, No. 1, 2008, pp. 24-32.

[16] M. Thaha, M. Yogiantoro and Y. Tomino, "Intravenous N-Acetylcysteine during Haemodialysis Reduces the Plasma Concentration of Homocysteine in Patients with End-Stage Renal Disease," *Clinical Drug Investigation*, Vol. 26, 2006, pp. 195-202.

[17] L. Jones, C. Tran, J. Leiper, A. Hingorani and P. Vallance, "Common Genetic Variation in a Basal Promoter Element Alters DDAH 2 Expression in Endothelial Cells," *Biochemical and Biophysical Research Communications*, Vol. 310, No. 3, 2003, pp. 836-843.

[18] R. Maas, J. Erdmann, N. Luneburg, J. Stritzke, E. Schwedhelm, C. Meisinger, *et al.*, "Polymorphisms in the Promoter Region of the Dimethylarginine Dimethylaminohydrolase 2 Gene Are Associated with Prevalence of Hypertension," *Pharmacological Research*, Vol. 60, No. 6, 2009, pp. 488-493.

[19] J. Wang, A. Sim, X. Wang, C. Salonikas, D. Naidoo and D. Wilcken, "Relations between Plasma Asymmetric Dimethylarginine (ADMA) and Risk Factors for Coronary Disease," *Atherosclerosis*, Vol. 184, No. 2, 2006, pp. 383-388.

[20] P. Vallance and J. Leiper, "Asymmetric Dimethylarginine and Kidney Disease—Marker or Mediator?" *Journal of the American Society of Nephrology*, Vol. 16, No. 8, 2005, pp. 2254-2256.

[21] J. T. Kielstein, S. R. Salpeter, S. M. Bode-Boeger, J. P. Cooke and D. Fliser, "Symmetric Dimethylarginine (SDMA) as Endogenous Marker of Renal Function—A Meta-Analysis," *Nephrology Dialysis Transplantation*, Vol. 21, No. 9, 2006, pp. 2446-2451.

[22] V. Achan, M. Broadhead, M. Malaki, G. Whitley, J. Leiper, R. MacAllister, *et al.*, "Asymmetric Dimethylar-

ginine Causes Hypertension and Cardiac Dysfunction in Humans and Is Actively Metabolized by Dimethylarginine Dimethylaminohydrolase," *Arteriosclerosis, Thrombosis, and Vascular Biology*, Vol. 23, No. 8, 2003, pp. 1455-1459.

[23] M. Feng, L. Liu, Z. Guo and Y. Xiong, "Gene Transfer of Dimethylarginine Dimethylaminohydrolase-2 Improves the Impairments of DDAH/ADMA/NOS/NO Pathway in Endothelial Cells Induced by Lysophosphatidylcholine," *European Journal of Pharmacology*, Vol. 584, No. 1, 2008, pp. 49-56.

[24] H. Dayoub, V. Achan, S. Adimoolam, J. Jacobi, M. C. Stuehlinger, B.-Y. Wang, *et al.*, "Dimethylarginine Dimethylaminohydrolase Regulates Nitric Oxide Synthesis," *Circulation*, Vol. 108, No. 24, 2003, pp. 3042-3047.

[25] J. Leiper, J. Santa Maria, A. Chubb, R. MacAllister, I. Charles, G. Whitley, *et al.*, "Identification of Two Human Dimethylarginine Dimethylaminohydrolases with Distinct Tissue Distributions and Homology with Microbial Arginine Deiminases," *Biochemical Journal*, Vol. 341, 1999, pp. 209-214. doi:10.1042/0264-6021:3430209

[26] J. Leiper and M. Nandi, "The Therapeutic Potential of Targeting Endogenous Inhibitors of Nitric Oxide Synthesis," *Nature Reviews Drug Discovery*, Vol. 10, No. 4, 2011, pp. 277-291.

[27] A. Tojo, W. Welch, V. Bremer, M. Kimoto, K. Kimura, M. Omata, *et al.*, "Colocalization of Demethylating Enzymes and NOS and Functional Effects of Methylarginines in Rat Kidney," *Kidney International*, Vol. 52, No. 6, 1997, pp. 1593-1601.

[28] M. E. Widlansky, N. Gokce, J. F. Keaney Jr. and J. A. Vita, "The Clinical Implications of Endothelial Dysfunction," *Journal of the American College of Cardiology*, Vol. 42, No. 7, 2003, pp. 1149-1160.

[29] N. Dhalla, R. Temsah and T. Netticadan, "Role of Oxidative Stress in Cardiovascular Diseases," *Journal of Hypertension*, Vol. 18, No. 6, 2000, pp. 655-673.

[30] C. Tran, M. Fox, P. Vallance and J. Leiper, "Chromosomal Localization, Gene Structure, and Expression Pattern of DDAH 1: Comparison with DDAH 2 and Implications for Evolutionary Origins," *Genomics*, Vol. 68, No. 1, 2000, pp. 101-105.

[31] A. Ito, K. Egashira, T. Narishige, K. Muramatsu and A. Takeshita, "Renin-Angiotensin System Is Involved in the Mechanism of Increased Serum Asymmetric Dimethylarginine in Essential Hypertension," *Japanese Circulation Journal*, Vol. 65, No. 9, 2001, pp. 775-778.

[32] F. Perticone, A. Sciacqua, R. Maio, M. Perticone, R. Maas, R. H. Boger, *et al.*, "Asymmetric Dimethylarginine, L-Arginine, and Endothelial Dysfunction in Essential Hypertension," *Journal of the American College of Cardiology*, Vol. 46, No. 3, 2005, pp. 518-523.

[33] J. Leiper and P. Vallance, "New Tricks from an Old Dog : Nitric Oxide-Independent Effects of Dimethylarginine Dimethylaminohydrolase," *Arteriosclerosis, Thrombosis, and Vascular Biology*, Vol. 26, No. 7, 2006, pp. 1419-1420.

[34] T. Ogawa, M. Kimoto and K. Sasaoka, "Purification and Properties of a New Enzyme, NG,NG-Dimethylarginine Dimethylaminohydrolase, from Rat Kidney," *Journal of Biological Chemistry*, Vol. 264, No. 17, 1989, pp. 10205-10209.

[35] T. Teerlink, "ADMA Metabolism and Clearance," *Vascular Medicine*, Vol. 1, Suppl. 1, 2005, pp. S73-S81.

[36] J. Jacobi, K. Sydow, G. von Degenfeld, Y. Zhang, H. Dayoub, B. Wang, *et al.*, "Overexpression of Dimethylarginine Dimethylaminohydrolase Reduces Tissue Asymmetric Dimethylarginine Levels and Enhances Angiogenesis," *Circulation*, Vol. 111, No. 11, 2005, pp. 1431-1438.

[37] C. Smith, G. Birdsey, S. Anthony, F. Arrigoni, J. Leiper and P. Vallance, "Dimethylarginine Dimethylaminohydrolase Activity Modulates ADMA Levels, VEGF Expression, and Cell Phenotype," *Biochemical and Biophysical Research Communications*, Vol. 308, No. 4, 2003, pp. 984-989.

[38] V. Achan, C. T. L. Tran, F. Arrigoni, G. S. J. Whitley, J. M. Leiper and P. Vallance, "All-Trans-Retinoic Acid Increases Nitric Oxide Synthesis by Endothelial Cells," *Circulation Research*, Vol. 90, No. 7, 2002, pp. 764-769.

[39] R. H. Böger, S. M. Bode-Böger, K. Sydow, D. D. Heistad and S. R. Lentz, "Plasma Concentration of Asymmetric Dimethylarginine, an Endogenous Inhibitor of Nitric Oxide Synthase, Is Elevated in Monkeys with Hyperhomocyst(e)inemia or Hypercholesterolemia," *Arteriosclerosis, Thrombosis, and Vascular Biology*, Vol. 20, No. 6, 2000, pp. 1557-1564.

Factors Influencing Behavior of Taking Medicine in Elderly Patients Undergoing Hemodialysis

Kumiko Ozawa[1], Setsuko Niki[1], Seiko Yamanouchi[1], Hideaki Yamabe[2], Toshiko Tomisawa[2], Maiko Kitajima[2], Mayumi Urushizaka[2], Kumiko Kawasaki[2], Chieko Itaki[2], Yuka Noto[2], Morito Endo[3]

[1]School of Nursing, Hachinohe Junior College, Hachinohe, Japan
[2]Hirosaki University Graduate School of Health Sciences, Hirosaki, Japan
[3]Faculty of Human Health Science, Hachinohe University, Hachinohe, Japan
Email: yamabe@cc.hirosaki-u.ac.jp

ABSTRACT

Purpose: The elderly are often faced with multiple diseases, in particular hemodialysis (HD) which requires many kinds of medication. This study examined the factors influencing the behavior of taking medicine in elderly patients undergoing HD. **Subjects and Methods:** The subjects comprised 70 outpatients >65 years undergoing HD (48 male and 22 fe- male). The mean age of the patients was 72.5 ± 4.4 years. The mean duration of dialysis history was 6.1 ± 5.2 years. We performed a questionnaire survey using Medication Assessment Tool, The Kidney Disease Quality of Life (QOL) —Short Form and Acceptance for Dialysis Instrument. **Result:** Two factors related to poor behavior of taking medicine: dialysis history <2 years and poor acceptance of dialysis. The multiple regression analysis showed patient satisfaction ($\beta = -0.329$, $p < 0.01$) and symptoms/problems ($\beta = -0.273$, $p < 0.05$) as significant independent variables relating to behavior of taking medicine. **Conclusion:** Poor behavior of taking medicine is related to a short dialysis period, poor acceptance and poor satisfaction of dialysis therapy in elderly patients.

Keywords: Behavior of Taking Medicine; Hemodialysis; Adherence; Elderly Patient

1. Introduction

The number of patients undergoing hemodialysis (HD) for chronic kidney disease is increasing every year. The mortality rate of HD patients is also increasing. In Japan, the total number of dialysis patients was 297,126 and the number of patients newly inducted to HD was 37,532 in 2010. For the causative diseases, the first position of the new dialysis patient was diabetic nephropathy. In particularly, elderly patients newly inducted to HD are increasing (mean age: 67.8 ± 13.3); the ratio of the patients older than 65 years was 63.5% and older than 75 years was 34.9% [1].

The elderly are often faced with multiple diseases, such as diabetes mellitus, hypertension, heart disease, and cerebrovascular disease. The processes of excretion of waste material, adjustment of water and electrolyte balance, hormonal resolution and excretion and activation of vitamin D work poorly in HD patients, requiring elderly HD patients to take many kinds of medicine. Graveley *et al.* have reported that the incidences of side effects and interactions of medicines occur 2 - 3 times more often in elderly people than in young people [2].

Other studies [3-6] have reported that adherence to medicine is influenced by several factors: lifestyle, effect of treatment, side effects, anxiety about the disorder, confidence in treatment, simple explanation of the medicine, presence of social or family support, and relationship between nurses and patients. Moreover, poor adherence to medicine is frequent in elderly patients [7]. Nurses also have a role in ensuring patients carry out self-care adequately. Therefore, we thought that the behavior of taking medicine should be properly evaluated.

There are few studies on the behavior of taking medicine in elderly HD patients. The purpose of this study was to elucidate the factors influencing the behavior of taking medicine in elderly patients undergoing HD.

His template, created in MS Word 2003 and saved as "Word 97-2003 & 6.0/95-RTF" for the PC, provides authors with most of the formatting specifications needed for preparing electronic versions of their papers. All standard paper components have been specified for three reasons: 1) ease of use when formatting individual papers; 2) automatic compliance to electronic requirements that facilitate the concurrent or later production of electronic products; and 3) conformity of style throughout a journal paper. Margins, column widths, line spacing, and type styles are builtin; examples of the type styles are provided throughout this document and are identified in italic type, within parentheses, following the example. Some components, such as multi-leveled equations, graphics, and tables are not prescribed, although the various table text styles are provided. The formatter will need to create these components, incorporating the applicable criteria that follow.

2. Subjects and Methods

2.1. Subjects

Subjects were 70 patients >65 years undergoing HD. Inclusion criteria were more than three months since the induction of HD, no major change in treatment content within the past three months and diagnosis of psychosis or dementia.

We collected individual clinical records and carried out a questionnaire survey. The questionnaire survey was carried out either during dialysis or after dialysis. When it was difficult for the patient to complete the survey in-house, we had them complete it at home, and collected it by collection box within a week. When it was difficult for the patients to write by themselves, the survey was taken verbally. The clinical record includes causative disease, dialysis history, weight gain rate between dialyses, clinical data, presence of diabetes, treatment content and type of oral medication. Clinical data was the most recently obtained data before the dialysis.

2.2. Behaviors of Taking Medicine

Medication Assessment Tool (MAT) [8] was used to study the behavior of taking medicine by the patients. MAT was developed to evaluate whether an outpatient understands how to take oral medicine and it consists of 11 items (**Table 1**). As for the evaluation, each item was evaluated on a 4-point scale from 1 to 4 with a total score between 11 and 44. A high score indicates problems in acceptance of taking the medicine.

2.3. Measuring QOL

The Kidney Disease Quality of Life-Short Form instrument (KDQOL-SF™; version 1.3) was used for this study.

Table 1. The items of the MAT.

1	Is it easy to understand how to take medicine?
2	Are you worried about side effect of the medicine taking now?
3	Do you understand why medicine is necessary by oneself?
4	Is the explanation of the medicine helpful to understand medicine?
5	Do you feel an effect of the medicine?
6	Is the medicine helpful to prevent sick deterioration?
7	Do you think that it is not good to depend on medicine?
8	Is the expense of the medicine a burden?
9	Do you think that there may be less medicine than now?
10	Is the work to take the medicine troublesome?
11	Does the taking medicine go well generally?
	One item marks from 1 to 4 points.

It was developed to evaluate the quality of life of patients with chronic kidney disease; its reliability and validity have been confirmed [9]. It consists of the kidney disease-specific instrument of 43 items and the Short-Form Health Survey of 36 items (SF-36), which is a generic instrument. It takes around 15 - 20 min to answer, which is a burden for elderly people. Therefore, we changed the SF-36 to the Short-Form Health Survey of 8 items (SF-8™), which can measure the same health concept with a shortened questionnaire, reducing the burden on elderly patients [10]. The score of all variables is high when QOL is good. The content of KDQOL-SF™ and SF-8™ is shown in **Table 2**.

Twenty eight items of KDQOL-SF™ consist of four variables: symptoms/problems (KD1), effect of kidney disease (KD2), burden of kidney disease (KD3) and sleep (KD6); and six items consist of two variables: cognitive function (KD4) and quality of social interaction (KD5). There are also two items of social support (KD7) in KDQOL-SF™ that evaluate the relationship between patients and their family or friends, and three items, which consist of two variables, dialysis staff encouragement (KD8) and patient satisfaction (KD9), to evaluate the relationship between the patient with medical staff.

Six items of SF-8™ consist of general health perceptions (SF8GH), physical functioning (SF8PF), role functioning physical (SF8RP), bodily pain (SF8BP), vitality (SF8VT), and social functioning (SF8SF) to evaluate the physical state of the patient. The other two items of SF-8™ consist of mental health (SF8MH) and role functional emotional (SF8RE) to evaluate the psychological state of the patient.

Table 2 .Variables in SF-8™ and KDQOL-SF™.

Variable
SF-8™
General Health Perceptions (SF8GH)
Physical Functioning (SF8PF)
Role Functioning Physical (SF8RP)
Bodily Pain (SF8BP)
Vitality (SF8VT)
Social Functioning (SF8SF)
Mental Health (SF8MH)
Role Functional Emotional (SF8RE)
Physical Component Summary (PCS-8)
Mental Component Summary (MCS-8)
KDQOL-SF™
Symptoms/Problems (KD1)
Effect of kidney disease (KD2)
Burden of kidney disease (KD3)
Cognitive function (KD4)
Quality of social interaction (KD5)
Sleep (KD6)
Social support (KD7)
Dialysis staff encouragement (KD8)
Patient satisfaction (KD9)

2.4. Evaluation of Acceptance of Dialysis

Acceptance of the dialysis instrument [11] consists of ten items and was developed to evaluate the psychological adjustment level of patients with chronic kidney disease, from dialysis induction to the maintenance period (**Table 3**). In the evaluation, each item was evaluated on a 4-point scale 1 to 4, with a total score between 10 and 40. A high score indicates that the receptive level is low.

2.5. Statistical Analysis

All data were expressed as means ± SD and the comparison between the mean of each item was carried out using t-test, analysis of variance, U-test of Mann-Whitney. The data were analyzed using SPSS Statistics 18.0 software (SPSS, Chicago, IL, USA). We considered $p < 0.05$ as statistical significant.

2.6. Ethical Consideration

This study was approved by the Committee of Medical Ethics of Hirosaki University Graduate School of Medicine, Hirosaki, Japan. The subjects gave us informed consent.

3. Results

3.1. Relationship between Patients' Characteristics and Total MAT Score

The α trust coefficient of Cronbach's of the total MAT score was 0.777.

We examined the relationship between patients' characteristics and MAT. The MAT score of the patients with a dialysis history of less than 2 years was significantly higher than those with more 2 years of history ($p < 0.05$). The MAT score showed no relation with other characteristics (**Table 4**).

3.2. Relationship between Patients' Characteristics and Each Item on MAT

We compared the mean value of each item on MAT with the patients' characteristics. For the question, "Is it easy

Table 3. The items of the acceptance for dialysis instrument.

1	Are you afraid that you think that you must undergo dialysis all the time in future
2	Are you anxious whether you can live by dialysis more how many years?
3	Are you anxious whether a physical complication does not occur?
4	Are you anxious in future whether you can continue work (housework)?
5	Are you anxious in future whether you can do life (economic aspects)?
6	Are you angry when you think why oneself must undergo dialysis?
7	Do you realize the situation to have to undergo dialysis?
8	Do you think that you had better die if you undergo dialysis, or you do not want to undergo dialysis?
9	How long do you receive explanation about the dialysis by the chief physician?
10	How long do you understand dialysis?
	One item marks from 1 to 4 points.

Table 4. The comparison between mean value of the total MAT score and the patients' characteristics.

Characteristic	Group	N (%)	Mean ± SD	p Value
Sex	Male	48 (68.6)	21.7 ± 4.4	ns
	Female	22 (31.4)	21.9 ± 5.3	
Age (years)	65 ~ 74	46 (65.7)	21.8 ± 4.2	ns
	≧75	24 (34.3)	21.5 ± 5.6	
Housemate	Lodger	61 (87.1)	21.6 ± 4.9	ns
	No	9 (12.9)	22.7 ± 3.0	
Education level	Elementary school or Junior high school graduation	37 (52.9)	22.0 ± 4.9	ns
	University or High school graduation	33 (47.1)	21.5 ± 4.5	
Causative disease	Glomerulonephritis chronic	12 (17.1)	22.2 ± 2.0	ns
	Diabetic nephropathy	37 (52.9)	21.7 ± 5.2	
	Nephrosclerosis	4 (5.7)	23.0 ± 5.7	
	A multiple cystic kidney	3 (4.3)	18.3 ± 7.0	
	Others	14 (20.0)	21.7 ± 4.4	
Dialysis history (years)	<2	17 (24.3)	24.0 ± 3.9	*
	≧2	53 (75.7)	21.1 ± 4.8	
Weight gain rate between the dialysis	A water well-controlled group	55 (78.6)	21.4 ± 4.9	ns
	A water poor-controlled group	15 (21.4)	23.0 ± 3.5	
Presence or absence of diabetes	Presence	37 (52.9)	21.7 ± 5.2	ns
	Absence	33 (47.1)	21.7 ± 4.1	
Diabetic treatment contents	An insulin injection	23 (62.2)	22.3 ± 5.4	ns
	An oral antidiabetic drug	4 (10.8)	17.2 ± 7.0	
	Only as for the diet	10 (27.0)	22.4 ± 3.4	

Continued

HbA1c (%)	<6	15(40.5)	20.8 ± 4.5	ns
	6.0 - 6.9	13(35.1)	22.4 ± 6.6	
	≧7	9(24.3)	22.4 ± 4.5	
The kind of the oral medicine(kinds)	<5	22(31.4)	20.6 ± 5.2	ns
	≧6	48(68.6)	22.3 ± 4.5	
Ht (%)	<30	15(21.4)	22.3 ± 5.2	ns
	30 - 32	22(31.4)	20.7 ± 5.8	
	≧33	33(47.1)	22.2 ± 3.6	

$^{*}p < 0.05$, ns: not-significant. Data analysis: An U-test of Mann-Whitney (Age), A t-test(Sex, Housemate, Dialysis history, Weight gain rate between the dialysis, Diabetic presence, The kind of the oral medicine), An analysis of variance (Education level, Causative disease, Diabetic treatment contents, HbA1c, Ht).

to understand how to take the medicine?" the water well-controlled group showed a significantly lower score than the water poor-controlled group ($p < 0.01$). For "Are you worried about side effects of the medicine your taking now?" the group that had graduated university or high school (continued education) showed a significantly lower score than the group that had only graduated elementary school or junior high school (limited education) ($p < 0.05$). The group with a dialysis history of ≥2 years showed a significantly lower score than the <2 year group ($p < 0.05$). For "Do you understand why you must take medicine by yourself?" the continued education group showed a significantly lower score than the limited education group ($p < 0.001$). Moreover, for "Is the explanation of the medicine helpful to understand the medicine?" the continued education group showed a significantly lower score than the limited education group ($p < 0.05$). For "Is the medicine helpful to prevent the worsening of your illness?" the group with a housemate showed a significantly lower score than the group without a housemate ($p < 0.01$). For "Is the expense of the medicine a burden?" women showed a significantly lower score than men ($p < 0.05$). For "Does taking the medicine generally go well?" the group of the dialysis history of ≥2 years showed a significantly lower score than the <2 year group ($p < 0.05$). There was no significant difference between the scores regarding age, causative disease and the number of types of oral medication.

3.3. Relationship between QOL and MAT Score

Relationship between QOL and MAT score was examined. The mean value of the total MAT score showed significant negative correlations with SF8RE ($r = -0.24$, $p < 0.05$), MCS-8 ($r = -0.29$, $p < 0.05$) in the SF-8^{TM}, KD1 ($r = -0.38$, $p < 0.01$), KD2 ($r = -0.30$, $p < 0.01$), KD4 ($r = -0.32$, $p < 0.01$), KD5 ($r = -0.30$, $p < 0.05$), KD6 ($r = -0.31$, $p < 0.01$), KD7 ($r = -0.35$, $p < 0.01$), KD8 ($r = -0.33$, $p < 0.01$), and KD9 ($r = -0.38$, $p < 0.01$) on the KDQOL-SF^{TM} (**Table 5**). The multiple regression analysis was used for the variables with a coefficient of correlation of more than 0.3 to determine variables significantly associated with MAT. Factors that influence MAT based on the multiple regression analysis are shown in **Table 6**. The mean value of the total MAT score showed significant negative correlations with KD9 ($\beta = -0.329$, $p < 0.01$) and KD1 ($\beta = -0.273$, $p < 0.05$) (**Figure 1**).

3.4. Relationship between MAT Score and Acceptance of Dialysis Instrument

The mean value of the total MAT score showed a significant positive correlation with the acceptance of the dialysis instrument ($r = 0.24$, $p < 0.05$) (**Figure 2**). This result means poor behavior of taking medicine relates to the poor acceptance of the dialysis therapy.

Table 5. Factors of QOL influencing the MAT by the correlation analysis.

Variable (item)	r	p
Role Functional emotional (SF8RE)[a]	−0.24	*
Mental component summary (MCS-8)	−0.29	*
Symptoms/problems (KD1)	−0.38	**
Effect of kidney disease (KD2)	−0.30	**
Cognitive function (KD4)	−0.32	**
Quality of social interaction (KD5)[a]	−0.30	*
Sleep (KD6)	−0.31	**
Social support (KD7)	−0.35	**
Dialysis staff encouragement (KD8)[a]	−0.33	**
Patient satisfaction (KD9)[a]	−0.38	**

$^{*}p < 0.05$, $^{**}p < 0.01$. [a]: Pearson's product moment correlation coefficient, Others: Spearman's rank correlation coefficient.

Table 6. Factors of QOL influencing the MAT by the multiple regression analysis.

Variable	Standard β	p value
Patient satisfaction (KD9)	−0.329	**
Symptoms/problems (KD1)	−0.273	*
Cognitive function (KD4)	−0.189	ns
Sleep (KD6)	0.014	ns
Social support (KD7)	−0.139	ns
Dialysis staff encouragement (KD8)	−0.222	ns

Adjusted $R^2 = 0.219$, $^{*}p < 0.05$, $^{**}p < 0.01$, ns: not-significant.

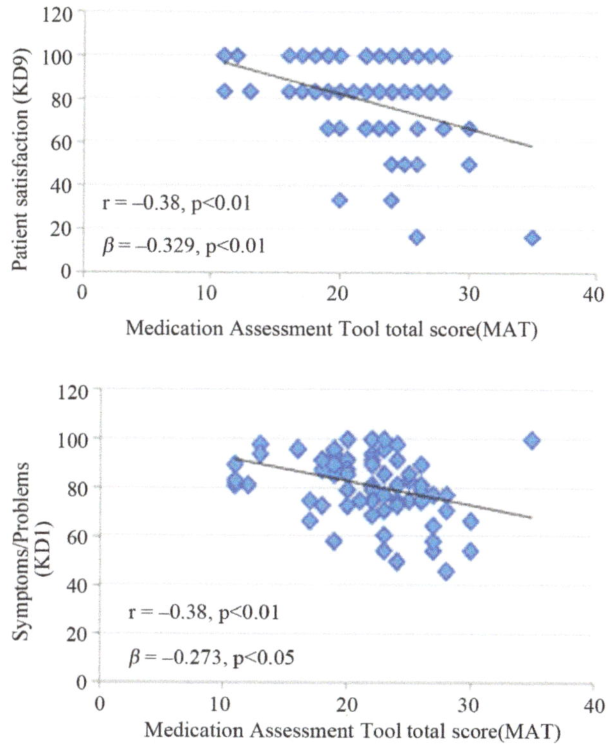

Figure 1. The mean value of the MAT score showed in particularly strong relation with Patient satisfaction (KD9) by multiple regression analysis ($\beta = -0.329$, $p < 0.01$). This result means poor behavior of taking medicine relates to the poor satisfaction of dialysis therapy. The mean value of the MAT score showed in particularly strong relation with Symptom/ Problem (KD1) by multiple regression analysis ($\beta = -0.273$, $p < 0.05$). This result means poor behavior of taking medicine relates to the poor healthy satisfaction of the symptom.

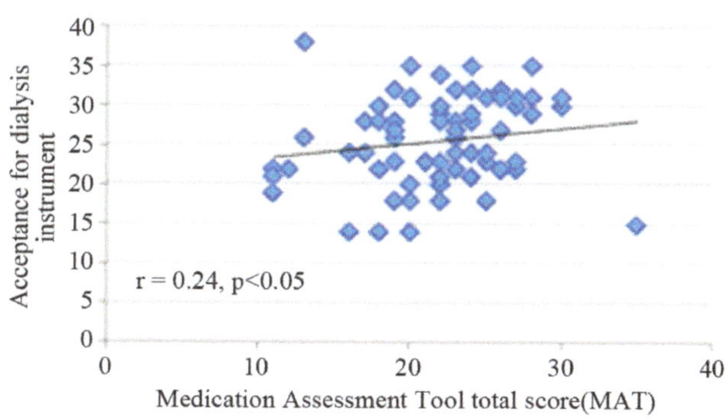

Figure 2. The mean value of the total MAT score showed a significant positive correlation with acceptance of the dialysis instrument ($r = 0.24$, $p < 0.05$). This result means poor behavior of taking medicine relates to the poor acceptance of dialysis therapy.

4. Discussion

The mean age of the patients in this study was 72.5 ± 4.4 years. The number of types of oral medication was 7.4 ± 3.1. Uejima *et al.* reported that patients older than 70 years take about five types of medication, which is twice that of patients younger than 40 years in Japan [12]. Elderly patients usually have multiple diseases and tend to take many medications; these rates increase for elderly HD patients. Moreover, elderly patients are more likely to forget to take their medicine, with noon being the most frequent time to forget [12].

We compared the mean value of the total MAT score relative to patients' characteristics. Patients with a dialysis history of more than 2 years, showed significantly better adherence to taking their medicine than those with less history. Siegal *et al.* have reported that an elapse of memory is more frequent in short-term HD patients than long-term HD patients [13]. Cukor *et al.* also noted memory lapse as a factor of worsened adherence of taking medicine in HD patients [14], as supported by our results.

We compared the score of each item in MAT relative to patients' characteristics. In regards to understanding how to take the medicine, water well-controlled patients had significantly better understanding than water poor-controlled patients. Lindberg *et al.* also reported that adherence of taking medicine is influenced by the avoidance of unnecessary fluid intake [15]. Water restrictions may therefore be a factor of poorer adherence to taking medicine.

Patients with less than 2 years of dialysis history also felt more apprehension of side effects of the medicine compared with those with more than 2 years of history, which was consistent with the total MAT score results. Patients with less than 2 years of dialysis history are thought to be unstable physically and psychologically, have poor disease acceptance, and apprehension for side effects of the medicine, which may worsen adherence. It is well known that side effects of medicine are associated with poor adherence [7,15-17].

Patients with a high school or university education had a better understanding of how to take their medicine than those with less education. This result suggests that patients are more likely to take their medicine after having understood the need of the medicine. We found no significant difference for the causative disease and MAT score, which is consistent with the results of Yuzawa [8].

The total MAT score showed significant negative correlations with SF8RE, MCS-8, KD1, KD2, KD4, KD5, KD6, KD7, KD8, and KD9. These results mean that if daily activity of HD patients for cognitive function and quality of social interaction are good, and the patients were satisfied with social support and the dialysis care, adherence is good in HD patients. Therefore, it is thought that the behavior of taking medicine is strongly associated with the QOL of HD patients.

In addition, the MAT score showed a particularly strong relationship with patient satisfaction and symptoms/problems by multiple regression analysis. Ferrans *et al.* have also reported that patient satisfaction of dialysis care is significantly correlated with the mental state, QOL, renal function and symptoms of the patient [18]. Therefore, it is important to improve patients' satisfaction, psychological adaptation and QOL.

As we showed a strong connection between behavior of taking medicine and patients' satisfaction for the dialysis care provided by medical staff, more attention should be placed on the consultation situation of medical staff when patients have doubts in taking medicine and questions about their health, for further understanding of the patient's relationship with medical staff.

Moreover, the total MAT score showed a significant positive correlation with acceptance of the dialysis instrument. Thus, more acceptable dialysis treatment may lead to improved adherence. Much effort is still needed to help patients accept dialysis therapy.

5. Conclusion

Poor behavior of taking medicine is related to a short dialysis period and the degree of patient satisfaction for dialysis therapy. It is important to improve patient satisfaction for dialysis care, increase healthy satisfaction regarding symptoms, and allow patients to better accept their disease.

REFERENCES

[1] Japanese Society for Dialysis Therapy, "An Overview of Regular Dialysis Treatment in Japan as of December 31, 2010," Tokyo, 2011.

[2] E. A. Graveley and C. S. Oseasohn, "Multiple Drug Regimens Medication Compliance among Veterans 65 Years and Older," *Resarch in Nursing & Health*, Vol. 14, No. 1, 1991, pp. 51-58. doi:10.1002/nur.4770140108

[3] J. M. Cargill, "Medication Compliance in Elderly People, Influencing Variables and Interventions," *Journal of Advanced Nursing*, Vol. 17, No. 4, 1992, pp. 422-426. doi:10.1111/j.1365-2648.1992.tb01925.x

[4] A. W. Deborah, "Evaluation of Medication Interventions for the Elderly," *Home Healthcare Nurse*, Vol. 16, No. 9, 1998, pp. 612-617. doi:10.1097/00004045-199809000-00008

[5] T. T. Fulmer, P. H. Feldman, T. S. Kim, B. Carty, M. Beers, M. Molina and M. Putnam, "An Intervention Study to Enhance Medication Compliance in Community-Dwelling Elderly Individuals," *Journal of Gerontology Nursing*, Vol. 25, No. 8, 1999, pp. 6-13.

[6] A. A. Ryan, "Medication Compliance and Older People: A Review of the Literature," *International Journal of Nursing Study*, Vol. 36, No. 2, 1999, pp. 153-162. doi:10.1016/S0020-7489(99)00003-6

[7] J. Petermans, A. S. Suarez and T. V. Hees, "Therapeutic Adherence in Elderly," *Revue Medical of Liege*, Vol. 65, No. 5-6, 2010, pp. 261-266.

[8] Y. Yuzawa, "Making and the Usefulness of the Medication Assessment Tool of the Outpatient," *Ochanomizu Medical Journal*, Vol. 50, No. 3, 2002, pp. 133-143.

[9] Y. Miura, J. Green and S. Fukuhara, "Manual of the KDQOL Japanese Version 1.3," Institute for Health Outcomes & Process Evaluation Research, Kyoto, 2004.

[10] S. Fukuhara and Y. Suzukamo, "Manual of the SF-8 Japanese Version," Institute for Health Outcomes & Process Evaluation Research, Kyoto, 2004.

[11] I. Fukunishi, "Development of the Measure of the Psychological Acceptance Level of the Dialysis Treatment," OFF TIME Chugai Pharmaceutical, Tokyo, 2002, p. 67.

[12] E. Uegima, S. Mikami and H. Morimoto, "Drug Compliance in the Elderly," *Nippon Ronen Igakkai Zasshi*, Vol. 29, No. 1, 1992, pp. 855-863. doi:10.3143/geriatrics.29.855

[13] B. R. Siegal, R. J. Calsyn and R. M. Cuddihee, "The Relationship of Social Support to Psychological Adjustment in End-Stage Renal Disease Patient," *Journal of Chronic Disease*, Vol. 40, No. 4, 1987, pp. 337-344.

[14] D. Cukor, D. S. Rosenthal, R. M. Jindal, C. D. Brown and P. L. Kimmel, "Depression Is an Important Contributor to Low Medication Adherence in Hemodialyzed Patients and Transplant Recipients," *Kidney International*, Vol. 75, No. 11, 2009, pp. 1223-1229. doi:10.1038/ki.2009.51

[15] M. Lindberg and P. Lindberg, "Overcoming Obstacles for Adherence to Phosphate Binding Medication in Dialysis Patients: A Qualitative Study," *Pharmacy World & Science*, Vol. 30, No. 5, 2008, pp. 571-576. doi:10.1007/s11096-008-9212-9

[16] C. M. Hughes, "Medication Non-Adherence in the Elderly," *Drugs & Aging*, Vol. 21, No. 12, 2004, pp. 793-811.

[17] R. Horne and J. Weinman, "Patients' Beliefs about Prescribed Medicines and Their Role in Adherence to Treatment in Chronic Physical Illness," *Journal of Psychosomatic Research*, Vol. 47, No. 6, 1999, pp. 555-567.

[18] C. E. Ferranns, M. J. Powers and C. R. Kasch, "Satisfaction with Health Care of Hemodialysis Patients" *Research of Nursing & Health*, Vol. 10, No. 6, 1987, pp. 367-374.

Anti-Neutrophil Cytoplasmic Antibody Vasculitis in Pediatric Patients: Is the Incidence Rising?*

Christine Sethna[1], Rachel Frank[1], Lulette Infante[1], Beth Gottlieb[2], Anne Eberhard[2], Xiaotong Wang[3], Howard Trachtman[4#]

[1]Department of Pediatrics, Division of Nephrology, Cohen Children's Medical Center of New York, New York, USA
[2]Department of Pediatrics, Division of Rheumatology, Cohen Children's Medical Center of New York, New York, USA
[3]Department of Pathology, North Shore University Hospital of the North Shore—LIJ Health System, New York, USA
[4]Department of Pediatrics, Division of Nephrology, NYU Langone Medical Center, New York, USA
Email: #howard.trachtman@nyumc.org

ABSTRACT

Objectives: Anti-neutrophil cytoplasmic antibody (ANCA)-associated vasculitis is an autoimmune disease usually seen in middle-aged and older adults but which is rare in children and adolescents. We sought to determine if there has been a change in the incidence of this disorder. **Methods:** Single-center, retrospective review. **Results:** Over the last 2 years, we have encountered a striking increase in the frequency of this disease in pediatric patients. All eight patients seen during this period had renal involvement and 5 patients rapidly progressed to end stage kidney disease. The prognosis was worse in younger patients, those with microscopic polyangiitis, and those with chronic kidney damage in the diagnostic renal biopsy. **Conclusions:** We report these observations to highlight this change in the epidemiology of ANCA-associated vasculitis and to promote earlier recognition and treatment of this severe form of glomerulonephritis.

Keywords: Anti-Neutrophil Cytoplasmic Antibody (ANCA); Vasculitis; Epidemiology

1. Introduction

Anti-neutrophil cytoplasmic antibody (ANCA)-associated vasculitis is an autoimmune disorder that usually presents with sudden onset disease. The organ systems that are primarily affected include the kidney and lung [1]. There are two main subtypes based on the identity of the causative antibody—granulomatosis with polyangiitis (GPA) [Wegener's] and microscopic polyangiitis (MPA). The former is associated with elevated titers of antibody to proteinase 3 and is characterized by cytoplasmic staining of neutrophils (cANCA) while the later is marked by antibodies to myeloperoxidase that stain neutrophils in a perinuclear pattern (pANCA) [1,2]. The kidney injury is characterized by necrotizing vasculitis and glomerular inflammation with minimal immune complex deposition. GPA and MPA require timely recognition and initiation of induction therapy in order to prevent permanent organ damage [2].

Both subtypes of ANCA-associated disease are rare and generally occur in middle-aged and elderly patients. Although it does occur in children, in most large patient series, less than 10% of all cases occur in the pediatric age range [3]. Over the last 2 years we have encountered an unexpected surge in the number of cases of ANCA-associated disease, well above the occurrence of at most one case annually at our referral center. We report our experience in order to promote heightened awareness of this condition in children in the hope that earlier case definition and prompt implementation of effective treatments will lead to improved clinical outcomes.

2. Patients and Methods

Patients were identified by a review of a clinical database maintained in the Division of Nephrology with cross referencing with the Division of Rheumatology to ensure inclusion of all cases. Out-patient charts and hospital records were retrieved and reviewed and the following data were recorded: age at diagnosis, gender, race and ethnicity, presenting symptoms and physical findings, CBC, serum BUN, creatinine, cholesterol, albumin, C3, and C4 levels, ANCA and ANA titers, and urinary protein excretion expressed as the protein:creatinine ratio (mg:mg) in a first morning urine sample. The kidney biopsy findings were described including the active and chronic changes in the kidney tissue. The renal functional

*Financial Disclosures: None. No payment of any type was made to anyone to produce the manuscript. **Conflict of Interest Declarations**: None.
#Corresponding author.

status at baseline and the last follow-up visit and the induction and maintenance treatment regimens were tabulated. The retrospective chart review was approved by the North Shore-LIJ Institutional Review Board.

3. Results

The demographic features, treatment and clinical outcomes of our patients are summarized in **Table 1**. The diagnosis was confirmed both serologically and by renal histopathology in all of the cases. Five patients had MPA and 3 (all male) had GPA (formerly called Wegener's). There were no children with Churg-Strauss disease. All three patients with GPA had pulmonary involvement. In one case, there was acute pulmonary hemorrhage that prompted urgent initiation of plasmapheresis. There was evidence of concomitant gastrointestinal disease in one child, central nervous system involvement in 2, dermatological findings in 2, and cardiac manifestations (non-infectious intraventricular mass) in 1 patient. None of the patients had documented sinusitis, subglottic stenosis, or nasal deformity (saddle nose).

All patients received intravenous "pulse" methylprednisolone, 7 were given intravenous cyclophosphamide, 3 rituximab, and 3 were treated with plasmapheresis. The later three cases were characterized by severe renal insufficiency and the need for dialysis at the time of presentation.

Maintenance therapy included oral prednisone with mycophenolate mofetil or methotrexate. The outcomes for kidney function were poor. All five patients with MPA progressed to end stage kidney disease (ESKD); 2 are on chronic dialysis and 3 received a kidney transplant. Allograft function is normal without recurrent disease in the later subgroup. Two patients on maintenance medications have normal kidney function and 1 is still receiving induction therapy and steadily improving.

The number of cases in this series is limited. However, reviewing our recent experience with ANCA-associated disease, it would appear that pediatric patients with GPA tend to be older (≥16 years of age) and to have a better prognosis for preservation of kidney compared to those with MPA. In addition, most of the patients displayed active glomerular inflammation and their clinical outcomes ranged from development of ESKD to recovery of kidney function. In contrast, three patients had evidence of chronic kidney injury with glomerulosclerosis, interstitial fibrosis, and tubular atrophy in the diagnostic biopsy that was done at the time of presentation and they all required renal replacement therapy.

4. Discussion

The diagnosis of ANCA-associated vasculitis and nephritis was confirmed in all 8 cases based on positive serological test results and the presence of characteristic histopathological findings in the kidney biopsy tissue. Misclassification of the disease is unlikely in view of the normal C3, ANA and double-stranded DNA antibody titers in all cases and the lack of alternative pathology findings that would suggest a different glomerular disorder. The only cause of glomerulonephritis that might resemble MPA/GPA in children and adolescents is Henoch Schonlein purpura nephritis; however, this diagnosis is excluded by the absence of mesangial IgA deposition in all patients [4].

In most previous reports of ANCA-associated vasculitis, less than 10% of cases are documented in childhood [3]. There is one previous report from Canada that, similar to our case series, describes a rising incidence of ANCA-associated disease and which suggests that it is a generalized phenomenon [5]. The diagnostic criteria for the disease are equally valid in children and adults, implying that atypical signs and symptoms at presentation are unlikely to explain the lower incidence that has been reported in childhood (6). Serological testing for ANCA

Table 1. Clinical features of pediatric patients with ANCA-associated nephritis.

Pt #	Age (yr) at Onset/Gender	Ethnicity	Disease Type	Glomerular Lesions, Active	Glomerular Lesions, Chronic	Interstitial Fibrosis/Tubular Atrophy	Treatments	Outcome
1	6 F	W	MPA	N/A	N/A	N/A	S, C	Transplant
2	12 F	H	MPA	100	0	0	S, C	Transplant
3	6 M	H	MPA	10% - 21%	80% - 90%	20% - 30%	S, C	Dialysis (Peritoneal)
4	12 F	W	MPA	0	60%	20%	S, C	Transplant
5	18 M	W	GPA	90% - 100%	0	0	S, C, R, PE	Scr 1.39, eGFR 95
6	16 M	B	GPA	26% - 32%	0	0	S, C,	Scr 1.27, eGFR 98
7	12 F	B	MPA	23% - 37%	50% - 60%	30% - 40%	S, C, R, PE	Dialysis (Hemo)
8	16 M	W	GPA	67% - 73%	0	0	S, R, PE	Scr 2.56, eGFR 49

The numbers in the columns detailing the pathology findings indicate the percentage of glomeruli affected by the abnormality or the interstitial area displaying the specific lesion. MPA: microscopic polyangiitis; GPA: granulomatosis with polyangiitis; S: solumedrol; C: cyclophosphamide; R: rituximab; PE: plasmapheresis.

may occasionally be negative in children and a positive result is not required for diagnosis. Therefore, a kidney biopsy may be required to confirm pauciimmune glomerulonephritis with vasculitic or necrotizing lesions [7]. All of our cases had characteristic features of ANCA-associated disease and positive serology. The trend shows no evidence of abating and a new case was encountered during the preparation of this report. The patient was not included in this series because she was 21 years of age and would be considered an adult even though she was cared for by pediatric subspecialists. Thus, we propose that the increased incidence encountered over the last 2 years reflects a true change in the frequency of this complex illness in pediatric patients. At present, the cause for the sudden change in the epidemiology of ANCA-associated disease remains a mystery.

Recent studies suggest that ANCA may develop due to molecular mimicry with fimbrial protein antigens in bacteria [8]. Although there is a follow-up report that has shed some doubt on this association [9], it raises the possibility that altered environmental exposure may account for the surge in pediatric cases of ANCA-associated disease over the last few years.

ANCA-associated vasculitis is usually abrupt and severe in onset and requires early identification to achieve optimal outcomes. The present cases, several of whom had irreversible kidney damage at the time of diagnosis, may heighten awareness of ANCA-associated vasculitis in pediatric patients so that serological testing is performed promptly and aggressive therapy is administered in a timely manner. It is worth noting that our outcomes for kidney function were much worse than in a series of 8 children with ANCA-associated vasculitis (7 GPA, 1 MPA), of whom only 1 developed ESKD over a follow-up period ranging from 11 - 30 years [10]. This suggests that both the incidence and severity of ANCA-associated vasculitis in childhood may be changing. A younger age, the diagnosis of MPA, and the presence of chronic glomerular and interstitial damage appear to be indicators of a poor prognosis for maintenance of normal kidney function. However, children who have significant active glomerular inflammation can respond to therapy with a return of renal function. The logistical difficulties in implementing effective but costly therapies such as plasmapheresis and rituximab that are required to achieve rapid remission underscore the urgency of establishing the diagnosis of GPA/MPA in an accurate and timely manner [11-13].

In conclusion, ANCA-associated vasculitis is not a new entity, but a change in epidemiology of this severe illness warrants concern among physicians who care for individual patients and public health officials. We encourage the formation of a registry through established societies in pediatric nephrology and rheumatology to monitor the incidence and outcomes of patients with these rare diseases.

REFERENCES

[1] R. J. Falk and J. C. Charles Jennette, "ANCA Disease: Where Is This Field Heading?" *Journal of the American Society of Nephrology*, Vol. 21, No. 5, 2010, pp. 745-752. doi:10.1681/ASN.2009121238

[2] A. E. Berden, F. Ferrario, E. Christian Hagen, D. R. Jayne, J. Charles Jennette, K. Joh, I. Neumann, L. H. Noël, C. D. Pusey, R. Waldherr, J. A. Bruijn and I. M. Bajema, "Histopathologic Classification of ANCA-Associated Glomerulonephritis," *Journal of the American Society of Nephrology*, Vol. 21, No. 10, 2010, pp. 1628-1636. doi:10.1681/ASN.2010050477

[3] C. E. Rodrigues, M. R. Callado, C. A. Nobre, F. E. Moura, R. M. Vieira, L. A. de Albuquerque and W. P. Vieira, "Wegener's Granulomatosis: Prevalence of the Initial Clinical Manifestations—Report of Six Cases and Review of the Literature," *Revista Brasileira de Reumatologia*, Vol. 50, No. 2, 2010, pp. 150-164. doi:10.1590/S0482-50042010000200005

[4] R. Coppo, P. Cirina, A. Amore, R. A. Sinico, A. Radice and C. Rollino, "Properties of Circulating IgA Molecules in Henoch Schonlein Purpura Nephritis with Focus on Neutrophil Cytoplasmic Antigen IgA Binding (IgA-ANCA): New Insight into a Debated Issue. Italian Group of Renal Immunopathology Collaborative Study on Henoch Schonlein Purpura in Adults and Children," *Nephrology Dialysis Transplantation*, Vol. 12, No. 11, 1997, pp. 2269-2276. doi:10.1093/ndt/12.11.2269

[5] S. Grisaru, G. W. Yuen, P. M. Miettunen and L. A. Hamiwka, "Incidence of Wegener's Granulomatosis in Children," *The Journal of Rheumatology*, Vol. 37, No. 2, 2010, pp. 440-442. doi:10.3899/jrheum.090688

[6] D. A. Cabral, A. G. Uribe, S. Benseler, K. M. O'Neil, P. J. Hashkes, G. Higgins, A. S. Zeft, D. J. Lovell, D. J. Kingsbury, A. Stevens, *et al.*, "Classification, Presentation, and Initial Treatment of Wegener's Granulomatosis in Childhood," *Arthritis Rheum*, Vol. 60, No. 11, 2009, pp. 3413-3424. doi:10.1002/art.24876

[7] M. Shimizu, T. Sekiguchi, *et al.*, "A Case of a 6-Year Old Girl with Anti-Neutrophil Cytoplasmic Antibody- Negative Pauci-Immune Crescentic Glomerulonephritis," *Clinical and Experimental Nephrology*, Vol. 15, No. 4, 2011, pp. 596-601. doi:10.1007/s10157-011-0423-3

[8] R. Kain, M. Exner, R. Brandes, *et al.*, "Molecular Mimicry in Pauci-Immune Focal Necrotizing Glomerulonephritis," *Nature Medicine*, Vol. 14, No. 10, 2008, pp. 1088-1096. doi:10.1038/nm.1874

[9] A. J. Roth, M. C. Brown, R. N. Smith, A. K. Badwar, *et al.*, "Anti-LAMP-2 Antibodies Are Not Prevalent in Patients with Antineutrophil Cytoplasmic Autoantibody Glomerulonephritis," *Journal of the American Society of Nephrology*, Vol. 23, No. 5, 2012, pp. 545-555.

[10] N. Arulkumaran, S. Jawad, S.W. Smith, L. Harper, P. Brogan, C. D. Pusey and A. D. Salama, "Long-Term Outcome of Paediatric Patients with ANA Vasculitis," *Pe-*

diatric Rheumatology Online Journal, Vol. 9, 2011, p. 12. doi:10.1186/1546-0096-9-12

[11] A. Casian and D. Jayne, "Plasma Exchange in the Treatment of Wegener's Granulomatosis, Microscopic Polyangiitis, Churg-Strauss Syndrome and Renal Limited Vasculitis," *Current Opinion in Rheumatology*, Vol. 23, No. 1, 2011, pp. 12-17. doi:10.1097/BOR.0b013e32834120c1

[12] R. B. Jones, J. Willem Cohen Tervaert, T. Hauser, R. Luqmani, M. D. Morgan, C. A. Peh, *et al.*, "Rituxamab Versus Cyclophosphamide in ANCA-Associated Renal Vasculitis," *The New England Journal of Medicine*, Vol. 363, 2010, pp. 211-220. doi:10.1056/NEJMoa0909169

[13] J. H. Stone, P. A. Merkel, *et al.*, "Rituximab Versus Cyclophosphamide for ANCA-Associated Vasculitis," *The New England Journal of Medicine*, Vol. 363, 2010, pp. 221-232. doi:10.1056/NEJMoa0909905

Abbreviations

ANA, anti-nuclear antibody
ANCA, Anti-neutrophil cytoplasmic antibody
  cANCA, cytoplasmic ANCA
  pANCA, perinuclear ANCA
BUN, blood urea nitrogen
C3, C4, complement component 3, 4
CBC, complete blood count
ESKD, end stage kidney disease
GPA, granulomatosis with polyangiitis [Wegener's]
MPA, microscopic polyangiitis

Renal Allograft Thrombosis in the Early Post Transplant Period

M. Budruddin[1*], Issa Al Salmi[2], R. Shilpa[2]
[1]Nephrology Department, Tawam Hospital, Al Ain, UAE
[2]Nephrology Department, Royal Hospital, Muscat, Oman
Email: *drbudruddin@gmail.com, isa.al.salmi@gmail.com, ramaiah_shilpa@yahoo.co.in

ABSTRACT

Renal allograft thrombosis involving either the renal artery or the veins is a well known entity in clinical practice. This complication of the renal transplant surgery is more common in the early part of the post transplant period and it is usually associated with acute antibody mediated rejection. This more commonly occurs in the paediatric renal transplant and also seems to have some relation to the duration of peritoneal dialysis pretransplant. However, the occurrence of graft thrombosis in isolation without clinical or histological graft rejection is not rare. We encountered a patient in whom the renal allograft thrombosis occurred after 6 weeks of commercial renal transplantation without any histological evidence of rejection.

Keywords: Allograft Thrombosis; Immunosuppression; Cyclosporine; OKT3; Hemodialysis; Renogram; Rejection and Pyelonephritis

1. Introduction

Renal allograft thrombosis is not an uncommon complication of renal transplantation. It usually occurs in the early post renal transplant period. Several factors have been implicated with this notorious complication. Thrombosis can even occur in the late part of the post transplant period. Irrespective of the time of development of thrombosis the outcome is equally bad.

2. Case Summary

A 58-year-old Omani male with background of long standing type I diabetes along with its complications of diabetic retinopathy, Nephropathy, Neuropathy, Ischemic heart disease and paroxysmal atrial fibrillation. He was initiated on haemodialysis in late 2009. He received commercial renal transplantation in October 2010 from Pakistan and was put on triple immunosuppression with Cyclosporin, Mycophenolate and prednisolone. Details of induction immunosuppression were not available in the discharge notes.

On the 8th post operative day on his arrival in our hospital he had mild leucocytosis, surgical wound infection, uncontrolled blood sugars and the renal functions were deranged with e-GFR 21 ml/min. He was started empirically on Tazocbactam after sending the samples for cultures and blood sugars were controlled with insulin. At this stage graft kidney biopsy was proposed but patient and his relatives did not agree. An impression of delayed graft function was made and he was treated for infection. Ultrasound of the graft kidney showed good blood flow in the graft kidney and the resistive index was 0.6 - 0.8 and there were no collection around the renal allograft. The renal functions gradually improved with decrease in the serum creatinine from 255 umol/l on presentation to 190 umol/l on discharge. DTPA renogram was planned but we could not get it done as the family wanted to take him to the peripheral Nephrology Unit close to their home, for further care.

During his stay there in hospital after a week he developed tenderness over the graft and the Doppler ultrasound of the graft showed perinephric collection of 5.7 × 2.9 × 1.4 cm with high suspicion of bleed (**Figure 1**). In the mean time he developed Symptomatic atrial fibrillation. Apart from the rate control drugs he was also warfarinised on the suggestion of cardiologist. Subsequent three days were uneventfull with the serum creatinine improving further to 119 umol/l and also with improvement in the graft tenderness. He was hence discharged with follow up appointment in the cardiology and Trans-

*Corresponding author.

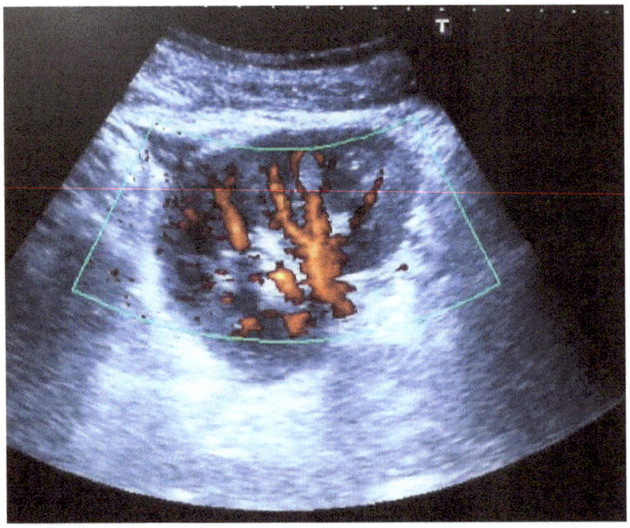

Figure 1. Perigraft haematoma shown by colour Doppler ultrasound.

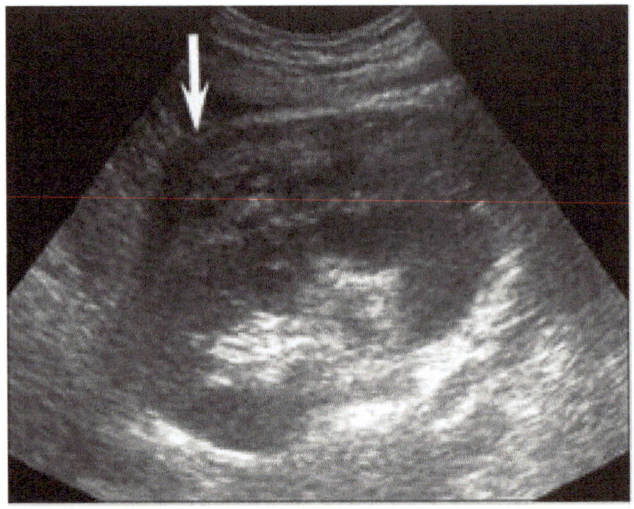

Figure 2. Perigraft Haematoma shown by arrow on ultrasound.

plant clinic. There his medications on discharge included Ciclosporin 150 mg bid, MMF 1gm bid, prednisolone 20 mg bid, warfarin 2 mg od, amlodepine 10mg od and isosorbid 10 mg tid.

Five days later he again presented to the emergency of that hospital with history of fever associated with chills, decreased urine output and loss of consciousness. Examination revealed hypotension blood pressure 80/50 mmhg, congested chest, bluish discolouration associated with tenderness over the right iliac fossa. Immediate resuscitation was done and the laboratory investigations showed serum creatinine of 230 umol/l, Hb of 7.6 gm% which was earlier 9.4 gm% on discharge, leucocytosis of 14000 cumm and INR of 3. Urgent ultrasound of the abdomen showed increase in the size of Haematoma to 11.7 × 7 × 9.1 cm (**Figure 2**). He was admitted under surgical team and started on antibiotics, fresh frozen plasma along with one dose of Vit K. Sequential ultrasound assesment of the collection was planned and the second ultrasound done the following day alarmingly showed no parenchymal blood flow and the renal functions worsened with exponential rise in serum creatinine to >800 umol/l and anuria. He was started on haemodialysis and CT scan of the abdomen was done there showed large perinephric collection with necrotic renal allograft and air bubbles suggestive of emphysematous pyelonephritis. He was shifted to our centre on 31st October for graft Nephrectomy. On admission in our centre he was septic with abdominal distention and severe tenderness over the Right side of the abdomen. There was leucocytosis, thrombocytopenia and the coagulation was deranged with fibrinogen degradation products (FDP) elevated. There was no evidence of Deep vein thrombosis of the lower limbs by Doppler ultrasound. He was urgently taken for exploration which showed pale looking necrotic graft

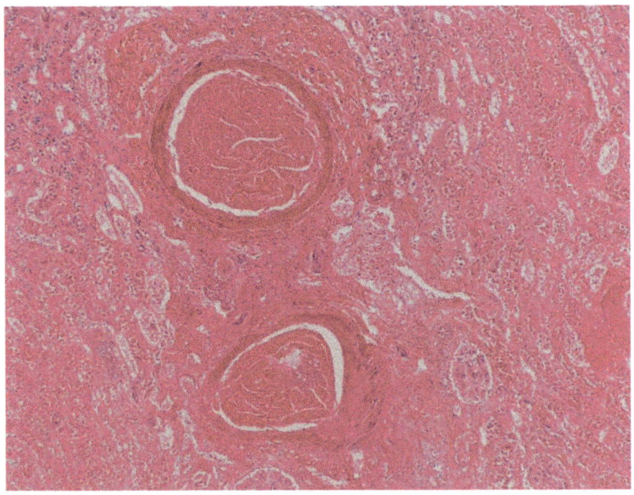

Figure 3. Slide showing the blood vessels with thrombi. (magnification ×400).

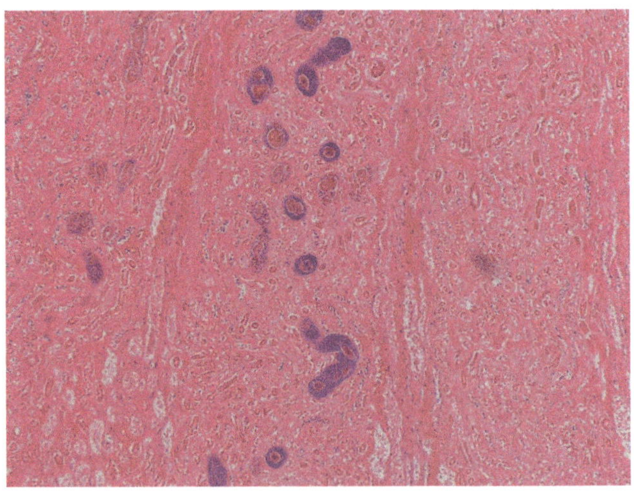

Figure 4. Tissue from the infracted kidney showing tubules with bacterial colonies (magnification ×400).

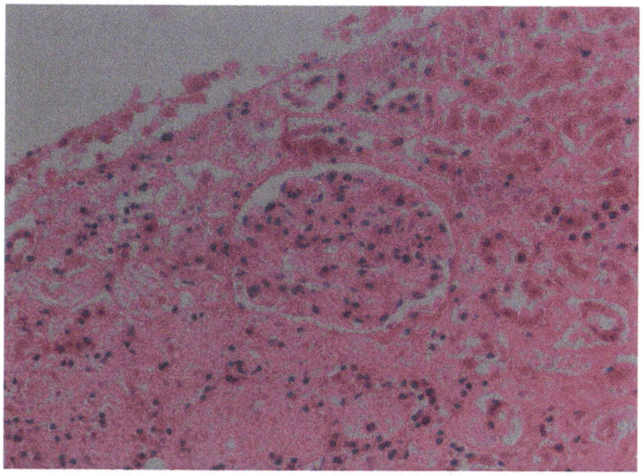

Figure 5. Infarcted tubules and glomeruli. Some of the tubules show bacterial colonies (blue-purple areas) magnification ×600.

kidney with large collection of slough and thrombosis of the vascular pedicles. Graft Nephrectomy was performed. Histopathology of the specimen (**Figures 3-5**) showed thrombus in the blood vessels with infracted tissue containing few viable glomeruli and tubules in the periphery, blood vessels showing wide spread thrombi with necrosis of the vessel wall and interstitium showing haemorhage. The tubules were showing bacterial colonies of gram negative bacilli. There were no features of acute rejection. Patient recovered from surgery and subsequently he was discharged home on maintenance dialysis.

3. Discussion

Renal graft thrombosis is not a rare, complication of renal transplantation. It is a dreaded and catastrophic complication. Graft thrombosis within a month of transplantation occurs in 0.9% of transplants and account for 17% of early (within 30days of transplantation) graft failure [1].

Most common causes of renal artery thrombosis are antibody mediated rejection, hypercoagulable syndrome, technical problems associated with graft harvesting and perfusion. This is reported to be associated with small sized graft, misalignment, torsion or kinking of the renal artery. In vitro data also suggest that immunosuppressive drugs like cyclosporine and OKT3 may increase the risk of thrombosis [2]. In our patient we have no information on the use of OKT3.

Early renal vein thrombosis often results from poor surgical technique, perigraft fluid collection, compression of the common iliac veins and hypovolemia [3]. The reported incidence varies between 0.9% and 4.5% [4]. On the other hand late renal vein thrombosis have been reported in association with recurrent or denovo membranous nephropathy, ilio-femoral vein thrombosis and thrombophilic disorders [5,6].

Epidemiology data points towards increased risk of thrombosis in retransplant, those on peritoneal dialysis prior to transplantation compared to those on haemodialysis and those with atherosclerotic lesions [3,7,8].

Coming to the donor related risk factors for increased risk of thrombosis Amezquita *et al.* have proposed that probably the right kidney from the donor as opposed to the left is the risk factor for early graft vascular thrombosis. On this basis, they further suggested for prophylactic anticoagulation or platelets antiaggregation therapy for right donor kidney implantation [9].

However, Bakir and colleagues [8], in a larger series, from a single centre, comprising of more than 550 cadaveric renal transplant recipients, have shown no association between primary renal graft thrombosis and reciepients age, sex, number of transplants, type of dialysis, pretransplant treatment with erythropoietin, antiplatelet agents, oral anticoagulation, donors age, sex, number of graft vessels, warm and cold ischemia time, site of transplantation and even the type of immunosuppressive agents used for induction like cyclosporine A or OKT3.

In our case both the renal vein and artery were thrombosed on macroscopic examination during the nephrectomy along with extensive thrombi in the intrarenal blood vessels. The graft had undergone necrosis with presence of emphysematous pyelonephritis of the graft kidney. There was no evidence of deep vein thrombosis of the lower limbs by Doppler ultrasound.

The presence of thrombus in both the arteries and veins including the small intra-renal vessels as in our case would partially exclude the role of local factors contributing to thrombosis. The predominant factor operating here being infection and its consequences like Disseminated intravascular coagulation (DIC). This could be well supported by thrombocytopenia, elevated FDP on presentation (**Table 1**) and the finding of gram negative bacterial colonies in the graft kidney.

The incidence of hemorrhage is much increased in the patients who are on warfarin and develop DIC. Our patient was on warfarin due to cardiac reasons and developed emphysematous pyelonephritis. The events culminated in hemorrhage followed by extensive thrombosis in the renal allograft. This was seen in the graft biopsy specimen.

Early detection, of thrombosis of the ilio-femoral vein, graft renal artery and vein, with timely surgical intervention or thrombolysis with streptokinase helps in improving the long term graft outcome [3,10]. However attempts at salvaging the graft by thrombolyis or by using heparin carries the risk of haemorrhage [3].

4. Conclusion

Thrombosis of the renal graft can be attributed to various

Table 1. Showing the levels of Hb, WBC, platelets, Prothrombin time PT, Firinogen degradation products and serum creatinine over time.

Date	Hb gm/dl	WBC × 10 × 9/lit	Platelets × 10 × 9/lit	Prothrombin Time in seconds	Fibrinogen degradation products in mg/lit	Serum Creatinine in mmol/l
15 Oct	9.6	10.6	337	10.5	2.29	288 mmol/l
31 Oct	9.5	22.9	41	15.8	7.98	857 mmol/l
02 Nov	10.4	5.3	95	11.8	3.99	599 mmol/l
23 Nov	10.2	8.9	245	10.5	3.35	219 mmol/l

reasons. Once thrombosed, the loss of graft is inevitable. However, prompt diagnosis and immediate attempt to thrombolyse with streptokinase or surgical intervention with endoluminal extraction of the thrombus do bear a great promise in the immediate and long term survival of the renal allograft.

REFERENCES

[1] J. A Bertolatus, "Etiology of Renal Artery Thrombosis in Renal Transplantation," *Medscape Transplantation*, Vol. 1, No. 1, 2000.

[2] E. Carlsen, "Enhancement of Procoagulant Activity in Stimulated Mononuclear Blood Cells and Monocytes by Cyclosporine," *Transplantation*, Vol. 43, No. 4, 1987, pp. 543-548. doi:10.1097/00007890-198704000-00018

[3] S. Gang and M. Rajapurkar, "Vascular Complications Following Renal Transplantation" *JNRT*, Vol. 2, No. 1, 2009, pp. 122-132.

[4] P. Giustacchini, F. Pisanti, F. Citterio, A. M. De Gaetano, M. Castagneto and G. Nanni, "Renal Vein Thrombosis after Renal Transplantation: An Important Cause of Graft Loss," *Transplantation Proceedings*, Vol. 34, No. 6, 2002, pp. 2126-2127. doi:10.1016/S0041-1345(02)02876-2

[5] M. R. First, N. Mendoza, R. K. Maryniak and M. A. Weiss, "Membranous Glomerulopathy Following Kidney Transplantation. Association with Renal Vein Thrombosis in Two of Nine Cases," *Transplantation*, Vol. 38, No. 6, 1984, pp. 603-607. doi:10.1097/00007890-198412000-00011

[6] P. J. Ramirez, R. Y. Gohh, A. Kestin, A. P. Monaco and P. E. Morrissey, "Renal Allograft Loss Due to Proximal Extension of the Ileofemoral Deep Venous Thrombosis," *Clinical Transplantation*, Vol. 16, No. 4, 2002, pp. 310-313. doi:10.1034/j.1399-0012.2002.02006.x

[7] A. Sanni, C. H. Wilson, H. Wyrley-Birch, D. Vijayanand, A. Navarro, S. Sohrabi, B. Jaques, D. Rix, N. Soomro, D. Manas and D. Talbot, "Donor Risk Factor for Renal Graft Thrombosis," *Transplantation Proceedings*, Vol. 39, No. 1, 2007, pp. 138-139.

[8] N. Bakir, W. J. Sluiter, R. J. Ploeg, W. J. van Son and A. M. Tegzess, "Primary Renal Graft Thrombosis," *Nephrology Dialysis Transplantation*, Vol. 11, No. 1, 1996, pp. 140-147. doi:10.1093/oxfordjournals.ndt.a027030

[9] Y. Amezquita, C. Mendez, A. Fernandez, S. Caldes, J. Pascual, A. Muriel, F. J. Burgos, R. Marcen and J. Ortuno, "Risk Factors for Early Graft Thrombosis: A Case-Controlled Study in Grafts from the Same Donor," *Transplantation Proceedings*, Vol. 40, No. 9, 2008, pp. 2891-2893. doi:10.1016/j.transproceed.2008.09.014

[10] E. Renoult, L. Cormier, M. Claudon, T. Cao-Huu, L. Frimat, O. Gaucher, J. Hubert and M. Kessler, "Successful Surgical Thrombectomy of Renal Allograft Vein Thrombosis in the Early Postoperative Period," *American Journal of Kidney Diseases*, Vol. 35, No. 5, 2000, p. E21. doi:10.1016/S0272-6386(00)70286-1

40

Effectiveness of an Secondary Prevention Program in Chronic Kidney Disease

Carlos Enrique Yepes Delgado*, Yanett Marcela Montoya Jaramillo, Beatriz Elena Orrego Orozco, Paulina Bernal Ramírez, Luz Denise González, José Miguel Abad Echeverri, María Patricia Arbeláez Montoya

University of Antioquia, Hospital Pablo Tobón Uribe, EPS SURA, Medellín, Colombia

Email: *caenyede@gmail.com

ABSTRACT

Background: There are many programs which focus on late-stage chronic kidney disease (CKD), and it is considered that further evidence needs to be generated regarding the effectiveness of the programs used before renal replacement therapy. Study Design: A cohort study. Settings & Participants: Patients over 15 years of age who had been diagnosed with CKD according to the KDOQI (Kidney Disease Outcomes Quality Initiative) guidelines and who had undergone conventional treatment (CT) or a renal protection program (RPP). These were patients of two Colombian health insurance companies. Predictors: Age, sex, marital status, comorbidities, CKD stage, and clinical indicators. Outcomes: First CKD progression, and need for renal replacement therapy (RRT). Measures: Clinical marker. Results: The RPP is structurally and functionally different from the CT. It offers the interdisciplinary management of patients, a greater number of medical appointments, and patients start to receive treatment at younger ages and at earlier stages of their condition. The clinical markers of the patients following the RPP are within adequate ranges, and their renal function is less impaired, despite the differences in basal conditions. Upon finishing the study, we found that patients who received CT had a higher risk of receiving nephrotoxic drugs and not receiving nephroprotective drugs. The explanatory variables for the first progression were age, stage, history of dyslipidemia, and hemoglobin, potassium, and albumin levels. These variables, together with glycemia levels were also valid for RRT, except for history of dyslipidemia, as it was not significant. Upon adjusting for the explanatory variables, it was found that belonging to the RPP and attending more appointments had a protective effect in the process of controlling renal damage. Limitations: A possible selection bias. Conclusions: Belonging to a structured renal protection program is an effective way to keeping the clinical markers associated with renal impairment within normal ranges.

Keywords: Chronic Kidney Disease; Renal Protection Program; Effectiveness; Clinical Markers; Progression of Renal Damage; Renal Replacement Program

1. Introduction

Due to the rapid increase in its prevalence, its close relationship with an increased risk of cardiovascular disease, and the high costs of treatment, chronic kidney disease (CKD) is now recognized as a public health problem that affects people of all ages and alters their quality of life [1,2]. Because of these characteristics, this disease is becoming a priority for healthcare systems. This has created an urgent need to develop effective ways of measuring interventions to prevent its progress [3,4].

According to the calculations of the National Health and Nutrition Examination Survey (NHANES) III, it is estimated that twenty million adults have CKD in the United States. Currently, approximately 360,000 patients have undergone renal replacement therapy (RRT) in the European Union. In developed countries, it is estimated that the number of people with end-stage CKD will continue to increase at an annual rate of around 5% to 8%. This growth is driven by population aging and the increased incidence of diseases related to renal failure [5].

In Colombia, there are over 20,000 individuals with stage 5 CKD, with an age-adjusted prevalence of 454

*Corresponding author.

patients per million people. This figure is lower than the prevalence observed in the United States and higher than the average prevalence in Latin American countries in 2005. Nevertheless, the prevalence of early-stage CKD is only 0.87%. This figure is lower than the one reported in other studies conducted on population samples and is thought to be the result of underreporting [6].

In order to delay CKD progression in Colombia, the Ministry of Social Protection implemented a model for its prevention and treatment in 2006. The model aimed to address the growing demand for services related to this condition [7,8]. Furthermore, Act 1122 of 2007 created the Cuenta de Alto Costo agency (CAC), a non-governmental technical agency forming part of the Colombian General System for Health-Related Social Security. This is a strategy involving both public and private institutions and seeking to address the high costs generated by the condition itself, an issue that has a significant impact on Colombia [9]. However, before the appearance of such provisions, a Colombian health insurance company (EPS) designed and implemented a renal protection program (RPP) that was structurally and functionally capable of providing its users with a particular type of medical care that was very different from the conventional treatment (CT) that other institutions continued to offer.

Although a number of national health institutions from across the world claim that it is important to reduce morbidity and mortality rates in the proactive management of CKD by making early referrals of patients to a multidisciplinary team, there are scant data within the current literature to support such a recommendation [10]. The authors of a meta-analysis published in April 2010 concerning evidence regarding the clinical and cost effectiveness of early referral strategies for managing people with markers of renal damage reported that, in the last two decades, only two studies in the world had focused on assessing the effectiveness of interventions carried out at early stages of CKD [11].

Not enough reports were found in the scientific literature that assessed RPPs which continuously monitored patients for at least four years and observed the relationship between the delay in kidney function impairment, and the behavior of variables such as clinical parameters (blood pressure, glycemia, lipid profile, etc.) and nutritional treatment [12-16].

Since the mechanisms for identifying CKD patients in the stages prior to RRT are not very effective, we are missing out many opportunities to implement strategies to reduce the progression speed of renal failure and thus reduce the incidence of terminal renal failure [6]. That is why this study aims to assess the effectiveness of the renal protection program in monitoring the clinical markers and their relationship with the progression of renal damage.

2. Methods

2.1. Type of Study

An analytic cohort study with ambispective follow-up given to two dynamic cohorts of patients over 15 years old and diagnosed with CKD. Individuals were classified by stage (according to the KDOQI guidelines) [17] in order to compare the behavior of the clinical and renal impairment indicators of the patients exposed to the RPP and those of the patients undergoing CT.

2.2. Population

The study was conducted with patients from two health insurance companies belonging to the same type of social security regime and operating in Antioquia, Colombia. Data was collected retrospectively from electronic medical records from April 1, 2004 (the starting date of the RPP) to the first half of 2007. After that date, information was collected prospectively until April 30, 2008. The total treatment time was 49 months. **Figure 1** describes the participant selection process.

2.3. Treatment Comparison

The RPP is an interdisciplinary healthcare program based on a protocol involving periodic appointments and moni-toring of clinical and laboratory tests accompanied by continuous education. The RPP is aimed at CKD patients from the initial stages of their condition and it is divided into several levels. The first level is aimed at patients in stages 1 and 2. It offers medical appointments

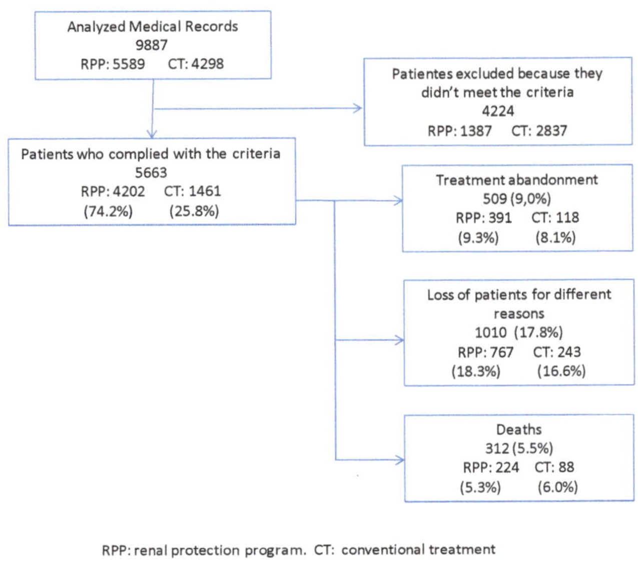

Figure 1. Flowchart depicting the CKD patient selection process in two Colombian private health insurance companies. Medellin 2004-2008.

with interists and nutritionists on an annual and biannual basis, respectively. The second level is for patients in stages 3 and 4, and it offers medical appointments with internists, nephrologists, and nutritionists on a three-per-year and bimonthly basis, respectively. Laboratory tests are per-ormed one month prior to the medical appointment with a specialist.

When patients request a medical appointment because they feel the need to do it, conventional treatment (CT) either provides primary level attention or refers patients to a specialist, depending on the general practitioner's criteion.

No significant differences were found between the RPP and CT groups in terms of treatment abandonment, loss of patients for different reasons, and death ($p = 0.157$; $p = 0.163$; $p = 0.318$ respectively).

2.4. Variables

The variables considered as criteria for CKD diagnosis were: creatinine clearance of less than 60 ml/min, alrations observed in renal ultrasound tests, proteinuria levels higher than 150 mg/day, alterations in urinary deposits, and -for diabetic patients- micro-albuminuria levels higher than 30 mg.

The variables included in the study were: age, sex, comorbidities, marital status, CKD stage according to the KDOQI guidelines, and clinical and laboratory variables as measured upon diagnosis and whenever stage progression took place. Some quantitative variables were categorized based on the clinical definitions for cutoff in accordance with the values reported in the literature

2.5. Analysis Technique

A comparison was carried out between the guidelines for clinical monitoring and care of patients with renal alterations used by the institution offering the RPP, and the treatment process used by the institution offering CT. The objective was to identify differences in the healthcare process, tests carried out, frequency of tests and appointments, types of professionals involved in the process, etc.

The population was characterized when CKD was diagnosed through frequency distributions and proportions for the qualitative variables. Quantitative variables were characterized via measures of dispersion and descriptive statistics. The Kolmogorov-Smirnov or Shapiro Wilk tests were also used. The qualitative variables of the two groups under study were then compared using the Pearson Chi2 test or the Chi2 test for trends, depending on the case. If the quantitative variables had a normal distribution, they were compared using the t-Student test. If the distribution was not normal, then the U Mann-Whitney test was used. The odds ratios (OR) and their corresponding confidence intervals were calculated to be 95%.

A propensity score (PS) was used to assess effectiveness in maintaining the values for clinical markers and exposure to nephrotoxic and nephroprotective drugs within normal ranges. This statistical technique calculates the conditional probability of having been exposed to the variable of interest based on the subject's baseline features [18]. The PS is composed of the following variables: age (>65 years/<=65 years), sex (female/male), marital status (no partner/ with permanent partner), arterial hypertension (yes/no), diabetes mellitus (yes/no) and dyslipidemia (yes/no). The PS created with these variables shows how they explain the probability of joining a RPP or undergoing CT by means of a logistic regression model that aims to predict exposure, and manages to group the various confounding variables into a single one [19]. These models also included the initial values of each variable.

Finally, two logistic regression models were created. Their dependent variables were the first progression into a later stage and the need for RRT. The variables included in the models were selected based on the Hosmer Lemeshow test. The quantity of data available for each variable was determined using the stepwise technique to obtain the final model. These models excluded patients who joined the study at stage 5 of their condition.

2.6. Avoidance of Bias

A potential bias could have arisen when we were forming the cohort and encountered participants with different features which increased the probability of having any of the outcomes. We therefore conducted multivariate analyses that adjusted for the features and basal conditions of the subjects. To avoid selection bias, we ensured that patients complied with the inclusion criteria. Possible migration bias could have occurred when the conditions of those who abandoned treatment were different from the conditions of those who stayed in it, and when such conditions were associated with the outcome itself. To prevent this, we inquired about censoring, either by reviewing the records of the health insurance companies or by asking via telephone. We thus located 80% of the patients and found no differences between the groups.

A possible reporting bias might have occurred when it was more likely to find more cases in the cohort being monitored for a longer time period (the RPP). Another bias resulted from the fact that the RPP actively searches for patients, thus its clinical records had more data than those of the patients following CT (underreporting). This bias was avoided by triangulating information and crossing the records for the missing data when possible.

3. Results

When comparing the number of appointments attended by patients from both programs, it was observed that patients belonging to the RPP had more appointments with internists, as well as educational and nutritional appointments. The highest percentage of appointments for patients following CT was with general practitioners and ophthalmologists, as shown in **Table 1**.

There was a proportional difference in CKD stage at the moment of diagnosis between the patients from the two health insurance companies. More than 30% of the patients who joined the RPP were in the first two stages of the condition, compared to only 16.7% of patients who underwent CT. In other words, CT had a higher number of patients in the final stages of CKD. Patients undergoing CT are more likely to be diagnosed with CKD when the condition is already in the final stages of its development, as shown by the OR represented in **Table 2**. According to this, a patient following CT is approximately 50% more likely to be diagnosed with late-stage CKD (stages 4 and 5) than a patient from the RPP.

Additionally, CKD patients following CT were significantly older (Me:70 years old) than RPP patients (Me: 66 years old). This was observed in both males and females.

Upon comparing the morbidities of the patients following CT and those of the RPP patients, it was observed that prevalence values were similar for both groups (**Figure 2**), except for arterial hypertension ($p < 0.001$), dyslipidemia ($P = 0.023$), diabetes mellitus ($p = 0.014$), cerebrovascular disease (0.002) and obesity ($p = 0.017$).

After analyzing the values observed for the various clinical markers at the moment of diagnosis, we found significant differences between the CT and RPP patients regarding serum creatinine, creatinine clearance, triglycerides, and potassium. These values were less affected or even within normal ranges for the RPP patients. The values for the high- and low-density lipoproteins were more favorable for the patients undergoing CT. No significant differences were found between the values for systolic arterial pressure, glycated hemoglobin, 24-hour proteinuria, total cholesterol, hemoglobin, phosphorus, and parathyroid hormone.

Likewise, upon analyzing the values at the moment of diagnosis, we found that the risk of receiving nephrotoxic drugs such as non-steroidal anti-inflammatory drugs or aminoglycoside antibiotics is 1.7 times greater for patients following CT (CI95%: 1.4 - 2.1) than for patients in the RPP. We also found that the risk of not receiving nephroprotective drugs is 2.1 times higher (CI95%: 1.8 - 2.4) for patients with CT than for those following a RPP.

The risk of having out-of-range values for the clinical markers and for the variable "final exposure to nephrotoxic and nephroprotective drugs" at the end of the treatment period was analyzed (**Table 3**). It was then found that CT patients had a higher risk of having clinical markers which were out of range for SAP, fasting blood glucose, glycated hemoglobin, and potassium. The risk of having out-of-range clinical markers for the cholesterol variable was higher in the RPP patients. No differences were found in albumin, calcium, and hemoglobin. Similarly, the risk of receiving nephrotoxic drugs for patients undergoing CT was 0.63 times greater than that of the patients in the RPP. The risk of not receiving nephroprotective drugs was 0.35 times higher for CT patients.

The models described below show the effect of the "first progression" and "need for RRT" variables on renal function impairment. The variables are adjusted for patient features (**Table 4**).

Regarding the variable representing the first progression into the next stage of CKD, we found that the patients in the RPP and those who attended more than eight medical appointments had a lower risk of CKD progression. Their protective fraction was 51.7% and 71.3% respectively. Likewise, a history of dyslipidemia, together with out-of-range levels of hemoglobin, potassium, albumin, and glycemia, behaves as a risk factor for CKD progression. On the other hand, out-of-range hemoglobin and albumin levels represent the highest risk (2.91 and 1.53 respectively). The association was not significant for glycemia. In terms of age, we found that the older the patient, the higher the risk of CKD progression.

Regarding the risk of CKD progression based on the condition's stage at the moment of diagnosis (and taking stage 4 patients as a reference point) we found that the risk of having the first progression increases as the stage at the moment of diagnosis decreases. Hence, the risk of progression for patients in stage 1 is 38.75 times higher than the risk for those in stage 4.

The model used to analyze the need for RRT also showed that patients belonging to the RPP have 44.9% less probability of requiring renal replacement therapy. Similarly, attending more than 8 medical appointments means 66.2% less probability of requiring RRT.

Likewise, it was found that patients with out-of-range levels of glycemia, hemoglobin, potassium, and albumin had a higher risk of needing RRT than those with levels within the acceptable range. Out-of-range hemoglobin posed the highest risk for needing RRT (3.64), followed by albumin (2.06). Similarly, patients with a history of dyslipidemia had a higher risk of needing RRT, but the association was not significant. Additionally, it was found that being younger is a protective factor against the risk of requiring RRT.

Regarding the CKD stage at the moment of diagnosis, it was observed that patients in stage 4, had a 9.35 times greater risk of requiring RRT than patients in stages 1, 2, and 3.

Table 1. Number of appointments for CKD patients in the RPP. Appointments are arranged by appointment type and treating professional. Medellín 2004-2008.

Clinical Indicators	RPP		CT	
	N (%)	Md (Q1 - Q3)	N (%)	Md (Q1 - Q3)
Educational appointments	450 (10.7)	4 (2 - 8)	55 (3.8)	1 (1 - 1)
Nutritional appointments	1630 (38.8)	2 (1 - 3)	320 (21.9)	1 (1 - 2)
Ophthalmological appointments	226 (5.4)	1 (1 - 2)	184 (12.6)	1 (1 - 1)
Psychological appointments	10 (0.2)	1 (1 - 6)	22 (1.5)	1 (1 - 3)
General practitioner	2401 (57.1)	3 (1 - 5)	1022 (70.0)	3 (1 - 5)
Internist	3909 (93.0)	4 (2 - 6)	773 (52.9)	3 (1 - 5)
Nephrologist	1925 (45.8)	3 (1 - 5)	4 (0.3)	3.5 (1.3 - 6.5)
Total appointments	**4186 (99.6)**	**8 (4 - 15)**	**1316 (90.1)**	**8 (4 - 13)**

Table 2. Percentage distribution and probability of belonging to each CKD stage among patients benefiting from two types of intervention. Medellín, 2004-2008.

Stage of the condition upon diagnosis	RPP		CT		OR	CI 95%
	n (%)		n (%)			
1	403	(9.6)	148	(10.1)	1.00	
2	885	(21.1)	96	(6.6)	0.30	(0.22 - 0.4)
3	2354	(56.0)	911	(62.4)	1.05	(0.86 - 1.3)
4	493	(11.7)	267	(18.3)	1.47	(1.17 - 1.91)
5	67	(1.6)	39	(2.7)	1.59	(1 - 2.51)
P value of the Chi-square test for tendency <0.001						

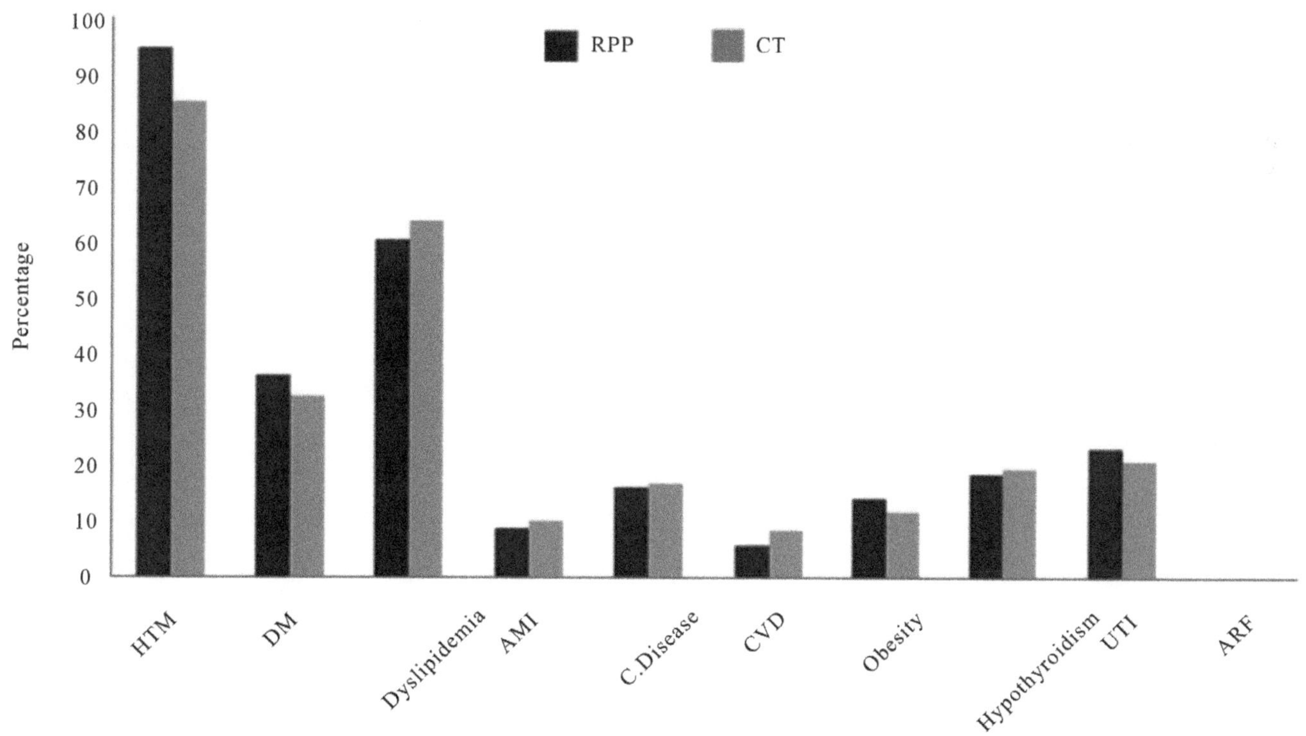

Figure 2. Comorbidities of the groups of CKD patients following a RPP and undergoing conventional treatment TC. Medellín, 2004-2008. HTN: arterial hypertension, DM: diabetes mellitus, AMI: acute myocardial infarction, C. Disease: Coronary disease, CVD: cerebrovascular disease, UTI: urinary tract infection, ARF: acute renal failure.

Table 3. Clinical conditions and exposure to nephrotoxic and nephroprotective drugs at the end of the treatment for the CKD patients in the renal protection program, RPP, and for those undergoing conventional treatment, CT. These variables are adjusted for the basal conditions (Propensity Score). Medellín, 2004-2008.

Clinical Markers	B	S.E.	Wald	gl	P value	OR	CI 95.0%	
							IL	SL
SAP								
Intervention through CT	0.180	0.072	6	1	0.013	1.197	1.039	1.379
Initial systolic arterial pressure outside of normal range	1.013	0.063	259	1	0.000	2.754	2.434	3.116
PS	−0.745	0.285	7	1	0.009	0.475	0.272	0.830
Constant	−0.713	0.080	78	1	0.000	0.490		
Fasting blood glucose								
Intervention through CT	0.264	0.130	4	1	0.042	1.302	1.010	1.680
Initial glycemia outside of normal range	2.424	0.131	342	1	0.000	11.291	8.734	14.595
PS	−0.965	0.560	3	1	0.085	0.381	0.127	1.143
Constant	−1.742	0.151	134	1	0.000	0.175		
Hba1c								
Intervention through CT	1.322	0.244	29	1	0.000	3.751	2.327	6.046
Initial Hba1c levels outside of normal range	2.911	0.202	209	1	0.000	18.377	12.380	27.276
PS	−1.650	0.965	3	1	0.087	0.192	0.029	1.274
Constant	−1.995	0.282	50	1	0.000	0.136		
Total cholesterol								
Intervention through CT	−0.252	0.116	5	1	0.030	0.778	0.620	0.975
Initial total cholesterol level outside of normal range	2.064	0.097	452	1	0.000	7.879	6.514	9.530
PS	−0.962	0.437	5	1	0.028	0.382	0.162	0.901
Constant	−1.473	0.131	126	1	0.000	0.229		
Hemoglobin								
Intervention through CT	−0.228	0.120	4	1	0.056	0.796	0.630	1.006
Initial hemoglobin level outside of normal range	2.376	0.151	248	1	0.000	10.763	8.005	14.470
PS	1.450	0.466	10	1	0.002	4.262	1.710	10.619
Constant	−1.391	0.127	120	1	0.000	0.249		
Albumin								
Intervention through CT	0.694	0.460	2	1	0.131	2.001	0.813	4.930
Initial albumin level outside of normal range	2.925	0.220	176	1	0.000	18.639	12.101	28.708
PS	−0.299	1.094	0	1	0.785	0.742	0.087	6.333
Constant	−2.960	0.293	102	1	0.000	0.052		
Calcium								
Intervention through CT	−0.111	0.248	0	1	0.656	0.895	0.551	1.455
Initial calcium level outside of normal range	1.827	0.177	107	1	0.000	6.218	4.399	8.788
PS	1.258	0.715	3	1	0.078	3.519	0.867	14.285
Constant	−1.985	0.203	95	1	0.000	0.137		
Potassium								
Intervention through CT	0.391	0.161	6	1	0.015	1.479	1.078	2.029
Initial potassium level outside of normal range	1.523	0.169	81	1	0.000	4.586	3.295	6.384
PS	0.268	0.548	0	1	0.625	1.307	0.447	3.825
Constant	−1.642	0.147	124	1	0.000	0.194		
Nephrotoxic drugs								
Intervention through CT	0.491	0.123	16	1	0.000	1.633	1.283	2.080
Initial nephrotoxic drug consumption	2.811	0.118	564	1	0.000	16.624	13.182	20.966
PS	0.590	0.485	1	1	0.224	1.803	0.697	4.668
Constant	−3.426	0.144	567	1	0.000	0.033		

Continued

Nephroprotective drugs								
Intervention through CT	0.300	0.099	9	1	0.002	1.350	1.112	1.638
No initial nephroprotective drug consumption	2.642	0.102	674	1	0.000	14.045	11.505	17.147
PS	3.365	0.359	88	1	0.000	28.935	14.325	58.442
Constant	-4.263	0.131	1.059	1	0.000	0.014		

Table 4. Logistic regression models for the variables "first progression" and "need for renal replacement therapy" amongst the CKD patients in the RPP and those following conventional treatment (CT), 2004-2008.

Variables in the model	First progression[1]				Need for RRT[2]			
	P value	OR	CI 95%		P value	OR	CI 95%	
			IL	SL			IL	SL
Treatment with RPP*	0.000	0.483	0.336	0.696	0.010	0.551	0.345	0.882
Attending more than 8 appointments	0.000	0.287	0.219	0.376	0.000	0.338	0.208	0.550
Age	0.000	1.032	1.023	1.041	0.020	0.984	0.972	0.997
History of dyslipidemia	0.010	1.354	1.078	1.701	0.250	1.243	0.857	1.801
Stage of the condition upon diagnosis								
Stage 4	0.000	1 (Reference)			0.000	10.354	7.02	15.273
Stage 3	0.000	2.018	1.468	2.775				
Stage 2	0.000	10.500	6.857	16.090	1 (Reference)**			
Stage 1	0.000	39.750	22.996	68.707				
Clinical Indicators								
Glycemia outside of normal range	0.870	1.025	0.757	1.389	0.010	1.899	1.212	2.977
Hemoglobin level outside of normal range	0.000	2.917	2.307	3.689	0.000	3.647	2.531	5.256
Potassium level outside of normal range	0.010	1.458	1.116	1.903	0.020	1.616	1.098	2.380
Albumin level outside of normal range	0.010	1.535	1.096	2.148	0.000	2.060	1.314	3.231
Constant	0.000	0.026			0.000	0.088		

1. First progression: ^{2}Nagelkerke R = 27.55%; 2. Need for RRT: ^{2} Nagelkerke R = 32.8%; *Reference intervention; **Stages 1, 2, and 3 were grouped as a reference in order to compare them with stage 4 in model 2.

4. Discussion

The Colombian healthcare system now considers CKD as a catastrophic and very costly pathology. Thanks to this, patients now have more and better access to the services designed to address it. This has also helped health insurance companies and other institutions reduce the impact of the costs associated with this condition. Consequently, improvements in users' health are expected, as well as a better use of the health system's resources [8].

However, a great deal of studies have focused on the final stages of CKD, both in the world and in Colombia, and it is considered that more evidence should be generated regarding the effectiveness of the programs used before RRT. In this sense, this study demonstrated the effect of a predialysis intervention program complying with strategies for generating scientific evidence [8,20], such as early patient uptake, comprehensive care, and treatment of comorbidities.

The fact that patients are started on the renal protection program when they are at the initial states of their condition (which is demonstrated by the fact that 30% of the patients join the program at stages 1 and 2 in comparison with CT patients) demonstrates the significant effect of this program's active search for patients, something which should be included in all secondary prevention strategies.

The results show that the RPP patients receive more interdisciplinary care. This is evidenced by the proportion of patients seen by doctors and by the higher number of medical appointments involving different health professionals. This is compliant with the interdisciplinarity proposed by a number of studies, which show differences in CKD outcomes when comorbidities are treated by multiple disciplines [21-23].

The higher percentage of educational appointments and the comprehensive care provided by the RPP show how it can be used for prevention. One of its positive effects could be a lower exposure to nephrotoxic drugs and higher rates of nephroprotective drugs usage.

The high number of general medical appointments for patients undergoing CT may be due to the particular characteristics of the on-demand type of health care provided by this kind of intervention. Additionally, the greater quantity of ophthalmology appointments observed in patients following CT may signify that this target organ is more affected in their case. This could be linked to the fact that their arterial hypertension, glycemia, or glycated hemoglobin levels were not within normal ranges at the end of their treatment.

The literature recommends that patients in stage 3 and onwards should be managed by nephrology professionals [24,25]. Despite this, only 4 individuals following CT had this kind of treatment, making it impossible to compare the groups studied.

In terms of clinical indicators, it's worth noting that, although the logistic regression model showed that having out-of-range hemoglobin and albumin levels represented a high risk of having the first CKD progression and needing RRT, no significant differences were found between the RPP and CT patients regarding the management of these markers upon adjusting for the basal levels and PS. This shows how necessary it is to implement or improve the actions aiming at keeping the levels of these indicators within normal ranges. This would greatly contribute to reducing the risk of renal function impairment [26].

Likewise, it is also worth mentioning that the RPP shows shortcomings regarding the management of total cholesterol when compared to CT—it is therefore necessary to identify the cause of such shortcomings, since inappropriate management of this indicator (*i.e.* high cholesterol values) is a risk factor for renal function impairment. Moreover, high cholesterol is also a risk factor for cardiovascular disease, which in turn is the main cause of morbidity and mortality among CKD patients [27].

Patients diagnosed with stage 4 CKD had a high risk of needing RRT compared with those diagnosed at earlier stages of their condition. This demonstrates the importance of early detection of CKD in order to prevent or slow down the deterioration of renal function and the resulting deterioration of patients' quality of life, 1-2 as well as the economic consequences for the various elements of the General System for Health-Related Social Security [28,29].

Although the results obtained in this study in most cases showed differences favoring the RPP, it can also be observed that the proportion of patients attending appointments offered by the program and having clinical markers within the normal ranges could be improved. However, the findings regarding the protection levels provided by the RPP against the studied outcomes exceed 50% and explain more than 25% of its variability, thus suggesting that it is possible to have more effectiveness and a higher effect on the delay of CKD progression.

Implementing strategies for early intervention for CKD patients is an effective contribution to help keep the clinical markers associated with renal damage within normal ranges. It also has a positive effect on the treatment of the condition. Therefore, encouraging the implementation of such strategies optimizes the use of resources and improves patient prognosis.

5. Acknowledgements

The authors would like to thank Colciencias, the University of Antioquia, the EPS Sura health insurance company, and the insurance company offering CT. Study sponsor not had any role in study design; collection, analysis, and interpretation of data; writing the report; and the decision to submit the report for publication. We, the authors, declare that there were no conflicts of interest during this study.

REFERENCES

[1] R. C. Atkins, "The Epidemiology of Chronic Kidney Disease," *Kidney International Supplement*, Vol. 94, 2005, pp. S14-18. doi:10.1111/j.1523-1755.2005.09403.x

[2] R. C. Atkins, "The Changing Patterns of Chronic Kidney Disease: The Need to Develop Strategies for Prevention Relevant to Different Regions and Countries," *Kidney International Supplement*, Vol. 98, 2005, pp. S83-85. doi:10.1111/j.1523-1755.2005.09815.x

[3] R. S. Barsoum, "Chronic Kidney Disease in the Developing World," *The New England Journal of Medicine*, Vol. 354, No. 10, 2006, pp. 997-999. doi:10.1056/NEJMp058318

[4] S. L. White, A. Cass, R. C. Atkins and S. J. Chadban, "Chronic Kidney Disease in the General Population," *Advances in Chronic Kidney Disease*, Vol. 12, No. 1, 2005, pp. 5-13. doi:10.1053/j.ackd.2004.10.009

[5] N. Lameire, K. Jager, W. Van Biesen, D. de Bacquer and R. Vanholder, "Chronic Kidney Disease: A European Perspective," *Kidney International Supplement*, Vol. 99, 2005, pp. S30-38. doi:10.1111/j.1523-1755.2005.09907.x

[6] Cuenta de Alto Costo, "Contenidos Mínimos Indispensables Para la Gestión Del Riesgo Renal en un Programa de Atención a Pacientes Adultos con Enfermedad Renal Crónica, Sin Terapia de Reemplazo Renal en Colombia, Definiciones Técnicas Basadas en Evidencias," 2011. http://www.cuentadealtocosto.org/patologias/ERC/docs/consenso/programas_ERC.pdf

[7] Ministerio de la Protección Social, República de Colombia, "Guía Para el Manejo de la Enfermedad Renal Crónica y Modelo de Prevención y Control de la Enfermedad Renal Crónica. Componente de un Modelo de Salud Re-

nal," 2011.
http://pos.gov.co/Documents/Archivos/ERC.pdf

[8] F. Martínez and M. Valencia "Modelo en Prevención y Control de la Enfermedad Renal Crónica. Componente de un Modelo de Salud Renal," Bogotá, 2005.

[9] Ministerio de Protección Social, República de Colombia, "Cuenta de Alto Costo," 2011.
http://www.cuentadealtocosto.org/CAC.html

[10] B. M. Curtis, P. Ravani, F. Malberti, F. Kennett, P. A. Taylor, O. Djurdjev and A. Levin, "The Short- and Long-Term Impact of Multi-Disciplinary Clinics in Addition to Standard Nephrology Care on Patient Outcomes," *Nephrology Dialysis Transplantation*, Vol. 20, No. 1, 2005, pp. 147-154. doi:10.1093/ndt/gfh585

[11] C. Black, P. Sharma, G. Scotland, K. McCullough, D. McGurn, L. Robertson, N. Fluck, A. MacLeod, P. McNamee, G. Prescott and C. Smith, "Early Referral Strategies for Management of People with Markers of Renal Disease: A Systematic Review of the Evidence of Clinical Effectiveness, Cost-Effectiveness and Economic Analysis," *Health Technology Assessment*, Vol. 14, No. 21, 2010, pp. 1-184.

[12] R. Pellicano, P. G. Kerr and R. C. Atkins, "What Have We Learned from Clinical Trials on Prevention?" *Kidney International Supplement*, Vol. 94, 2005, pp. 101-106. doi:10.1111/j.1523-1755.2005.09424.x

[13] L. D. B. Gray, "Outcomes Research in Nutrition and Chronic Kidney Disease: Perspectives, Issues in Practice, and Processes for Improvement," *Advances in Chronic Kidney Disease*, Vol. 12, No. 1, 2005, pp. 96-106. doi:10.1053/j.ackd.2004.10.012

[14] M. M. Slowik, "Early Education of Patients with Chronic Renal Insufficiency: The Healthy Start program. Case Study of the Anemic Patient," *Nephrology Nursing Journal*, Vol. 28, No. 6, 2001, pp. 643-646.

[15] K. Tungsanga, C. Ratanakul, W. Pooltavee, N. Mahatanan, A. I. Na Ayuthaya and S. Rodpai, "Experience with Prevention Programs in Thailand," *Kidney International Supplement*, Vol. 94, 2005, pp. 68-69. doi:10.1111/j.1523-1755.2005.09417.x

[16] R. T. Gansevoort, Van der Heij, C. A. Stegeman, F. T. De Charro, M. G. Nieuwenhuizen and D. De Zeeuw, "Trends in the Incidence of Treated End-Stage Renal Failure in the Netherlands: Hope for the Future?" *Kidney International Supplement*, Vol. 92, 2004, pp. 7-10. doi:10.1111/j.1523-1755.2004.09202.x

[17] National Kidney Foundation, "K/DOQI Clinical Practice Guidelines for Chronic Kidney Disease: Evaluation, Classification, and Stratification," Recommendations for clinical Performance Measures, 2007.
http://www.kidney.org/professionals/kdoqi/guidelines_ckd/p8_cpm.htm

[18] M. Katz, "Multivariable Analysis. A Practical Guide for Clinicians," 2nd Edition, Cambridge, 2006.

[19] A. Ruiz and L. Morillo, "Epidemiología Clínica. Investigación Clínica Aplicada," Editorial Panamericana, Bogotá, 2004.

[20] H. Tazeen, "The Growing Burden of Chronic Kidney Disease in Pakistan," *The New England Journal of Medicine*, Vol. 9, No. 10, 2006, pp. 995-997.

[21] B. J. Barrett, "Applying Multiple Interventions in Chronic Kidney Disease," *Seminars in Dialysis*, Vol. 16, No. 2, 2003, pp. 157-164.
doi:10.1046/j.1525-139X.2003.16032.x

[22] D. C. Mendelssohn, "Coping with the CKD Epidemic: The Promise of Multidisciplinary Team-Based Care," *Nephrology Dialysis Transplantation*, Vol. 20, No. 1, 2005, pp. 10-12. doi:10.1093/ndt/gfh636

[23] R. Pellicano, R. C. Atkins and P. G. Kerr, "What Have We Learned from Clinical Trials on Prevention?" *Kidney International Supplement*, Vol. 94, 2005, pp. 101-106. doi:10.1111/j.1523-1755.2005.09424.x

[24] B. J. Pereira, "Overcoming Barriers to the Early Detection and Treatment of Chronic Kidney Disease and Improving Outcomes for End-Stage Renal Disease," *American Journal of Managed Care*, Vol. 8, No. 4, 2002, pp. S122-S135.

[25] "Chronic Kidney Disease: Stating the Managed Care Case for Early Treatment Discussion and Consensus of Presentations of Economic Analyses, Managed Care Organization Case Studies, and Opportunities for Intervention in a Managed Care Setting," *American Journal of Managed Care*, Vol. 8, No. 4, 2002, pp. S114-S120.

[26] A. Levin, "The Need for Optimal and Coordinated Management of CKD," *Kidney International*, Vol. 68, No. 99, 2005, pp. S7-S10.

[27] W. F. Owen, "Patterns of Care for Patients with Chronic Kidney Disease in the United States: Dying for Improvement," *Journal of the American Society of Nephrology*, Vol. 14, No. 2, 2003, pp. 76-80.
doi:10.1097/01.ASN.0000070145.00225.EC

[28] Grupo de Economía de la Salud, "Evaluación Económica en Salud: Tópicos Teóricos y Aplicaciones en Colombia," Observatorio de la Seguridad Social, 2006.

[29] B. Manns, B. Hemmelgan, M. Tonelli, Au Flora, T. C. Chiasson, J. Dong and S. Klarenbach, "Population Based Screening for Chronic Kidney Disease: Cost Effectiveness Study," *BMJ*, Vol. 341, 2010, p. 5869.

Patient with Churg Strauss Syndrome and Myocarditis Treated with Cyclophosphamide

Liam Mullen, Janice Harper, Sukumaran Binukrishnan
Royal Liverpool University Hospital, Liverpool Heart and Chest Hospital, Liverpool, UK
Email: Liam.Mullen@nhs.net

ABSTRACT

Cardiac involvement in Churg Strauss Syndrome is common and a poor prognostic indicator. Myocarditis in Churg Strauss Syndrome can present in different ways. It has been shown that basic cardiac investigations including echocardiography can be normal even in symptomatic patients. More recently cardiac magnetic resonance imaging (MRI) has been shown to be more sensitive in its diagnosis. Our case report describes a 45 year old male who presented with palpitations and breathlessness. Echocardiography was normal but cardiac MRI demonstrated abnormalities consistent with Myocarditis. He was treated with Cyclophosphamide and follow up MRI imaging demonstrated complete resolution of these abnormalities which was accompanied by resolution of symptoms. This case therefore supports the use of cardiac MRI in Churg Strauss Syndrome as a sensitive diagnostic tool and as a means of monitoring response to therapy. It also supports the therapeutic effectiveness of Cyclophosphamide therapy in Churg Strauss related Myocarditis, something that has yet to be assessed on a large scale.

Keywords: Cardiac MRI; Cyclophosphamide; Myocarditis; Churg Strauss Syndrome

1. Introduction

Cardiac involvement in Churg Strauss Syndrome is common, with a prevalence of up to 62% [1]. It is the leading cause of mortality in this disease [2]. The necrotising granulomatous Myocarditis associated with Churg Strauss can manifest in different ways. Clear diagnosis is difficult without myocardial biopsy. Unlike patients with renal disease, patients with cardiac involvement are usually ANCA (perinuclear type) negative [3,4]. Furthermore traditional cardiac investigations including echocardiography can be normal even in symptomatic patients. More recently cardiac MRI has been proposed as a useful diagnostic and monitoring tool in this condition. Here we present a case of Churg Strauss Myocarditis in which cardiac MRI was utilised to good effect.

2. Case Report and Methods

A 45 year old man, recently diagnosed with Churg Strauss Syndrome, presented with a two week history of palpitations, presyncope and breathlessness on exertion. He had been taking Prednisolone since 1999 when he had been initially diagnosed with chronic eosinophilic pneumonia, and was currently prescribed 30mg daily.

He was admitted in January 2010 for investigation of his symptoms. Electrocardiography and serum Troponin *T* were normal. A 24 hour tape showed sinus rhythm with 22 isolated ventricular ectopics and 962 episodes of ventricular bigeminy. An echocardiogram demonstrated normal biventricular size and function, and no significant abnormalities.

He was incidentally prescribed Myfortic (Mycophenolic Acid) 720 mg twice a day in February 2010, in addition to Prednisolone, on the basis of persistent sinus symptoms.

Based on his ongoing cardiac symptoms he subsequently underwent cardiac MRI in April. This demonstrated a mildly reduced left ventricular ejection fraction (LVEF) of 46%. There was mild hypokinesia of the basal septum with late contrast hyper-enhancement; consistent with Myocarditis (see **Figure 1**). There was no evidence of endocardial disease or myocardial hypertrophy.

Based on the MRI findings he was commenced on Cyclophosphamide in May and Myfortic therapy was withdrawn. He received 12 doses (at 15 mg/Kg body weight) as an intravenous infusion every 2 weeks.

A cardiac MRI was repeated in August after 6 doses of Cyclophosphamide. This demonstrated clear improvement with a LVEF of 62%. There was very subtle hyper-enhancement in the basal septum but significantly less than previously. He was also now asymptomatic.

He received his last Cyclophsophamide dose in October 2010 and was then commenced on Azathioprine therapy at 150 mg a day. A third MRI was performed two months after conversion to maintenance immunosuppression in December 2010. He remained symptom free at this time. This demonstrated preserved LV function, with an ejection fraction of 61%. There was now no evidence of the previously noted abnormalities (see **Figure 2**).

In summary; a 45 year old man with Churg Strauss syndrome, on long term oral corticosteroid therapy, developed symptoms of palpitations and breathlessness. Echocardiography was normal but cardiac MRI demonstrated mildly impaired LVEF and basal hypokinesia; consistent with Myocarditis. His symptoms were successfully treated with Cyclophosphamide and repeat cardiac MRI was able to demonstrate resolution of the abnormalities.

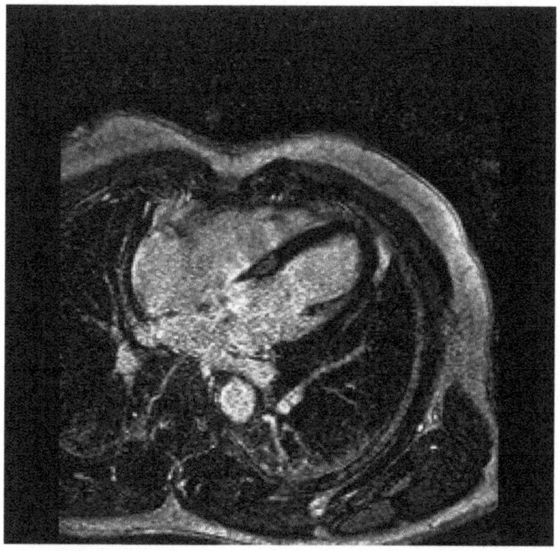

Figure 1. MRI April 2010. 2D Horizontal Long Axis view demonstrating hyper-enhancement in basal septum after gadolinium administration.

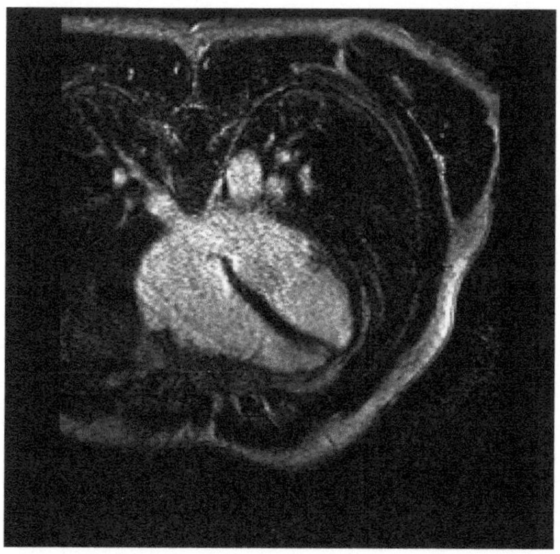

Figure 2. MRI December 2010. 2D Horizontal Long Axis view showing no hyper-enhancement in basal septum after gadolinium administration.

3. Discussion

Cardiac MRI has been shown to be more sensitive than basic echocardiography in diagnosing Myocarditis [5]. MRI can demonstrate delayed enhancement in affected myocardial segments which has been shown to correlate with histologically proven myocardial inflammation or fibrosis [6]. One study showed such abnormalities to occur even in some asymptomatic patients [5]. Cardiac MRI has also been advocated for monitoring in patients who receive immunosuppressive treatment [7]. Follow up cardiac MRI in some of these patients showed resolution of abnormalities after treatment which correlated with clinical improvement. Our case report further supports the use of cardiac MRI as a diagnostic tool. Without evidence of myocardial disease on MRI it would have been difficult to justify the increment in immunosuppressive therapy. Cardiac MRI therefore appears to be very useful in Churg Strauss Syndrome patients presenting with cardiac symptoms, particularly when other investigations are normal. This case also supports its use in monitoring for expected resolution after immunosuppressive therapy. The resolution of MRI abnormalities indicates they were due to myocardial inflammation, rather than fibrosis. The potential role of cardiac MRI as a screening tool for cardiac involvement in asymptomatic patients is less clear and requires further research. Nonetheless it could be argued that baseline imaging is useful given the high lifetime prevalence and mortality of cardiac disease in Churg Strauss Syndrome. It would allow for easier diagnosis in the event of the future development of symptoms.

This case also supports the therapeutic effectiveness of Cyclophosphamide in Churg Strauss Myocarditis. To our knowledge there have, as of yet, been no large scale trials to support its use. Its prescription is largely on an empirical basis but case reports have shown benefit. One of the largest studies of its kind to date showed a clinical or radiological improvement (demonstrated on cardiac MRI) in 6 of 8 patients with Myocarditis treated with Cyclophosphamide [8]. The patient in our case report showed radiological and clinical resolution of his Myocarditis with Cyclophosphamide. He developed cardiac disease despite long term steroid treatment and his symptoms did not improve with Myfortic therapy. Our case would therefore support the use of Cyclophosphamide in Churg Strauss Myocarditis above these other therapies.

4. Conclusion

In conclusion, we would advocate the use of cardiac MRI in Churg Strauss Syndrome Myocarditis; both as a sensitive diagnostic tool and as a means of monitoring response to immunosuppressive therapy. Our case also supports the therapeutic effectiveness of Cyclophosphamide in this condition.

REFERENCES

[1] R. M. Dennert, *et al.*, "Cardiac Involvement in Churg-Strauss Syndrome," *Arthritis and Rheumatism*, Vol. 62, No. 2, 2010, pp. 627-634.

[2] G. Pela, G. Tirabassi, P. Pattoneri, L. Pavone, G. Garini and G. Bruschi, "Cardiac Involvement in the Churg-Strauss Syndrome," *American Journal of Cardiology*, Vol. 97, No. 10, 2006, pp. 1519-1524. doi:10.1016/j.amjcard.2005.11.088

[3] J. Vinit, *et al.*, "Heart Involvement in Churg-Strauss Syndrome: Retrospective Study in French Burgundy Population in Past 10 years," *European Journal of Internal Medicine*, Vol. 21, No. 4, 2010, pp. 341-346. doi:10.1016/j.ejim.2010.05.004

[4] R. Sablé-Fourtassou, P. Cohen, A. Mahr, C. Pagnoux, L. Mouthon, D. Jayne, D. Blockmans, J. F. Cordier, P. Delaval, X. Puechal, D. Lauque, J. F. Viallard, A. Zoulim and L. Guillevin, "The French Vasculitis Study Group. Antineutrophil Cytoplasmic Antibodies and the Churg-Strauss Syndrome," *Annals of Internal Medicine*, Vol. 143, No. 9, 2005, pp. 632-638.

[5] J. Marmursztejn, O. Vignaux, P. Cohen, P. Guilpain, C. Pagnoux, H. Gouya, L. Mouthon, P. Legmann, D. Duboc and L. Guillevin, "Impact of Cardiac Magnetic Resonance Imaging for Assessment of Churg-Strauss Syndrome: A Cross-Sectional Study in 20 Patients," *Clinical and Experimental Rheumatology*, Vol. 27, Suppl. 52, 2009, pp. S70-S76.

[6] H. Mahrholdt, C. Goedecke, A. Wagner, *et al.*, "Cardiovascular Magnetic Resonance Assessment of Human Myocarditis: A Comparison to Histology and Molecular Pathology," *Circulation*, Vol. 109, No. 10, 2004, pp. 1250-1258. doi:10.1161/01.CIR.0000118493.13323.81

[7] H. Baccouche, A. Yilmaz, D. Alscher, K. Klingel, J. F. Val-Bernal and H. Mahrholdt, "Images in Cardiovascular Medicine. Magnetic Resonance Assessment and Therapy Monitoring of Cardiac Involvement in Churg-Strauss Syndrome," *Circulation*, Vol. 117, No. 13, 2008, pp. 1745-1749. doi:10.1161/CIRCULATIONAHA.107.721738

[8] J. Marmursztejn, P. Cohen, D. Duboc, C. Pagnoux, L. Mouthon, P. Guilpain, P. Legmann, L. Guillevin and O. Vignaux, "Cardiac Magnetic Resonance Imaging in Churg-Strauss-Syndrome. Impact of Immunosuppressants on Outcome Assessed in a Prospective Study on 8 Patients," *Clinical and Experimental Rheumatology*, Vol. 28, Suppl. 57, 2010, pp. 8-13.

Therapeutic Modalities in Diabetic Nephropathy: *Future Approaches*[*]

William Brian Reeves[1], Bishal B. Rawal[1], Emaad M. Abdel-Rahman[2], Alaa S. Awad[1]
[1]Department of Medicine, Division of Nephrology, Penn State Hershey Medical Center, Hershey, USA
[2]Department of Medicine, Division of Nephrology, University of Virginia, Charlottesville, USA
Email: asa17@psu.edu

ABSTRACT

Diabetes mellitus is the leading cause of end stage renal disease and is responsible for more than 40% of all cases in the United States. Several therapeutic interventions for the treatment of diabetic nephropathy have been developed and implemented over the past few decades with some degree of success. However, the renal protection provided by these therapeutic modalities is incomplete. More effective approaches are therefore urgently needed. Recently, several novel therapeutic strategies have been explored in treating DN patients including Islet cell transplant, Aldose reductase inhibitors, Sulodexide (GAC), Protein Kinase C (PKC) inhibitors, Connective tissue growth factor (CTGF) inhibitors, Transforming growth factor-beta (TGF-β) inhibitors and bardoxolone. The benefits and risks of these agents are still under investigation. This review aims to summarize the utility of these novel therapeutic approaches.

Keywords: Markers; Albuminuria; Diabetes; Therapy

1. Introduction

Diabetes mellitus (DM) is a leading cause of morbidity and mortality in the United States. DM is often complicated by micro- and macrovascular involvement which contribute to damage to one or more target organs. Diabetic nephropathy (DN) is a well-known microvascular complication of diabetes and is responsible for 40% - 50% of all cases of end stage renal disease (ESRD) in the U.S. adult population [1,2].

DN is defined by the presence of persistent pathologic albuminuria of greater than 300 mg/24 hrs (macroalbuminuria) accompanied by abnormally elevated plasma creatinine or diminished glomerular filtration rate (GFR) [2]. Histologically, DN manifests as diffuse or nodular mesangial expansion, tubular and glomerular basement membrane thickening, as well as interstitial fibrosis.

DN is usually preceded by microalbuminuria (urinary albumin excretion > 30 mg but <300 mg/24 hrs) which is the earliest clinical manifestation of renal involvement in diabetic patients [3]. The onsets of microalbuminuria and overt nephropathy are variable in DM type 1 (DMT1) and type 2 (DMT2). Patients with DMT1 have a more predictable natural history and may present with microalbuminuria 7 - 10 years after being diagnosed with diabetes. About 20% - 45% of these patients progress to DN over the next 10 years (almost 20 years after the diagnosis of DMT1) [4]. On the other hand, patients with DMT2, which comprise approximately 80% of all diabetics, may have overt DN at the time of diagnosis since the duration of diabetes is often not precisely known in this population. The rate of progression of DN towards ESRD is influenced by complex interactions between genetic predisposition, dietary and lifestyle factors as well as therapeutic interventions. Compared to patients with normoalbuminuria (urine albumin excretion < 30 mg/24 hrs), patients with persistent macroalbuminuria (overt DN) have an almost 10-fold higher risk of developing ESRD [5]. Overt proteinuria is also an independent predictor of cardiovascular morbidity and death in diabetic patients [6].

Current therapeutic options directed at delaying the progression of diabetic nephropathy (DN) include intensive blood glucose control, improved blood pressure control, interruption of the RAAS using angiotensin-converting enzyme (ACE) inhibitors and/or angiotensin type 1 (AT_1) receptor blockers (ARB) along with dietary modification and cholesterol-lowering agents (for review please see: [7]). Despite aggressive multifactorial interventions, (DN) remains the single leading cause of ESRD in the United States. The cost of ESRD care for these patients exceeds $10 billion/year. Therefore, more effective approaches are urgently needed.

In this article, we will review several novel therapeutic strategies that have been explored recently in patients with DN which may stop or even reverse disease pro-

[*]Conflict of interest: None.

gression.

2. Diabetic Nephropathy Markers

Early diagnosis of DN is crucial for its effective management. Thus, the search for reliable markers for this disease has been the focus of many studies. Traditionally, GFR has been considered the gold standard in the evaluation of overt nephropathy. Several markers have been used to measure GFR including inulin, iohexol, and iothalamate. However these methods require complex measurements and are expensive, time consuming and not readily feasible in clinical practice. The clearance of endogenous creatinine is another index for GFR. However, it requires timed urine collections and tends to overestimate GFR due to tubular creatinine secretion. This has led to the development of several equations for GFR based on serum creatinine such as the Cockcroft-Gault formula (C-G) [8], the Modification of Diet in Renal Disease four-variable (MDRD-4) formula [9], and the CKD-EPI formula [10] and the measurement of serum cystatin C as an alternative to serum creatinine [11]. A study of patients with DMT2 found that serum cystatin C more accurately identified those with a GFR < 60 ml/min/1.73 m^2 than did serum creatinine, MDRD-4 and C-G formulas [12]. Therefore, cystatin C may be regarded as a superior measure of GFR, especially at lower GFR levels, than serum creatinine. Unfortunately, cystatin C measurements are more expensive than creatinine and may yield falsely low GFR in certain circumstances such as inflammation, steroid therapy and hyperthyroidism.

Urine albumin excretion has received considerable attention and has achieved widespread clinical use as a marker of early DN and as a target for intervention. Increased urinary albumin excretion is the hallmark of DN and estimating urinary albumin excretion is now considered the most reliable marker for assessing disease progression and determining efficacy of treatment in diabetic patients. Nonetheless, urine microalbumin measurements are subject to several limitations relating to specimen collection, indexing to urine creatinine or volume, intrasubject variability and influences of medications, diet and activity which confound its interpretation [11-15]. Thus, a prospective longitudinal study of 232 patients with DM found that the positive predictive value of microalbuminuria as a marker of risk for DN was 43% and the negative predictive value was 77% [13]. Therefore, microalbuminuria may not serve as a strong predictor of DN [14]. On the other hand, macroalbuminuria (overt proteinuria) develops at advanced stage of DN when attempts to prevent progression to ESRD can be very challenging. The discovery of better markers for early detection of DN is an area of active investigation.

3. Candidate Markers in Future

Recently, certain cytokines, such as connective tissue growth factor (CTGF), transforming growth factor-β (TGF-β), and tumor necrosis factor-α (TNF-α) have emerged as potential markers of progression of DN (**Table 1**). For instance, the number of CTGF messenger RNA positive cells in the kidney biopsy was closely related to the renal biopsy fibrosis score and urinary CTGF levels in 65 subjects, three of whom had diabetes [15]. Additional studies have suggested that the urinary excretion of CTGF is related to both albuminuria and GFR in DMT1 [16]. Jaffa and colleagues measured the circulating and urinary levels of CTGF in 1050 subjects with DMT1 from the DCCT/Epidemiology of Diabetes Interventions and Complications (EDIC) study [17]. They showed that significantly higher levels of plasma CTGF are apparent in advanced kidney disease as measured by increased urinary albumin excretion rate (AER), concluding that plasma CTGF is a risk marker of diabetic renal and vascular disease. More recently, urinary TGF-β excretion was shown to be attenuated by ACE inhibition in DMT2 patients with nephropathy [18].

In animal models of DMT1, the renal TNF-α level (renal interstitial fluid and urinary TNF-α) showed an early rise after the induction of diabetes [19], which preceded the rise in urinary albumin excretion by about 2 weeks suggesting a possible contribution of TNF-α in the complicated pathogenic process resulting in microalbuminuria in diabetes. Further studies are necessary to assess value of urinary CTGF, TGF-β and TNF-α as markers of DN progression.

Podocyte loss, effacement, and alterations of the podocyte cytoskeleton and structural proteins play a pivotal role in the pathogenesis of DN. Podocytes have been shown in the urine of diabetic patients with microalbuminuria (53%) and with macroalbuminuria (80%) using immunofluorescence microscopy [20]. The number of podocytes in the urine of patients with macroalbuminuria was significantly greater than in patients with microal-

Table 1. Diabetic nephropathy markers.

Current markers	Candidate markers in future
1. Creatinine, Cystatin C (estimated GFR).	1. Urinary podocytes
2. Microalbuminuria	2. NGAL
3. Macroalbuminuria or Proteinuria	3. KIM-1
	4. Smad 1
	5. CTGF
	6. TGF-β
	7. TNF-α

NGAL = Neutrophil Gelatinase-Associated Lipocalin; KIM-1 = Kidney Injury Molecule 1; CTGF = Connective tissue growth factor; TGF-β = Transforming growth factor beta; TNF-α = Tumor necrosis factor alpha.

buminuria ($p < 0.01$). Preliminary studies in animal models of diabetes show that flow cytometry is a feasible and less expensive method for assessing urinary podocytes (Awad AS, unpublished data). Whether the measurement of urinary podocytes may serve as a surrogate marker not only for the progression of DN, but also for the efficacy of potential therapies, is not clear at this point. Additional research is needed to explore this possibility.

More recently, Mima *et al.* demonstrated the critical role of Smad1 in the development of mesangial matrix expansion in the early phase of DN in Streptozotocin-induced diabetic rats [21]. Under diabetic conditions, Smad1 regulates the genetic expression of type IV collagen (Col4) which is a key component involved in mesangial expansion. They also showed a direct correlation between urinary Smad1 levels and the severity of mesangial expansion [22].

Additional promising biomarkers include neutrophil gelatinase-associated lipocalin (NGAL) and kidney injury molecule 1 (KIM-1). NGAL is a small, 25-kD protein that belongs to the lipocalin protein family and is produced in epithelial cells and neutrophils. NGAL is an established novel biomarker for early diagnosis of acute kidney injury (AKI) [23-27]. It has also been linked as an independent biomarker for predicting chronic kidney disease progression [28]. In a cohort of 56 patients with DMT2, serum and urinary NGAL levels were evaluated in 3 groups of varying degrees of proteinuria: normoalbuminuria, microalbuminuria and overt DN [28]. The results revealed that all groups had increased NGAL levels as compared to controls and both serum and urinary NGAL levels correlated with the severity of renal disease reaching highest levels in patients with overt DN. The presence of elevated NGAL levels even in normoalbuminuric patients, who had no signs of glomerular damage, raised the possibility that NGAL may be a useful, non-invasive tool for early detection of incipient DN.

Urinary KIM-1 has also been proposed to be a novel biomarker of AKI in humans [29,30]. KIM-1 is a transmembrane protein exclusively located in the proximal tubules of the kidney and is markedly upregulated in ischemic kidney damage. Nielsen *et al.* [31] studied both NGAL and KIM-1 in DMT1 patients with different levels of albuminuria (normo-, micro- and macroalbuminuria) compared to non-diabetic control subjects. They also evaluated the effect of ACE inhibition (lisinopril) on urinary NGAL excretion in patients with DN. The results of the study showed both urinary NGAL and KIM-1 to be elevated in all groups of diabetic patients compared to non-diabetics, reflecting possible utility of both NGAL and KIM-1 as independent biomarkers of early diabetic kidney disease. They also found a reduction, albeit not statistically significant, of urinary NGAL with ACE inhibition. However, these biomarkers did not provide additional prognostic information to that of known traditional markers in predicting the decline of kidney function in diabetic patients who have already developed overt nephropathy [32].

Until more studies are available, periodic measurements of microalbuminuria and serum creatinine (for estimated GFR) still remain the standard of care for screening of DN in the diabetic population.

4. Potential Future Therapeutic Agents for Diabetic Nephropathy

Currently available measures to control DN are mostly preventative. Recently, several emerging as well as potential therapies for future have been proposed for treating DN based on both animal and human studies (**Table 2**). Emerging therapeutic agents include thiazolidinediones/PPAR-gamma agonists, angiotensin converting enzyme-2 (ACE-2), endothelin receptor blockers, advanced glycation endproduct (AGE) inhibitors, and selective vitamin D activation which have been suggested to have a protective role in DN by causing a reduction or even reversal of proteinuria (for review please see: [7]).

In this article, we will review some of the potential future therapeutic agents for treating DN (**Figure 1**) as

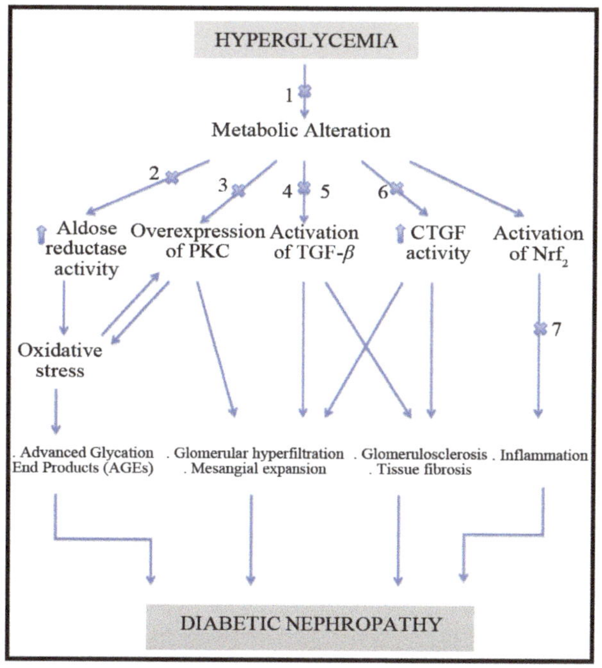

Targets for potential therapy in future: 1 = Islet cell transplant; 2 = Aldose reductase inhibitor; 3 = Protein kinase C (PKC) inhibitor; 4 = Suldexide; 5 = Transforming growth factor-beta (TGF-β) inhibitor; 6 = Connective tissue growth factor (CTGF) inhibitor; 7 = Bardoxolone methyl.

Figure 1. Pathogenesis of Diabetic Nephropathy (DN) and potential future therapeutic measures for treatment and/or reversal of DN.

Table 2. Therapeutic modalities in diabetic nephropathy.

Current therapy	Emerging therapy	Potential therapy for future
1. Intensive glycemic control.	1. Thiazolidinediones/PPAR-gamma agonists.	1. Islet cell transplant.
- Pharmacologic measures.	2. ACE-2.	2. Aldose reductase inhibitors.
- Pancreas transplant.	3. Endothelin receptor blockers.	3. Sulodexide (GAG).
2. Blood pressure control.	4. AGE inhibitors.	4. Protein kinase C (PKC) inhibitors.
- Drugs affecting RAAS:	5. Vitamin D activation.	5. Connective tissue growth factor (CTGF) inhibitors.
. ACE inhibitor		6. Transforming growth factor beta (TGF-B) inhibitors.
. ARB		7. Bardoxolone.
. Direct renin inhibitor		
. Aldosterone antagonist		
- Drugs not affecting RAAS:		
. NDHP CCB		
. B-blocker		
. Diuretics		
3. Lipid lowering agents.		
4. Lifestyle modification.		

follows.

4.1. Islet Cell Transplant

Several studies have shown that islet transplantation is associated with improved diabetic control with a possibility of protection against diabetic complications. Warnok *et al.* [33] performed a prospective crossover, cohort study of 42 patients with DM for more than 5 years and with established diabetic complications such as retinopathy and mild nephropathy. All patients were initially enrolled in group I and treated with intensive medical therapy. Thirty one patients from group I subsequently received islet cell transplants and crossed over to group II. After almost 3 years of follow up, group II patients showed better glycemic control (HBA1c 7.5% (I) vs. 6.6% (II); $p < 0.01$) and less progression on retinopathy. However, both groups showed similar declines in kidney function suggesting no additional benefit of islet cell transplantation in preserving GFR (eGFR = –0.45 ml/min (I) vs. –0.12 ml/min (II); $p = 0.1$). While islet cells are typically obtained from a deceased organ donor, another technique involving transplant of autologous islets has been developed. The basic technique requires total pancreatectomy, fragmentation of the pancreas followed by collagenase digestion and then differential centrifugation. The isolated islets are then re-implanted in the patient's liver via the portal vein [34]. Webb *et al.* [34] studied 46 patients who received auto islet transplantation. After 10 years of follow up, the median serum creatinine increased very little from 0.8 mg/dl to 0.87 mg/dl, suggesting a role for auto islet cell transplantation in possible protection against diabetic complications.

4.2. Aldose Reductase Inhibitors

Aldose reductase catalyzes the first and rate-limiting step of the polyol pathway of glucose metabolism [35]. Activation of the polyol pathway is implicated in diabetes induced renal dysfunction via *de novo* synthesis of diacylglycerol (DAG), activation of protein kinase C (PKC) with increased production of TGF-β, extracellular matrix proteins and prostaglandins. Increased aldose reductase activity also results in depletion of NADPH, a decrease in cellular levels of reduced glutathione, and increased oxidative stress. The complex interaction between hyperglycemia-induced oxidative stress from aldose reductase activation, increased formation of advanced glycation endproducts (AGEs) and activation of vascular PKC isoforms ultimately result in microvascular diabetic complications. Increased aldose reductase expression has been shown in DMT2 patients [36]. A number of studies have shown a decrease in urinary albumin excretion in animals treated with aldose reductase inhibitors [37-39]. For instance, the aldose reductase inhibitor, sorbinil, was found to reduce albuminuria and glomerular basement membrane thickening in STZ diabetic rats treated for five months [38]. These actions were attributed to a reduction in the renal cortical activity of glucosyl-galactosyl-hydroxylysyl-glucohydrolase, an enzyme involved in the catabolism of collagen disaccharide units [39].

Small clinical trials have assessed the efficacy of aldose reductase inhibitors in the treatment of DN in both DMT1 [40] and DMT2 [41]. Both studies showed reduced urinary albumin excretion rate after aldose reductase inhibitor treatment for 6 months [40] or 5 years [41]. In contrast to these results, McAuliffe *et al.* reported that aldose reductase inhibitors had no effect on proteinuria in

16 diabetic subjects treated for 12 months [42]. Drugs which block aldose reductase activity include spirohydantoins (sorbinil), carboxylic acid derivatives (tolrestat, epalrestat, ponalrestat) and flavonoids. Sorbinil and tolrestat have been withdrawn from the worldwide market because of severe toxicity (hepatotoxic). Taken together, these studies of aldose reductase inhibitors have not shown convincing evidence of benefit in the treatment of DN.

4.3. Sulodexide (GAG)

Sulodexide is an oral formulation of a highly purified mixture of glycosaminoglycans. It is composed of 80% fast-moving heparin sulfate and 20% dermatan sulfate and is the most extensively studied glycosaminoglycan for diabetic patients. It bears strong chemical similarity to heparin but does not have anticoagulation properties when given orally [43]. Sulodexide has emerged as a potential treatment of DN as multiple studies have demonstrated reductions in urinary albumin excretion with glycosaminoglycan therapy [44-47].

The precise physiology of the sulodexide-mediated renoprotection in DN is not clear, but several mechanisms have been proposed. Sulodexide has been shown to block heparinase-1 activity [48,49], an enzyme that is upregulated in hyperglycemia and can degrade heparin sulfate molecules of the glomerular basement membrane. As sulodexide is a mixture of glycosaminoglycans, it may help in restoring the glycoproteins present in the GBM and mesangium. Another mechanism involves restoring the anionic heparin sulfate charge on the GBM. Finally, sulodexide may suppress high-glucose induced overexpression of TGF-$\beta 1$ that is responsible for enhanced expression of mesangial matrix and collagens [50]. In a study of the *db*/*db* mouse model of diabetes, sulodexide was shown to reduce proteinuria significantly in early stage kidney disease but not late kidney disease (12 weeks and after) [51].

The efficacy of sulodexide in diabetes was also evaluated in the DiNAS study [52]. DiNAS was a randomized, double blind and placebo controlled trial involving 223 patients with DMT1 or DMT2 and microalbuminuria or macroalbuminuria. Patients were randomized to receive sulodexide (50 to 200 mg daily) or placebo for 4 months. After 4 months of therapy, albuminuria decreased by as much as 74% compared with the placebo group. Four months after drug discontinuation, albuminuria remained 69% lower in those randomized to 200 mg of sulodexide compared with the placebo group. This sustained response suggests that some anatomical or structural changes had occurred with sulodexide treatment. Sulodexide was well tolerated in that study. Another study showed a significant reduction in albuminuria with long term use of oral sulodexide at a moderate dose in patients with DN [53]. In this study, thirty patients (both DMT1 and DMT2) treated with 50 mg per day of oral sulodexide for 12 months were compared with thirty matched diabetic patients in the control group. The degree of albuminuria was greatly reduced in patients treated with sulodexide at the end of 12 months but was increased in the control group (–260% and +29% respectively; $p = 0.0001$).

Another recent study included 149 patients with DMT2 and microalbuminuria [54] who were randomized to receive 200 or 400 mg of sulodexide versus placebo. The primary endpoint at 6 months was a 50% reduction in albuminuria or return to normoalbuminuria. This was achieved in 33.3% of the sulodexide 200 mg group and 18.4% of the sulodexide 400 mg group as compared to 15.4% of the placebo group ($p = 0.075$ and 0.781 respectively) [54]. Based on the experience gained from these smaller studies, two large multicenter double-blinded, randomized placebo controlled trials were designed to establish the renoprotective potential of sulodexide. The results, unfortunately, were disappointing. The first study was the Sulodexide Microalbuminuria (SUN-micro) Trial, which examined the efficacy of sulodexide given over 26 weeks in 1000 patients with DMT2, hypertension and microalbuminuria [55]. The second study was the Sulodexide Overt Nephropathy (SUN-macro) Trial which aimed to examine the efficacy of sulodexide in 2240 patients with DMT2, hypertension and proteinuria ≥ 900 mg/24 h [55]. Both SUN-micro and SUN-macro trials used Sulodexide 200 mg daily vs. placebo in patients being treated with maximum approved or tolerated dose of ACE inhibitor or ARB in both arms. The primary outcome of the SUN-micro Trial was the conversion to normoalbuminuria and at least a 25% decrease in the urinary albumin creatinine ratio (UACR) or at least a 50% reduction in UACR. The primary outcome of the SUN-macro Trial was time to a composite end point of doubling of serum creatinine or ESRD. However, the SUN-micro trial failed to show a reduction of albuminuria in DN. With the failure of the SUN-micro trial, the SUN-macro trial was cancelled.

4.4. Protein Kinase C (PKC) Inhibitors

Activation of PKC is one of the key metabolic pathways involved in the pathogenesis of the DN. PKC is a family of at least 12 serine-threonine protein kinases that play an important role in intracellular signal transduction [56]. Hyperglycemia-induced oxidative stress has been strongly implicated in microvascular complications from diabetes. High ambient blood glucose levels increase diacylglycerol levels, advanced glycation end products, and enhance mitochondrial synthesis of reactive oxygen species, thereby activating protein kinase C (PKC), particularly in organs that are susceptible to developing diabetic micro- and macro-vascular complications [57]. Activated PKC causes kidney damage through a number of mechanisms including NADPH oxidase-dependent generation of oxidants, signaling TGF-β to induce extracellular matrix production and increased secretion of vasodilatory prostanoids which contribute to glomerular hyperfiltration [58,59]. Ruboxistaurin mesylate (RTX) (previously known as LY333531) is a bisindolylmaleimide with a high degree of specificity for inhibiting PKC-β1 and –β2 isoforms [60] which has been studied in animal models of DM [61-63].

Ruboxistaurin was shown to have several positive impacts on the pathogenesis of DN. It was able to normalize glomerular hyperfiltration, reduce extracellular matrix protein production and TGF-β1, reduce mesangial expansion, glomerulosclerosis and tubulointerstitial fibrosis and decrease albuminuria.

A randomized, double blind, placebo-controlled, multicenter, pilot study was conducted to evaluate the effect of LY333531 in type 2 DN patients [64]. In this study, 123 patients with DN and macroalbuminuria were randomized to either 32 mg daily of RTX or placebo for 1 year [64]. Patients in both arms were continued on ACEIs or ARBs during the trial. The primary endpoint was a reduction in ACR. After one year, active treatment was associated with a reduction in albuminuria and stabilization of GFR whereas the placebo group experienced no change in albuminuria and worsening of GFR. The reduction in albuminuria appeared as early as 1 month following treatment initiation. Although the study showed beneficial effects of LY333531 in DN (reduction in albuminuria and prevention in loss of eGFR), this study had some limitations. It was underpowered to detect any significant differences in albumin-creatinine ratio and eGFR. Another limitation of this study was its short duration of follow-up that limited conclusions about safety of RTX. Unfortunately, the PKC diabetic retinopathy study 2 (PKC-DRS 2) seemed to show an increased frequency of the adverse event of "diabetic nephropathy" in ruboxistaurin-treated patients compared with placebo-treated patients [65]. Furthermore, Tuttle *et al.* analyzed results from studies investigating the effects of ruboxistaurin on renal outcomes and found that the rate of kidney outcomes was similar in ruboxistaurin-treated patients and individuals receiving placebo [66].

4.5. Connective Tissue Growth Factor (CTGF) Inhibitors

CTGF is a recently identified potent profibrotic peptide that has been shown to play a role in the pathogenesis of kidney diseases, micro- and macrovascular complications of diabetes [67,68]. Several agents regulate CTGF expression such as TGF-β, high glucose and fibroblast growth factor [69].

CTGF stimulates cell adhesion and migration, production and deposition of extracellular matrix (ECM) proteins, and angiogenesis [70,71]. Zhou *et al.* showed that AGE-induced CTGF expression plays a critical role in renal ECM accumulation leading to DN [72]. CTGF has been implicated in promoting tissue fibrosis in DN by activating several intracellular signaling molecules in human mesangial cells (HMC) including receptor tyrosine kinases (TrkA) and induction of transcription factor TGF-B-inducible early gene [73]. Multiple *in vitro* and animal studies have demonstrated that inhibition of CTGF prevents the production of key proteins that compose scar [74] and prevents development of renal fibrosis [75, 76]. Several animal and human studies have been undertaken to evaluate the role of CTGF inhibition using a monoclonal antibody that targets CTGF (FG-3019). Flyvbjerg and colleagues investigated the effects of FG-3019 in obese mice with DMT2 [77]. FG-3019 reduced urinary albumin excretion, GBM thickening and normalized hyperfiltration in these mice. A similar study in rats showed that FG-3019 reduced diabetic proteinuria [78].

Likewise, encouraging results were noted in human studies examining FG-3019 as a therapeutic agent in patients with DN. Adler and colleagues studied 24 microalbuminuric subjects (21% with DMT1 and 79% with DMT2) who received 3 or 10 mg/kg FG-3019 (total 4 doses 2 weeks apart) with one year follow up. The results showed that FG-3019 was associated with a significant reduction of urinary albumin/creatinine ratio (mean pretreatment value of 48 mg/g to a mean post-treatment value of 20 mg/g, p = 0.027) without evidence for a dose-response relationship [79]. Similarly, Schwartz and colleagues showed that FG-3019 reduced microalbuminuria in patients with diabetes [80]. These preliminary results suggest that CTGF does play a role in the pathogenesis of DN, a role that needs further clarification. Inhibition of CTGF is promising as a therapeutic target for patients with DN.

4.6. Transforming Growth Factor-Beta (TGF-β) Inhibitors

TGF-β1 is a powerful cytokine that plays several roles in the kidney; including cell proliferation, migration, differentiation, immunomodulation and ECM turnover regulation [81]. The role of TGF-β in diabetic nephropathy has been examined in both animal and human studies. Langham *et al.* [18] extracted RNA from 12 human renal biopsies taken from participants in the Diabiopsies study, a randomized controlled 2-year trial that reported a reduction in proteinuria and cortical matrix expansion in DMT2 patients treated with perindopril (an ACE inhibitor) vs. placebo. The study showed a substantial diminution in TGF-β mRNA gene expression (mean 83% reduction, $p < 0.05$) in patients who had reduced proteinuria, reflecting a potential role of TGF-β inhibition in the treatment of DN. Therapeutic strategies were developed to block the production/activity of the renal TGF-β1 system to limit DN. Among these strategies are indirect approaches to decrease the TGF-β effects using renin-angiotensin inhibition, tight glycemic control, statin therapy and/or tight blood pressure control. Other direct approaches decrease TGF-β effect using neutralizing anti-TGF-β antibodies and antisense or using novel antifibrotic agents such as Pirfenidone [82].

Several animal studies have been performed to evaluate the therapeutic role of TGF-β blockers in DN. Sharma and colleagues administered TGF-β neutralizing antibodies to diabetic rats and showed that TGF-β antibodies prevented glomerular enlargement and suppressed the expression of genes encoding ECM components [83]. Ziyadeh and colleagues further showed that administration of anti-TGF-β antibody could attenuate progressive diabetic kidney disease in diabetic mice by preventing pathological changes of glomerulosclerosis [84]. Pirfenidone (PFD; 5-methyl-1-phenyl-2-(1H)-pyridone), a novel antifibrotic agent, is a low molecular weight synthetic molecule that inhibits TGF-β production and exerts antifibrotic properties in cell culture and various animal models of fibrosis [85,86]. Recently RamachandraRao and colleagues evaluated the therapeutic efficacy of PFD in *db/db* diabetic mice [87]. DN developed in the *db/db* mice as evidenced by albuminuria and mesangial matrix expansion by 12 to 16 wk of age. PFD was then given to the *db/db* mice from week 17 to week 21. Four weeks of PFD treatment led to a significant reduction in the degree of mesangial matrix expansion. They concluded that PFD can promote resolution of mesangial matrix when administered after the onset of nephropathy. They also showed that PFD did not worsen renal blood flow, lower BP, affect glycemic parameters, or cause hyperkalemia [87].

Several clinical studies have confirmed that TGF-β is increased in the kidneys of diabetic patients. Glomerular expression of TGF-β is also increased in early [85,88] and late stages [86,89] of DMT1 and DMT2 and correlates with the degree of glycemic control in these patients [88]. These data were the grounds for a recent clinical trial to evaluate the role of TGF-β inhibitors on the course of DN. A double blind, placebo-controlled study with 77 subjects of DN were randomized to treatment with placebo, low dose (1200 mg daily) or high dose (2400 mg daily) PFD for one year [90]. Treatment with low dose, but not high dose of PFD resulted in an improvement in GFR with no change in albuminuria. The major side effects were gastrointestinal symptoms and fatigue. The results of the study suggested that PFD could be a potential promising therapeutic agent in patients with DN. Additional studies in larger numbers of patients, ideally with histologic assessment of the kidneys, appear to be warranted to support this benefit.

4.7. Anti-Inflammatory Agents—Bardoxolone

Recently, an orally available synthetic triterpenoid, Bardoxolone methyl, has shown promising results in DN. Bardoxolone methyl exerts potent anti-oxidant and anti-inflammatory activity via induction of the Nrf2 transcription factor. A Phase 2 trial of bardoloxone methyl treatment for 8 weeks in 20 patients with moderate-severe CKD and DMT2 demonstrated improved renal function as evidenced by increased eGFR paralleled by a significant reduction in serum creatinine and BUN [91]. A subsequent trial examined the effect of bardoloxone methyl (25 - 150 mg/d) administered for 52 weeks to 227 patients with moderate to severe CKD and DMT2 [92]. Bardoloxone methyl produced a significant increase in GFR of 8 - 11 ml/min/1.73 m^2. The improvement in GFR was evident by 8 - 12 weeks of treatment and persisted for the entire 52 week treatment period. Likewise, bardoloxone treatment reduced the proportion of patients who experienced a 25% fall in GFR from 13% in the placebo group to only 2% in treatment group. Although hard outcomes, such as dialysis dependency and death, were not evaluated, these results are very encouraging and justify further study of bardoxolone methyl and related compounds.

5. Summary and Conclusions

There is clear evidence that optimal glycemic control [93-99] and blood pressure control [100-109] are of paramount importance in preventing progression of DN. The renoprotective benefits of agents that block reninangiotensin aldosterone system (RAAS) in preventing progression of DN is well-established [110-121]. Non-dihydropyrdine CCBs (diltiazem, verapamil), that do not affect RAAS, have also been shown to reduce proteinuria and slow progression of kidney disease in diabetics [122-127]. Similarly, lipid lowering agents (such as statins) have been shown to slow the rate of progression of DN [128], but the data supporting this are scant. Even so, it is important to understand that currently available strategies are geared towards limiting or slowing the rate of progression of DN to ESRD. These modalities do not actually stop the progression of DN. In this modern era of medical advancement, we are in dire need of novel strategies that can halt or even reverse the disease progression.

While pancreas transplantation [129] is an effective approach in preventing DN in patients with DMT1, islet cell transplantation appears to be a reasonable alternative to improve glycemic control but has questionable benefit in terms of preserving GFR in patients with established DN. Aldose-reductase is a rate-limiting enzyme in glucose metabolism pathway, and its activation leads to increased oxidative stress, formation of AGE products and activation of protein kinase C, ultimately resulting in micro-vascular complications such as DN. Although aldose-reductase inhibitors have been shown to reduce albuminuria and prevent glomerular basement membrane thickening in animal studies, their efficacy in humans has been inconclusive. Sulodexide, an oral formulation of a purified mixture of glycosaminoglycans reduced proteinuria by uncertain mechanisms. It produced sustained reductions in albuminuria in both animal and human studies even after discontinuation of the drug, suggesting the possibility for anatomical or structural changes with long term protection against DN. Unfortunately, larger multi-center studies (SUN-micro and SUN-macro trials) failed to confirm these benefits. Protein kinase C inhibitors (Ruboxistaurin) have shown promising results with respect to improving glomerular hyperfiltration, reducing mesangial expansion and reduction of albuminuria in diabetic animal models as well as humans. They have been associated with a reduction in albuminuria and prevention of loss of GFR in a few randomized pilot studies, although large scale prospective studies have yet to confirm their beneficial effects on renal outcomes. CTGF is a potent profibrotic peptide that has been implicated in extracellular matrix deposition and promotion of tissue fibrosis. Therefore, CTGF inhibition is a promising therapeutic target in patients with DN. FG-3019, a CTGF-inhibitor, has been shown to reduce glomerular basement membrane thickening and normalize hyperfiltration diabetic mice and reduce albuminuria in humans. Similarly, pirfenidone is a TGF-β inhibitor that is recognized as a novel anti-fibrotic agent. In humans, at a low treatment dose, it was shown to improve GFR without improvement in albuminuria. Similarly, the use of bardoxalone is encouraging and justifies its further study.

In summary, these data indicate that there are several promising therapeutic targets that could potentially be utilized to treat patients with established DN. While currently available measures to control DN are largely preventative, there is hope that therapies capable of stopping, or even reversing progression of DN will soon become available. The current cost of ESRD care exceeds $10 billion per year, much of which is devoted to care of DN. In addition, overt proteinuria in DN is a known independent risk factor for cardiovascular events, including death. Therefore, the potential ability to halt or reverse DN with these candidate markers in future may offer significant benefits in terms of minimizing cardiovascular morbidity and mortality and also reducing tremendous health-care spending. However, additional human studies are warranted to prove the effectiveness of these agents in treating DN.

6. Acknowledgements

This work was supported by NIH Grant DK077444.

REFERENCES

[1] United States Renal Data System (USRDS), "The National Institutes of Diabetes and Digestive and Kidney Diseases," Annual Data Report, Bethesda, 2005.

[2] G. Eknoyan, T. Hostetter, G. L. Bakris, L. Hebert, A. S. Levey, H. H. Parving, M. W. Steffes and R. Toto, "Proteinuria and Other Markers of Chronic Kidney Disease: A Position Statement of the National Kidney Foundation (NKF) and the National Institute of Diabetes and Digestive and Kidney Diseases (NIDDK)," *Journal of Kidney Diseases*, Vol. 42, No. 4, 2003, pp. 617-622. doi:10.1016/S0272-6386(03)00826-6

[3] C. E. Mogensen, "Microalbuminuria as a Predictor of Clinical Diabetic Nephropathy," *Kidney International*, Vol. 31, 1987, pp. 673-689. doi:10.1038/ki.1987.50

[4] A. S. Krolewski, J. H. Warram, L. I. Rand and C. R. Kahn, "Epidemiologic Approach to the Etiology of Type I Diabetes Mellitus and Its Complications," *The New England Journal of Medicine*, Vol. 317, No. 22, 1987, pp. 1390-1398. doi:10.1056/NEJM198711263172206

[5] A. M. Berhane, E. J. Weil, W. C. Knowler, R. G. Nelson and R. L. Hanson, "Albuminuria and Estimated Glomerular Filtration Rate as Predictors of Diabetic End-Stage Renal Disease and Death," *Clinical Journal of the American Society of Nephrology*, Vol. 6, No. 10, 2011, pp. 2444-2451. doi:10.2215/CJN.00580111

[6] H. C. Gerstein, J. F. Mann, Q. Yi, B. Zinman, S. F. Dinneen, B. Hoogwerf, J. P. Halle, J. Young, A. Rashkow, C. Joyce, S. Nawaz and S. Yusuf, "Albuminuria and Risk of Cardiovascular Events, Death, and Heart Failure in Diabetic and Nondiabetic Individuals," *The Journal of the American Medical Association*, Vol. 286, No. 4, 2001, pp. 421-426. doi:10.1001/jama.286.4.421

[7] E. M. Abdel-Rahman, L. Saadulla, W. B. Reeves and A. S. Awad, "Therapeutic Modalities in Diabetic Nephropathy: Standard and Emerging Approaches," *Journal of General Internal Medicine*, Vol. 27, No. 4, 2011, pp. 458-468.

[8] D. W. Cockcroft and M. H. Gault, "Prediction of Creatinine Clearance from Serum Creatinine," *Nephron*, Vol. 16, No. 1, 1976, pp. 31-41. doi:10.1159/000180580

[9] A. S. Levey, J. Coresh, E. Balk, A. T. Kausz, A. Levin, M. W. Steffes, R. J. Hogg, R. D. Perrone, J. Lau and G. Eknoyan, "National Kidney Foundation Practice Guidelines for Chronic Kidney Disease: Evaluation, Classification, and Stratification," *Annals of Internal Medicine*, Vol. 139, No. 2, 2003, pp. 137-147.

[10] A. S. Levey, L. A. Stevens, C. H. Schmid, Y. L. Zhang, A. F. Castro, H. I. Feldman, J. W. Kusek, P. Eggers, F. Van Lente, T. Greene and J. Coresh, "A New Equation to Es-

timate Glomerular Filtration Rate," *Annals of Internal Medicine*, Vol. 150, No. 9, 2009, pp. 604-612.

[11] B. A. Perkins, R. G. Nelson, B. E. Ostrander, K. L. Blouch, A. S. Krolewski, B. D. Myers and J. H. Warram, "Detection of Renal Function Decline in Patients with Diabetes and Normal or Elevated GFR by Serial Measurements of Serum Cystatin C Concentration: Results of a 4-Year Follow-Up Study," *Journal of the American Society of Nephrology*, Vol. 16, No. 5, 2005, pp. 1404-1412. doi:10.1681/ASN.2004100854

[12] R. J. Macisaac, C. Tsalamandris, M. C. Thomas, E. Premaratne, S. Panagiotopoulos, T. J. Smith, A. Poon, M. A. Jenkins, S. I. Ratnaike, D. A. Power and G. Jerums, "The Accuracy of Cystatin C and Commonly Used Creatinine-Based Methods for Detecting Moderate and Mild Chronic Kidney Disease in Diabetes," *Diabetic Medicine*, Vol. 24, No. 4, 2007, pp. 443-448. doi:10.1111/j.1464-5491.2007.02112.x

[13] B. P. Tabaei, A. S. Al-Kassab, L. L. Ilag, C. M. Zawacki and W. H. Herman, "Does Microalbuminuria Predict Diabetic Nephropathy?" *Diabetes Care*, Vol. 24, No. 9, 2001, pp. 1560-1566. doi:10.2337/diacare.24.9.1560

[14] B. A. Perkins, L. H. Ficociello, B. E. Ostrander, K. H. Silva, J. Weinberg, J. H. Warram and A. S. Krolewski, "Microalbuminuria and the Risk for Early Progressive Renal Function Decline in Type 1 Diabetes," *Journal of the American Society of Nephrology*, Vol. 18, No. 4, 2007, pp. 1353-1361.

[15] Y. Ito, J. Aten, R. J. Bende, B. S. Oemar, T. J. Rabelink, J. J. Weening and R. Goldschmeding, "Expression of Connective Tissue Growth Factor in Human Renal Fibrosis," *Kidney International*, Vol. 53, 1998, pp. 853-861. doi:10.1111/j.1523-1755.1998.00820.x

[16] T. Q. Nguyen, L. Tarnow, S. Andersen, P. Hovind, H. H. Parving, R. Goldschmeding and F. A. van Nieuwenhoven, "Urinary Connective Tissue Growth Factor Excretion Correlates with Clinical Markers of Renal Disease in a Large Population of Type 1 Diabetic Patients with Diabetic Nephropathy," *Diabetes Care*, Vol. 29, No. 1, 2006, pp. 83-88. doi:10.2337/diacare.29.01.06.dc05-1670

[17] A. A. Jaffa, W. R. Usinger, M. B. McHenry, M. A. Jaffa, S. R. Lipstiz, D. Lackland, M. Lopes-Virella, L. M. Luttrell and P. W. Wilson, "Connective Tissue Growth Factor and Susceptibility to Renal and Vascular Disease Risk in Type 1 Diabetes," *The Journal of Clinical Endocrinology & Metabolism*, Vol. 93, No. 5, 2008, pp. 1893-1900. doi:10.1210/jc.2007-2544

[18] R. G. Langham, D. J. Kelly, R. M. Gow, Y. Zhang, D. J. Cordonnier, N. Pinel, P. Zaoui and R. E. Gilbert, "Transforming Growth Factor-β in Human Diabetic Nephropathy: Effects of ACE Inhibition," *Diabetes Care*, Vol. 29, No. 12, 2006, pp. 2670-2675. doi:10.2337/dc06-0911

[19] K. Kalantarinia, A. S. Awad and H. M. Siragy, "Urinary and Renal Interstitial Concentrations of TNF-α Increase Prior to the Rise in Albuminuria in Diabetic Rats," *Kidney International*, Vol. 64, 2003, pp. 1208-1213. doi:10.1046/j.1523-1755.2003.00237.x

[20] T. Nakamura, C. Ushiyama, S. Suzuki, M. Hara, N. Shimada, I. Ebihara and H. Koide, "Urinary Excretion of Podocytes in Patients with Diabetic Nephropathy," *Nephrology Dialysis Transplantation*, Vol. 15, No. 9, 2000, pp. 1379-1383. doi:10.1093/ndt/15.9.1379

[21] T. Matsubara, H. Abe, H. Arai, K. Nagai, A. Mima, H. Kanamori, E. Sumi, T. Takahashi, M. Matsuura, N. Iehara, A. Fukatsu, T. Kita and T. Doi, "Expression of Smad1 Is Directly Associated with Mesangial Matrix Expansion in Rat Diabetic Nephropathy," *Laboratory Investigation*, Vol. 86, 2006, pp. 357-368. doi:10.1038/labinvest.3700400

[22] A. Mima, H. Arai, T. Matsubara, H. Abe, K. Nagai, Y. Tamura, K. Torikoshi, M. Araki, H. Kanamori, T. Takahashi, T. Tominaga, M. Matsuura, N. Iehara, A. Fukatsu, T. Kita and T. Doi, "Urinary Smad1 Is a Novel Marker to Predict Later Onset of Mesangial Matrix Expansion in Diabetic Nephropathy," *Diabetes*, Vol. 57, No. 6, 2008, pp. 1712-1722. doi:10.2337/db07-1726

[23] J. Mishra, C. Dent, R. Tarabishi, M. M. Mitsnefes, Q. Ma, C. Kelly, S. M. Ruff, K. Zahedi, M. Shao, J. Bean, K. Mori, J. Barasch and P. Devarajan, "Neutrophil Gelatinase-Associated Lipocalin (NGAL) as a Biomarker for Acute Renal Injury after Cardiac Surgery," *The Lancet*, Vol. 365, No. 9466, 2005, pp. 1231-1238. doi:10.1016/S0140-6736(05)74811-X

[24] C. R. Parikh, J. Mishra, H. Thiessen-Philbrook, B. Dursun, Q. Ma, C. Kelly, C. Dent, P. Devarajan and C. L. Edelstein, "Urinary IL-18 Is an Early Predictive Biomarker of Acute Kidney Injury after Cardiac Surgery," *Kidney International*, Vol. 70, 2006, pp. 199-203. doi:10.1038/sj.ki.5001527

[25] M. Bennett, C. L. Dent, Q. Ma, S. Dastrala, F. Grenier, R. Workman, H. Syed, S. Ali, J. Barasch and P. Devarajan, "Urine NGAL Predicts Severity of Acute Kidney Injury after Cardiac Surgery: A Prospective Study," *Clinical Journal of the American Society of Nephrology*, Vol. 3, No. 3, 2008, pp. 665-673. doi:10.2215/CJN.04010907

[26] W. Ling, N. Zhaohui, H. Ben, G. Leyi, L. Jianping, D. Huili and Q. Jiaqi, "Urinary IL-18 and NGAL as Early Predictive Biomarkers in Contrast-Induced Nephropathy after Coronary Angiography," *Nephron Clinical Practice*, Vol. 108, No. 3, 2008, pp. 176-181. doi:10.1159/000117814

[27] T. L. Nickolas, M. J. O'Rourke, J. Yang, M. E. Sise, P. A. Canetta, N. Barasch, C. Buchen, F. Khan, K. Mori, J. Giglio, P. Devarajan and J. Barasch, "Sensitivity and Specificity of a Single Emergency Department Measurement of Urinary Neutrophil Gelatinase-Associated Lipocalin for Diagnosing Acute Kidney Injury," *Annals of Internal Medicine*, Vol. 148, No. 11, 2008, pp. 810-819.

[28] D. Bolignano, A. Lacquaniti, G. Coppolino, V. Donato, S. Campo, M. R. Fazio, G. Nicocia and M. Buemi, "Neutrophil Gelatinase-Associated Lipocalin (NGAL) and Progression of Chronic Kidney Disease," *Clinical Journal of the American Society of Nephrology*, Vol. 4, No. 2, 2009, pp. 337-344. doi:10.2215/CJN.03530708

[29] W. K. Han, V. Bailly, R. Abichandani, R. Thadhani and J. V. Bonventre, "Kidney Injury Molecule-1 (KIM-1): A Novel Biomarker for Human Renal Proximal Tubule Injury," *Kidney International*, Vol. 62, 2002, pp. 237-244. doi:10.1046/j.1523-1755.2002.00433.x

[30] M. M. van Timmeren, M. C. van den Heuvel, V. Bailly, S. J. Bakker, H. van Goor and C. A. Stegeman, "Tubular Kidney Injury Molecule-1 (KIM-1) in Human Renal Disease," *The Journal of Pathology*, Vol. 212, No. 2, 2007, pp. 209-217. doi:10.1002/path.2175

[31] S. E. Nielsen, K. J. Schjoedt, A. S. Astrup, L. Tarnow, M. Lajer, P. R. Hansen, H. H. Parving and P. Rossing, "Neutrophil Gelatinase-Associated Lipocalin (NGAL) and Kidney Injury Molecule 1 (KIM1) in Patients with Diabetic Nephropathy: A Cross-Sectional Study and the Effects of Lisinopril," *Diabetic Medicine*, Vol. 27, No. 10, 2010, pp. 1144-1150. doi:10.1111/j.1464-5491.2010.03083.x

[32] S. E. Nielsen, S. Andersen, D. Zdunek, G. Hess, H. H. Parving and P. Rossing, "Tubular Markers Do Not Predict the Decline in Glomerular Filtration Rate in Type 1 Diabetic Patients with Overt Nephropathy," *Kidney International*, Vol. 79, No. 10, 2011, pp. 1113-1118. doi:10.1038/ki.2010.554

[33] G. L. Warnock, D. M. Thompson, R. M. Meloche, R. J. Shapiro, Z. Ao, P. Keown, J. D. Johnson, C. B. Verchere, N. Partovi, I. S. Begg, M. Fung, S. E. Kozak, S. O. Tong, K. M. Alghofaili and C. Harris, "A Multi-Year Analysis of Islet Transplantation Compared with Intensive Medical Therapy on Progression of Complications in Type 1 Diabetes," *Transplantation*, Vol. 86, No. 12, 2008, pp. 1762-1766. doi:10.1097/TP.0b013e318190b052

[34] M. A. Webb, S. C. Illouz, C. A. Pollard, R. Gregory, J. F. Mayberry, S. G. Tordoff, M. Bone, C. J. Cordle, D. P. Berry, M. L. Nicholson, P. P. Musto and A. R. Dennison, "Islet Auto Transplantation Following Total Pancreatectomy: A Long-Term Assessment of Graft Function," Pancreas, Vol. 37, No. 3, 2008, pp. 282-287. doi:10.1097/mpa.0b013e31816fd7b6

[35] D. L. Vander Jagt, B. Robinson, K. K. Taylor and L. A. Hunsaker, "Aldose Reductase from Human Skeletal and Heart Muscle. Interconvertible Forms Related by Thiol-Disulfide Exchange," *The Journal of Biological Chemistry*, Vol. 265, No. 34, 1990, pp. 20982-20987.

[36] H. Kasajima, S. Yamagishi, S. Sugai, N. Yagihashi and S. Yagihashi, "Enhanced *in Situ* Expression of Aldose Reductase in Peripheral Nerve and Renal Glomeruli in Diabetic Patients," *Virchows Archiv*, Vol. 439, No. 1, 2001, pp. 46-54. doi:10.1007/s004280100444

[37] R. G. Tilton, K. Chang, G. Pugliese, D. M. Eades, M. A. Province, W. R. Sherman, C. Kilo and J. R. Williamson, "Prevention of Hemodynamic and Vascular Albumin Filtration Changes in Diabetic Rats by Aldose Reductase Inhibitors," *Diabetes*, Vol. 38, No. 10, 1989, pp. 1258-1270. doi:10.2337/diabetes.38.10.1258

[38] W. G. Robison Jr., T. N. Tillis, N. Laver and J. H. Kinoshita, "Diabetes-Related Histopathologies of the Rat Retina Prevented with an Aldose Reductase Inhibitor," *Experimental Eye Research*, Vol. 50, No. 4, 1990, pp. 355-366. doi:10.1016/0014-4835(90)90136-I

[39] J. P. Kassab, R. Guillot, J. Andre, N. Claperon, G. Bellon, G. Feldmann, J. Peyroux and M. Sternberg, "Renal and Microvascular Effects of an Aldose Reductase Inhibitor in Experimental Diabetes. Biochemical, Functional and Ultrastructural Studies," *Biochemical Pharmacology*, Vol. 48, No. 5, 1994, pp. 1003-1008. doi:10.1016/0006-2952(94)90371-9

[40] N. Passariello, J. Sepe, G. Marrazzo, A. de Cicco, A. Peluso, M. C. Pisano, S. Sgambato, P. Tesauro and F. D'Onofrio, "Effect of Aldose Reductase Inhibitor (Tolrestat) on Urinary Albumin Excretion Rate and Glomerular Filtration Rate in Iddm Subjects with Nephropathy," *Diabetes Care*, Vol. 16, No. 5, 1993, pp. 789-795. doi:10.2337/diacare.16.5.789

[41] K. Iso, H. Tada, K. Kuboki and T. Inokuchi, "Long-Term Effect of Epalrestat, an Aldose Reductase Inhibitor, on the Development of Incipient Diabetic Nephropathy in Type 2 Diabetic Patients," *Journal of Diabetes and Its Complications*, Vol. 15, No. 5, 2001, pp. 241-244. doi:10.1016/S1056-8727(01)00160-X

[42] A. V. McAuliffe, B. A. Brooks, E. J. Fisher, L. M. Molyneaux and D. K. Yue, "Administration of Ascorbic Acid and an Aldose Reductase Inhibitor (Tolrestat) in Diabetes: Effect on Urinary Albumin Excretion," *Nephron*, Vol. 80, No. 3, 1998, pp. 277-284. doi:10.1159/000045187

[43] G. Andriuoli, R. Mastacchi and M. Barbanti, "Antithrombotic Activity of a Glycosaminoglycan (Sulodexide) in Rats," *Thrombosis Research*, Vol. 34, No. 1, 1984, pp. 81-86. doi:10.1016/0049-3848(84)90108-7

[44] C. A. Solini A, Barzon I and Crepaldi G, "Therapy with Glycosaminoglycans Lowers Albumin Excretion Rate in Non-Insulin Dependent Diabetic Patients with Microalbuminuria," *Diabetes, Nutrition & Metabolism*, Vol. 7, 1994, pp. 304-307.

[45] J. Skrha, J. Perusicova, P. Pontuch and A. Oksa, "Glycosaminoglycan Sulodexide Decreases Albuminuria in Diabetic Patients," *Diabetes Research and Clinical Practice*, Vol. 38, No. 1, 1997, pp. 25-31. doi:10.1016/S0168-8227(97)00076-4

[46] M. Velussi, *et al.*, "Glycosaminoglycans Oral Therapy Reduces Microalbuminuria, Blood Fibrinogen Levels and Limb Arteriopathy Clinical Signs in Patients with Non-Insulin Dependent Diabetes Mellitus," *Diabetes*, *Nutrition & Metabolism*, Vol. 9, 1996, pp. 53-58.

[47] A. Solini, L. Vergnani, F. Ricci and G. Crepaldi, "Glycosaminoglycans Delay the Progression of Nephropathy in NIDDM," *Diabetes Care*, Vol. 20, No. 5, 1997, pp. 819-823. doi:10.2337/diacare.20.5.819

[48] X. Xu, *et al.*, "Mechanism of Action of Sulodexide-Mediated Control of Diabetic Proteinuria: Inhibition of Heparanase-1 Activity," *Journal of the American Society of Nephrology*, Vol. 16, 2005, p. 673.

[49] J. B. Maxhimer, M. Somenek, G. Rao, C. E. Pesce, D. Baldwin, P. Gattuso, M. M. Schwartz, E. J. Lewis, R. A. Prinz and X. Xu, "Heparanase-1 Gene Expression and Regulation by High Glucose in Renal Epithelial Cells: A Potential Role in the Pathogenesis of Proteinuria in Diabetic Patients," *Diabetes*, Vol. 54, No. 7, 2005, pp. 2172-2178. doi:10.2337/diabetes.54.7.2172

[50] G. Gambaro, A. O. Cavazzana, P. Luzi, A. Piccoli, A. Borsatti, G. Crepaldi, E. Marchi, A. P. Venturini and B. Baggio, "Glycosaminoglycans Prevent Morphological Renal Alterations and Albuminuria in Diabetic Rats," *Kid-*

ney International, Vol. 42, 1992, pp. 285-291. doi:10.1038/ki.1992.288

[51] M. Rossini, T. Naito, H. Yang, M. Freeman, E. Donnert, L. J. Ma, S. R. Dunn, K. Sharma and A. B. Fogo, "Sulodexide Ameliorates Early But Not Late Kidney Disease in Models of Radiation Nephropathy and Diabetic Nephropathy," *Nephrology Dialysis Transplantation*, Vol. 25, No. 6, 2010, pp. 1803-1810. doi:10.1093/ndt/gfp724

[52] G. Gambaro, I. Kinalska, A. Oksa, P. Pontuch, M. Hertlova, J. Olsovsky, J. Manitius, D. Fedele, S. Czekalski, J. Perusicova, J. Skrha, J. Taton, W. Grzeszczak and G. Crepaldi, "Oral Sulodexide Reduces Albuminuria in Microalbuminuric and Macroalbuminuric Type 1 and Type 2 Diabetic Patients: The Di.N.A.S. Randomized Trial," *Journal of the American Society of Nephrology*, Vol. 13, No. 6, 2002, pp. 1615-1625. doi:10.1097/01.ASN.0000014254.87188.E5

[53] A. Achour, M. Kacem, K. Dibej, H. Skhiri, S. Bouraoui and M. El May, "One Year Course of Oral Sulodexide in the Management of Diabetic Nephropathy," *Journal of Nephrology*, Vol. 18, No. 5, 2005, pp. 568-574.

[54] H. L. Heerspink, T. Greene, J. B. Lewis, I. Raz, R. D. Rohde, L. G. Hunsicker, S. L. Schwartz, S. Aronoff, M. A. Katz, G. M. Eisner, J. H. Mersey and T. B. Wiegmann, "Effects of Sulodexide in Patients with Type 2 Diabetes and Persistent Albuminuria," *Nephrology Dialysis Transplantation*, Vol. 23, No. 6, 2008, pp. 1946-1954. doi:10.1093/ndt/gfm893

[55] H. J. Lambers Heerspink, *et al.*, "Rationale for and Study Design of the Sulodexide Trials in Type 2 Diabetic, Hypertensive Patients with Microalbuminuria or Overt Nephropathy," *Diabetic Medicine*, Vol. 24, No. 11, 2007, pp. 1290-1295. doi:10.1111/j.1464-5491.2007.02249.x

[56] P. G. Goekjian and M. R. Jirousek, "Protein Kinase C in the Treatment of Disease: Signal Transduction Pathways, Inhibitors and Agents in Development," *Current Medicinal Chemistry*, Vol. 6, No. 9, 1999, pp. 877-903.

[57] K. R. Tuttle, "Protein Kinase C-β Inhibition for Diabetic Kidney Disease," *Diabetes Research and Clinical Practice*, Vol. 82, Suppl. 1, 2008, pp. 70-74. doi:10.1016/j.diabres.2008.09.041

[58] S. Yamagishi, K. Fukami, S. Ueda and S. Okuda, "Molecular Mechanisms of Diabetic Nephropathy and Its Therapeutic Intervention," *Current Drug Targets*, Vol. 8, No. 8, 2007, pp. 952-959. doi:10.2174/138945007781386884

[59] M. Kunisaki, S. E. Bursell, F. Umeda, H. Nawata and G. L. King, "Normalization of Diacylglycerol-Protein Kinase C Activation by Vitamin E in Aorta of Diabetic Rats and Cultured Rat Smooth Muscle Cells Exposed to Elevated Glucose Levels," *Diabetes*, Vol. 43, No. 11, 1994, pp. 1372-1377. doi:10.2337/diabetes.43.11.1372

[60] M. R. Jirousek, J. R. Gillig, C. M. Gonzalez, W. F. Heath, J. H. McDonald, D. A. Neel, C. J. Rito, U. Singh, L. E. Stramm, A. Melikian-Badalian, M. Baevsky, L. M. Ballas, S. E. Hall, L. L. Winneroski and M. M. Faul, "(*S*)13-[(Dimethylamino)methyl]-10,11,14,15-tetrahydro-4,9:16,21-dimetheno-1*H*,13*H*-dibenzo[*e*,*k*]pyrrolo[3,4-h][1,4,13]oxadiazacyclohexadecene-1,3(2*H*)-dione (LY333531) and Related Analogues: Isozyme Selective Inhibitors of Protein Kinase Cβ," *Journal of Medicinal Chemistry*, Vol. 39, No. 14, 1996, pp. 2664-2671. doi:10.1021/jm950588y

[61] H. Ishii, M. R. Jirousek, D. Koya, C. Takagi, P. Xia, A. Clermont, S. E. Bursell, T. S. Kern, L. M. Ballas, W. F. Heath, L. E. Stramm, E. P. Feener and G. L. King, "Amelioration of Vascular Dysfunctions in Diabetic Rats by an Oral PKC β Inhibitor," *Science*, Vol. 272, No. 5262, 1996, pp. 728-731. doi:10.1126/science.272.5262.728

[62] D. Koya, M. Haneda, H. Nakagawa, K. Isshiki, H. Sato, S. Maeda, T. Sugimoto, H. Yasuda, A. Kashiwagi, D. K. Ways, G. L. King and R. Kikkawa, "Amelioration of Accelerated Diabetic Mesangial Expansion by Treatment with a PKC β Inhibitor in Diabetic db/db Mice, a Rodent Model for Type 2 Diabetes," *The FASEB Journal*, Vol. 14, No. 3, 2000, pp. 439-447.

[63] D. J. Kelly, Y. Zhang, C. Hepper, R. M. Gow, K. Jaworski, B. E. Kemp, J. L. Wilkinson-Berka and R. E. Gilbert, "Protein Kinase Cβ Inhibition Attenuates the Progression of Experimental Diabetic Nephropathy in the Presence of Continued Hypertension," *Diabetes*, Vol. 52, No. 2, 2003, pp. 512-518. doi:10.2337/diabetes.52.2.512

[64] K. R. Tuttle, G. L. Bakris, R. D. Toto, J. B. McGill, K. Hu and P. W. Anderson, "The Effect of Ruboxistaurin on Nephropathy in Type 2 Diabetes," *Diabetes Care*, Vol. 28, No. 11, 2005, pp. 2686-2690. doi:10.2337/diacare.28.11.2686

[65] L. P. Aiello, M. D. Davis, A. Girach, K. A. Kles, R. C. Milton, M. J. Sheetz, L. Vignati and X. E. Zhi, "Effect of Ruboxistaurin on Visual Loss in Patients with Diabetic Retinopathy," *Ophthalmology*, Vol. 113, No. 12, 2006, pp. 2221-2230. doi:10.1016/j.ophtha.2006.07.032

[66] K. R. Tuttle, J. B. McGill, D. J. Haney, T. E. Lin and P. W. Anderson, "Kidney Outcomes in Long-Term Studies of Ruboxistaurin for Diabetic Eye Disease," *Clinical Journal of the American Society of Nephrology*, Vol. 2, No. 4, 2007, pp. 631-636. doi:10.2215/CJN.00840207

[67] F. A. van Nieuwenhoven, L. J. Jensen, A. Flyvbjerg and R. Goldschmeding, "Imbalance of Growth Factor Signalling in Diabetic Kidney Disease: Is Connective Tissue Growth Factor (CTGF, CCN2) the Perfect Intervention Point?" *Nephrology Dialysis Transplantation*, Vol. 20, No. 1, 2005, pp. 6-10. doi:10.1093/ndt/gfh570

[68] N. A. Wahab, N. Yevdokimova, B. S. Weston, T. Roberts, X. J. Li, H. Brinkman and R. M. Mason, "Role of Connective Tissue Growth Factor in the Pathogenesis of Diabetic Nephropathy," *Biochemical Journal*, Vol. 359, Pt. 1, 2001, pp. 77-87. doi:10.1042/0264-6021:3590077

[69] L. F. Lau and S. C. Lam, "The CCN Family of Angiogenic Regulators: The Integrin Connection," *Experimental Cell Research*, Vol. 248, No. 1, 1999, pp. 44-57. doi:10.1006/excr.1999.4456

[70] B. L. Riser, M. Denichilo, P. Cortes, C. Baker, J. M. Grondin, J. Yee and R. G. Narins, "Regulation of Connective Tissue Growth Factor Activity in Cultured Rat Mesangial Cells and Its Expression in Experimental Diabetic Glomerulosclerosis," *Journal of the American Society of Nephrology*, Vol. 11, No. 1, 2000, pp. 25-38.

[71] S. M. Twigg, A. H. Joly, M. M. Chen, J. Tsubaki, H. S.

Kim, V. Hwa, Y. Oh and R. G. Rosenfeld, "Connective tissue Growth Factor/IGF-Binding Protein-Related Protein-2 Is a Mediator in the Induction of Fibronectin by Advanced Glycosylation End-Products in Human Dermal Fibroblasts," *Endocrinology*, Vol. 143, No. 4, 2002, pp. 1260-1269. doi:10.1210/en.143.4.1260

[72] G. Zhou, C. Li and L. Cai, "Advanced Glycation End-Products Induce Connective Tissue Growth Factor-Mediated Renal Fibrosis Predominantly through Transforming Growth Factor β-Independent Pathway," *American Journal of Pathology*, Vol. 165, No. 6, 2004, pp. 2033-2043. doi:10.1016/S0002-9440(10)63254-3

[73] N. A. Wahab, B. S. Weston and R. M. Mason, "Connective Tissue Growth Factor CCN2 Interacts with and Activates the Tyrosine Kinase Receptor TrkA," *Journal of the American Society of Nephrology*, Vol. 16, No. 2, 2005, pp. 340-351. doi:10.1681/ASN.2003100905

[74] P. Roestenberg, F. A. van Nieuwenhoven, J. A. Joles, C. Trischberger, P. P. Martens, N. Oliver, J. Aten, J. W. Hoppener and R. Goldschmeding, "Temporal Expression Profile and Distribution Pattern Indicate a Role of Connective Tissue Growth Factor (CTGF/CCN-2) in Diabetic Nephropathy in Mice," *American Journal of Physiology*, Vol. 290, No. 6, 2006, pp. 1344-1354. doi:10.1152/ajprenal.00174.2005

[75] H. Yokoi, M. Mukoyama, T. Nagae, K. Mori, T. Suganami, K. Sawai, T. Yoshioka, M. Koshikawa, T. Nishida, M. Takigawa, A. Sugawara and K. Nakao, "Reduction in Connective Tissue Growth Factor by Antisense Treatment Ameliorates Renal Tubulointerstitial Fibrosis," *Journal of the American Society of Nephrology*, Vol. 15, No. 6, 2004, pp. 1430-1440. doi:10.1097/01.ASN.0000130565.69170.85

[76] H. Okada, T. Kikuta, T. Inoue, Y. Kanno, S. Ban, T. Sugaya, M. Takigawa and H. Suzuki, "Dexamethasone Induces Connective Tissue Growth Factor Expression in Renal Tubular Epithelial Cells in a Mouse Strain-Specific Manner," *American Journal of Pathology*, Vol. 168, No. 3, 2006, pp. 737-747. doi:10.2353/ajpath.2006.050656

[77] A. Flyvbjerg, *et al.*, "Long-Term Renal Effects of a Neutralizing Connective Tissue Growth Factor (Ctgf)-Antibody in Obese Type 2 Diabetic Mice," *Journal of the American Society of Nephrology*, Vol. 15, 2004, p. 261.

[78] Q. Wang, *et al.*, "Amelioration of Diabetic Nephropathy (DN) Incused by Renal Ischemia-Reperfusion (IR) in Rats with Diabetes Mellitus (DM) by Treatment with FG-3019, a Monoclonal Antibody Against Connective Tissue Growth Factor (CTGF)," *Journal of the American Society of Nephrology*, 2004, p. 731.

[79] S. G. Adler, S. Schwartz, M. E. Williams, C. Arauz-Pacheco, W. K. Bolton, T. Lee, D. Li, T. B. Neff, P. R. Urquilla and K. L. Sewell, "Phase 1 Study of Anti-CTGF Monoclonal Antibody in Patients with Diabetes and Microalbuminuria," *Clinical Journal of the American Society of Nephrology*, Vol. 5, No. 8, 2010, pp. 1420-1428. doi:10.2215/CJN.09321209

[80] S. Schwartz, "Phase 1 Study of FG-3019, an Anti-CTGF Monoclonal Antibody, in Type 1/2 Diabetes Mellitus with Microalbuminuria," *Diabetes*, Vol. 56, 2007, p. 151.

[81] W. Qi, X. Chen, P. Poronnik and C. A. Pollock, "Transforming Growth Factor-β/Connective Tissue Growth Factor Axis in the Kidney," *The International Journal of Biochemistry & Cell Biology*, Vol. 40, No. 1, 2008, pp. 9-13. doi:10.1016/j.biocel.2007.01.006

[82] T. A. McGowan, Y. Zhu and K. Sharma, "Transforming Growth Factor-β: A Clinical Target for the Treatment of Diabetic Nephropathy," *Current Diabetes Reports*, Vol. 4, No. 6, 2004, pp. 447-454. doi:10.1007/s11892-004-0055-z

[83] K. Sharma, Y. Jin, J. Guo and F. N. Ziyadeh, "Neutralization of TGF-β by Anti-TGF-β Antibody Attenuates Kidney Hypertrophy and the Enhanced Extracellular Matrix Gene Expression in STZ-Induced Diabetic Mice," *Diabetes*, Vol. 45, 1996, pp. 522-530. doi:10.2337/diabetes.45.4.522

[84] F. N. Ziyadeh, B. B. Hoffman, D. C. Han, M. C. Iglesias-de la Cruz, S. W. Hong, M. Isono, S. Chen, T. A. McGowan and K. Sharma, "Long-Term Prevention of Renal Insufficiency, Excess Matrix Gene Expression and Glomerular Mesangial Matrix Expansion by Treatment with Monoclonal Antitransforming Growth Factor-β Antibody in db/db Diabetic Mice," *Proceedings of the National Academy of Sciences*, Vol. 97, No. 14, 2000, pp. 8015-8020. doi:10.1073/pnas.120055097

[85] K. Sharma, F. N. Ziyadeh, B. Alzahabi, T. A. McGowan, S. Kapoor, B. R. Kurnik, P. B. Kurnik and L. S. Weisberg, "Increased Renal Production of Transforming Growth Factor-β1 in Patients with Type II Diabetes," *Diabetes*, Vol. 46, No. 5, 1997, pp. 854-859. doi:10.2337/diabetes.46.5.854

[86] T. Yamamoto, T. Nakamura, N. A. Noble, E. Ruoslahti and W. A. Border, "Expression of Transforming Growth Factor β Is Elevated in Human and Experimental Diabetic Nephropathy," *Proceedings of the National Academy of Sciences*, Vol. 90, No. 5, 1993, pp. 1814-1818. doi:10.1073/pnas.90.5.1814

[87] S. P. RamachandraRao, Y. Zhu, T. Ravasi, T. A. McGowan, I. Toh, S. R. Dunn, S. Okada, M. A. Shaw and K. Sharma, "Pirfenidone Is Renoprotective in Diabetic Kidney Disease," *Journal of the American Society of Nephrology*, Vol. 20, No. 8, 2009, pp. 1765-1775.

[88] M. Iwano, A. Kubo, T. Nishino, H. Sato, H. Nishioka, Y. Akai, H. Kurioka, Y. Fujii, M. Kanauchi, H. Shiiki and K. Dohi, "Quantification of Glomerular TGF-β1 mRNA in Patients with Diabetes Mellitus," *Kidney International*, Vol. 49, 1996, pp. 1120-1126. doi:10.1038/ki.1996.162

[89] T. Yamamoto, N. A. Noble, A. H. Cohen, C. C. Nast, A. Hishida, L. I. Gold and W. A. Border, "Expression of Transforming Growth Factor-β Isoforms in Human Glomerular Diseases," *Kidney International*, Vol. 49, 1996, pp. 461-469. doi:10.1038/ki.1996.65

[90] K. Sharma, J. H. Ix, A. V. Mathew, M. Cho, A. Pflueger, S. R. Dunn, B. Francos, S. Sharma, B. Falkner, T. A. McGowan, M. Donohue, S. Ramachandrarao, R. Xu, F. C. Fervenza and J. B. Kopp, "Pirfenidone for Diabetic Nephropathy," *Journal of the American Society of Nephrology*, Vol. 22, No. 6, 2011, pp. 1144-1151. doi:10.1681/ASN.2010101049

[91] P. E. Pergola, M. Krauth, J. W. Huff, D. A. Ferguson, S.

Ruiz, C. J. Meyer and D. G. Warnock, "Effect of Bardoxolone Methyl on Kidney Function in Patients with T2D and Stage 3b-4 CKD," *American Journal of Nephrology*, Vol. 33, No. 5, 2011, pp. 469-476. doi:10.1159/000327599

[92] P. E. Pergola, P. Raskin, R. D. Toto, C. J. Meyer, J. W. Huff, E. B. Grossman, M. Krauth, S. Ruiz, P. Audhya, H. Christ-Schmidt, J. Wittes and D. G. Warnock, "Bardoxolone Methyl and Kidney Function in CKD with Type 2 Diabetes," *The New England Journal of Medicine*, Vol. 365, 2011, pp. 327-336. doi:10.1056/NEJMoa1105351

[93] "Retinopathy and Nephropathy in Patients with Type 1 Diabetes Four Years after a Trial of Intensive Therapy. The Diabetes Control and Complications Trial/Epidemiology of Diabetes Interventions and Complications Research Group," *The New England Journal of Medicine*, Vol. 342, 2000, pp. 381-389. doi:10.1056/NEJM200002103420603

[94] "Sustained Effect of Intensive Treatment of Type 1 Diabetes Mellitus on Development and Progression of Diabetic Nephropathy: The Epidemiology of Diabetes Interventions and Complications (EDIC) Study," *The Journal of the American Medical Association*, Vol. 290, No. 16, 2003, pp. 2159-2167. doi:10.1001/jama.290.16.2159

[95] D. M. Nathan, P. A. Cleary, J. Y. Backlund, S. M. Genuth, J. M. Lachin, T. J. Orchard, P. Raskin and B. Zinman, "Intensive Diabetes Treatment and Cardiovascular Disease in Patients with Type 1 Diabetes," *The New England Journal of Medicine*, Vol. 353, 2005, pp. 2643-2653. doi:10.1056/NEJMoa052187

[96] I. M. Stratton, A. I. Adler, H. A. Neil, D. R. Matthews, S. E. Manley, C. A. Cull, D. Hadden, R. C. Turner and R. R. Holman, "Association of Glycaemia with Macrovascular and Microvascular Complications of Type 2 Diabetes (UKPDS 35): Prospective Observational Study," *British Medical Journal*, Vol. 321, 2000, pp. 405-412. doi:10.1136/bmj.321.7258.405

[97] R. R. Holman, S. K. Paul, M. A. Bethel, D. R. Matthews and H. A. Neil, "10-Year Follow-up of Intensive Glucose Control in Type 2 Diabetes," *The New England Journal of Medicine*, Vol. 359, 2008, pp. 1577-1589. doi:10.1056/NEJMoa0806470

[98] UK Prospective Diabetes Study (UKPDS) Group, "Intensive Blood-Glucose Control with Sulphonylureas or Insulin Compared with Conventional Treatment and Risk of Complications in Patients with Type 2 Diabetes (UKPDS 33)," *The Lancet*, Vol. 352, No. 9131, 1998, pp. 837-853. doi:10.1016/S0140-6736(98)07019-6

[99] A. Patel, S. MacMahon, J. Chalmers, B. Neal, L. Billot, M. Woodward, M. Marre, M. Cooper, P. Glasziou, D. Grobbee, P. Hamet, S. Harrap, S. Heller, L. Liu, G. Mancia, C. E. Mogensen, C. Pan, N. Poulter, A. Rodgers, B. Williams, S. Bompoint, B. E. de Galan, R. Joshi and F. Travert, "Intensive Blood Glucose Control and Vascular Outcomes in Patients with Type 2 Diabetes," *The New England Journal of Medicine*, Vol. 358, 2008, pp. 2560-2572. doi:10.1056/NEJMoa0802987

[100] C. E. Mogensen, "Long-Term Antihypertensive Treatment Inhibiting Progression of Diabetic Nephropathy," *British Medical Journal*, Vol. 285, 1982, pp. 685-688. doi:10.1136/bmj.285.6343.685

[101] R. W. Schrier, R. O. Estacio, A. Esler and P. Mehler, "Effects of Aggressive Blood Pressure Control in Normotensive Type 2 Diabetic Patients on Albuminuria, Retinopathy and Strokes," *Kidney International*, Vol. 61, 2002, pp. 1086-1097. doi:10.1046/j.1523-1755.2002.00213.x

[102] UK Prospective Diabetes Study Group, "Tight Blood Pressure Control and Risk of Macrovascular and Microvascular Complications in Type 2 Diabetes: UKPDS 38," *British Medical Journal*, Vol. 317, 1998, pp. 703-713. doi:10.1136/bmj.317.7160.703

[103] UK Prospective Diabetes Study Group, "Cost Effectiveness Analysis of Improved Blood Pressure Control in Hypertensive Patients with Type 2 Diabetes: UKPDS 40," *British Medical Journal*, Vol. 317, 1998, pp. 720-726. doi:10.1136/bmj.317.7160.720

[104] A. Patel, S. MacMahon, J. Chalmers, B. Neal, M. Woodward, L. Billot, S. Harrap, N. Poulter, M. Marre, M. Cooper, P. Glasziou, D. E. Grobbee, P. Hamet, S. Heller, L. S. Liu, G. Mancia, C. E. Mogensen, C. Y. Pan, A. Rodgers and B. Williams, "Effects of a Fixed Combination of Perindopril and Indapamide on Macrovascular and Microvascular Outcomes in Patients with Type 2 Diabetes Mellitus (the ADVANCE trial): A Randomised Controlled Trial," *The Lancet*, Vol. 370, No. 9590, 2007, pp. 829-840. doi:10.1016/S0140-6736(07)61303-8

[105] B. E. de Galan, V. Perkovic, T. Ninomiya, A. Pillai, A. Patel, A. Cass, B. Neal, N. Poulter, S. Harrap, C. E. Mogensen, M. Cooper, M. Marre, B. Williams, P. Hamet, G. Mancia, M. Woodward, P. Glasziou, D. E. Grobbee, S. MacMahon and J. Chalmers, "Lowering Blood Pressure Reduces Renal Events in Type 2 Diabetes," *Journal of the American Society of Nephrology*, Vol. 20, No. 4, 2009, pp. 883-892. doi:10.1681/ASN.2008070667

[106] A. V. Chobanian, G. L. Bakris, H. R. Black, W. C. Cushman, L. A. Green, J. L. Izzo, D. W. Jones, B. J. Materson, S. Oparil, J. T. Wright and E. J. Roccella, "Seventh Report of the Joint National Committee on Prevention, Detection, Evaluation and Treatment of High Blood Pressure," *Hypertension*, Vol. 42, 2003, pp. 1206-1252. doi:10.1161/01.HYP.0000107251.49515.c2

[107] American Diabetes Association, "Standards of Medical Care in Diabetes," *Diabetes Care*, Vol. 28, Suppl. 1, 2005, pp. 4-36. doi:10.2337/diacare.28.suppl_1.S4

[108] Kidney Disease Outcomes Quality Initiative (K/DOQI), "K/DOQI Clinical Practice Guidelines on Hypertension and Antihypertensive Agents in Chronic Kidney Disease," *American Journal of Kidney Disease*, Vol. 43, No. 5, 2004, pp. 1-290. doi:10.1053/j.ajkd.2003.11.027

[109] The ACCORD Study Group, "Effects of Intensive Blood-Pressure Control in Type 2 Diabetes Mellitus," *The New England Journal of Medicine*, 2010, Vol. 362, pp. 1575-1585. doi:10.1056/NEJMoa1001286

[110] The EUCLID Study Group, "Randomised Placebo-Controlled Trial of Lisinopril in Normotensive Patients with Insulin-Dependent Diabetes and Normoalbuminuria or Microalbuminuria," *Lancet*, Vol. 349, No. 9068, 1997, pp. 1787-1792. doi:10.1016/S0140-6736(96)10244-0

[111] M. Ravid, D. Brosh, Z. Levi, Y. Bar-Dayan, D. Ravid and R. Rachmani, "Use of Enalapril to Attenuate Decline in Renal Function in Normotensive, Normoalbuminuric Patients with Type 2 Diabetes Mellitus," *Annals of Internal Medicine*, Vol. 128, No. 12, 1998, pp. 982-988.

[112] R. O. Estacio, B. W. Jeffers, N. Gifford and R. W. Schrier, "Effect of Blood Pressure Control on Diabetic Microvascular Complications in Patients with Hypertension and Type 2 Diabetes," *Diabetes Care*, Vol. 23, Suppl. 2, 2000, pp. 54-64.

[113] M. Ravid, H. Savin, I. Jutrin, T. Bental, B. Katz and M. Lishner, "Long-Term Stabilization of Angiotensin-Converting Enzyme Inhibition on Plasma Creatinine and on Proteinuria in Normotensive Type II Diabetic Patients," *Annals of Internal Medicine*, Vol. 118, 1993, pp. 577-581.

[114] S. Andersen, L. Tarnow, P. Rossing, B. V. Hansen and H. H. Parving, "Renoprotective Effects of Angiotensin II Receptor Blockade in Type 1 Diabetic Patients with Diabetic Nephropathy," *Kidney International*, Vol. 57, 2000, pp. 601-606. doi:10.1046/j.1523-1755.2000.00880.x

[115] B. M. Brenner, M. E. Cooper, D. de Zeeuw, W. F. Keane, W. E. Mitch, H. H. Parving, G. Remuzzi, S. M. Snapinn, Z. Zhang and S. Shahinfar, "Effects of Losartan on Renal and Cardiovascular Outcomes in Patients with Type 2 Diabetes and Nephropathy," *The New England Journal of Medicine*, Vol. 345, 2001, pp. 861-869. doi:10.1056/NEJMoa011161

[116] E. J. Lewis, L. G. Hunsicker, W. R. Clarke, T. Berl, M. A. Pohl, J. B. Lewis, E. Ritz, R. C. Atkins, R. Rohde and I. Raz, "Renoprotective Effect of the Angiotensin-Receptor Antagonist Irbesartan in Patients with Nephropathy Due to Type 2 Diabetes," *The New England Journal of Medicine*, Vol. 345, 2001, pp. 851-860. doi:10.1056/NEJMoa011303

[117] H. H. Parving, H. Lehnert, J. Brochner-Mortensen, R. Gomis, S. Andersen and P. Arner, "The Effect of Irbesartan on the Development of Diabetic Nephropathy in Patients with Type 2 Diabetes," *The New England Journal of Medicine*, Vol. 345, 2001, pp. 870-878. doi:10.1056/NEJMoa011489

[118] Y. Uresin, A. A. Taylor, C. Kilo, D. Tschope, M. Santonastaso, G. Ibram, H. Fang and A. Satlin, "Efficacy and Safety of the Direct Renin Inhibitor Aliskiren and Ramipril Alone or in Combination in Patients with Diabetes and Hypertension," *Journal of the Renin-Angiotensin-Aldosterone System*, Vol. 8, No. 4, 2007, pp. 190-198. doi:10.3317/jraas.2007.028

[119] H. H. Parving, F. Persson, J. B. Lewis, E. J. Lewis and N. K. Hollenberg, "Aliskiren Combined with Losartan in Type 2 Diabetes and Nephropathy," *The New England Journal of Medicine*, Vol. 358, 2008, pp. 2433-2446. doi:10.1056/NEJMoa0708379

[120] M. J. Dunn, "Prostaglandins, Angiotension II, and Proteinuria," *Nephron*, Vol. 55, Suppl. 1, 1990, pp. 30-37. doi:10.1159/000186032

[121] W. R. Melchior, V. Bindlish and L. A. Jaber, "Angiotensin-Converting Enzyme Inhibitors in Diabetic Nephropathy," *The Annals of Pharmacotherapy*, Vol. 27, 1993, pp. 344-350.

[122] G. L. Bakris, M. R. Weir, M. Secic, B. Campbell and A. Weis-McNulty, "Differential Effects of Calcium Antagonist Subclasses on Markers of Nephropathy Progression," *Kidney International*, Vol. 65, 2004, pp. 1991-2002. doi:10.1111/j.1523-1755.2004.00620.x

[123] G. Remuzzi, P. Ruggenenti and A. Benigni, "Understanding the Nature of Renal Disease Progression," *Kidney International*, Vol. 51, 1997, pp. 2-15. doi:10.1038/ki.1997.2

[124] H. J. Kloke, A. J. Branten, F. T. Huysmans and J. F. Wetzels, "Antihypertensive Treatment of Patients with Proteinuric Renal Diseases: Risks or Benefits of Calcium Channel Blockers?" *Kidney International*, Vol. 53, 1998, pp. 1559-1573. doi:10.1046/j.1523-1755.1998.00912.x

[125] R. T. Gansevoort, W. J. Sluiter, M. H. Hemmelder, D. de Zeeuw and P. E. de Jong, "Antiproteinuric Effect of Blood-Pressure-Lowering Agents: A Meta-Analysis of Comparative Trials," *Nephrology Dialysis Transplantation*, Vol. 10, 1995, pp. 1963-1974.

[126] G. L. Bakris, "Effects of Diltiazem or Lisinopril on Massive Proteinuria Associated with Diabetes Mellitus," *Annals of Internal Medicine*, Vol. 112, No. 9, 1990, pp. 707-708.

[127] G. L. Bakris, J. B. Copley, N. Vicknair, R. Sadler and S. Leurgans, "Calcium Channel Blockers Versus Other Antihypertensive Therapies on Progression of NIDDM Associated Nephropathy," *Kidney International*, Vol. 50, 1996, pp. 1641-1650. doi:10.1038/ki.1996.480

[128] G. Tonolo, M. Velussi, E. Brocco, C. Abaterusso, A. Carraro, G. Morgia, A. Satta, R. Faedda, A. Abhyankar, H. Luthman and R. Nosadini, "Simvastatin Maintains Steady Patterns of GFR and Improves AER and Expression of Slit Diaphragm Proteins in Type II Diabetes," *Kidney International*, Vol. 70, 2006, pp. 177-186. doi:10.1038/sj.ki.5001515

[129] R. W. Bilous, S. M. Mauer, D. E. Sutherland, J. S. Najarian, F. C. Goetz and M. W. Steffes, "The Effects of Pancreas Transplantation on the Glomerular Structure of Renal Allografts in Patients with Insulin-Dependent Diabetes," *The New England Journal of Medicine*, Vol. 321, No. 2, 1989, pp. 80-85. doi:10.1056/NEJM198907133210204

Antihypertensive Therapy in Non-Diabetic Chronic Kidney Disease Associated with Proteinuria in Adults

Khawar Maqsood[1], Adeel Siddiqui[2], Geoffrey Teehan[2*]
[1]Department of Medicine, Baystate Medical Center, Tufts University School of Medicine, Springfield, USA
[2]Department of Nephrology, Lankenau Medical Center, Lankenau Institute for Medical Research, Wynnewood, USA
Email: *gteehan@comcast.net

ABSTRACT

Controlling blood pressure and reducing proteinuria are common goals in Chronic Kidney Disease associated with hypertension and proteinuria and lead to fewer cardiovascular outcomes. This review summarizes the available literature.

Keywords: Hypertension; Proteinuria; Chronic Kidney Disease

1. Introduction

Proteinuria is a risk factor for progression of chronic kidney disease (CKD) and is associated with adverse cardiovascular outcomes. Controlling blood pressure particularly with strongly anti-proteinuric agents slows the progression of chronic kidney disease (CKD) and delays/ prevents cardiovascular outcomes. Angiotensin converting enzyme inhibitors (ACE-I) and angiotensin receptor antagonists (ARBs) have a blood pressure-independent antiproteinuric effect and are considered first line agents in this scenario [1]. This review will apprise the literature to date on antihypertensive agents studied in non-diabetic proteinuric kidney disease. **Table 1** summarizes these trials.

2. ACE Inhibitors

Captopril was the first ACE-I approved by Food and Drug Administration (FDA) in 1981 followed by enalapril which was marketed two years later. Since then at least twelve other ACE-I have been marketed. Multiple trials have identified a preferential benefit of ACE-I in reducing proteinuria when compared with other antihypertensive drugs. The basis of all these studies was the observation that protein excretion varies directly with the intra-glomerular pressure in animals with structural glomerular disease [2].

Apart from the reduction in intra-glomerular pressure, a variety of other mechanisms may contribute to ACE-I induced reduction in proteinuria. These include:

- The hemodynamic effects of ACE inhibition occur rapidly but then become stable, whereas protein excretion progressively decreases over weeks to several months [3].
- Acute administration of angiotensin II increases intraglomerular pressure by causing renal and systemic vasoconstriction but does not reverse the antiproteinuric effect of ACE-I [4].
- Nephrin is a major component of the podocyte slit pore membrane and an important contributor to the glomerular filtration barrier. Angiotensin II reduces the expression of nephrin [5]. In contrast, ACE-I increase expression of nephrin [6].
- ACE-I may contribute to slowing of renal disease by their possible anti fibrotic properties.
- ACE-I related reduction in proteinuria may be associated with a reduction in serum lipid level which may have a beneficial effect on progression of renal disease and systemic atherosclerosis.

Multiple clinical trials have demonstrated a beneficial effect of antihypertensive therapy with renin-angiotensin system (RAS) inhibitors, mostly ACE-I in patients with proteinuric non-diabetic chronic kidney disease (CKD).

Jafar *et al* studied 1860 patients with CKD in 11 randomized controlled trials (RCT) and the response to ACE-I versus other antihypertensives or placebo [7]. ACE-I use was associated with significant reductions in the rate of progression to end-stage renal disease (ESRD) (7.4% versus 11.6%, RR 0.69, 95% CI 0.51 - 0.94), while that for doubling of the baseline serum creatinine concentration or ESRD was 13.2 versus 20.5 percent (RR 0.70, 95% CI 0.55 - 0.88) independent of blood pressure

*Corresponding author.

Table 1. Studies of antihypertensive treatment in patients with chronic kidney disease.

Study	Design/Intervention	Effect on GFR	Effect on Proteinuria	Cardiovascular outcomes	Others
Maione et al[9]	SR of 85 RCT. 21,708 patients. ACE-I, ARBs and combination therapy in patients with albuminuria and other cardiovascular risk factors.	ACE-I better than placebo. ARB better than placebo. Combination not better than monotherapy.	ACE-I better than placebo. ARB better than placebo. Combination not better than monotherapy	Better with ACE-I versus placebo only.	N/A
Benazepril trial[10]	583 patients, 300 patients received benazepril and 283 received placebo. Primary end point: doubling of the baseline Cr or the need for HD.	Benazepril better than placebo for primary end point.	Benazepril therapy reduced protein excretion by 25 percent compared with placebo.	N/A	Outcomes better in patients with glomerular diseases, diabetic nephropathy and those with baseline urinary protein excretion >1 g/24 hr.
REIN trial[11]	Prospective double-blind trial, 352 patients were classified according to baseline proteinuria • 1 - 3 g/24 h • ≥ 3 g/24 h Randomly assigned to ramipril or placebo plus conventional antihypertensive therapy targeted at achieving diastolic blood pressure under 90 mm Hg. Primary end point: rate of GFR decline.	Significantly lower rate of GFR decline with ramipril.	In patients with baseline proteinuria of 3 g/24 h or higher, ramipril was more Reno protective than placebo	N/A	More benefits seen with higher proteinuria.
REIN-2 trial[13]	Multicenter RCT, 338 patients on ramipril were randomized to intensified control with felodipine vs conventional blood pressure control. Primary outcome was progression to ESRD.	No benefit seen with intensified BP control with felodipine.	N/A	N/A	No Reno protection in patients with nondiabetic proteinuric renal disease with dihydropyridine calcium channel blockers.
AASK trial[14]	1094 African American patients with hypertensive renal disease. Randomly assigned to ramipril, amlodipine or metoprolol Primary outcome: rate of change in GFR. Secondary outcome: composite endpoint of r eduction in GFR of more than 50% or more than 25 mL/min per 1.73 m^2; ESRD; or death.	At 3 years, ramipril significantly reduced the relative risk of the composite endpoint but not primary outcome. Beneficial effect of ramipril was seen in patients with urine protein-to-Cr ratio >0.22 (300 mg protein/24 hr).	N/A	Ramipril showed benefit in patients with urine protein-to-Cr ratio >0.22.	N/A
ONTARGET[19]	ACE-I and ARB combination versus monotherapy. 5623 patients with estimated GFR less than 60 mL/min per 1.73 m^2 and/or proteinuria.	ACE + ARB resulted in a small but significant increase in the incidence of ESRD and a non significant increase in ESRD alone.	N/A	Combination therapy not better than monotherapy.	Higher potassium level with combination therapy.

Abbreviations: SR systematic review, RCT randomized controlled trial, ACE-I angiotensin converting enzyme inhibitor, ARB angiotensin receptor blocker, Cr creatinine, GFR glomerular filtration rate, HD hemodialysis control. These benefits of ACE-I correlated with increasing baseline proteinuria but did not apply to those with proteinuria below 500 to 1000 mg/day [8].

Maione *et al.* conducted a systematic review of 85 RCTs (21,708 subjects) to look at ACE-I, ARBs and combination therapy in patients with microalbuminuria, macroalbuminuria and other cardiovascular risk factors [9]. Neither ACE I, ARB, nor the combination of the two was associated with a significant reduction in the risk of all-cause mortality or fatal cardiac-cerebrovascular events. ACE I, and not ARB, did however reduce the risk of nonfatal cardiovascular events. Development of ESRD disease and progression of microalbuminuria to macroalbuminuria were reduced significantly with ACE-I versus placebo, ARB versus placebo but not with combined therapy with ACE-I and ARB versus monotherapy. Authors concluded that ACE-I and ARB exert independent renal and nonfatal cardiovascular benefits while their effects on mortality and fatal cardiovascular disease are uncertain. Use of combination therapy was not supported by the evidence.

Maschio et al. performed a placebo-controlled RCT involving 583 patients with renal insufficiency (creatinine clearance 30 - 60 ml per minute) in which 300 patients received benazepril and 283 received placebo. The primary end point was a doubling of the baseline serum creatinine concentration or the need for dialysis. At three years the risk reduction attributed to benazepril was 53 percent overall (95% CI, 27% - 70%) and was particularly evident in milder kidney disease. The risk reduction was greatest among men; those with glomerular diseases, diabetic nephropathy, or miscellaneous or unknown causes of renal disease; and those with baseline urinary protein excretion above 1 g per 24 hours. Benazepril was not effective in patients with polycystic kidney disease [10].

The Ramipril Efficacy in Nephropathy (REIN) trial was a RCT in which patients (N = 352) with proteinuric non-diabetic CKD were randomized to ramipril or placebo plus other antihypertensive therapy to attain a diastolic pressure below 90 mmHg. It showed similar benefits as the Maschio trial [11]. Stratified by level of daily proteinuria, the primary endpoint was the rate of glomerular filtration rate (GFR) decline. The trial was terminated prematurely in patients excreting more than 3 grams of protein per day because of a significant benefit with ACE-I in ameliorating the rate of decline of renal function (0.53 versus 0.88 mL/min per month for placebo). Subsequently all patients with proteinuria of 3 g or more per 24 h either continued on ramipril or were shifted to ramipril.

A REIN follow-up study compared the rate of decline of renal function and the need for dialysis in patients who continued to receive ramipril (51 patients) and in those originally randomized to conventional antihypertensive therapy plus placebo who were switched to ramipril at the beginning of the observational follow-up (46 patients). At 20 months (and at 44 months for the trial phase and observational follow-up combined), mean rate of GFR decline slowed significantly and end of trial GFRs were significantly higher in the ramipril group (36 vs 24 ml per minute, P = 0.01). Progression to ESRD was more common in those receiving placebo (35 versus 19, P = 0.027) [12]. The original and follow-up ramipril studies strongly suggest that patients who particularly benefit are those with prominent proteinuria, but significant benefit was also seen in patients with sub-nephrotic proteinuria (1.0 to 2.9 g/day).

REIN-2 evaluated lowering blood pressure beyond usual targets in patients with chronic nephropathies using ACE I. Patients receiving ACE I (Ramipril 2.5 - 5 mg/d) with non-diabetic proteinuric CKD (mean baseline GFR 35 mL/min and mean proteinuria 2.9 g/day, N = 338) were enrolled in this RCT [13]. Subjects were randomly assigned to either conventional (diastolic < 90 mm Hg; n = 169) or intensified (systolic/diastolic < 130/80 mm Hg; n = 169) blood-pressure control with Felodipine (5 - 10 mg/day) added as needed to achieve the intensified blood-pressure level. The primary outcome measure, time to ESRD over 36 months did not differ between the two groups (20% vs 23%, P = 0.99). Further blood pressure reduction with Felodipine therefore is not warranted to slow progression to ESRD in this population. These findings are consistent with previous observations showing that dihydropyridine calcium channel blockers fail to provide renoprotection in patients with non-diabetic proteinuric renal disease.

Hypertension and ESRD are more prevalent among African Americans than Caucasians. Monotherapy with a calcium channel blocker or a diuretic may be superior in this population than ACE-I. The African American Study of Kidney Disease and Hypertension (AASK trial) [14] included 1094 African American patients with hypertensive renal disease. Mean GFR was 46 ml/min (range 20-65 mL/min per 1.73 m^2) and mean protein excretion was about 600 mg/day in men and 400 mg/day in women. Patients were randomly assigned to three different antihypertensive drugs and to two different blood pressure goals. The blood pressure target was a mean arterial pressure of 92 mm Hg or less in the intensive-control group (corresponds to lower than the traditional blood-pressure target of 130/80 mm Hg for CKD) and 102 to 107 mm Hg in the standard-control group (corresponds to the traditional blood-pressure target of 140/90 mm Hg). Patients were randomly assigned to treatment with an ACE inhibitor (ramipril, 2.5 - 10 mg/day), a calcium channel blocker (amlodipine, 5 - 10 mg/day), or a beta blocker (metoprolol, 50 - 200 mg day); other antihypertensive drugs were added to initial monotherapy to achieve the blood pressure goals. The primary outcome was the rate of change in GFR; the main secondary outcome was a composite endpoint of: reduction in GFR of more than 50 percent or more than 25 mL/min per 1.73 m^2; ESRD; or death.

Although the GFR decline with ramipril and amlodipine therapy were similar at 3 years, ramipril significantly reduced the relative risk of the composite endpoint by 38 percent. Additionally, ramipril was significantly better at slowing GFR decline among those with a urine protein-to creatinine ratio >0.22 (approximately equivalent to 300 mg protein in 24 hours). It also showed that sustained-release metoprolol has antiproteinuric effects nearly equal to that of ramipril ($P = 0.06$ for the comparison of total change over 4 years) and better than that of amlodipine. Proteinuria increased by 58% for the amlodipine group and declined by 14% in the sustained-release metoprolol group between baseline and 6 months ($P < 0.001$) [14].

After completion of the AASK trial, all of the participants were invited to enroll in a cohort phase during which ramipril was prescribed to everyone. After an additional five years of follow-up progression of nephropathy was significantly slowed but not stopped [15].

2.1. Use of ACEI/ARB in Advanced CKD

The pitfalls of using an ACE-I or ARBs in advanced CKD include an initial GFR decline and hyperkalemia, prompting many practitioners to avoid their use. Fan Fan Hou *et al.* enrolled 422 patients with non-diabetic CKD and randomly assigned them to benazepril or placebo plus other antihypertensive therapy to attain a systolic and diastolic pressure below 130 and 80 mmHg, respectively [16]. Patients were divided into two groups based on renal function: Group 1 (N = 141, Serum Creatinine 1.5 - 3.0 mg/dL; mean GFR 37 ml/min/1.73 m^2, mean proteinuria 1.6 g/d) and Group 2 (N = 281, Serum Creatinine 3.1 - 5.0 mg/dL, mean GFR 26 ml/min/1.73m^2, mean proteinuria 1.6 g/d).

After an eight-week run-in period in which they received benazepril at 10 mg/day for four weeks 104 patients remained in Group 1 and 224 remained in Group 2. Group 1 subjects then received benazepril (at 10 mg twice daily, since it was deemed unethical to administer placebo), while Group 2 participants were randomly assigned to benazepril (10 mg twice daily) or placebo. Additional antihypertensive therapy was administered to attain blood pressure goals. The primary endpoint was the composite of doubling of the serum creatinine level, ESRD, or death, while secondary endpoints were change in proteinuria and rate of progression of the renal disease.

At a mean follow up of 3.4 years, significantly fewer Group 2 patients (mean GFR of 26 mL/min per 1.73 m^2) treated with benazepril reached the primary endpoint (41 versus 60 percent with placebo), resulting in an overall risk reduction of 43 percent with active therapy. The primary endpoint was reached less often in group 1 patients (22 percent), who had less severe disease and were all treated with benazepril.

In group 2 doubling of the serum creatinine and reaching ESRD occurred in 51 and 40% fewer patients receiving Benazepril. Fall in proteinuria (52 versus 20 percent) and a slower rate of decline in GFR (6.8 versus 8.8 mL/min per 1.73 m^2 per year) were also noticed. The benefits with benazepril were independent of blood pressure. Benazepril conferred substantial renal benefits in highly selected patients without diabetes who had advanced renal insufficiency.

The *REIN* trial confirms the benefit from ACE-I in patients with advanced CKD. As previously mentioned, patients with an initial GFR within the lowest group (11 to 33 mL/min/1.73 m^2) had a 20 percent decrease in the rate of decline in GFR and a 33 percent reduction in the incidence of end-stage renal disease.

2.2. Use of ACE I in Elderly Patients

The benefits from RAS inhibition in proteinuric CKD patients older than 70 years are largely unknown. Most of the above trials did not include such individuals since older patients with CKD are less likely to have proteinuria. This is confirmed by an analysis of 1190 National Health and Nutrition Examination Survey (NHANES) participants who were over age 70 and had CKD, which was defined as an estimated GFR < 60 mL/min per 1.73 m^2 or an albumin-to-creatinine ratio >200 mg/g of creatinine (approximately 300 mg/day) [17]. This level of proteinuria was present in only 13 percent. There is no evidence of benefit from RAS inhibition in patients with protein excretion below 500 mg/day. It suggests that the great majority of patients over age 70 with CKD would not benefit from RAS inhibition for renal protection and may have harm from a higher rate of side effects. However, this does not fully apply on patients excreting more than 1 g/day. Treatment of proteinuric individuals over the age of 70 with CKD remains an area for investigation.

2.3. Combination of ACE Inhibitors and ARBs

A number of small trials have shown that combination ACE-I and ARB therapy has a greater antiproteinuric effect than either agent alone. A meta-analysis of 14 trials in non-diabetic renal disease found that combination therapy produced a significant 18% - 25% greater reduction in proteinuria compared with monotherapy [18]. These trials did not attempt to identify a maximum antiproteinuric dose, did not compare combination therapy to high dose monotherapy, and did not assess renal outcomes.

Combination therapy however may have adverse effects in proteinuric CKD. The *ONTARGET* trial evaluated combination therapy versus monotherapy in a subset of 5623 patients who, at baseline, had reduced renal function (defined as an estimated GFR less than 60 mL/min per 1.73 m^2) and/or proteinuria [19]. Combination therapy resulted in a small but significant increase in the incidence of ESRD or doubling of the serum creatinine (0.79 versus 0.56 percent per year), but a nonsignificant increase in ESRD alone (0.34 versus 0.27 percent per year) and caused more hyperkalemia while failing to reduce the risk of cardiovascular disease or death [20].

3. Other Antihypertensive Drugs

3.1. Calcium Channel Blockers

Numerous studies suggest that the dihydropyridine calcium antagonists (DCAs) and non-dihydropyridine calcium antagonists (NDCAs) have differential antiproteinuric effects. The NDCAs, such as diltiazem and verapamil are generally considered to have significant antiproteinuric effects while DCAs, such as amlodipine and nifedipine either have no effect or cause a small rise in protein excretion [21].

Bakris *et al.* systematically reviewed 23 studies of NDCA versus DCA and found NDCAs decreased mean proteinuria by 30 percent and DCAs increased proteinuria by 2 percent (95% CI 10% - 54% for the differences between the two drug classes). Similar observations were noted when these agents were used in combination with ACE-I or ARBs: despite similar reductions in blood pressure, the mean change in proteinuria was minus 39 and plus 2 percent for NDCAs and DCAs, respectively. They concluded that NDCA and DCAs lower blood pressure equivalently, but that NDCAs are superior to DCAs in reducing proteinuria in both diabetic and non-diabetic kidney disease [21].

3.2. Aldosterone Antagonists

Addition of aldosterone antagonists may provide renal benefits to proteinuric CKD patients over and above the inhibition of RAS blockers by virtue of partially eliminating secondary hyperaldosteronism. Navaneethan *et al.* performed a meta- analysis of 11 trials in which patients were treated with an ACE-I and/or ARB plus either spironolactone (usually 25 mg/day) or placebo and found a significantly greater reduction in proteinuria in the spironolactone group (weighted mean difference 800 mg/day, 95% CI 330 - 1270 mg/day). Short-term changes in GFR (less than one year of follow-up) were similar with spironolactone and placebo. However, most of these studies did not first maximize the dose of the ACE-I or ARB, and the aldosterone antagonist was associated with an increased risk of hyperkalemia (relative risk 3.1 in the meta-analysis) [22]. Longer-term data are lacking in this field.

3.3. Direct Renin Inhibitors

Aliskiren, being the first oral direct renin inhibitor (DRI) became available in the United States in March 2007. A number of studies have evaluated the blood pressure lowering effect of aliskiren in combination with other antihypertensive drugs [23-26]. Its novel mechanism of action, inhibition of catalytic activity of renin, the most proximal and rate-limiting step in RAS activation, makes it of particular interest. In the *AVOID trial*, aliskiren plus losartan was associated with a 20 percent greater reduction in proteinuria compared with losartan alone in patients with type-2 diabetes and nephropathy in the absence of a significantly greater effect on blood pressure [27]. However, this effect on proteinuria did not translate into a clinical benefit.

In the *ALTITUDE trial*, 8600 patients with type-2 diabetes and kidney disease already taking either an ACE-I or ARB were randomly assigned to additional therapy with aliskiren or placebo [28]. The trial was terminated early due to no benefit on the primary cardiovascular and renal outcomes and the preliminary analysis indicated that aliskiren therapy produced a higher rate of adverse events (i.e., non-fatal stroke, hypotension, hyperkalemia) [29]. Other studies also described an increased risk of hyperkalemia when aliskiren is combined with ACE-I or ARB [30]. Thus, aliskiren should not be combined with ACE-I or ARBs.

3.4. Drugs with Little or No Effect

Other antihypertensive drugs have little or no effect on protein excretion. As an example, beta blockers, diuretics, and the alpha-1-blockers (such as prazosin) typically have a lesser antiproteinuric effect than RAS inhibitors [31-33]. A meta-analysis showed that ACE-I lowered protein excretion by 40 percent compared with 16 percent for beta blockers and 14 percent for other non-calcium channel blocker antihypertensive drugs [31]. Methyldopa and Guanfacine, have little effect on protein excretion.

4. Conclusion

Proteinuria is associated with adverse renal and cardiovascular outcomes. Retarding proteinuria in CKD slows progression of CKD and can limit some cardiovascular outcomes. ACE-I and ARBs are the first line agents in this setting because they have a blood pressure-independent antiproteinuric effect and have shown to improve renal and cardiovascular outcomes. If proteinuria is not controlled with ACE-I or ARB, combination therapy is generally discouraged. We recommend the addition of an NDCA such as diltiazem or verapamil, long acting metoprolol or a mineralocorticoid antagonist as the next line agent. Aggressive measures must be taken to improve blood pressure and reduce proteinuria for better renal and cardiovascular outcomes.

REFERENCES

[1] P. A. Sarafidis, N. Khosla and G. L. Bakris, "Antihypertensive Therapy in the Presence of Proteinuria," *American Journal of Kidney Diseases*, Vol. 49, No. 1, 2007, pp. 12-26. doi:10.1053/j.ajkd.2006.10.014

[2] T. Yoshioka, H. G. Rennke, D. J. Salant, W. M. Deen and I. Ichikawa, "Role of Abnormally High Transmural Pressure in the Permselectivity Defect of Glomerular Capillary Wall: A Study in Early Passive Heymann Nephritis," *Circulation Research*, Vol. 61, No. 4, 1987, p. 531. doi:10.1161/01.RES.61.4.531

[3] R. T. Gansevoort, D. de Zeeuw and P. E. de Jong, "Dissociation between the Course of the Hemodynamic and Antiproteinuric Effects of Angiotensin I Converting Enzyme Inhibition," *Kidney International*, Vol. 44, No. 3, 1993, pp. 579-584. doi:10.1038/ki.1993.284

[4] J. E. Heeg, P. E. de Jong, G. K. van der Hem and D. de Zeeuw, "Angiotensin II Does Not Acutely Reverse the Reduction of Proteinuria by Long-Term ACE Inhibition," *Kidney International*, Vol. 40, No. 4, 1991, pp. 734-741. doi:10.1038/ki.1991.268

[5] F. N. Ziyadeh and G. Wolf, "Pathogenesis of the Podocytopathy and Proteinuria in Diabetic Glomerulopathy," *Current Diabetes Reviews*, Vol. 4, No. 1, 2008, pp. 39-45. doi:10.2174/157339908783502370

[6] R. G. Langham, D. J. Kelly, A. J. Cox, N. M. Thomson, H. Holthöfer, P. Zaoui, N. Pinel, D. J. Cordonnier and R. E. Gilbert, "Proteinuria and the Expression of the Podocyte Slit Diaphragm Protein, Nephrin, in Diabetic Nephropathy: Effects of Angiotensin Converting Enzyme Inhibition," *Diabetologia*, Vol. 45, No. 11, 2002, pp. 1572-1576. doi:10.1007/s00125-002-0946-y

[7] T. H. Jafar, C. H. Schmid, M. Landa, I. Giatras, R. Toto, G. Remuzzi, G. Maschio, B. M. Brenner, A. Kamper, P. Zucchelli, G. Becker, A. Himmelmann, K. Bannister, P. Landais, S. Shahinfar, P. E. de Jong, D. de Zeeuw, J. Lau and A. S. Levey, "Angiotensin-Converting Enzyme Inhibitors and Progression of Nondiabetic Renal Disease. A Meta-Analysis of Patient-Level Data," *Annals of Internal Medicine*, Vol. 135, No. 2, 2001, pp. 73-87. doi:10.7326/0003-4819-135-2-200107170-00007

[8] D. M Kent, T. H. Jafar, R. A. Hayward, H. Tighiouart, M. P. Landa, de Jong, D. de Zeeuw, G. Remuzzi, A. L. Kamper and A. S. Levey, "Progression Risk, Urinary Protein Excretion, and Treatment Effects of Angiotensin-Converting Enzyme Inhibitors in Nondiabetic Kidney Disease," *Journal of the American Society of Nephrology*, Vol. 18, No. 6, 2007, pp. 1959-1965. doi:10.1681/ASN.2006101081

[9] A. Maione, S. D. Navaneethan, G. Graziano, R. Mitchell, D. Johnson, J. F. Mann, P. Gao, J. C. Craig, G. Tognoni, V. Perkovic, A. Nicolucci, S. De Cosmo, A. Sasso, O. Lamacchia, M. Cignarelli, V. M. Manfreda, G. Gentile and G. F. Strippoli, "Angiotensin-Converting Enzyme Inhibitors, Angiotensin Receptor Blockers and Combined Therapy in Patients with Micro- and Macroalbuminuria and Other Cardiovascular Risk Factors: A Systematic Review of Randomized Controlled Trials," *Nephrology Dialysis Transplantation*, Vol. 26, No. 9, 2011, pp. 2827-2847. doi:10.1093/ndt/gfq792

[10] G. Maschio, D. Alberti, G. Janin, F. Locatelli, J. F. Mann, M. Motolese, C. Ponticelli, E. Ritz and P. Zucchelli, "Effect of the Angiotensin-Converting-Enzyme Inhibitor Benazepril on the Progression of Chronic Renal Insufficiency," *The New England Journal of Medicine*, Vol. 334, No. 15, 1996, pp. 939-945. doi:10.1056/NEJM199604113341502

[11] The GISEN Group "Randomised Placebo-Controlled Trial of Effect of Ramipril on Decline in glomerular Filtration Rate and Risk of Terminal Renal Failure in Proteinuric, Non-Diabetic Nephropathy," *Lancet*, Vol. 349, No. 9069, 1997, pp. 1857-1863. doi:10.1016/S0140-6736(96)11445-8

[12] P. Ruggenenti, A. Perna, G. Gherardi, F. Gaspari, R. Benini and G. Remuzzi, "Renal Function and Requirement for Dialysis in Chronic Nephropathy Patients on Long-Term Ramipril: REIN Follow-Up Trial," Gruppo Italiano di Studi Epidemiologici in Nefrologia (GISEN). Ramipril Efficacy in Nephropathy. *Lancet*, Vol. 352, No. 9136, 1998, pp. 1252-1256. doi:10.1016/S0140-6736(98)04433-X

[13] P. Ruggenenti, A. Perna, G. Loriga, M. Ganeva, B. Ene-Iordache, M. Turturro, M. Lesti, E. Perticucci, I. N. Chakarski, D. Leonardis, G. Garini, A. Sessa, C. Basile, M. Alpa, R. Scanziani, G. Sorba, C. Zoccali and G. Remuzzi, "REIN-2 Study Group Blood-Pressure Control for Reno Protection in Patients with Non-Diabetic Chronic Renal Disease (REIN-2): Multi Centre Randomized Controlled Trial," *Lancet*, Vol. 365, No. 9463, 2005, pp. 939-946. doi:10.1016/S0140-6736(05)71082-5

[14] J. T. Wright Jr, G. Bakris, T. Greene, L. Y. Agodoa, L. J. Appel, J. Charleston, D. Cheek, J. G. Douglas-Baltimore, J. Gassman, R. Glassock, L. Hebert, K. Jamerson, J. Lewis, R. A. Phillips, R. D. Toto, J. P. Middleton, S. G. Rostand and African American Study of Kidney Disease and Hypertension Study Group, "Effect of Blood Pressure Lowering and Antihypertensive Drug Class on Progression of Hypertensive Kidney Disease: Results from the AASK Trial," *Journal of the American Medical Association*, Vol. 288, No. 19, 2002, pp. 2421-2431. doi:10.1001/jama.288.19.2421

[15] L. J. Appel, J. T. Wright Jr., T. Greene, J. W. Kusek, J. B. Lewis, X. Wang, M. S. Lipkowitz, K. C. Norris, G. L. Bakris, M. Rahman, G. Contreras, S. G. Rostand, J. D. Kopple, F. B. Gabbai, G. I. Schulman, J. J. Gassman, J. Charleston and L. Y. Agodoa, "African American Study of Kidney Disease and Hypertension Collaborative Research Group Long-Term Effects of Renin-Angiotensin System-Blocking Therapy and a Low Blood Pressure Goal on Progression of hypertensive Chronic Kidney Disease in African Americans," *JAMA Internal Medicine*,

Vol. 168, No. 8, 2008, pp. 832-839. doi:10.1001/archinte.168.8.832

[16] F. F. Hou, X. Zhang, G. H. Zhang, D. Xie, P Y. Chen, W. R. Zhang, J. P. Jiang, M. Liang, G. B. Wang, Z. R. Liu and R. W. Geng, "Efficacy and Safety of Benazepril for Advanced Chronic Renal Insufficiency," *The New England Journal of Medicine*, Vol. 354, No. 2, 2006, pp. 131-140. doi:10.1056/NEJMoa053107

[17] A. M. O'Hare, J. S. Kaufman, K. E. Covinsky, C. S. Landefeld, L. V. McFarland and E. B. Larson, "Current Guidelines for Using Angiotensin-Converting Enzyme Inhibitors and Angiotensin II-Receptor Antagonists in Chronic Kidney Disease: Is the evidence Base Relevant to Older Adults?" *Annals of Internal Medicine*, Vol. 150, No. 10, 2009, pp. 717-724. doi:10.7326/0003-4819-150-10-200905190-00010

[18] R. Kunz, C. Friedrich, M. Wolbers and J. F. Mann, "Meta-Analysis: Effect of Monotherapy and Combination Therapy with Inhibitors of the Renin Angiotensin System on Proteinuria in Renal Disease," *Annals of Internal Medicine*, Vol. 148, No. 1, 2008, pp. 30-48. doi:10.7326/0003-4819-148-1-200801010-00190

[19] S. W. Tobe, C. M. Clase, P. Gao, M. McQueen, A. Grosshennig, X. Wang, K. K. Teo, S. Yusuf and J. F. Mann, "Cardiovascular and Renal Outcomes with Telmisartan, Ramipril, or Both in People at High Renal Risk: Results from the ONTARGET and TRANSCEND Studies," *Circulation*, Vol. 123, No. 10, 2011, pp. 1098-1107. doi:10.1161/CIRCULATIONAHA.110.964171

[20] M. MacKinnon, S. Shurraw, A. Akbari, G. A. Knoll, J. Jaffey and H. D. Clark, "Combination Therapy with an Angiotensin Receptor Blocker and an ACE Inhibitor in Proteinuric Renal Disease: A Systematic Review of the Efficacy and Safety Data," *American Journal of Kidney Diseases*, Vol. 48, No. 1, 2006, pp. 8-20. doi:10.1053/j.ajkd.2006.04.077

[21] G. L. Bakris, M. R. Weir, M. Secic, B. Campbell and A. Weis-McNulty, "Differential Effects of Calcium Antagonist Subclasses on Markers of Nephropathy Progression," *Kidney International*, Vol. 65, No. 6, 2004, pp. 1991-2002. doi:10.1111/j.1523-1755.2004.00620.x

[22] S. D. Navaneethan, S. U. Nigwekar, A. R. Sehgal and G. F. Strippoli, "Aldosterone Antagonists for Preventing the Progression of Chronic Kidney Disease: A Systematic Review and Meta-Analysis," *Clinical Journal of the American Society of Nephrology*, Vol. 4, No. 3, 2009, pp. 542-551. doi:10.2215/CJN.04750908

[23] B. H. Oh, J. Mitchell, J. R. Herron, J. Chung, M. Khan and D. L. Keefe, "Aliskiren, an Oral Renin Inhibitor, Provides Dose-Dependent Efficacy and Sustained 24-Hour Blood Pressure Control in Patients with Hypertension," *Journal of the American College of Cardiology*, Vol. 49, No. 11, 2007, pp. 1157-1163. doi:10.1016/j.jacc.2006.11.032

[24] J. L. Pool, R. E. Schmieder, M. Azizi, J. C. Aldigier, A. Januszewicz, W. Zidek, Y. Chiang and A. Satlin, "Aliskiren, an Orally Effective Renin Inhibitor, Provides Antihypertensive Efficacy Alone and in Combination with Valsartan," *American Journal of Hypertension*, Vol. 20, No. 1, 2007, pp. 11-20. doi:10.1016/j.amjhyper.2006.06.003

[25] A. Villamil, S. G. Chrysant, D. Calhoun, B. Schober, H. Hsu, L. Matrisciano-Dimichino and J. Zhang, "Renin Inhibition with Aliskiren Provides Additive Antihypertensive Efficacy When Used in Combination with Hydrochlorothiazide," *Journal of Hypertension*, Vol. 25, No. 1, 2007, pp. 217-226. doi:10.1097/HJH.0b013e3280103a6b

[26] M. M. Shafiq, D. V. Menon and R. G. Victor, "Oral Direct Renin Inhibition: Premise, Promise, and Potential Limitations of a New Antihypertensive Drug," *The American Journal of Medicine*, Vol. 121, No. 4, 2008, pp. 265-271. doi:10.1016/j.amjmed.2007.11.016

[27] H. H. Parving, F. Persson, J. B. Lewis, E. J. Lewis and N. K. Hollenberg, "AVOID Study Investigators Aliskiren Combined with Losartan in Type 2 Diabetes and Nephropathy," *The New England Journal of Medicine*, Vol. 358, No. 23, 2008, pp. 2433-2446. doi:10.1056/NEJMoa0708379

[28] H. H. Parving, B. M. Brenner, J. J. McMurray, D. de Zeeuw, S. M. Haffner, S. D. Solomon, N. Chaturvedi, M. Ghadanfar, N. Weissbach, Z. Xiang and J. Armbrecht, "Cardiorenal End Points in a Trial of Aliskiren for Type 2 Diabetes," *The New England Journal of Medicine*, Vol. 367, 2012, pp. 2204-2213. doi:10.1056/NEJMoa1208799

[29] M. Azizi and J. Ménard, "Renin Inhibitors and Cardiovascular and Renal Protection: An Endless Quest?" *Cardiovascular Drugs and Therapy*, 2012.

[30] Z. Harel, C. Gilbert, R. Wald, C. Bell, J. Perl, D. Juurlink, J. Beyene and P. S. Shah, "The Effect of Combination Treatment with Aliskiren and Blockers of the Renin-Angiotensin System on Hyperkalemia and Acute Kidney Injury: Systematic Review and Meta-Analysis," *British Medical Journal*, Vol. 344, 2012, p. e42. doi:10.1136/bmj.e42

[31] R. T. Gansevoort, W. J. Sluiter, M. H. Hemmelder, D. de Zeeuw and P. E. de Jong, "Antiproteinuric Effect of Blood-Pressure-Lowering Agents: A Meta-Analysis of Comparative Trials," *Nephrology Dialysis Transplantation*, Vol. 10, No. 11, 1995, p. 1963.

[32] A. J. Apperloo, D. de Zeeuw, H. E. Sluiter and P. E. de Jong, "Differential Effects of Enalapril and Atenolol on Proteinuria and Renal Hemodynamics in Non-Diabetic Renal Disease," *British Medical Journal*, Vol. 303, No. 6806, 1991, p. 821. doi:10.1136/bmj.303.6806.821

[33] M. E. Rosenberg and T. H. Hostetter, "Comparative Effects of Antihypertensives on Proteinuria: Angiotensin-Converting Enzyme Inhibitor versus Alpha 1-Antagonist," *American Journal of Kidney Diseases*, Vol. 18, No. 4, 1991, p. 472.

44

Prevalence of Restless Legs Syndrome in Patients Treated with Peritoneal Dialysis: Clinical and Biochemical Characteristics among Patients with and without Restless Legs Syndrome

Selda Korkmaz[1], Bulent Tokgoz[2], Sevda Ismailogullari[3], Ismail Kocyigit[2], Merva Kocyigit[3], Ozgur Berkay Aksu[4], Murat Aksu[3]

[1]Department of Neurology, Acibadem Hospital, Kayseri, Turkey
[2]Department of Nephrology, Erciyes University Medical School, Kayseri, Turkey
[3]Department of Neurology, Erciyes University Medical School, Kayseri, Turkey
[4]Medical Faculty, Near East University, Nicosia, Cyprus
Email: aksu@erciyes.edu.tr

ABSTRACT

Introduction and Aims: This is a prospective study identifying prevalence of Restless Legs Syndrome (RLS) in patients ongoing peritoneal dialysis (PD) due to end stage renal disease (ESRD) and comparing clinical and biochemical characteristics among patients with and without RLS. **Methods:** Two hundred ESRD patients who received PD at least six months assessed by neurologist and nephrologist with regards to presence of RLS. Also, clinical and biochemical features of these patients are determined. One hundred and forty four patients were excluded from study because they had other secondary causes of RLS except for ESRD. **Results:** Thirteen of 56 patients (23.2%) had RLS. The use of vitamin B + folic acid supplements was significantly lower in patients with RLS than in those without RLS (69.2% vs 97.7%; $p = 0.008$). There was no significant difference between patient groups with and without RLS in terms of age, gender, body mass index, cause of ESRD, peritoneal membrane transport characteristic, smoking, consuming alcohol, use of erythropoietin, duration of PD, hemoglobin, serum calcium, serum phosphorus, serum albumin, levels of serum iron, total iron binding capacity, ferritin, folic acid and vitamin B12, transferrin saturation, weekly Kt/V urea value, and amount of residual urine volume ($p > 0.05$). **Conclusion:** RLS is more common among PD patients than general population. Although essential cause is not exactly known, use of folic acid and vitamin B complex decrease the RLS prevalence in this particular patient group.

Keywords: Peritoneal Dialysis; Restless Legs Syndrome; Renal Failure

1. Introduction

Restless legs syndrome (RLS) is the most prevalent sensorimotor disorder during sleep. The prevalence of RLS is estimated to be 5% - 15% in general [1-3]. The diagnosis of RLS is based on history with standardized clinical criteria, defined by the International RLS Study Group (IRLSSG) [4]. RLS is defined in two categories: idiopathic RLS (iRLS), which refers to familial tendency and no-known background condition while secondary RLS refers to various co morbid conditions, such as iron deficiency, diabetes mellitus, pregnancy, multiple sclerosis (MS), Parkinson's disease and end stage renal disease (ESRD) [5-12]. Prevalence of RLS in patients undergoing dialysis therapy due to ESRD has a wide range between 6.6% and 83% [13-24] depending on the varying diagnostic criteria applied in those studies, before the final standardization by the IRLSSG criteria. Moreover, this variation has been explained by the improvement of dialytic techniques as well as the pharmacological treatment of the ESRD.

The pathophysiological mechanisms involved in the idiopathic RLS are multifactorial, including dopaminergic dysfunction, spinal cord disinhibiting and dysfunction in the iron metabolism [25-29]. Regarding the secondary RLS in ESRD, iron-vitamin B—folic acid deficiency, DM as well as inadequate peritoneal dialysis (PD) was suggested to be the main risk factors for this condition.

Most of previous prevalence studies among ESRD patients have been conducted in those undergoing hemodialysis (HD) therapy and the results were mainly explained by the known risk factors as described above. To date, only a few studies addressed the prevalence of RLS among ESRD patients undergoing PD. Moreover, the real prevalence of RLS in ESRD, after excluding the patients with other known risk factors, is still unknown.

The aim of the current study was to evaluate the prevalence of RLS in ESRD patients treated with PD without known risk factors and to compare the clinical and biochemical characteristics of RLS patients with subjects without this condition.

2. Methods

2.1. Patients

The study was performed on 200 patients who were on PD treatments due to ESRD for at least 6 months and were followed up by Nephrology Department of Erciyes University Medical Faculty. Patients were also evaluated for RLS in Sleep Disorders Unit of Neurology Department of Erciyes University Medical Faculty. The local ethics committee approved the study protocol. The study was conducted in accordance with the declaration of Helsinki and local laws depending on whichever afforded greater protection to the patients. All the patients gave their informed consent of participation in the study.

We excluded 144 patients from the study who are under 18 years, or have either diabetes mellitus, anemia which was defined as a hemoglobin level < 10 g/dL, iron deficiency which was defined as a transferrin saturation < 20% and a serum ferritin concentration < 100 ng/mL, Multiple Sclerosis, Parkinson's disease, pregnancy and/or acute peritonitis because these conditions are important risk factors for symptomatic RLS. Also, patients who have taken medications such as antidepressants, neuroleptics or hypnotics that are known to affect sleep structure and have the sensorimotor symptoms of RLS were excluded.

Finally, 56 patients who fulfilled the inclusion and exclusion criteria were included in the study.

2.2. Data Collection

Firstly, clinical and laboratorial data of 56 patients were collected by the nephrologist of the PD unit. These data contained age, gender, body mass index, etiology of ESRD, smoking, drinking alcohol, use of erythropoietin, use of B complex vitamins and folic acid, duration of peritoneal dialysis, weekly Kt/Vurea, amount of residual urine volume, hemoglobin, serum calcium level, serum phosphorus level, calcium × phosphorus product, serum albumin level, serum iron level, total iron binding capacity, transferrin saturation, serum ferritin level, serum vitamin B12 level and serum folic acid level.

Secondly, all patients were examined by neurologist who were experts in sleep disorders and were evaluated with regard to presence of four essential RLS criteria as defined by the IRLSSG.

2.3. Statistical Analysis

SPSS 15.0 statistic software was used for the statistical analysis. The Kolmogorov-Smirnov test was used to determine the normality of the distributions of the variables. Continuous variables with normal distribution were presented as mean ± standard deviation. Median value was used when normal distribution was absent. Statistical analysis for the parametric variables was performed by the Student's t test between two groups. The Mann-Whitney U test was used to compare nonparametric variables between two groups. The qualitative variables were given as percent and the chi-square test and Fisher's exact test were used to compare variables between the two groups. p value of <0.05 was considered to be significant.

3. Results

The mean age of the 56 patients was 47.10 ± 12.42 years. Thirty one of the 56 patients were male and the rest of them were female. RLS was found in 13 (23.2%) of 56 PD patients. The most frequent cause of the etiology of end-stage renal disease was hypertension. The most of the patients had average peritoneal transport characteristics. The demographic, clinical, and biochemical parameters of the patients are summarized in **Table 1**.

Demographic, clinical, and biochemical parameters of the 13 patients with RLS are compared to 43 patients without RLS in **Table 2**. The use of vitamin B complex + folic acid supplements was significantly lower in patients with RLS than in those without RLS (69.2% vs 97.7%; $p = 0.008$). Although there was no statistically significant difference between two groups, folic acid levels were found in lower levels in patients with RLS than in those without RLS. On the other hand, there was no significant difference between patients with RLS and those without RLS in regard to age, gender, body mass index, cause of ESRD, peritoneal membrane transport characteristic, smoking, drinking, use of erythropoietin, duration of PD, hemoglobin, serum calcium, serum phosphorus, serum albumin, levels of serum iron, total iron binding capacity, ferritin, and vitamin B12, transferrin saturation, weekly Kt/Vurea value, and amount of residual urine volume ($p > 0.05$).

4. Discussion

The prevalence of RLS in dialysis populations appears to be greater than in the general population although there is a wide variation, ranging between 6.6% and 83% [13-24]. Also, in previous studies which most of them were made in HD patients, no significant difference has been found between HD and PD patients in terms of RLS prevalence

Table 1. Demographic, clinical and biochemical characteristics of patients on peritoneal dialysis.

Age (year)	47.10 ± 12.42
Gender	
Male	31 (55.4%)
Female	25 (44.6%)
Body mass index (kg/m^2)	24.20 ± 3.96
Etiology of ESRD	
Hypertension	28 (50.0%)
Glomerulonephritis	4 (7.1%)
Polycystic kidney disease	3 (5.4%)
Amyloidosis	2 (3.6%)
Obstructive nephropathy	4 (7.1%)
Others	1 (1.8%)
Unknown	14 (25%)
Solute transport group according to PET	
High	7 (12.5%)
High-average	19 (33.9%)
Low-average	28 (50%)
Low	2 (3.6%)
Smoking	7 (12.5%)
Drinking alcohol	2 (3.6%)
Use of erythropoietin	33 (58.9%)
Use of B complex vitamins + folic acid	51 (91.1%)
Duration of peritoneal dialysis (month)	39.5 (3 - 165)
Hemoglobin (g/dL)	11.42 ± 1.29
Serum calcium (mg/dL)	8.82 ± 0.90
Serum phosphorus (mg/dl)	4.26 ± 1.17
Serum albumin level (g/dL)	3.41 ± 0.38
Iron (μg/dL)	75.92 ± 23.67
Total iron binding capacity (μg/dL)	243.21 ± 49.53
Transferrin saturation (%)	31.44 ± 10.19
Ferritin (ng/mL)	335 (107 - 2354)
Vitamin B12 (pg/mL)	546 (89 - 1500)
Folic acid (ng/mL)	24 (1 - 24)
Weekly Kt/Vurea	2.59 ± 0.93
Amount of residual urine volume (mL/day)	500 (0 - 2200)

ESRD: end-stage renal disease, PET: peritoneal equilibration test.

[13,17,30-32]. Our study group was constituted from under PD patients and prevalence of RLS was found 23.2 % when the other risk factors except for ESRD for secondary RLS were excluded. To date, only few studies evaluated the prevalence of RLS in PD patients [17,33, 34] and in those studies, RLS prevalence has been found between 19.7% [33] and 69.2% [34]. In the whole prevalence studies in uremic patients, RLS has been found more common than general population. This condition has been tried to be explained by increased frequency in presence of some risk factors such as iron deficiency, DM, vitamin and folic acid deficiencies in uremic patients. In present study, we studied the prevalence of RLS in ESRD patients treated with PD after risk factors that have been known to be frequently related with RLS were excluded. Consequently, prevalence of RLS in PD patients was found more common than general population even PD patients were applied to our exclusion criteria which are very strict to exclude any other possible factors that could be cause of secondary RLS. Although it is believed that RLS in PD patients evolve with different mechanism than RLS in general population, it is not clear what risk factors of RLS in PD patients are apart from known risk factors.

Although RLS pathophysiology are tried to be explained by different mechanism such as dopaminergic dysfunction, spinal disinhibiting and iron metabolism, it is still unclear. Also, pathophysiology of RLS in ESRD patients who are treated both HD and PD is unknown. One of mechanisms that are the most emphasized is anemia and iron deficiency. In fact, controversial results have been reported on the relationship between lower serum hemoglobin, ferritin, iron and RLS in ESRD patients, showing both the absence [16,19,30,35] and presence of this association [23,36]. Especially, more recent studies have failed to show this association, but this might be caused by the routine use of high-dose intravenous iron and erythropoietin in modern dialysis management [29]. In current study, no significant differences were found in hemoglobin level, iron and ferritin levels in serum, total iron binding capacity, transferrin saturation and use of erythropoietin between PD patients with and without RLS.

Although prevalence of RLS has been reported to be higher in female gender and advanced age in general population, relationship between presence of RLS and age, gender in ESRD patients has not been exactly known. Some authors [23] have suggested that RLS prevalence in uremic patients is more in female gender and related with advanced age whereas others [16] and the current study haven't shown this relation.

Relationship between smoking, alcohol consumption and RLS in ESRD patients is controversial. Some studies suggest negatively effect of smoking and alcohol consumption

Table 2. Comparison of demographic, clinical, and biochemical parameters between patients with RLS and those without RLS.

Characteristic	RLS group (n: 13)	Non-RLS group (n: 43)	p value
Age (year)	48.00 ± 11.95	46.83 ± 12.69	0.771
Gender			0.140
Female	8 (61.5%)	17 (39.5%)	
Male	5 (38.5%)	26 (60.5%)	
Body mass index (kg/m^2)	24.37 ± 3.00	24.14 ± 4.24	0.855
Etiology			0.270
Hypertension	7 (53.8%)	21 (48.8%)	
Glomerulonephritis	2 (15.4%)	2 (4.7%)	
Polycystic kidney disease	1 (7.7%)	2 (4.7%)	
Amyloidosis	-	2 (4.7%)	
Obstructive nephropathy	-	4 (9.3%)	
Others	1 (7.7%)	-	
Unknown	2 (15.4%)	12 (27.9%)	
Solute transport group according to PET			0.252
High	1 (7.7%)	6 (14.0%)	
High-average	2 (15.4%)	17 (39.5%)	
Low-average	9 (69.2%)	19 (44.2%)	
Low	1 (7.7%)	1 (2.3%)	
Smoking	2 (15.4%)	5 (11.6%)	0.519
Drinking alcohol	-	2 (4.7%)	0.586
Use of erythropoietin	8 (61.5%)	25 (58.1%)	0.545
Use of B complex vitamins + folic acid	9 (69.2%)	42 (97.7%)	0.008
Duration of peritoneal dialysis (month)	38 (3 - 165)	40 (6 - 144)	0.930
Hemoglobin (g/dL)	11.80 ± 1.44	11.30 ± 1.23	0.221
Serum calcium (mg/dL)	9.23 ± 1.13	8.70 ± 0.79	0.062
Serum phosphorus (mg/dl)	4.61 ± 1.44	4.15 ± 1.08	0.219
Serum albumin level (g/dL)	3.48 ± 0.28	3.38 ± 0.40	0.455
Iron (μg/dL)	72.61 ± 27.90	75.76 ± 23.36	0.685
Total iron binding capacity (μg/dL)	257.00 ± 45.30	239.04 ± 50.49	0.256
Transferrin saturation (%)	27.92 ± 8.09	32.24 ± 10.91	0.193
Ferritin (ng/mL)	160 (126 - 862)	337.5 (107 - 2354)	0.188
Vitamin B12 (pg/mL)	553 (265 - 1000)	546 (89 - 1500)	0.783
Folic acid (ng/mL)	20 (3 - 24)	24 (1 - 24)	0.070
Weekly Kt/Vurea	2.51 ± 0.71	2.61 ± 1.00	0.744
Amount of residual urine volume (mL/day)	500 (0 - 2000)	500 (0 - 2200)	0.549

RLS: Restless legs syndrome, PET: peritoneal equilibration test.

on RLS in ESRD patients [37] whereas the others and our study have not demonstrated this relation [30,38,39].

The role of serum calcium, phosphorus and intact parathormone levels in uremic RLS are controversial. Until today, relationship of RLS with high calcium [40], abnormal phosphorus [30], low [16] and high levels of PTH [21] have been described in uremic RLS patients. Moreover an anecdotal improvement of symptoms after parathyroidectomy have been described in uremic RLS [41].

On the other hand, there are also studies that lacked to show any significant difference on calcium, phosphorus and PTH levels [19,37]. In this study, no significant difference was found between ESRD patients with and without RLS in serum calcium, phosphorus and PTH levels.

It is not known which factors associated with dialysis play a role in the development of RLS in ESRD patients. For example, there are contradictory study results assessing affect of dialysis duration on presence of RLS [16,21,42]. The other dialysis parameter that is thought related to RLS is level of urea Kt/V. Urea Kt/V is accepted as the optimal method for assessing the adequacy of dialysis. Some studies have suggested that RLS might represent a marker of inadequate dialysis in ESRD patients [37,43]. However, results of the present study showed any correlation neither dialysis duration nor level of Kt/v urea between PD patients with and without RLS, concordant with some previous studies [32,44].

Although in previous studies it was shown that vitamin B12 and folic acid are associated with RLS, our study did not confirm that in PD patients with RLS. However, in this study RLS was found to be more common in patients who are not taking B complex vitamins + folic acid supplement.

This study is the first and unique study that evaluates the prevalence of RLS on PD patients and describes clinical and biochemical parameters which may be related to RLS in patients under PD due to ESRD in Turkish patients. In fact the most important aspect of the study is that a prevalence study after other risk factors for RLS are excluded.

RLS is a very important sleep related sensorimotor disorder that decreases life quality and increases morbidity and mortality rates in PD patients. Therefore RLS must be diagnosed and treated at early period. Also, vitamin B and folic acid supplements could be used to decrease RLS prevalence in PD patients.

REFERENCES

[1] K. A. Ekbom, "Restless Legs Syndrome," *Neurology*, Vol. 10, 1960, pp. 868-873. doi:10.1212/WNL.10.9.868

[2] G. J. Lavigne and J. Y. Montplaisir, "Restless Legs Syndrome and Sleep Bruxism: Prevalence and Association among Canadians," *Sleep*, Vol. 17, No. 8, 1994, pp. 739-743.

[3] B. Phillips, T. Young, L. Finn, *et al.*, "Epidemiology of Restless Legs Symptoms in Adults," *Archives of Internal Medicine*, Vol. 160, No. 14, 2000, pp. 2137-2141. doi:10.1001/archinte.160.14.2137

[4] R. P. Allen, D. Picchietti, W. A. Hening, *et al.*, "Restless Legs Syndrome: Diagnostic Criteria, Special Considerations and Epidemiology. A Report from the Restless Legs Syndrome Diagnosis and Epidemiology Workshop at the National Institutes of Health," *Sleep Medicine*, Vol. 4, No. 2, 2003, pp. 101-119.

[5] M. Zucconi and L. Ferini-Strambi, "Epidemiology and Clinical Findings of Restless Legs Syndrome," *Sleep Medicine*, Vol. 5, No. 3, 2004, pp. 293-299. doi:10.1016/j.sleep.2004.01.004

[6] R. P. Allen and C. J. Earley, "Restless Legs Syndrome: A Review of Clinical and Pathophysiologic Features," *Journal of Clinical Neurophysiology*, Vol. 18, No. 2, 2001, pp. 128-147. doi:10.1097/00004691-200103000-00004

[7] L. A. Lopes, C. M. Lins, V. G. Adeodato, *et al.*, "Restless Legs Syndrome and Quality of Sleep in Type 2 Diabetes," *Diabetes Care*, Vol. 28, No. 11, 2005, pp. 2633-2636. doi:10.2337/diacare.28.11.2633

[8] M. Manconi, V. Govoni, A. De Vito, *et al.*, "Pregnancy as a Risk Factor for Restless Legs Syndrome," *Sleep Medicine*, Vol. 5, No. 3, 2004, pp. 305-308. doi:10.1016/j.sleep.2004.01.013

[9] B. Phillips, T. Young, L. Finn, *et al.*, "Epidemiology of Restless Legs Symptoms in Adults," *Archives of Internal Medicine*, Vol. 160, No. 14, 2000, pp. 2137-2141. doi:10.1001/archinte.160.14.2137

[10] N. C. Moreira, R. S. Damasceno, C. A. Medeiros, *et al.*, "Restless Leg Syndrome, Sleep Quality and Fatigue in Multiple Sclerosis Patients," *Brazilian Journal of Medical and Biological Research*, Vol. 41, No. 10, 2008, pp. 932-937. doi:10.1590/S0100-879X2008001000017

[11] T. Nomura, Y. Inoue, M. Miyake, *et al.*, "Prevalence and Clinical Characteristics of Restless Legs Syndrome in Japanese Patients with Parkinson's Disease," *Movement Disorders*, Vol. 21, No. 3, 2006, pp. 380-384. doi:10.1002/mds.20734

[12] J. P. Bastos, R. B. Sousa, L. A. Nepomuceno, *et al.*, "Sleep Disturbances in Patients on Maintenance Hemodialysis: Role of Dialysis Shift," *Revista da Associação Médica Brasileira*, Vol. 53, No. 6, 2007, pp. 492-496. doi:10.1590/S0104-42302007000600014

[13] J. L. Holley, S. Nespor and R. Rault, "A Comparison of Reported Sleep Disorders in Patients on Chronic Hemodialysis and Continuous Peritoneal Dialysis," *American Journal of Kidney Diseases*, Vol. 2, 1992, pp. 156-161.

[14] S. L. Walker, A. Fine and M. H. Kryger, "Sleep Complaints Are Common in Dialysis Unit," *American Journal of Kidney Diseases*, Vol. 26, No. 5, 1995, pp. 751-756. doi:10.1016/0272-6386(95)90438-7

[15] J. W. Winkelman, G. M. Chertow and J. M. Lazarus, "Restless Legs Syndrome in End-Stage Renal Disease,"

American Journal of Kidney Diseases, Vol. 28, No. 3, 1996, pp. 372-378. doi:10.1016/S0272-6386(96)90494-1

[16] V. Collado-Seidel, R. Kohnen, W. Samtleben, *et al.*, "Clinical and Biochemical Findings in Uremic Patients with and without Restless Legs Syndrome," *American Journal of Kidney Diseases*, Vol. 31, No. 2, 1998, pp. 324-328. doi:10.1053/ajkd.1998.v31.pm9469505

[17] D. S. C. Hui, T. Y. H. Wong, F. W. S. Ko, *et al.*, "Prevalence of Sleep Disturbances in Chinese Patients with End-Stage Renal Failure on Continuous Ambulatory Peritoneal Dialysis," *American Journal of Kidney Diseases*, Vol. 36, No. 4, 2000, pp. 783-788. doi:10.1053/ajkd.2000.17664

[18] Q. Huiqi, L. Shan and Q. Mingcai, "Restless Legs Syndrome (RLS) in Uremic Patients Is Related to the Frequency of Hemodialysis Sessions," *Nephron*, Vol. 86, No. 4, 2000, p. 540. doi:10.1159/000045861

[19] M. Miranda, F. Araya, J. L. Castillo, *et al.*, "Restless Legs Syndrome: A Clinical Study in Chilean General Population and in Uremic Patients," *Revista Médica de Chile*, Vol. 129, 2001, pp. 179-186.

[20] M. L. Thorp, C. D. Morris and S. P. Bugby, "A Crossover Study of Gabapentin in Treatment of Restless Legs Syndrome among Hemodialysis Patients," *American Journal of Kidney Diseases*, Vol. 38, No. 1, 2001, pp. 104-108. doi:10.1053/ajkd.2001.25202

[21] M. Sabbatini, B. Minale, A. Crispo, *et al.*, "Insomnia in Maintenance Haemodialysis Patients," *Nephrology Dialysis Transplantation*, Vol. 17, No. 5, 2002, pp. 852-856. doi:10.1093/ndt/17.5.852

[22] D. S. C. Hui, T. Y. H. Wong, T. S. T. Li, *et al.*, "Prevalence of Sleep Disturbances in Chinese Patients with End Stage Renal Failure on Maintenenance Hemodialysis," *Medical Science Monitor*, Vol. 8, No. 5, 2002, pp. 331-336.

[23] J. Takaki, T. Nishi, M. Nangaku, *et al.*, "Clinical and Psychological Aspects of Restless Legs Syndrome in Uremic Patients on Hemodialysis," *American Journal of Kidney Diseases*, Vol. 41, No. 4, 2003, pp. 833-839. doi:10.1016/S0272-6386(03)00031-3

[24] D. Bhowmik, M. Bhatia, S. Gupta, *et al.*, "Restless Legs Syndrome in Hemodialysis Patients in India: A Case Controlled Study," *Sleep Medicine*, Vol. 4, No. 2, 2003, pp. 143-146. doi:10.1016/S1389-9457(03)00005-4

[25] S. Akpinar, "Treatment of Restless Legs with Levodopa plus Benserazide," *Archives of Neurology*, Vol. 39, No. 11, 1982, p. 739. doi:10.1001/archneur.1982.00510230065027

[26] J. Montplaisir, R. Godbout, G. Poirer, *et al.*, "Restless Legs Syndrome and Periodic Movements in Sleep; Physiology and Treatment with L-Dopa," *Clinical Neuropharmacology*, Vol. 9, No. 5, 1986, pp. 456-463. doi:10.1097/00002826-198610000-00006

[27] J. Winkelmann, J. Schadrack, T. Wetter, *et al.*, "Opioid and Dopamine Antagonist Drug Challenges in Untreated Restless Legs Syndrome Patients," *Sleep Medicine*, Vol. 2, No. 1, 2001, pp. 57-61. doi:10.1016/S1389-9457(00)00025-3

[28] M. Aksu and W. Bara-Jimenez, "State Dependent Excitability Changes of Spinal Flexor Reflex in Patients with Restless Legs Syndrome Secondary to Chronic Renal Failure," *Sleep Medicine*, Vol. 2, No. 1, 2002, pp. 427-430. doi:10.1016/S1389-9457(02)00073-4

[29] R. L. Benz, M. R. Pressman, E. T. Hovick, *et al.*, "A Preliminary Study of the Effects of Correction of Anemia with Recombinant Human Erythropoietin Therapy on Sleep, Sleep Disorders, and Daytime Sleepiness in Hemodialysis Patients (The SLEEPO Study)," *American Journal of Kidney Diseases*, Vol. 34, No. 6, 1999, pp. 1089-1095. doi:10.1016/S0272-6386(99)70015-6

[30] G. L. Gigli, M. Adorati, P. Dolso, *et al.*, "Restless Legs Syndrome in End-Stage Renal Disease," *Sleep Medicine*, Vol. 5, No. 3, 2004, pp. 309-315. doi:10.1016/j.sleep.2004.01.014

[31] N. G. Kutner, R. Zhang, Y. Huang, *et al.*, "Racial Differences in Restless Legs Symptoms and Serum Ferritin in an Incident Dialysis Patient Cohort," *International Urology and Nephrology*, Vol. 44, No. 6, 2012, pp. 1825-1831.

[32] G. Merlino, S. Lorenzut, G. Romano, *et al.*, "Restless Legs Syndrome in Dialysis Patients: A Comparison between Hemodialysis and Continuous Ambulatory Peritoneal Dialysis," *Neurological Sciences*, Vol. 33, No. 6, 2012, pp. 1311-1318.

[33] M. L. Unruh, A. S. Levey, C. D'Ambrosio, *et al.*, "Restless Legs Symptoms among Incident Dialysis Patients: Association with Lower Quality of Life and Shorter Survival. Choices for Healthy Outcomes in Caring for End-Stage Renal Disease (CHOICE) Study," *American Journal of Kidney Diseases*, Vol. 43, No. 5, 2004, pp. 900-909. doi:10.1053/j.ajkd.2004.01.013

[34] H. H. Al-Jahdali, W. A. Al-Qadhi, H. A. Khogeer, *et al.*, "Restless Legs Syndrome in Patients on Dialysis," *Saudi Journal of Kidney Diseases and Transplantation*, Vol. 20, No. 3, 2009, pp. 378-385.

[35] S. Siddiqui, M. Mak, D. Kavanagh, *et al.*, "Restless Legs Syndrome in Haemodialysis Patients," *Scottish Renal Association*, 9-10 May 2003.

[36] S. Roger, D. Harris and J. Stewart, "Possible Relation between Restless Legs and Anemia in Renal Dialysis Patients," *Lancet*, Vol. 337, No. 8756, 1991, p. 1551. doi:10.1016/0140-6736(91)93248-8

[37] W. C. Chen, P. S. Lim, W. C. Wu, *et al.*, "Sleep Behavior Disorders in a Large Cohort of Chinese (Taiwanese) Patients Maintained by Long-Term Hemodialysis," *American Journal of Kidney Diseases*, Vol. 48, No. 2, 2006, pp. 277-284. doi:10.1053/j.ajkd.2006.04.079

[38] S. M. Araujo, V. M. de Bruin, L. A. Nepomuceno, *et al.*, "Restless Legs Syndrome in End-Stage Renal Disease: Clinical Characteristics and Associated Comorbidities," *Sleep Medicine*, Vol. 11, No. 8, 2010, pp. 785-790. doi:10.1016/j.sleep.2010.02.011

[39] C. Quinn, M. Uzbeck, I. Saleem, *et al.*, "Iron Status and Chronic Kidney Disease Predict Restless Legs Syndrome in an Older Hospital Population," *Sleep Medicine*, Vol. 12, No. 3, 2011, pp. 295-301. doi:10.1016/j.sleep.2010.08.014

[40] A. Kawauchi, Y. Inoue, T. Hashimoto, *et al*., "Restless Legs Syndrome in Hemodialysis Patients: Health-Related Quality of Life and Laboratory Data Analysis," *Clinical Nephrology*, Vol. 66, No. 6, 2006, pp. 440-446.

[41] L. L. Lim, D. Dinner, K. W. Tham, *et al*., "Restless Legs Syndrome Associated with Primary Hyperparathyroidism," *Sleep Medicine*, Vol. 6, No. 3, 2005, pp. 283-285. doi:10.1016/j.sleep.2004.10.014

[42] N. Kutner and D. Bliwise, "Restless Legs Complaint in African-American and Caucasian Hemodialysis Patients," *Sleep Medicine*, Vol. 3, No. 6, 2002, pp. 497-500. doi:10.1016/S1389-9457(02)00025-4

[43] J. Perl, M. L. Unruh and C. T. Chan, "Sleep Disorders in End-Stage Renal Disease: 'Markers of Inadequate Dialysis'?" *Kidney International*, Vol. 70, 2006, pp. 1687-1693. doi:10.1038/sj.ki.5001791

[44] J. L. Holley, S. Nespor and R. Rault, "Characterizing Sleep Disorders in Chronic Hemodialysis Patients," *ASAIO Transactions*, Vol. 37, No. 3, 1991, pp. M456-M457.

Evidence-Based Therapy May Improve Outcome in Glomerulonephritis—A Prospective Field Survey

Norbert Braun[1], Anna Schweisfurth[2], Hermann-Josef Gröne[3], Guenther Kundt[4]
[1]Department of Internal Medicine, MediClin Müritz-Klinikum, Waren, Germany
[2]Department of Nephrology and Dialysis, HELIOS Hospital, Schwerin, Germany
[3]Department of Cellular and Molecular Pathology, German Cancer Research Centre, Heidelberg, Germany
[4]Institute for Biostatistics and Informatics in Medicine, University of Rostock, Rostock, Germany
Email: norbert.richard.braun@t-online.de

ABSTRACT

Introduction and Aims: Although glomerulonephritis is rare in the general population it is the second most important cause for end-stage renal failure. The therapy of glomerulonephritis is guided by a limited number of individual clinical trials and treatment recommendations are based on meta-analysis and Cochrane Systematic Reviews. The impact of such therapy standards on the prognosis of glomerulonephritis is not known. **Methods:** Between October 2002 and December 2008 patients with abnormal urine findings and/or decreasing renal function of unknown cause were referred for renal biopsy. In a collaboration of out-patient nephrologists with a major teaching hospital, all patients received treatment recommendations according to evidence-based therapy guidelines based on Cochrane Systematic Reviews. Patient charts were systematically reviewed and patients were re-examined for follow-up until November 2009. Cox Regression analysis was performed to identify independent prognostic factors. **Results:** Two hundred patients with primary or secondary glomerulonephritis were identified. Complete follow-up data were available from 196 patients with 324 therapeutic interventions. The mean follow-up was 2.8 ± 2.0 years. Among all patients, 37% remained unchanged ill, 13% died, 17% had progressing renal disease, while 19% had a complete and 14% a partial remission. Proteinuria declined in primary glomerulonephritis (5.0 ± 5.4 g/d to 2.1 ± 3.4 g/d, $p < 0.001$) and secondary glomerulonephritis (4.8 ± 4.6 g/d to 2.7 ± 3.1 g/d, $p = 0.004$). The highest rates of remission were observed in minimal change disease (83%) and membranous nephropathy (50%). Survival was lowest in MPGN and secondary rapid-progressive glomerulonephritis (33% and 50%, respectively). 70 (22%) interventions were complicated by adverse events resulting in treatment cessation in 25 cases. Cox univariate analyses identified the following parameters to improve outcome: Histology, no tubulointerstitial fibrosis, primary glomerulopathy, absence of hypertension at presentation, diabetes, ischemic heart disease, no diuretics or insulin, serum creatinine < 175 µmol/l, blood pressure < 160 mmHg, age < 60 ys, prednisolone, cyclosporin A, azathioprine, and follow-up by 24 hr urine. In a multivariate forward Cox regression analysis, tubulo-interstitial fibrosis had a hazard for the combined end-point of death, dialysis and progression of renal failure of 4.4 (95% confidence interval (95% CI: 1.8 - 10.6) while intensive follow-up by regular 24 hr urine collections reduced the risk to 0.3 (95% CI: 0.1 - 0.7), treatment with prednisolone had a hazard of 0.3 (95% CI: 0.1 - 0.9), and cyclosporin A therapy a hazard of 0.2 (95% CI: 0.02 - 1.4). Application of Cochrane review based therapy guidelines along with intensified monitoring of renal function prolonged dialysis-free survival by 1.7 years. **Conclusions:** In a multivariate model of standardised glomerulonephritis therapy the presence of tubulointerstitial fibrosis was associated with death or progressive renal disease, while prednisolone-based therapy regimens and intensified nephrological follow-up resulted in a significant delay of endstage-renal failure. This result should direct future health care policies because glomerulonephritis accounts for nearly 20% of the dialysis population.

Keywords: Glomerulonephritis; Therapy; Evidence-Based Medicine; Treatment Recommendation; Field Survey; Immunosuppression; Tubulointerstitial Fibrosis; Cox Regression Analysis

1. Introduction

Glomerulonephritis can be classified as a rare disease because the prevalence is less than 5 per 10,000 population [1]. Rare diseases are a threat to the health of EU citizens insofar as they are life-threatening or chronically debilitating diseases with a low prevalence and a high level of complexity [2]. Thus, glomerulonephritis is the underlying disease for 19% of all dialysis-dependent patients in Germany [3]. Similar numbers are reported from the United Kingdom [4] and the United States of America [5] making glomerulonephritis to the second most important cause for end-stage renal disease beside diabetes mellitus. Systematic diagnosis and therapeutic approaches were limited to individual research groups. The results of clinical trials are limited by the small number of included patients. During the last years, systematic Cochrane reviews have tried to summarize the results and give therapeutic recommendations. The validity of such recommendations is still pending and search in Health Technology Assessment databases [6] gives no answer to the question of treatment efficacy or cost absorption by this group of patients.

This paper presents data on the systematic application of recommendations from Cochrane systematic reviews about the therapy of glomerulonephritis in a well-defined population backed by epidemiological data.

2. Methods

The study was approved by the Ethical Board of the University of Rostock, ref # A 2009 33. Written consent was received from all patients.

2.1. Patients

Between October 2002 and December 2008 patients with abnormal urine findings and/or decreasing renal function of unknown cause in the state capital of Mecklen-burg-Lower Pomerania Schwerin and the surrounding counties Nordwestmecklenburg, Güstrow, Parchim, Prignitz, and Ludwigslust were referred for renal biopsy. For details of the patient cohort see Braun *et al.* [1].

2.2. Therapy

Following the establishment of a histopathological diagnosis all patients received treatment recommendations considering their individual clinical presentation. The recommendations were strictly based on evidence-based therapy guidelines as given in continuously updated and published Cochrane Systematic Reviews (cited in their latest version):

Minimal Change Nephropathy (MCN) with nephrotic syndrome: As the Cochrane review by Palmer *et al.* [7] was inconclusive with respect to the treatment of adults due to a lack of clinical studies, recommendations were deducted from one cited adult study [8] and analogous recommendations given in Cochrane Reviews for the treatment of children [9-11]. Patients received 1 mg/kgBW/day of oral prednisolone for 4 - 6 weeks. In the case of steroid-resistant nephrotic syndrome, cyclosporin A was given in an adult adjusted dose of 3.5 - 5 mg/kgBW/day in two divided doses aiming at a full blood through level between 80 - 140 ng/ml.

Focal and segmental glomerulosclerosis (FSGS): Patients with nephrotic syndrome treated with cyclosporin A (CSA) at an initial dose of 3.5 - 5 mg/kgBW/day in two divided doses in combination with oral prednisolone 0.15 mg/kgBW/day are more likely to achieve a partial remission of the nephrotic syndrome compared with symptomatic treatment or prednisolone alone [12]. Thus, patients initially received prednisolone 1 mg/kgBW/day for at least 6 weeks followed by cyclosporin A and prednisolone if still nephrotic. Non nephrotic patients received symptomatic treatment. In the case of cyclosporin resistance a trial with cyclophosphamide was offered [13].

Primary mesangioproliferative glomerulonephritis (MesGN) of the IgA type: Treatment was based on the Cochrane review by Samuels *et al.* [14] and stratified according to the suggestions by Floege *et al.* [15] In brief, patients with proteinuria $\geq$ 1 g/d and GFR $\geq$ 60 ml/min were treated according to Pozzi *et al.* [16] but when proteinuria was less than 1 g/d only oral prednisolone was prescribed. Patients with deteriorating renal function were treated with oral cyclophosphamide 1.5 mg/kgBW/day for three months followed by azathioprine and prednisolone 0.5 mg/kgBW/day [17].

Idiopathic membranous glomerulonephritis (MGN): Treatment was based on the Cochrane review by Schieppati *et al.* [18]. After stratification according to Cattran [19]. In brief, patients with mild proteinuria <4 g/d and normal renal function were treated symptomatically. Patients with persistent moderate proteinuria $\geq$4 g/d and <8 g/d with normal renal function for more than 6 months were treated with a modified Ponticelli scheme using methylprednisolone in combination with 1.5 mg/kgBW/day cyclophosphamide instead of chlorambucil for 6 months [20]. Patients with persistent proteinuria $\geq$8 g/d and/or deteriorating renal function were treated with an adjusted dose of 3.5 - 5 mg/kgBW/day cyclosporin A in two divided doses for at least 6 months. In the case of treatment-resistance an attempt to switch the primary therapy option was undertaken. Patients not responding to this treatment recommendation after one year could be treated experimentally with other immunosuppressants.

Necrotising glomerulonephritis with crescents (NGN): This histological entity presented clinically as rapidly progressive glomerulonephritis and patients were treated as an emergency according to the recommendations of Walters' Cochrane review [21]. Methylprednisolone, oral cyclophosphamide and plasmapheresis were applied for induction therapy and azathioprine was used for maintenance therapy. Antibiotics were not routinely administered to prevent relapse, although in single cases rheumatologists prescribed such medication.

Secondary immune complex nephritis without necrotising glomerulonephritis: These patients who suffered mainly from pauci-immune complex glomerulonephritis were treated according to the recommendations of the Cochrane review by Walters *et al.* [21].

Lupus nephritis: Patients with lupus nephritis class II were treated for non major organ involvement according to the current guidelines of the American College of Rheumatology, *i.e.* primarily with oral prednisolone 0.5 mg/kgBW/day, hydrochloroquine, and if appropriate with azathioprine or cyclosporin A [22]. Patients with class III - IV lupus nephritis were treated according the recommendations of the Cochrane review by Flanc *et al.* [23] with monthly IV cyclophosphamide and methylprednisolone/prednisolone for six months followed by azathioprine. Patients with class V lupus nephritis were treated with cyclophosphamide only if severe proteinuria ≥8 g/d and/or deteriorating renal function were present.

Symptomatic treatment: Patients with nephrotic range proteinuria were recommended to take a diet reduced in salt (3 g/d sodium chloride) and protein (0.8 g/kgBW/d) content. Medication consisted in loop diuretics in combination with ACE inhibitors and angiotensin receptor blockers [24]. For hypertension, additional calcium receptor blockers and β receptor blockers were prescribed. Target blood pressure was 125/75 mmHg but diastolic blood pressure in patients with impaired renal function should be at least below 90 mmHg [25].

2.3. Definitions

Patients with nephrotic syndrome were regarded to have complete remission if proteinuria was ≤0.3 g/d with normal renal function and a serum creatinine ≤ 110 µmol/l. Partial remission was defined for all types of glomerulonephritis except MesGN as proteinuria ≤2.0 g/d (MesGN ≤ 1.0 g/d) and normal renal function. Patients with persistent proteinuria and stable renal function were classified "diseased". Patients with doubling of serum creatinine were considered to have progressive renal disease. A combined end-point of progressive renal failure or death of any cause until last follow-up was defined for statistical analysis.

2.4. Patient Follow-Up and Patient Adherence

All patients were offered a personal counselling once the histological diagnosis was established. An interpretation of the histology in association with the clinical presentation and laboratory results were given together with a treatment advice according to the most recent Cochrane Review recommendations. The referring nephrologist then was responsible for the further treatment and data on applied treatment, blood pressure, renal function and proteinuria were monitored prospectively. All patients were advised to collect 24 hrs urine samples in regular intervals for the estimation of endogeneous creatinine clearance and proteinuria by a written instruction sheet. For most patients and medical practitioners, 24 hrs urine collection is a cumbersome procedure and was not standard before this programme. However, our hypothesis was that regular 24 hrs urine collections demands cooperation of the patient and could increased the patient's insight into the pathomechanism of nephritis and thus, increase the acceptance of correct intake of symptomatic and specific medications.

2.5. Data Acquisition

Collection of individual patients' data, biopsy report and treatment recommendation were performed prospectively in a central registry, while treatment and follow-up responsibility was transferred to the referring physician. In the year 2009, records of all patients biopsied between October 2002 and December 2008 were again systematiccally reviewed by a structured form for the following data: Patient identification and pseudonym, age at the time of biopsy, gender, histological diagnosis and percentage of tubulo-interstitial fibrosis in the renal cortex, referring nephrologist or general practitioner, comorbidity (coronary heart disease, peripheral arterial occlusive disease, arterial hypertension, diabetes mellitus), medication with ACE inhibitors, angiotensin receptor blockers, diuretics, HMG CoA inhibitors, insulin, oral antidiabetics, oral anticoagulation or anti-platelet drugs, serum creatinine, MDRD-GFR, endogeneous creatinine clearance, 24 hrs proteinuria or alternatively, spot urinary protein-createnine quotient and dip-stick proteinuria. Blood pressure monitoring was recommended for all patients if possible by ambulatory automatic blood pressure measurement. For statistical analysis mean of systolic and diastolic blood pressure measurements were calculated at the beginning and end of the follow-up. If 24 hrs ambulatory blood pressure recordings were performed, mean of all systolic and diastolic blood pressure measurements were used. Mean arterial blood pressure was calculated according to the formula MAD = diastolic blood pressure + (systolic – diastolic blood pressure)/3.

2.6. Statistics

For quantitative parameters we present the results as mean ± standard deviation (SD) for normally distributed variables or as median and information about the range. Qualitative measurements were given as absolute and relative frequencies. Testing for differences of continuous variables between two independent groups was accomplished by the two-sample t-test or the Mann-Whitney U test by ranks as appropriate. Test selection was based on evaluating the variables for normal distribution employing the Kolmogorov-Smirnov test. Intraindividual changes were tested by using Student's paired t-test. Survival for the combined end-point of progressive renal disease or dialysis or death was calculated and graphically displayed according to Kaplan-Meyer method. Differences between curves were assessed by Mantel's log-rank test for censored survival data.

The Cox proportional hazards model [26] was used to identify relevant variables influencing the combined endpoint progressive renal failure or dialysis or death. Thereafter, variables yielding p-values ≤ 0.20 in the univariate analyses were entered in the multivariate model to highlight some adjusted associations between the outcome and covariates [27]. All p-values are two-sided, and $p \leq 0.05$ was considered to be significant. All calculations were performed with PASW Statistics 18 for Microsoft Windows, a courtesy gift by SPSS Munich, Germany (www.spss.com).

3. Results

3.1. Patients and Treatment

The demographics of the patient cohort is described elsewhere (see "Incidence and prevalence of glomerulonephritis in Northern Germany"). In summary, 200 patients (123 males, 77 females, mean age 53 ± 16 years) with either primary (n = 130) or secondary glomerulonephritis (n = 70) were diagnosed between October 2002 and December 2008. Over this time period, 324 different therapies in 195 patients were analysed. Ninety seven patients (49%) received a specific immunosuppressant therapy and 13 patients (7%) were not started on their recommended specific treatment. The mean follow-up was 2.8 ± 2.0 years (median 2.6 years, range 0.008 - 7.1 years). Number of patients in the different glomerulonephritis subtypes, follow-up and their specific first-line therapy recommendations are given in **Table 1**. Symptomatic treatment was prescribed in 191 patients (96%), predominantly ACE inhibitors (72%) and diuretics (71%). Details are given in **Table 2**.

3.2. Outcome

The highest rate of complete remission was seen in MCN (50%) followed by MGN (22%) and MesGN (18%).

Table 1. Glomerulonephritis subtypes, follow-up and first-line therapy recommendation.

GN Type	N	Follow-up	Therapy according to recommendation	Therapy not begun
MCN	12	12 (100%)	7 P, 1 CsA, 2 S	2
FSGS	42	42 (100%)	12 P, 3 CsA, 27 S*	
MesGN	82	78 (85%)	17 MP, 13 P, 1 CyP, 47 S	2
MGN	19	18 (95%)	7 CsA, 6 CyP, 2 S	3
MPGN	3	3 (100%)	1 MMF, 2 S	
NGN	20	20 (100%)	17 Px/MP/CyP, 1 MP, 1 P	1
ICN	7	7 (100%)	1 P, 1 CyP, 3 MMF, 1 Aza, 1 S	0
Other	15	15 (100%)	1 CyP, 3 P, 11 S	
Total	200	195 (98%)		13

MCN = minimal change nephropathy; FSGS = focal and segmental glomerulosclerosis; MesGN = mesangioproliferative glomerulonephritis; MGN = membranous glomerulonephritis; MPGN = membranoproliferative glomerulonephritis; NGN = necrotising glomerulonephritis; ICN = secondary immune complex nephritis; P = prednisolone; CsA = cyclosporin A; S = symptomatic treatment; MP = methylprednisolone; CyP = cyclophosphamide; MMF = mycophenolate mofetil; Px = plasmapheresis; Aza = azathioprine, *Patients with secondary FSGS were treated symptomatically only.

Table 2. Supportive therapy according to glomerulonephritis subtype.

Diagnosis	N	Supp	ACE-I	ARB	Diuretics	CSE-I	Insulin	Coumarin	Plt-I
MCN	12	12	10	3	10	7	1	4	0
FSGS	42	42	33	15	34	27	8	5	10
MesGN	82	77	63	30	52	34	12	5	15
MPGN	3	3	3	1	3	3	2	0	1
MGN	19	19	17	9	17	14	2	4	4
NGN	20	20	8	5	16	8	6	2	2
ICN	7	7	3	2	4	3	3	3	1
Others	15	11	7	3	6	4	4	1	3
Total	200	191	144	68	142	100	38	24	36

N = number of patients; Supp = supportive therapy; ACE-I ACE inhibitors; ARB = angiotensin receptor blockers; CSE-I cholesterin synthesis enzyme inhibitors; Plt-I = platelet inhibitors.

In all patients, complete remission was achieved in 19.4%. Partial remission was found in one third of the patients with MCN, in 28% of patients with MGN and in 17% of patients with FSGS. Complete and partial remission was seen in 33.2% of all patients. The worst prognosis with respect to progressive renal failure and dialysis was found for FSGS patients (31%). Patients with NGN and MesGN had progressive renal failure in 20 and 18%, respectively. At the end of follow-up 17.3% of all patients had either dialysis dependent renal failure or doubling of serum creatinine. Twenty-five patients had died (12.8%) whereas MPGN and NGN had the worst prognosis. One third of the patients remained unchanged diseased despite specific and symptomatic treatment. Summary of all outcomes is displayed in **Table 3**.

3.3. Renal Function and Proteinuria

Patients with secondary glomerulonephritis had a significantly lower MDRD-GFR (45 ± 26 ml/min/1.73 m^2) compared with patient diagnosed to have primary glomerulonephritis (59 ± 24 ml/min/1.73 m^2, two-sample t-test: $p < 0.001$). In patients undergoing 24 hrs urine collection endogeneous creatinine clearance did not change over time in the primary glomerulonephritis (initial creatinine clearance 78 ± 42 ml/min, end of follow-up 84 ± 48 ml/min, paired t-test: $p = 0.14$) nor in the secondary glomerulonephritis group of patients (45 ± 26 ml/min, 54 ± 36 ml/min, $p = 0.76$). This was confirmed for the whole cohort by analysis of the changes in MDRD-GFR in primary glomerulonephritis (end of follow-up: 55 ± 28 ml/min/1.73 m^2) and secondary glomerulonephritis (43 ± 29 ml/min/1.73m^2). 24 hrs proteinuria declined significantly in primary (5.0 ± 5.4 g/d to 2.1 ± 3.4 g/d, paired t-test: $p < 0.001$) and secondary glomerulonephritis (4.8 ± 4.6 g/d to 2.7 ± 3.1 g/d, paired t-test: $p = 0.004$).

3.4. Blood Pressure Control

In primary glomerulonephritis initial systolic, diastolic and mean arterial blood pressure were 134 ± 16, 82 ± 11, and 99 ± 12 mmHg at the time of biopsy and 134 ± 21, 78 ± 12, and 97 ± 14 mmHg at the final visit, reaching significance only for the diastolic blood pressure (paired t-test: $p = 0.004$). In secondary glomerulonephritis, systolic, diastolic and mean arterial blood pressures at the time of biopsy were 131 ± 17, 76 ± 12, 94 ± 14 mmHg. At the end of follow-up, no significant differences were observed (129 ± 19, 75 ± 10, and 93 ± 12 mmHg).

3.5. Adverse Events

Among the 324 therapeutic interventions which included symptomatic treatment recommendations, 70 (22%) adverse events were recorded and treatment had to be stopped in 25 cases. Newly diagnosed steroid-induced diabetes in 23 cases and haematological disorders (19 cases) were most frequently reported. Musculoskeletal complaints and Cushing were diagnosed in 13 cases, each.

3.6. Factors Influencing Outcome

In **Figure 1** we present the result of survival analysis for all 200 patients. The combined end-point of progressive

Table 3. Outcome summery according to glomerulonephritis subtype.

Diagnosis		Outcome					Total
		Disease	Death	RF	CR	PR	
MCN	N	2	0	0	6	4	12
	%	16.7%	0%	0%	50%	33.3%	100.0%
FSGS	N	16	1	13	5	7	42
	%	38.1%	2.4%	31.0%	11.9%	31.7%	100.0%
MesGN	N	38	3	14	14	9	78
	%	48.7%	3.8%	17.9%	17.9%	11.5%	100.0%
MPGN	N	1	2	0	0	0	3
	%	33.3%	66.7%	0%	0%	0%	100.0%
MGN	N	5	3	1	4	5	18
	%	27.8%	16.7%	5.6%	22.2%	27.8%	100.0%
NGN	N	4	10	4	2	0	20
	%	20.0%	50.0%	20.0%	10.0%	0%	100.0%
ICN	N	3	2	0	1	1	7
	%	42.9%	28.6%	0%	14.3%	14.3%	100.0%
Others	N	3	4	2	5	1	15
	%	18.8%	25.0%	12.5%	33.3%	6.3%	100.0%
Total	N	72	25	34	38	27	195
	%	36.9%	12.8%	17.4%	19.0%	13.9%	100.0%

RF = progressive renal failure; CR = complete remission; PR = partial remission; for other abbreviations see **Table 1**.

renal failure or death was seen in 59 patients until the end of follow-up (**Figure 1 (a)**). In an univariate Cox regression analysis the following parameters were tested: Gender, age, presence or absence of tubulointerstital fibrosis, primary or secondary glomerulonephritis, initial blood pressure, initial renal function, proteinuria at the time of biopsy, comorbidities, supportive therapy, specific immunomodulatory therapy, and patient adherence to 24 hrs urine analysis. The comparison between the curves of patients with secondary glomerulonephritis and patients diagnosed to have primary glomerulonephritis by using the logrank test results in $p < 0.001$ (hazard ratio (seconddary vs. primary) 2.52, 95% CI: 1.51 to 4.21) (**Figure 1 (b)**).

The risk for progressive renal failure or death was highest in patients with an initial serum creatinine >175 µmol/l. For the Kaplan-Meier curves of patients whose biopsy report indicated substantial tubulo-interstitial fibrosis of more than 30% versus patients with tu-bulo-interstitial fibrosis of at most 30% we received $p < 0.001$ (hazard ratio (more than 30% vs. at most 30%) 4.71, 95% CI: 2.03 to 11.0) (**Figure 1(c)**).

Further risk factors were the association with higher age, coronary heart disease or peripheral artery occlusive disease, the development of diabetes mellitus and arterial hypertension. Patients with poor controlled hypertension and systolic blood pressure > 160 mmHg had a significantly higher rate of progression compared to patients with controlled hypertension. Among the tested specific therapy recommendations, prednisolone and cyclosporin A treatment had an advantage over symptomatic and cyclophosphamide treatment (**Figure 1(d)**). The complete univariate analysis is given in **Table 4**.

Independent variables whose hazard ratio test had an error probability of less than 0.2 (see **Table 4**) were further investigated in a Cox multivariate model with forward regression analysis. After three regression steps no further variables with a p-value < 0.05 by likelihood ratio testing was found (see **Table 5**).

The strongest impact on the prognosis of patients with glomerulonephritis was found for the presence of more than 30% of tubulointerstitial fibrosis in renal cortex as classified by the histopathologist ($p = 0.001$). Tubulointersitital fibrosis had a hazard ratio of 4.37 (95% confidence interval 1.79 - 10.6) for the combined endpoint of progressive renal disease or death. Monitoring the patients renal function with 24 hrs urine sampling decreased the hazard ratio to 0.298 (95% CI: 0.139 - 0.64, $p = 0.002$; **Figure 1(e)**)

Kaplan-Meier curves of the combined endpoint death, renal failure or progress to renal failure were compared for the group of patients considered compliant with 24 hr urine sampling and the group of patients not being fol lowed up by this method. Mean time to reach the combined endpoint was 5.5 years in the 24 hr urine group and 3.8 years in others. The difference was 1.7 years. Finally, prednisolone or cyclosporin A therapy had a lower hazard ratio in comparision to symptomatic or cyclophosphamide treatment. Overall treatment effect was significant ($p = 0.008$).

4. Discussion

Nowadays, randomised controlled trials are the gold-standard to evaluate a treatment for a specific disease in a well-defined population of patients [28]. However, this approach reaches its limits in so call "orphan" diseases where it is unlikely to design and perform clinical trials with sufficient numbers of patients. Published trials in this area are usually of poor quality, seldom reach significance and do not find the support by the pharmaceutical industry due to the time and money consuming process of performing such a trial. Nevertheless, patients demand treatment and health care officials recognise its importance because of the immense financial burden. In recent years, meta-analysis and Cochrane systematic reviews collecting all available information about the treatment of glomerulonephritis attempted to overcome these problems. However, their results can only be as good as the underlying data which—as stated above—is generally poor. Treatment recommendations derived from such systematic reviews need to be evaluated in daily practice. In this context, glomerulonephritis can be a good example to investigate the role of such gained evidence-based treatment recommendations and its impact on a regional health care policy for various reasons: Firstly, glomerulonephritis is regarded as an orphan disease. Secondly, treatment recommendations on the basis of Cochrane systematic reviews have been published at the beginning of the millennium. Thirdly, glomerulonephritis is a chronically debilitating disease resulting in an extreme cost load for the patient and the health care system all over the world while at the same time physicians and medical industry earn billions of Euros year by year in keeping those patients with end-stage renal disease at life. The latter may be responsible for the low investment made into clinical research for the prevention of end-stage disease.

In this paper the impact of the implementation of treatment recommendations based on Cochrane systematic reviews for a variety of glomerulonephritis subtypes in a well-defined population of Northern Germany was investigated. Three independent factors influencing the outcome of patients among a multitude of different variables were identified in a Cox mulitvariate model: Tubulointerstitial fibrosis, the application of prednisolone or cyclosporin A, and close follow-up by the responsible physician using 24 hrs urine collection technique. Tubulointerstial fibrosis and immunosuppression are well

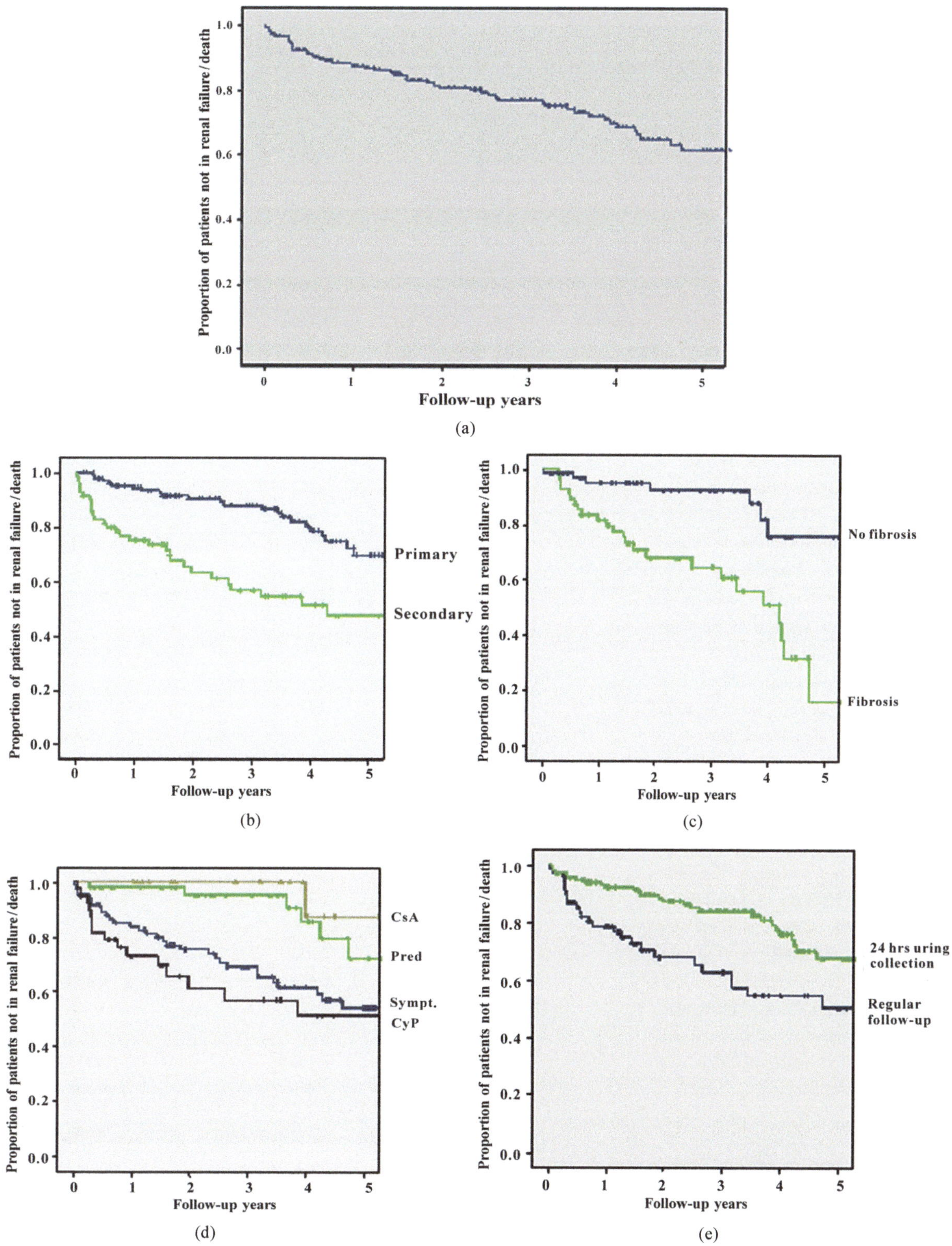

Figures 1. (a) Cumulative survival of all patients without progressive renal failure; (b) Cumulative survival of patients without progressive renal failure subclassified into primary (upper line) or secondary glomerulonephritis (lower line); (c) Cumulative survival of patients without progressive renal failure subclassified into patients with (lower line) or without (upper line) substantial tubulo-interstital fibrosis of more than 30%; (d) Cumulative survival of patients without progressive renal failure subclassified according to treatment (CsA = cyclosporin A, Pred = prednisolone only, Sympt. = symptomatic treatment only, CyP = cyclophosphamide based treatment regimen); (e) Cumulative survival of patients without progressive renal failure according to follow-up with or without 24 hrs urine sampling.

Table 4. Cox univariate model.

Variable	p-value	Non adjusted Hazard-Ratio (HR)	95%-confidence-interval for HR
Gender:			
male vs. female*	0.833	0.944	0.553 - 1.612
Histopathology:	<0.001		
MesGN vs. MCN + FSGS*	0.270	0.669	0.327 - 1.368
MPGN vs. MCN + FSGS*	0.058	4.242	0.952 - 18.904
MGN vs. MCN + FSGS*	0.504	0.674	0.212 - 2.143
NGN vs. MCN + FSGS*	<0.001	3.912	1.856 - 8.243
ICN vs. MCN + FSGS*	0.892	1.108	0.251 - 4.884
Others vs. MCN + FSGS*	0.988	0.993	0.378 - 2.605
Tubulointerstitial fibrosis: > 30% vs. < 30%*	<0.001	4.712	2.026 - 10.958
Primary/secondary GN: sec. GN vs. prim. GN*	<0.001	2.521	1.509 - 4.213
Hypertension: Arterial hypertension vs. normotension*	0.018	3.416	1.233 - 9.461
Diabetes mellitus: Diabetes vs. no diabetes*	0.006	2.100	1.238 - 3.564
Peripheral arterial occlusive disease: PAOD vs. no PAOD*	0.001	4.088	1.830 - 9.133
Coronary heart disease: CHD vs. no CHD*	<0.001	3.058	1.725 - 5.420
ACE inhibitors: ACE-I vs. no ACE-I*	0.129	0.658	0.384 - 1.129
ARB: ARB vs. no ARB*	0.259	0.718	0.404 - 1.277
Diuretics: Diuretics vs. no diuretics*	0.003	3.267	1.481 - 7.207
CSE-I: CSE-I vs. no CSE-I*	0.575	0.869	0.518 - 1.441
Insulin: Insulin vs. no insulin*	0.001	2.537	1.461 - 4.405
Coumarine:			
Coumarine vs. no coumarine*	0.327	0.652	0.277 - 1.534
Platelet aggregation inhibitors			
Plt-I vs. no Plt-I*	0.120	1.599	0.885 – 2.886
24 hrs urine collection			
24 hrs urine vs. no 24 hrs urine*	0.002	0.432	0.256 - 0.728
Initial creatinine	<0.001		
110 - 175 µmol/l vs. <110 µmol/l*	0.165	1.945	0.760 - 4.980
>175 µmol/l vs. <110 µmol/l*	<0.001	12.466	5.661 - 27.450
Initial proteinuria	0.258		
1 - 3.5 g/24hrs vs. <1 g/24hrs*	0.76	1.99	0.930 - 4.255
>3.5 - 5 g/24hrs vs. <1 g/24hrs*	0.675	1.26	0.427 - 3.717
>5 g/24hrs vs. <1 g/24hrs*	0.138	1.767	0.832 - 3.750
Initial systolic blood pressure	0.003		
120 - 140 mmHg vs. <120 mmHg*	0.182	0.631	0.321 - 1.240
140 - 160 mmHg vs. <120 mmHg*	0.953	0.978	0.460 - 2.076
>160 mmHg vs. <120 mmHg*	0.023	2.722	1.146 - 6.467
Initial diastolic blood pressure	0.098		
85 - 95 mmHg vs. <85 mmHg*	0.311	0.673	0.313 - 1.448
>95 mmHg vs. 85 mmHg*	0.98	1.850	0.893 - 3.833
Initial mean arterial pressure >100 mmHg vs. <100 mmHg*	0.7	1.115	0.640 - 1.941
Age	<0.001		
30 - 60 y vs. <30 y*	0.242	0.590	0.244 - 1.428
>60 y vs. >30 y	0.042	2.364	1.032 - 5.416
Therapy	0.004		
Prednisolone vs. symptomatic treatment*	0.013	0.376	0.173 - 0.817
Cyclosporin A vs. symptomatic treatment*	0.030	0.206	0.049 - 0.862
Cyclophosphamide vs. symptomatic treatment*	0.645	1.157	0.623 - 2.147

HR = hazard ratio; MCN = minimal change nephropathy; FSGS = focal and segmental glomerulonephritis; MesGN = mesangioproliferative glomerulonephritis; MPGN = membranoproliferative glomerulonephritis; MGN = membranous glomerulonephritis; NGN = necrotising glomerulonephritis; ICN = secondary immune complex nephritis; PAOD = peripheral artery occlusive disease; CHD = coronary heart disease; ACE-I = angiotensin receptor inhibitor; ARB = angiotensin receptor blocker; CSE-I = cholesterin synthesis enzyme inhibitor; Plt-I = platelet aggregation inhibitor; y = years; asterix denotes reference category.

Table 5. Cox multivariate model with forward regression analysis.

		p-value	Adjusted Hazard-Ratio (HR)	95%-confidence interval for HR
Step 1	24 hrs urine sampling			
	24 hrs urine vs. no 24 hrs urine*	0.002	0.298	0.139 - 0.640
Step 2	Tubulointerstitial fibrosis			
	>30% vs. <30%*	0.003	3.73	1.57 - 8.84
	24 hrs urine sampling			
	24 hrs urine vs. no 24 hrs urine*	0.002	0.293	0.135 - 0.635
Step 3	Tubulointerstitial fibrosis			
	>30% vs. <30%*	0.001	4.37	1.79 - 10.6
	24 hrs urine sampling			
	24 hrs urine vs. no 24 hrs urine*	0.005	0.283	0.116 - 0.687
	Therapy	0.008		
	Prednisolone vs. sympt.*	0.037	0.320	0.110 - 0.934
	CyA. vs. sympt.*	0.099	0.182	0.024 - 1.38
	CyP vs. sympt.*	0.121	2.48	0.786 - 7.84

HR = hazard ratio; sympt. = symptomatic therapy; CyA = cyclosporin A therapy; CyP = cyclophosphamide based therapy; asterix denotes reference category.

known to direct patients into end-stage renal failure [29,30] or induce remission [16,31-34]. The application of cyclophosphamide was not associated with a better survival. This may be due to the negative selection of patients. As shown in the univariate model, secondary glomerulonephritis has a poor outcome. Many of these patients suffered from necrotising glomerulonephritis with severe renal involvement and half of them died or ended on dialysis which is comparable to other recent reports [35]. It was surprising that a simple measure such as 24 hrs urine collection also had a strong impact on the outcome. Previously, it was suggested to replace the 24 hrs urine collection by a spot urine test for proteinuria/urine creatinine ratio [36]. We admit that 24 hrs urine collection may be a process affected by some errors (sampling error, calculation error). Nevertheless, we assume that the process of explaining the collection method and its reason to the patient may contribute to an intensified physician-patient contact and might increase patient and probably physician adherence to recommended therapy strategies by the referral centre. Beside these three main factors, other variables have been shown to improve or worsen outcome. As almost all patients received antihypertensive medication with ACE inhibitors or angiotensin receptor blockers by the end of follow-up, the control of systolic blood pressure is an important determinant for renal progressive disease. On the other hand, the use of diuretics as a poor prognostic factor can be interpreted as a necessary treatment modality for severe nephrotic syndrome which cannot be avoided.

In summary, this paper shows that the application of knowledge derived from Cochrane systematic reviews can be successfully implemented in a region of mainly independently working nephrologists. Treatment recommendations—although widely but not completely followed—showed efficacy in prevention of progression of renal disease. In order to improve patient outcome patients require early renal biopsy, evidence-based treatment recommendation, close renal care including monitoring of their disease status, and strict symptomatic treatment with renin angiotensin blockade aiming at recommended blood pressure targets. If one regards 24 hrs urine collections as an indirect measure of adherence to the recommendations given by the referral centre a prolongation of the time to dialysis can be estimated to approximately 1.7 years. The costs of one year of haemodialysis in Germany are currently 26,200 EUR. Consequently, adherence to treatment recommendations could possibly save 45,000 EUR per treated patient.

5. Acknowledgements

We are grateful for the cooperation with the following nephrologists, rheumatologists and general practitioners who submitted data for this analysis:

Dr. Eberhard Schmitt, Dr. Achim Selck, and Jens Freytag, Krückmannstr. 4 - 5, 18273 Güstrow; Dipl.-Med. Cornelia Brenning, Ziegendorfer Chaussee 7, 19370 Parchim; Dr. Kristin Nöhring, Einsteinstr. 12, 17192 Waren; Andreas Morawietz, Reinhard Schodrok, and Dipl.-Med. Maren Paukstat, Kieler Str. 31 a, 19057 Schwerin; Dr. Bernd Gohlke and Dipl.-Med. Niels Baumann, Parkstr. 16, 19230 Hagenow; Michael Pollok and Beate Bley, Bahnhofstr. 29, 19288 Ludwigslust; Dr. Wolfgang Haaf, Kuratorium für Dialyse und Transplantation Wismar, Am Friedenshof, 23966 Wismar; Dr. Margitta Oppermann and Dr. Ilona Lange, K.-Liebknecht-Str. 13a, 19348 Perleberg; Dr. Helge Mentzel and Dr. Astrid Ohlmann, Klützer Str. 6, Grevesmühlen; Frau Inge Selmikat, Dr. Raimar Steinbeck and Dr. Gerd Oehme, Johannes-R.-Becher Str. 20, 19059 Schwerin; Dr. Elisabeth Ständer, Beethovenstr. 3, 19053 Schwerin; Dr. Cathleen Bauer and Dipl.-Med. Rainer Kubbutat, Obotritenring 117, 19053 Schwerin; Dr. Roland Schünding, Kieler Str. 31a, 19057 Schwerin; Dirk Gutsmuths, Körnerstr. 22, 19055 Schwerin; Dr. Malte Ganssauge, Alte Dorfstr. 20, 19069 Lübstorf; Dipl.-Med. Jens-Rüdeger Kastorff, Kieber Damm 21, 19300 Grabow; Dr. Rosita Krellenberg, Am Wallhotel 1, 19370 Parchim.

REFERENCES

[1] N. Braun, A. Schweisfurth, C. Lohofener, *et al.*, "Epidemiology of Glomerulonephritis in Northern Germany," *International Urology and Nephrology*, Vol. 43, No. 4, 2011, pp. 1117-1126. doi:10.1007/s11255-011-9955-4

[2] Council of the European Union, "Council Recommendation on an Action in the Field of Rare Diseases," Interinstitutional File 2008/0218 (CNS).

[3] U. Frei and H.-J. Schober-Halstenberg, "Nierenersatztherapie in Deutschland 2006/2007," Quasi-Niere gGmbH, Schöneberg, 2008.

[4] K. Farrington, A. Hodsman, A. Casula, D. Ansell and J. Feehally, "UK Renal Registry 11th Annual Report (December 2008): Chapter 4 ESRD Prevalent Rates in 2007 in the UK: National and Centre-Specific Analyses," *Nephron Clinical Practice*, Vol. 111, Suppl. 1, 2009, pp. c43-c68

[5] S. C. Chen, "United States Renal Data System—The Concise 2008 Annual Data Report," 2008. www.usrds.org.

[6] A. Rüther, H. P. Dauben and H. Schweim, "Die Deutsche Agentur für Health Technology Assessment (HTA) Beim DIMDI (DAHTA@DIMDI)," *Bundesgesundheitsbl-Gesundheitsforsch-Gesundheitsschutz*, Vol. 44, No. 9, 2001, pp. 865-869.

[7] S. C. Palmer, K. Nand and G. F. Strippoli, "Interventions for Minimal Change Disease in Adults with Nephrotic Syndrome," *Cochrane Database of Systematic Reviews*, Vol. 23, No. 1, Article No. CD001537.

[8] C.-K. Yeung, K.-L. Wong and W. L. Ng, "Intravenous Methylprednisolone Pulse Therapy in Minimal Change Nephrotic Syndrome," *Australian and New Zealand Journal of Medicine*, Vol. 13, No. 4, pp. 349-351. doi:10.1111/j.1445-5994.1983.tb04479.x

[9] E. M. Hodson, N. S. Willis and J. C. Craig, "Corticosteroid Therapy for Nephrotic Syndrome in Children," *Cochrane Database of Systematic Reviews*, No. 4, 2007, Article No. CD001533.

[10] E. M. Hodson, D. Habashy and J. C. Craig, "Interventions for Idiopathic Steroid-Resistant Nephrotic Syndrome in Children," *Cochrane Database of Systematic Reviews*, Vol. 19, No. 2, 2006, Article No. CD003594.

[11] E. M. Hodson, N. S. Willis and J. C. Craig, "Non-Corticosteroid Treatment for Nephrotic Syndrome In Children," *Cochrane Database of Systematic Reviews*, No. 4, 2008, Article No. CD002290.

[12] N. Braun, F. Schmutzler, C. Lange, *et al.*, "Immunosuppressive Treatment for Focal Segmental Glomerulosclerosis in Adults (Review), Non-Corticosteroid Treatment for Nephrotic Syndrome in Children," *Cochrane Database of Systematic Reviews*, No. 3, 2008, Article No. CD003233.

[13] G. Banfi, M. Moriggi, E. Sabadini, G. Fellin, G. D'Amico and C. Ponticelli, "The Impact of Prolonged Immunosuppression on the Outcome of Idiopathic Focal-Segmental Glomerulosclerosis with Nephrotic Syndrome in Adults. A Collaborative Retrospective Study," *Clinical Nephrology*, Vol. 36, No. 2, 1991, pp. 53-59.

[14] J. A. Samuels, G. F. Strippoli, J. C. Craig, F. P. Schena and D. A. Molony, "Immunosuppressive Agents for Treating IgA Nephropathy," *Cochrane Database of Systematic Reviews*, No. 4, 2003, Article No. CD003965.

[15] J. Floege and H. J. Grone, "IgA-Nephropathie," *Der Internist*, Vol. 44, No. 9, 2002, pp. 1131-1139. doi:10.1007/s00108-003-1026-1

[16] C. Pozzi, P. G. Bolasco, G. B. Fogazzi, *et al.*, "Corticosteroids in IgA Nephropathy: A Randomised Controlled Trial," *Lancet*, Vol. 353, No. 9156, 1999, pp. 883-887. doi:10.1016/S0140-6736(98)03563-6

[17] F. W. Ballardie and I. S. D. Roberts, "Controlled Prospective Trial of Prednisolone and Cytotoxis in Progressive IgA Nephropathy," *Journal of the American Society of Nephrology*, Vol. 13, No. 1, 2002, pp. 42-148.

[18] A. Schieppati, A. Perna, J. Zamora, G. A. Giuliano, N. Braun and G. Remuzzi, "Immunosuppressive Treatment for Idiopathic Membranous Nephropathy in Adults with Nephrotic Syndrome," *Cochrane Database of Systematic Reviews*, No. 4, 2004, Article No. CD004293.

[19] D. Cattran, "Management of Membranous Nephropathy: When and What for Treatment," *Journal of the American Society of Nephrology*, Vol. 16, No. 5, 2005, pp. 1188-1194. doi:10.1681/ASN.2005010028

[20] C. Ponticelli, P. Altieri, F. Scolari, *et al.*, "A Randomized Study Comparing Methylprednisolone Plus Chlorambucil versus Methylprednisolone Plus Cyclophosphamide in Idiopathic Membranous Nephropathy," *Journal of the American Society of Nephrology*, Vol. 9, No. 3, 1998, pp. 444-450.

[21] G. Walters, N. S. Willis and J. C. Craig, "Interventions for Renal Vasculitis in Adults," *Cochrane Database of Systematic Reviews*, No. 3, 2008, Article No. CD003232.

[22] American College of Rheumatology Ad Hoc Committee on Systemic Lupus Erythematosus Guidelines, "Guidelines for Referral and Management of Systemic Lupus Erythematosus in Adults," *Arthritis & Rheumatism*, Vol. 42, 1999, pp. 1785-1796.

[23] R. S. Flanc, M. A. Roberts, G. F. Strippoli, S. J. Chadban, P. G. Kerr and R. C. Atkins, "Treatment for Lupus Nephritis," *Cochrane Database of Systematic Reviews*, No. 1, 2004, Article No. CD002922.

[24] C. S. Wilcox, "New Insights into Diuretic Use in Patients with Chronic Renal Disease," *Journal of the American Society of Nephrology*, Vol. 13, No. 2002, pp. 798-805.

[25] G. Maschio, D. Alberti, F. Locatelli, *et al.*, "Angiotensin-

Converting Enzyme Inhibitors and Kidney Protection: The AIPRI Trial. The ACE Inhibition in Progressive Renal Insufficiency (AIPRI) Study Group," *Journal of Cardiovascular Pharmacology*, Vol. 33, Suppl. 1, 1999, pp. S16-S20. doi:10.1097/00005344-199900001-00004

[26] D. Cox, "Regression Models and Life Tables," *Journal of the Royal Statistical Society. Series B*, Vol. 34, No. 2, 1972, pp. 187-220.

[27] R. Muecke, O. Micke, B. Reichl, *et al.*, "Demographic, Clinical and Treatment Related Predictors for Event-Free Probability Following Low-Dose Radiotherapy for Painful Heel Spurs—A Retrospective Multicenter Study of 502 Patients," *Acta Oncologica*, Vol. 46, No. 2, 2007, pp. 239-246. doi:10.1080/02841860600731935

[28] D. L. Sackett, S. E. Straus, W. S. Richardson, W. Rosenberg and R. B. Haynes, "Evidence-Based Medicine: How to Practic and Teach EBM," Churchill Livingstone, Edinburgh, 2000.

[29] A. Bohle, S. Mackensen-Haen and G. H. Von, "Significance of Tubulointerstitial Changes in the Renal Cortex for the Excretory Function and Concentration Ability of the Kidney: A Morphometric Contribution," *American Journal of Nephrology*, Vol. 7, No. 6, 1987, pp. 421-433. doi:10.1159/000167514

[30] D. C. Cattran, R. Coppo, H. T. Cook, *et al.*, "The Oxford Classification of IgA Nephropathy: Rationale, Clinicopathological Correlations, and Classification," *Kidney International*, Vol. 76, No. 5, 2009, pp. 534-545. doi:10.1038/ki.2009.243

[31] "Safety and Tolerability of Cyclosporin a (Sandimmun) in Idiopathic Nephrotic Syndrome. Collaborative Study Group of Sandimmun in Nephrotic Syndrome," *Clinical Nephrology*, Vol. 35, Suppl. 1, 1991, pp. S48-S60

[32] D. C. Cattran, G. B. Appel, L. A. Hebert, *et al.*, "A Randomized Trial of Cyclosporine in Patients with Steroid-Resistant Focal Segmental Glomerulosclerosis. North America Nephrotic Syndrome Study Group," *Kidney International*, Vol. 56, 1999, pp. 2220-2226. doi:10.1046/j.1523-1755.1999.00778.x

[33] E. Imbasciati, R. Gusmano, A. Edefonti, *et al.*, "Controlled Trial of Methylprednisolone Pulses and Low Dose Oral Prednisone for the Minimal Change Nephrotic Syndrome," *British Medical Journal* (*Clinical Research Edition.*), Vol. 291, No. 6505, 1985, pp. 1305-1308. doi:10.1136/bmj.291.6505.1305

[34] D. J. Wallace, D. Goldfinger, G. Savage, *et al.*, "Predictive Value of Clinical, Laboratory, Pathologic, and Treatment Variables in Steroid/Immunosuppressive Resistant Lupus Nephritis," *Journal of Clinical Apheresis*, Vol. 4, No. 1, 1988, pp. 30-34. doi:10.1002/jca.2920040107

[35] D. R. Jayne, G. Gaskin, N. Rasmussen, *et al.*, "Randomized Trial of Plasma Exchange or High-Dosage Methylprednisolone as Adjunctive Therapy for Severe Renal Vasculitis," *Journal of the American Society of Nephrology*, Vol. 18, No. 7, 2007, pp. 2180-2188. doi:10.1681/ASN.2007010090

[36] NKF K/DOQI Clinical Practice Guidelines on Hypertension and Antihypertensive Agents in Chronic Kidney Disease," *American Journal of Kidney Diseases*, Vol. 43, Suppl. 291, 2004, pp. S1-S290. doi:10.1053/S0272-6386(04)00369-5

Permissions

All chapters in this book were first published by Scientific Research Publishing; hereby published with permission under the Creative Commons Attribution License or equivalent. Every chapter published in this book has been scrutinized by our experts. Their significance has been extensively debated. The topics covered herein carry significant findings which will fuel the growth of the discipline. They may even be implemented as practical applications or may be referred to as a beginning point for another development.

The contributors of this book come from diverse backgrounds, making this book a truly international effort. This book will bring forth new frontiers with its revolutionizing research information and detailed analysis of the nascent developments around the world.

We would like to thank all the contributing authors for lending their expertise to make the book truly unique. They have played a crucial role in the development of this book. Without their invaluable contributions this book wouldn't have been possible. They have made vital efforts to compile up to date information on the varied aspects of this subject to make this book a valuable addition to the collection of many professionals and students.

This book was conceptualized with the vision of imparting up-to-date information and advanced data in this field. To ensure the same, a matchless editorial board was set up. Every individual on the board went through rigorous rounds of assessment to prove their worth. After which they invested a large part of their time researching and compiling the most relevant data for our readers.

The editorial board has been involved in producing this book since its inception. They have spent rigorous hours researching and exploring the diverse topics which have resulted in the successful publishing of this book. They have passed on their knowledge of decades through this book. To expedite this challenging task, the publisher supported the team at every step. A small team of assistant editors was also appointed to further simplify the editing procedure and attain best results for the readers.

Apart from the editorial board, the designing team has also invested a significant amount of their time in understanding the subject and creating the most relevant covers. They scrutinized every image to scout for the most suitable representation of the subject and create an appropriate cover for the book.

The publishing team has been an ardent support to the editorial, designing and production team. Their endless efforts to recruit the best for this project, has resulted in the accomplishment of this book. They are a veteran in the field of academics and their pool of knowledge is as vast as their experience in printing. Their expertise and guidance has proved useful at every step. Their uncompromising quality standards have made this book an exceptional effort. Their encouragement from time to time has been an inspiration for everyone.

The publisher and the editorial board hope that this book will prove to be a valuable piece of knowledge for researchers, students, practitioners and scholars across the globe.

List of Contributors

Jan M. Fertmann, Helmut P. Arbogast, Wolf-D. Illner, Walter Land and Karl-W. Jauch
Department of Surgery, Klinikum Grosshadern, Ludwig-Maximilians University of Munich, Munich, Germany

Johannes N. Hoffmann
Department of Surgery, Klinikum Grosshadern, Ludwig-Maximilians University of Munich, Munich, Germany
Department of Surgery, University of Duisburg-Essen, Duisburg and Essen, Germany

Neil Smart and James McFarlane
Department of Exercise Science, University of New England, Armidale, Australia

Veronique Cornelissen
Department of Rehabilitation Sciences, University of Leuven, Leuven, Belgium

Supatra Lohsiriwat
Department of Physiology, Faculty of Medicine Siriraj Hospital, Mahidol University, Bangkok, Thailand

Mickael Coupé, Marc-Antoine Custaud and Nastassia M. Navasiolava
CNRS UMR 6214, INSERM U1083, Angers University, Angers, France
Associated French-Russian Laboratory CaDyWEC, Angers, France & Moscow, Russia

Elena Tomilovskaya and Inesa B. Kozlovskaya
Institute of Biomedical Problems RAS SSC, Moscow, Russia

Françoise Larcher
Biochemistry Laboratory, Angers University Hospital, Angers, France

Bertrand Diquet
Pharmacokinetics Laboratory, Angers University Hospital, Angers, France

Liudmila Kh. Pastushkova and Irina M. Larina
Associated French-Russian Laboratory CaDyWEC, Angers, France & Moscow, Russia
Institute of Biomedical Problems RAS SSC, Moscow, Russia

Guillemette Gauquelin-Koch
French Space Agency (CNES), Paris, France

Vladimir A. Kulchitsky
Institute of Physiology, National Academy of Sciences, Minsk, Belarus

Maria Delia Colombo
Novartis Farma S.p.A., Origgio (VA), Italy
Department of Dermatology, Marchesi Hospital, Inzago (MI), Italy

Renata Perego
Department of Dermatology, Marchesi Hospital, Inzago (MI), Italy

Gilberto Bellia
Novartis Farma S.p.A., Origgio (VA), Italy

Rolf Bambauer
Institute for Blood Purification, Homburg, Germany

Ralf Schiel
Inselklinik Heringsdorf GmbH, Seeheilbad Heringsdorf, Germany

Carolin Bambauer
Main Hospital Darmstadt, Darmstadt, Germany

Reinhard Latza
Laboratorium of Medicine, St. Ingbert, Germany

Nand K. Wadhwa
Division of Nephrology, Stony Brook School of Medicine, Stony Brook, New York, USA

Catherine R. Messina
Department of Preventive Medicine, Stony Brook School of Medicine, Stony Brook, New York, USA

Nasser M. Hebah
Corporate Home Dialysis, Dialysis Clinic Inc., Nashville, USA

Tajamul H. Shah, Ajaz N. Koul, Sonaullah Shah, Umar H. Khan, Parvaiz A. Koul, Fayaz A. Sofi and Mufti S., Rafi Ahmed Jan
Intrenal & Pulmonary Medicine, Sheri Kashmir Institute of Medicine, Srinagar, India

Mohammad Budruddin
Nephrology Department, Tawam Hospital, Al Ain, UAE

Muhammad Yasir Khalil, Issa Al Salmi and Ramaiah Shilpa
Nephrology Department, Royal Hospital, Muscat, Oman

Md Shihamul Islam and Jerzy Szpunar
Department of Mechanical Engineering, University of Saskatchewan, Saskatoon, Canada

Satoru Kuriyama, Naoki Sugano, Kohki Takane, Akimitsu Kobayashi, Yasushi Otsuka and Tatsuo Hosoya
Division of Kidney & Hypertension, Department of Internal Medicine, School of Medicine, Jikei University, Tokyo, Japan

Nasim Shahbazi
Department of Medicine, Division of Nephrology, Thunder Bay Regional Health Sciences Centre, Thunder Bay, Canada

Pierre A. Brown
Department of Medicine, Division of Nephrology, Ottawa Hospital, Ottawa, Canada

Ayub Akbari and Deborah L. Zimmerman
Kidney Research Centre, Ottawa Hospital Research Institute, Ottawa, Canada

Annette Lennerling
Transplant Institute, Sahlgrenska University Hospital, Gothenburg, Sweden
Institute of Health and Care Sciences, University of Gothenburg, Gothenburg, Sweden

Abdul Rashid Qureshi
Baxter Novum, CLINTEC, Karolinska Institute, Stockholm, Sweden

Ingela Fehrman-Ekholm
Transplant Institute, Sahlgrenska University Hospital, Gothenburg, Sweden
Renal Department, Karolinska University Hospital, Stockholm, Sweden

Shadi Hassan
Internal Medicine Department, Carmel Medical Center, Haifa, Israel

Batya Kristal and Kamal Hassan
Faculty of Medicine in the Galilee, Bar-Ilan University, Safed, Israel
Nephrology and Hypertension Department, Western Galilee Hospital, Nahariya, Israel

Khalid Khazim
Nephrology and Hypertension Department, Western Galilee Hospital, Nahariya, Israel

Fadi Hassan
Sackler Faculty of Medicine, Tel Aviv University, Tel Aviv, Israel

Dunia Hassan
The Ruth and Bruce Faculty of Medicine, Technion Israel Institute of Technology, Haifa, Israel

Ioannis Koulouridis and Efstathios Koulouridis
Department of Nephrology, General Hospital of Corfu, Corfu, Greece

Dong-Su Jeon, Tae-Hee Kim and Hae-Hyeog Lee
Department of Obstetrics and Gynecology, Soonchunhyang University Bucheon Hospital, Bucheon, South Korea

Dong Won Byun
Division of Endocrinology and Metabolism, Department of Internal Medicine, Soonchunhyang University Hospital, Bucheon, South Korea

Absar Ali
Department of Medicine, Aga Khan University, Karachi, Pakistan

Naila Asif and Zunaira Rais
Liaquat National Hospital, Karachi, Pakistan

Mekdess Abebe, Wing Mu, Heesuck Suh, Edward P. Nord and Nand K. Wadhwa
Division of Nephrology, Department of Medicine, School of Medicine, State University of New York at Stony Brook, Stony Brook, USA

Jason R. DeGuire and Hope A. Weiler
School of Dietetics and Human Nutrition, McGill University, Montreal, Canada

Anil Kumar Mohanty, Deepti Damayanty Pradhan, Bijay Kumar Meher and Pradeep Sivraj
Department of Paediatrics, Sardar Vallavbhai Patel Post Graduate Institute of Paediatrics (SCB Medical College), Cuttack, India

Leopoldo Muniz da Silva, Pedro Thadeu Galvão Vianna, Mariana Takaku, Glênio Bittencourt Mizubuti and Yara Marcondes Machado Castiglia
Department of Anaesthesiology, Botucatu School of Medicine, São Paulo State University (UNESP), São Paulo, Brazil

Roberto Sanchez and Luis Zegarra
Surgery and Urology Unit, Department of Surgery, Cayetano Heredia Hospital, Lima, Peru
Renal Transplant Unit, Cayetano Heredia Hospital, Lima, Peru

Reyner Loza
Renal Transplant Unit, Cayetano Heredia Hospital, Lima, Peru
Paediatric Nephrology Unit, Department of Pediatrics, Cayetano Heredia Hospital, Lima, Peru

Cesar Loza
Renal Transplant Unit, Cayetano Heredia Hospital, Lima, Peru
Nephrology Service, Department of Medicine, Cayetano Heredia Hospital, Lima, Peru

Olivier Mat and Rim Kada
Department of Nephrology of EpiCURA, Ath, Belgium

Patrick Philippart, Quentin Mat and Steffy Larroze
Department of Surgery of EpiCURA, Ath, Belgium

Myriam Remmelink
Department of Lung Pathology, Hopital Erasme, Université Libre de Bruxelles, Brussels, Belgium

Selda Aydin
Department of Renal Pathology, Cliniques Universitaires St-Luc, Université Catholique de Louvain, Brussels, Belgium

Vincent Colombie
Department of Infectious Diseases of EpiCURA, Ath, Belgium

Richard Fuquay
Health Science Center Division of Renal Diseases and Hypertension, University of Colorado Denver, Aurora, USA

James Eric Cooper
Health Science Center Division of Renal Diseases and Hypertension, Transplant Center, University of Colorado Denver, Aurora, USA

Reiko Sato and Teruhiko Kido
Graduate School of Medical Science, Kanazawa University, Kanazawa, Japan

Hideaki Nakagawa, Muneko Nishijo and Ryumon Honda
Kanazawa Medical University, Uchinada, Japan

Etsuko Kobayashi and Yasushi Suwazono
Graduate School of Medical Science, Chiba University, Chiba, Japan

Mostapha Habib Allah, Nour Houda Bassit, Wafaa Fadili and Inass Laouad
Department of Nephrology, Transplantation UHC Mohammed VI, Marrakesh, Morocco

Sertac Cimen and Ian Alwayn
The Division of General Surgery, Dalhousie University, Queen Elizabeth II Health Sciences Centre, Halifax, Canada

Sanem Guler
Atlantic Centre for Transplantation Research, Dalhousie University, Halifax, Canada

Joseph Lawen
Department of Urology, Dalhousie University, Queen Elizabeth II Health Sciences Centre, Halifax, Canada

Bryce Kiberd
Faculty of Medicine, Dalhousie University, Queen Elizabeth II Health Sciences Centre, Halifax, Canada

Edward P. Nord, Deep Patel, Heesuck Suh and Nand K. Wadhwa
Division of Nephrology, Department of Medicine, School of Medicine, State University of New York at Stony Brook, Stony Brook, USA

Tobias A. Marsen
Nephrology Center and KfH Kidney and Dialysis Center Köln-Lindenthal, Köln, Germany

Iqbal Masood and Geoffrey Teehan
Department of Nephrology, Lankenau Medical Center and Lankenau Institute for Medical Research, Wynnewood, USA

Cai-Mei Zheng, Yung-Ho Hsu and Yuh-Feng Lin
Division of Nephrology, Department of Medicine, Taipei Medical University-Shuang Ho Hospital, Taipei Medical University, Chinese Taipei

Min-Tser Liao
Department of Pediatrics, Taoyuan Armed Forces General Hospital, Chinese Taipei
Department of Pediatrics, Tri-Service General Hospital, National Defense Medical Center, Chinese Taipei

Mei-Yu Lin, Lan Lo and Kuo-Cheng Lu
Department of Medicine, Cardinal Tien Hospital, School of Medicine, Fu Jen Catholic University, New Taipei City, Chinese Taipei

Chia-Chao Wu
Division of Nephrology, Department of Medicine, Tri-Service General Hospital, National Defense Medical Center, Chinese Taipei

Kolitha H. Sellahewa
Department of Medicine, Melaka Manipal Medical College, Melaka, Malaysia

Abdul Halim Abdul Gafor, Azrina Abdul Kadir, Rizna Abdul Cader, Rozita Mohd, Kong Wei Yen, and Norella C. T. Kong
Department Nephrology Unit, Department of Medicine, University Kebangsaan Malaysia Medical Centre, Kuala Lumpur, Malaysia

Rohana Abdul Ghani
Endocrine Unit, Department of Medicine, University Kebangsaan Malaysia Medical Centre, Kuala Lumpur, Malaysia

Shamsul Azhar Shah
Department of Epidemiology and Biostatistics, University Kebangsaan Malaysia Medical Centre, Kuala Lumpur, Malaysia

Laura Connor
Department of Internal Medicine, Lankenau Medical Center, Wynnewood, USA

Geoffrey Teehan
Department of Nephrology, Lankenau Medical Center, Wynnewood, USA
Lankenau Institute of Medical Research, Wynnewood, USA

Mochamad Yusuf
Cardiology and Vascular Medicine Department, Faculty of Medicine, Airlangga University, Surabaya, Indonesia
Tropical Disease Center, Airlangga University, Surabaya, Indonesia
Division of Nephrology, Departement of Internal Medicine, Juntendo University Faculty of Medicine, Tokyo, Japan

Raden Mohammad Yogiarto and Muhammad Aminuddin
Cardiology and Vascular Medicine Department, Faculty of Medicine, Airlangga University, Surabaya, Indonesia

Mochammad Thaha
Division of Nephrology, Departement of Internal Medicine, Juntendo University Faculty of Medicine, Tokyo, Japan
Nephrology-Hypertension Division, Internal Medicine Departement, Faculty of Medicine, Airlangga University, Surabaya, Indonesia

Raden Mohammad Yogiantoro
Nephrology-Hypertension Division, Internal Medicine Departement, Faculty of Medicine, Airlangga University, Surabaya, Indonesia

Retno Handajani
Tropical Disease Center, Airlangga University, Surabaya, Indonesia

Yasuhiko Tomino
Division of Nephrology, Departement of Internal Medicine, Juntendo University Faculty of Medicine, Tokyo, Japan

Kumiko Ozawa, Setsuko Niki and Seiko Yamanouchi
School of Nursing, Hachinohe Junior College, Hachinohe, Japan

Hideaki Yamabe, Toshiko Tomisawa, Maiko Kitajima, Mayumi Urushizaka, Kumiko Kawasaki, Chieko Itaki and Yuka Noto
Hirosaki University Graduate School of Health Sciences, Hirosaki, Japan

Morito Endo
Faculty of Human Health Science, Hachinohe University, Hachinohe, Japan

Christine Sethna, Rachel Frank and Lulette Infante
Department of Pediatrics, Division of Nephrology, Cohen Children's Medical Center of New York, New York, USA

Beth Gottlieb and Anne Eberhard
Department of Pediatrics, Division of Rheumatology, Cohen Children's Medical Center of New York, New York, USA

Xiaotong Wang
Department of Pathology, North Shore University Hospital of the North Shore—LIJ Health System, New York, USA

Howard Trachtman
Department of Pediatrics, Division of Nephrology, NYU Langone Medical Center, New York, USA

M. Budruddin
Nephrology Department, Tawam Hospital, Al Ain, UAE

Issa Al Salmi and R. Shilpa
Nephrology Department, Royal Hospital, Muscat, Oman

Carlos Enrique Yepes Delgado, Yanett Marcela Montoya Jaramillo, Beatriz Elena Orrego Orozco, Paulina Bernal Ramírez, Luz Denise González, José Miguel Abad Echeverri and María Patricia Arbeláez Montoya
University of Antioquia, Hospital Pablo Tobón Uribe, EPS SURA, Medellín, Colombia

Liam Mullen, Janice Harper and Sukumaran Binukrishnan
Royal Liverpool University Hospital, Liverpool Heart and Chest Hospital, Liverpool, UK

William Brian Reeves, Bishal B. Rawal and Alaa S. Awad
Department of Medicine, Division of Nephrology, Penn State Hershey Medical Center, Hershey, USA

Emaad M. Abdel-Rahman
Department of Medicine, Division of Nephrology, University of Virginia, Charlottesville, USA

Khawar Maqsood
Department of Medicine, Baystate Medical Center, Tufts University School of Medicine, Springfield, USA

Adeel Siddiqui and Geoffrey Teehan
Department of Nephrology, Lankenau Medical Center, Lankenau Institute for Medical Research, Wynnewood, USA

Selda Korkmaz
Department of Neurology, Acibadem Hospital, Kayseri, Turkey

Bulent Tokgoz and Ismail Kocyigit
Department of Nephrology, Erciyes University Medical School, Kayseri, Turkey

Sevda Ismailogullari, Murat Aksu and Merva Kocyigit
Department of Neurology, Erciyes University Medical School, Kayseri, Turkey

Ozgur Berkay Aksu
Medical Faculty, Near East University, Nicosia, Cyprus

Norbert Braun
Department of Internal Medicine, MediClin Müritz-Klinikum, Waren, Germany

Anna Schweisfurth
Department of Nephrology and Dialysis, HELIOS Hospital, Schwerin, Germany

Hermann-Josef Gröne
Department of Cellular and Molecular Pathology, German Cancer Research Centre, Heidelberg, Germany

Guenther Kundt
Institute for Biostatistics and Informatics in Medicine, University of Rostock, Rostock, Germany